Musculoskeletal Repair and Regeneration

New Tools, Technology and Techniques

Musculoskeletal Repair and Regeneration

New Tools, Technology and Techniques

Editors

Melanie Coathup
University of Central Florida, USA

Mehdi Razavi
University of Central Florida, USA

Thomas J Kean
University of Central Florida, USA

Aadil Mumith
Basingstoke and North Hampshire Hospital, UK

Liza Osagie-Clouard
Solice Health, UK

World Scientific

NEW JERSEY • LONDON • SINGAPORE • BEIJING • SHANGHAI • HONG KONG • TAIPEI • CHENNAI • TOKYO

Published by

World Scientific Publishing Co. Pte. Ltd.
5 Toh Tuck Link, Singapore 596224
USA office: 27 Warren Street, Suite 401-402, Hackensack, NJ 07601
UK office: 57 Shelton Street, Covent Garden, London WC2H 9HE

British Library Cataloguing-in-Publication Data
A catalogue record for this book is available from the British Library.

MUSCULOSKELETAL REPAIR AND REGENERATION
New Tools, Technology and Techniques

ISBN 978-981-98-1963-8 (hardcover)
ISBN 978-981-98-1964-5 (ebook for institutions)
ISBN 978-981-98-1965-2 (ebook for individuals)

For any available supplementary material, please visit
https://www.worldscientific.com/worldscibooks/10.1142/14490#t=suppl

Typeset by Stallion Press
Email: enquiries@stallionpress.com

https://doi.org/10.1142/9789819819645_fmatter

Preface

The dramatic increase in average life expectancy during the 20th century ranks as one of society's greatest achievements. Advances in public health and medicine have reduced deaths earlier in life, allowing more of us to reach old age than ever before. While further significant leaps in human life expectancy are not anticipated in this century, the global proportion of the oldest-old (>85 years of age) and the number of centenarians continues to rise nonetheless. Aging is accompanied by a natural decline in the capacity of our tissues to repair and regenerate. Because more of us are living longer, this means the burden of age-onset non-communicable diseases is also rising. Amongst these, aging significantly increases the risk and prevalence of degenerative non-fatal musculoskeletal disorders, including osteoarthritis, osteoporosis, and sarcopenia. Satisfactory musculoskeletal health is essential to enable mobility and wellness in our older adults. Thus these conditions become major causes of frailty, pain, and disability, which burden healthcare systems. Thus, a significant and growing burden of global musculoskeletal diseases has been forecasted into the future. Also, while contemporary evidence confirms we are living longer, whether we are living "better" remains a complex question to answer. Presently, significant challenges persist in the clinical treatment of musculoskeletal disorders, and this has spurred the development of diverse tools, technologies, and techniques to augment and accelerate tissue repair — each carrying its own advantages and drawbacks. To address current limitations and facilitate future discovery, this book primarily aims to highlight scientific and medical knowledge gaps and the cutting-edge technologies engineered to resolve them. The reader is guided through contemporary insights into the common disorders that affect the patient, molecular targets, and smart biomaterials in early chapters, to the use of artificial intelligence and CRISPR technology to combat disease in latter sections. This makes it an ideal book for physicians, surgeons, research scientists, medical and allied health students, and university students.

Dr. Melanie J. Coathup
Professor of Medicine and Lead of the Biionix Cluster,
University of Central Florida, USA.

https://doi.org/10.1142/9789819819645_fmatter

Contents

https://doi.org/10.1142/9789819819645_0001

Chapter 1

The Burden of Musculoskeletal Disease

Hilal Memis, Hatice Feyzan Ay, Hande Maden, Hilal Calik, Rabia Cakir*

Department of Bioengineering, Faculty of Chemical and Metallurgical Engineering, Yıldız Technical University, Istanbul, Turkey

Chapter Outline

Abstract

Musculoskeletal diseases include a wide range of conditions that affect motor organs, tendons, muscles, cartilage, bone, nerves, and ligaments, resulting in loss of function and pain. They were identified as the second leading cause of nonfatal disability in 2020, impacting more than 1.63 billion people worldwide. Although many of these disorders

***Corresponding author:** Rabia Cakir, Department of Bioengineering, Faculty of Chemical and Metallurgical Engineering, Yıldız Technical University, Istanbul, Turkey; E-mail: rabiacakir@gmail.com

primarily reduce quality of life, certain musculoskeletal diseases are directly associated with mortality. In 2020, reports revealed that musculoskeletal disease was responsible for 83,100 deaths worlwide. These conditions also have significant socioeconomic impacts that directly or indirectly result in costs for individuals and society, including physiotherapy, surgery, hospital admissions and referrals, materials, and medications used. The management of musculoskeletal diseases should involve a multidisciplinary strategy comprising a variety of medical professionals and therapies, ranging from pharmaceutical therapy to invasive procedures and noninvasive rehabilitation methods. Depending on the severity of the disease, physical therapy, pharmacological and nonpharmacological drug systems, and surgical intervention are recommended for treatment. In recent years, alternative strategies such as ozone treatments, phototherapies, nuclear and molecular approaches, development of biomaterials, and engineering and genetic approaches have been developed. The major difficulties include offering treatments to patients while taking into consideration each patient's specific requirements and preferences, as well as providing patients with ongoing and coordinated care during rehabilitation therapy. Recent therapeutic strategies have been shown to effectively enhance musculoskeletal function both in the preoperative period and throughout postoperative rehabilitation. However, despite the availability of numerous effective preventive and therapeutic strategies, no fully effective method for the complete treatment of musculoskeletal conditions has been identified.

1. Introduction

As the age of our population increases rapidly around the world, many researchers continue to investigate our ability to live long, healthy lives. People need to have good musculoskeletal health in order to maintain their social, economic, and functional freedom throughout their lives. However, the importance of musculoskeletal disease is underestimated because these diseases are considered age-related and, although rarely fatal, cause irreversible conditions [1]. The accepted but not entirely correct idea about musculoskeletal disease is that it mostly affects the elderly. Although the incidence of these diseases is higher in the elderly, some conditions begin during youth and manifest themselves with increasing effects and various conditions over time [2]. Musculoskeletal system disorders are the totality of diseases that affect motor organs, tendons, muscles, cartilage, bone, nerves, and ligaments that result in loss of function and pain. These are classified into many kinds based on the afflicted parts. Table 1 summarizes some of the major categories [3]. These conditions include rheumatoid

Table 1. A summary of musculoskeletal system diseases by affected areas.

Category	Condition	Description
Joint conditions	Gout	Inflammatory arthritis causes swelling, stiffness, and pain in joints, typically affecting lower limbs.
	Osteoarthritis	Disease where the cartilage in joints breaks down, leading to pain, swelling, and stiffness.
	Psoriatic arthritis	Autoimmune disease. Causes fatigue, pain, stiffness, and swelling in the joints.
	Rheumatoid arthritis	Autoimmune disease. Characterized by swelling, pain, and stiffness in joints, often affecting hands, wrists, and feet.
	Bursitis	Inflammation of the bursa, causing pain and reduced mobility.
Bone conditions	Osteoporosis	Gradual weakening of the bones, making them more vulnerable to fractures and breaks.
	Osteopenia	Decrease in bone mineral density, not severe enough for a diagnosis of osteoporosis.
	Osteomalacia	Softening and weakening of the bones due to improper hardening after formation.
Muscle and tendon conditions	Muscular dystrophy	A group of genetic conditions causing muscles to weaken over time.
	Sarcopenia	Loss of muscle size and strength.
	Myasthenia gravis	A rare condition where voluntary muscles weaken and tire easily.
	Rotator cuff tear	Torn tendon around the shoulder joint causing pain and reduced mobility.
	Tendinitis	Inflammation of a tendon, causing pain, swelling, and reduced mobility.
Other health conditions	Fibromyalgia	Causes widespread musculoskeletal pain in the body.
	Systemic lupus erythematosus	An autoimmune condition where the immune system mistakenly attacks healthy tissues.

arthritis (RA), osteoarthritis (OA), low back pain (LBP), neck pain (NP), and gout. The remaining conditions are grouped as "other musculoskeletal system disorders" [4]. As such, musculoskeletal system diseases cover a wide range of conditions, from acute short-term illnesses to lifelong illnesses that negatively affect life. These diseases can target joints and cause OA, but they can also be caused by autoimmune diseases, leading to RA, and genetic diseases, such as ankylosing spondylitis [2]. Arthritis is defined as inflammation of the joints and can not only affect daily life but also cause irreversible joint damage, leading to depression, cardiovascular diseases, and high blood pressure [5].

Musculoskeletal diseases were identified as the second leading cause of nonfatal disability in 2020, affecting more than 1.63 billion people worldwide. According to the data obtained in 2020, an estimated 494 million people were living with a musculoskeletal disease, while it was determined that there were 221 million people with these diseases in 1990. The number of people living with musculoskeletal disease has increased significantly by 123.4% from 1990 to 2020 [6]. The onset of musculoskeletal disease ranged between the ages of 35 and 39 years in 1990, with the mean age increasing to 50–54 years in 2019 [4]. At the same time, the prevalence of musculoskeletal disease was found to be 47.4% higher in women than in men [6]. Another study found that death rates due to musculoskeletal disease were higher in women than in men and increased with age after the age of 60 years [1].

The prevalence of musculoskeletal diseases worldwide has been examined according to different categories, with LBP having the highest rate of incidence (36.8%), while RA was reported to have the lowest rate of 1.3%. When these percentages were compared with the data measured in 1990, no significant differences were observed. According to the prevalent cases, the highest incidence of LBP is seen in Central Europe, with 59.7% of the population affected, and the lowest was reported in East Asia, with 21.6% [1]. Despite a higher rate and greater number of rural residents in Africa compared to economically developed regions, Africa is a region that is least affected by the disease burden. This may be because the prevalence rates of those who are overweight (34.5%) and obese (12.7%) in Africa are lower than those in the Americas (64.2% are overweight and 28.3% are obese). In 2019, there were over 37.23 million instances of gout worldwide among the older population [7]. The global incidence of gout has risen by 63.44% in the last two decades [8]. Bursitis accounted for 400 out of every 100,000 visits to a primary care clinic [9]. Bursitis rarely coincides with a high death rate, although complications such as septic bursitis can raise the risk [10]. Sarcopenia affects around 10% of men and women aged 60 years and over worldwide [11]. The frequency rises with age, affecting up to half of those over the age of 80 years [12]. People with sarcopenia have a two times higher risk of death than those without [13]. Sarcopenia was estimated to affect 10.87 million people in Europe in 2016 and is projected to increase to 18.74 million by 2045, representing a 72.4% increase [14]. Rotator cuff tears are more common as people get older. According to studies, rotator cuff tears affect 13% of people in their fifth decade, 20% in their sixth decade, and 31% in their seventh decade [15]. Full-thickness tears occur in 22.2% of the general population, and the percentage rises with age [16]. Rotator cuff therapy costs vary greatly. For example, arthroscopic surgery costs roughly $7,000, but open shoulder surgery might cost over $17,450 [17].

The significant health and economic consequences of musculoskeletal disease have been associated with a higher body mass index (BMI). Morbidity associated with a high BMI has resulted in a global productivity loss of $120.2 billion. This economic burden varies across regions. The highest loss was recorded in the Americas, reaching $64.0 billion, followed by Europe at $34.3 billion, the Western Pacific at $16.1 billion, the Eastern Mediterranean at $2.5 billion, Southeast Asia at $2.3 billion, and Africa at $1.1 billion. Interestingly, the economic burden is not directly proportional to population size and morbidity rates. For example, the Americas, home to 13.2% of the world's population (1.0 billion people), account for 56.8% ($34.4 billion) of global healthcare costs, 53.3% ($64.0 billion) of morbidity-related costs, and 26.6% (2.0 million) of global years lost due to disability (YLD). In contrast, Southeast Asia, which hosts a quarter of the world's population (2.0 billion people, 25.9%), contributes only 1.4% ($838 million) to global healthcare costs, 1.9% ($2.3 billion) to morbidity-related costs, and 13.1% (1.0 million) to global YLD. These figures indicate that regional healthcare expenditures and productivity losses are influenced not only by population size but also by economic conditions, healthcare systems, and disease burden [18]. Musculoskeletal diseases have significant socioeconomic impacts that directly or indirectly result in costs for individuals and society. Direct costs include physiotherapy, surgery, hospital admissions and referrals, materials, and medications used. According to the calculated data reported in the United Kingdom (UK), approximately two million applications were made to the rheumatology outpatient clinic between 2019 and 2020, and the cost of these applications is estimated to be £304,057,289 [19]. Indirect costs include lost productivity at work associated with poor health, sick leave (absenteeism), and early retirement [19]. More than 30 million days off due to illness are reportedly taken annually in the UK due to musculoskeletal diseases, costing employers an estimated 5.6 billion sterling [20]. In the United States, the annual healthcare expenditure for OA is estimated to be $81 billion, whereas RA costs around $19.3 billion. Osteoporosis-related fractures are estimated to cost $19 billion in healthcare costs each year, while fibromyalgia costs around $12 billion. Furthermore, the annual healthcare costs for systemic lupus erythematosus are anticipated to be around $20,000 per patient. These expenditures encompass costs associated with medications, hospitalizations, and outpatient visits. The economic burden of sarcopenia-related disability in Iran has been estimated at $257.1 million. Comparable financial impacts are projected in other countries with aging populations [18]. Musculoskeletal problems are expected to grow by 115% between 2020 and 2050, with an estimated 1.06 billion cases. The aging population will make a considerable contribution to the growing burden of musculoskeletal illnesses, with older persons facing greater rates of disability and healthcare expenses. The requirement for therapeutic and rehabilitative services is predicted to increase dramatically, putting further strain on healthcare systems [21, 22].

In 2020, 595 million people, 7.6% of the global population, were reported to be suffering from OA. Also in 2020, the global prevalence of LBP was estimated to affect 619 million individuals. It is anticipated that this will increase to 843 million cases by 2050 [23]. Further, health expenditures to treat musculoskeletal disease in the United States reached 380.9 billion dollars, and health care costs in the European region have reached 240 billion euros [21]. Furthermore, musculoskeletal diseases often lead to mental health problems and increase the risk of varying chronic health problems. Moreover, it reduces mental and physical capacity, which threatens healthy aging. In addition, musculoskeletal disease accounts for 1/3 of workers' compensation claims and is a cause of disability that leads to more than 200 million workforce losses. It also increases the need for rehabilitation services [23]. Musculoskeletal disorders and common mental health disorders are among the leading causes of sick leave and work disability worldwide. These conditions not only affect individuals' physical and psychological health but also significantly impact their social interactions and economic participation. In this context, promoting return-to-work (RTW) for individuals with musculoskeletal disorders or mental health conditions is crucial, as it not only improves the quality of life for individuals but also makes a significant contribution to the economic growth and social well-being of industrialized societies. Facilitating the RTW process helps ensure the sustainability of the workforce, enhances workplace productivity, and reduces healthcare costs [24]. Despite the implementation of various policies, guidelines, and best practices aimed at reducing days lost due to sick leave, high absenteeism rates due to musculoskeletal disorders continue to persist. Musculoskeletal conditions significantly reduce an individual's ability to work and participate in society. Additionally, musculoskeletal disorders tend to have high recurrence rates and can become chronic. Therefore, to mitigate the economic and societal impacts of musculoskeletal disorders, it is crucial to focus on early diagnosis, effective treatment approaches, and the development of strategies to improve RTW processes [10]. Therefore, workplaces and healthcare systems should develop and implement more effective policies to support the return to work of individuals after the onset of disability. This process not only minimizes workforce loss but also plays a critical role in ensuring the long-term economic stability of communities [24].

2. Risk Factors for Musculoskeletal Disease

Many vital, behavioral, metabolic, environmental, and occupational conditions and their combinations constitute risk factors for musculoskeletal diseases [25]. The main risk factors for these disorders include gender and age [26]. For instance, the higher prevalence of musculoskeletal diseases in women is believed to result from a combination of genetic and hormonal factors, such as relaxin, which increases ligament laxity, as well as estrogen and progesterone, along with life events like pregnancy and menopause, and environmental and social influences, including physical activity levels and occupational conditions [4, 27]. Joint deterioration, muscle weakening, and inactivity that occurs with old age lead to deterioration of the musculoskeletal system and, as a result, to the emergence of diseases [28]. Moreover, improper actions, such as poor posture, incorrect sitting positions, and unsafe techniques for lifting or carrying objects, are considered major contributors to the development of these diseases. Therefore, these risk factors can be prevented by providing and developing ergonomic workplace practices and designs [29, 30]. Occupational ergonomic factors, smoking, and high BMI are other important risk factors for musculoskeletal disease. Since smoking, which is a major risk factor for many diseases, causes oxidative stress, systemic proinflammation, autoantibody formation, epigenetic alterations, and synovial hyperplasia, it may have an impact on some musculoskeletal illnesses, particularly low back pain, osteoporosis, and RA. Also, high BMI is reported to cause OA, LBP, and gout occurrence and progression [4]. In addition, other risk factors for musculoskeletal disease depend on lifestyle, genetic predisposition, and ethnicity. In some cases, nteractions between ethnicity and socioeconomic status may further raise the risk of disease. Some musculoskeletal diseases, such as RA and gout, tend to occur as inherited conditions in some families. This could be due to a genetic predisposition and/or related environmental influences [26, 31]. Also, possible risk factors for musculoskeletal disorders include factors related to social life and psychological reasons such as insomnia and sleep diseases, anxiety, and depression [28]. Furthermore, the presence of other diseases might be associated with musculoskeletal disease. For example, the initiation of musculoskeletal diseases can be associated with an increased risk of other chronic consequences, including depression and cardiovascular disease, as well as extended disease exposure [25]. Also, obesity is an important risk factor for other musculoskeletal diseases, including RA and gout. As obesity rates grow, the prevalence of these diseases rises [26, 31]. In addition, an important risk factor for gout is kidney dysfunction. Kidney dysfunction prevents urate excretion and uric acid accumulation in intra- and extra-articular structures, which forms tophus and so causes gout [4]. Therefore, research on all mentioned risk factors is crucially important for developing preventive and therapeutic strategies to take proactive measures against diseases and to reduce the burden of diseases.

3. Current Strategies and Challenges to Manage the Musculoskeletal Disease Burden

While there are no effective therapies for many musculoskeletal diseases, various analgesics, medications, and therapeutic interventions can improve symptoms and pain, delay outcomes, and prevent further damage. Healthy lifestyle habits such as weight loss, exercise, and sports are recommended as preventive measures for some musculoskeletal diseases [32]. Musculoskeletal diseases can be prevented by improving the quality of life and eliminating possible risk factors. One of the primary preventive strategies is to avoid actions that generate occupational risk factors, attach importance to occupational health and safety, and implement its measures. Another important preventive strategy is to reduce body injuries and disability to overcome muscle weakness and exercise to improve muscle control, which causes disease progression [33]. For musculoskeletal diseases, home exercises, physical therapy, and rehabilitation treatments are recommended for patients in the first stage of disease and/or with symptoms [34] (**Figure 1**). In addition to physical therapy, non-pharmacological treatments also include cryotherapy, heat therapy, acupuncture, and electrical nerve stimulation therapy can also be applied [28]. For patients in advanced stages, treatment options, including medication, adjuvant therapies, and surgical intervention are selected according to the disease and its progression [34]. Therapeutic use of bone-forming agents is also an important therapeutic strategy for musculoskeletal disease [33]. In addition, aromatherapy, which uses herbal medicines and natural products and their essential oils and extracts, is one of the traditional approaches. Many medicinal plants and herbal extracts contain active ingredients, essential oils, terpenoids, alkaloids, flavonoids, phenolic acids, and vitamins. Thus, they have the potential to be used as a muscle relaxant, reduce musculoskeletal pain and inflammation, and relieve physical symptoms. Several

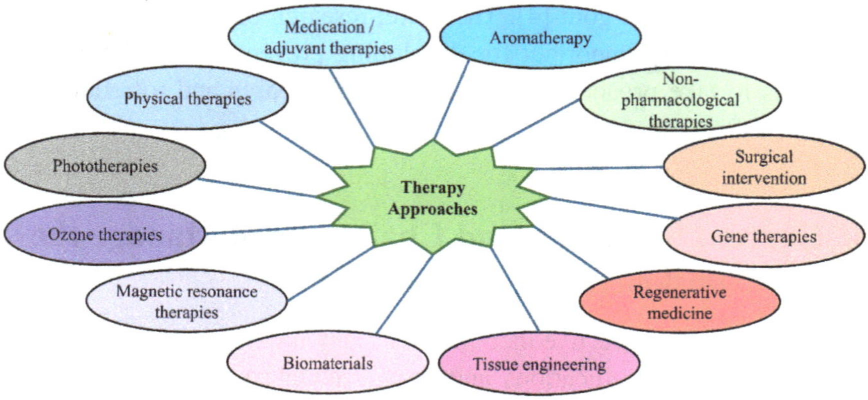

Figure 1. Current therapy approaches to reduce the musculoskeletal disease burden.

studies investigated the use of herbs, such as ginger, lavender, peppermint, rosemary, eucalyptus, chamomile, and jasmine as therapeutic options for the treatment of musculoskeletal diseases and relieve their symptoms [35–43].

In addition to these conventional methods, the efficacy of novel approaches is being researched for musculoskeletal disease treatment. As part of these approaches, hydrogels are being studied extensively for musculoskeletal applications. The injectable hydrogels are commercially approved or in trial stages for use in clinical applications. Some examples of these products include: Gel-One® (Zimmer Biomet), GelrinC® (Regentis Biomaterials), Emdogain® (Straumann), Actifuse® (Baxter), Tactoset® (Anika Therapeutics), Kinex® Bioactive Gel (Globus Medical), etc. These can be used in several ways to treat various diseases or tissue lesions. Viscosupplementation, a good treatment strategy for OA, can provide temporary pain relief and functional improvement and support tissue regrowth in joints but cannot regenerate functional cartilage. In research investigating the effectiveness of biomaterials, there are large differences in the responses between *in vitro* tests using single cell types and *in vivo* tests where different cell types interact. Despite advancements in organ-on-chip systems or co-culture models, the native tissue response to biomaterials has not yet been fully replicated [41]. Regional gene therapy, which involves local implantation of nucleic acids or genetically modified cells to direct specific protein expression, holds promise for bone repair. In preclinical studies in animal models, regional gene therapy is effective in healing critical-sized bone defects [42]. Also, phototherapy, a noninvasive technique that includes photothermal therapy and photodynamic therapy methods, has been proposed as an important treatment approach for musculoskeletal diseases. Phototherapy techniques can regulate bone, cartilage, and muscle regeneration and treat conditions such as bone tumors, bone infections, and arthritis [43]. Recently, researchers have investigated the potential of molecular biophysical stimulation therapy (MBST), specifically nuclear magnetic resonance therapy. In the treatment of musculoskeletal diseases, including OA, osteoporosis, and chronic back pain, the effectiveness of MBST has been evaluated, and successful results have been obtained in promoting bone and cartilage healing [44]. Moreover, the investigation of ozone and oxygen-ozone therapy as an alternative treatment has become significant in recent years. Oxygen-ozone treatments have been reported to have antalgic, antioxidant, anti-inflammatory, and immunomodulatory properties. They have been recommended for several years as an effective treatment for some musculoskeletal diseases such as LBP, knee OA, carpal tunnel syndrome, cervical diseases, and meniscus injuries [45, 46]. Biomaterials, tissue engineering, regenerative medicine, and gene therapy strategies are increasingly important in the treatment of musculoskeletal disease to promote muscle and bone regeneration [47, 48]. However, there is still no proven method for completely treating musculoskeletal diseases, despite many beneficial preventive and therapeutic strategies. The management of musculoskeletal diseases should involve a multidisciplinary strategy comprising a variety of medical professionals and therapies, ranging from pharmaceutical therapy to invasive procedures and noninvasive rehabilitation methods. The major difficulties include offering treatments to patients while taking into consideration each patient's specific requirements and preferences, as well as providing patients with ongoing and coordinated care during rehabilitation therapy [49].

4. Conclusions

Musculoskeletal diseases are severe conditions that impose a considerable health and economic burden on patients and have a profound impact on their lives. Among musculoskeletal diseases worldwide, the most prevalent are lower back and NP, followed by OA, RA, and gout. Risk factors of musculoskeletal problems are typically associated with lifestyle and standards of living. This is followed by old age and adverse conditions related to aging, genetic predisposition, environmental factors, and side effects of another disease or treatment. The most important preventive treatment strategy for musculoskeletal diseases is to improve the quality of life to eliminate the defined risk factors. In addition, depending on the severity of the disease, physical therapy, pharmacological and nonpharmacological therapies, and surgical intervention are recommended. In recent years, in addition to these traditional approaches, alternative strategies such as ozone treatments, phototherapies, and molecular approaches; the development of biomaterials, and engineering and genetic approaches have been developed. To summarize, the significant burden of musculoskeletal diseases, caused by multiple risk factors, emphasizes the urgent need for comprehensive prevention methods and innovative treatments to address these issues and enhance patient outcomes in the future.

References

1. Safiri S, Kolahi A-A, Cross M, Hill C, Smith E, Carson-Chahhoud K, et al. Prevalence, deaths, and disability-adjusted life years due to musculoskeletal disorders for 195 countries and territories 1990–2017. *Arthritis & Rheum.* 2021 Apr;73(4):702–14.
2. Summers K, Jinnett K, Bevan S. Musculoskeletal disorders, workforce health and productivity in the United States. 2015.
3. Belluzzi E, Pozzuoli A, Ruggieri P. Musculoskeletal diseases: From molecular basis to therapy. *Biomedicines.* 2023 Dec 22;12(1):32.
4. Liu S, Wang B, Fan S, Wang Y, Zhan Y, Ye D. Global burden of musculoskeletal disorders and attributable factors in 204 countries and territories: A secondary analysis of the global burden of disease 2019 study. *BMJ Open.* 2022;12(6):e062183.
5. Gibson DS, Rooney ME. Musculoskeletal diseases. *Proteomics Clin. Appl.* 2016;10(6):623–4.
6. Gill TK, Mittinty MM, March LM, Steinmetz JD, Culbreth GT, Cross M, et al. Global, regional, and national burden of other musculoskeletal disorders, 1990–2020, and projections to 2050: A systematic analysis of the Global Burden of Disease Study 2021. *Lancet Rheumatol.* 2023;5(11):e670–e82.

7. Li Y, Chen Z, Xu B, Wu G, Yuan Q, Xue X, et al. Global, regional, and national burden of gout in elderly 1990–2021: An analysis for the global burden of disease study 2021. *BMC Public Health*. 2024 Nov 27;24(1):3298.
8. He Q, Mok T-N, Sin T-H, Yin J, Li S, Yin Y, et al. Global, regional, and national prevalence of gout from 1990 to 2019: Age-period-cohort analysis with future burden prediction. *JMIR Public Health Surveill.* 2023 Jun 7;9:e45943.
9. McAfee JH, Smith DL. Olecranon and prepatellar bursitis. Diagnosis and treatment. *West. J. Med.*1988 Nov;149(5):607–10.
10. Lieber SB, Fowler ML, Zhu C, Moore A, Shmerling RH, Paz Z. Clinical characteristics and outcomes of septic bursitis. *Infection*. 2017 Dec;45(6):781–6.
11. Shafiee G, Keshtkar A, Soltani A, Ahadi Z, Larijani B, Heshmat R. Prevalence of sarcopenia in the world: A systematic review and meta-analysis of general population studies. *J. Diabetes Metab. Disord.* 2017 May 16;16:21.
12. Morley JE, Anker SD, von Haehling S. Prevalence, incidence, and clinical impact of sarcopenia: Facts, numbers, and epidemiology-update 2014. *J. Cachexia Sarcopenia Muscle*. 2014 Dec;5(4):253–9.
13. Xu J, Wan CS, Ktoris K, Reijnierse EM, Maier AB. Sarcopenia is associated with mortality in adults: A systematic review and meta-analysis. *Gerontology*. 2022;68(4):361–76.
14. Ethgen O, Beaudart C, Buckinx F, Bruyère O, Reginster JY. The future prevalence of sarcopenia in Europe: A claim for public health action. *Calcif. Tissue Int.* 2017 Mar;100(3):229–234.
15. Gumina S, Passaretti D, Candela V. Epidemiology and demographics of the rotator cuff tear. In: Gumina S. (eds) *Rotator Cuff Tear*. Cham: Springer, 2017.
16. Hinsley H, Ganderton C, Arden NK, Carr AJ. Prevalence of rotator cuff tendon tears and symptoms in a Chingford general population cohort, and the resultant impact on UK health services: A cross-sectional observational study. *BMJ Open*. 2022;12:e059175.
17. Pierami R, Antonioli E, Oliveira I, Castro IQ, Manente F, Fairbanks P, et al. Clinical outcomes and cost-utility of rotator cuff repair surgery by open and arthroscopic techniques: Study protocol for a randomised clinical trial. *BMJ Open*. 2020;10:e043126.
18. Chen N, Fong DYT, Wong JYH. Health and economic outcomes associated with musculoskeletal disorders attributable to high body mass index in 192 countries and territories in 2019. *JAMA Netw. Open*. 2023;6(1):e2250674.

19. Humphreys JH, Verstappen SMM. The burden of musculoskeletal disease. *Medicine*. 2022;50(2):82–4.
20. Hartfiel N, Clarke G, Havenhand J, Phillips C, Edwards RT. Cost-effectiveness of yoga for managing musculoskeletal conditions in the workplace. *Occup Med (Lond)*. 2017;67(9):687–95.
21. ScienceDaily. *New Insights into the Role of Gut Microbiota in Health and Disease*. 2023, November 20.
22. Jiang F, Lu C, Zeng Z, Sun Z, Qiu Y. Global burden of disease for musculoskeletal disorders in all age groups, from 2024 to 2050, and a bibliometric-based survey of the status of research in geriatrics, geriatric orthopedics, and geriatric orthopedic diseases. *J. Orthop. Surg. Res*. 2025 Feb 19;20(1):179.
23. Nguyen AT, Aris IM, Snyder BD, Harris MB, Kang JD, Murray M, et al. Musculoskeletal health: An ecological study assessing disease burden and research funding. *Lancet Reg. Health Am.* 2024;29:100661.
24. Gragnano A, Villotti P, Larivière C, Negrini A, Corbière M. A systematic search and review of questionnaires measuring individual psychosocial factors predicting return to work after musculoskeletal and common mental disorders. *J. Occup. Rehabil.* 2021;31(3):491–511.
25. Guan S-Y, Zheng J-X, Sam NB, Xu S, Shuai Z, Pan F. Global burden and risk factors of musculoskeletal disorders among adolescents and young adults in 204 countries and territories, 1990–2019. *Autoimmun. Rev*. 2023;22(8):103361.
26. Ingram M, Symmons DPM. The burden of musculoskeletal conditions. *Medicine*. 2018;46(3):152–5.
27. Wolf JM, Cannada L, Van Heest AE, O'Connor MI, Ladd AL. Male and female differences in musculoskeletal disease. *J. Am. Acad. Orthop. Surg.* 2015;23(6):339–47.
28. El-Tallawy SN, Nalamasu R, Salem GI, LeQuang JAK, Pergolizzi JV, Christo PJ. Management of musculoskeletal pain: An update with emphasis on chronic musculoskeletal pain. *Pain Ther.* 2021;10:181–209.
29. Oakman J, Lambert KA, Rogerson S, Bell A. We know it doesn't work: Why do we still use how to lift training for the prevention of musculoskeletal disorders? *Int. J. Ind. Ergon.* 2024;100:103542.
30. Odebiyi DO, Okafor UAC. *Musculoskeletal disorders, workplace ergonomics and injury prevention*. Ergonomics-new insights: IntechOpen, 2023.
31. Parsons S, Symmons DPM. The burden of musculoskeletal conditions. *Medicine* 2014 Apr;42(4):190–2.

32. Storheim K, Zwart J-A. Musculoskeletal disorders and the Global Burden of Disease study. *Ann. Rheum. Dis.* 2014;73(6): 949–50.
33. Mody GM, Woolf AD, Bearel A. The global burden of musculoskeletal disorders. *Bus. Brief. Eur. Pharmacother.* 2003:1–5.
34. Qaseem A, Wilt TJ, McLean RM, Forciea MA, Clinical Guidelines Committee of the American College of Physicians, Denberg TD, et al. Noninvasive treatments for acute, subacute, and chronic low back pain: A clinical practice guideline from the American College of Physicians. *Ann. Intern. Med.* 2017;166(7):514–30.
35. Bakó E, Fehérvári P, Garami A, Dembrovszky F, Gunther EE, Hegyi P, et al. Efficacy of topical essential oils in musculoskeletal disorders: Systematic review and meta-analysis of randomized controlled trials. *Pharmaceuticals.* 2023;16(2):144.
36. El Sayed EM, Al Sebaee HA, Mohammed HA, Nawito ZO. Effect of lavender oil massage on pain among patients with knee osteoarthritis. *Indian J. Public Health Res. Dev.* 2020;11(1):304–9.
37. Rahbardar MG, Hosseinzadeh H. Therapeutic effects of rosemary (Rosmarinus officinalis L.) and its active constituents on nervous system disorders. *Iran. J. Basic Med. Sci.* 2020;23(9):1100–12.
38. Saud Gany SL, Chin K-Y, Tan JK, Aminuddin A, Makpol S. Preventative and therapeutic potential of tocotrienols on musculoskeletal diseases in ageing. *Front. Pharmacol.* 2023;14:1290721.
39. Song J-A, Bae IL. Effects of aromatherapy on pain in patients with musculoskeletal disease: A systematic literature review. 2021:8(5):2427–44.
40. Varkaneh ZK, Karampourian A, Oshvandi K, Basiri Z, Mohammadi Y. The effect of eucalyptus inhalation on pain and the quality of life in rheumatoid arthritis. *Contemp. Clin. Trials Commun.* 2022;29:100976.
41. Øvrebø Ø, Perale G, Wojciechowski JP, Echalier C, Jeffers JRT, Stevens MM, et al. Design and clinical application of injectable hydrogels for musculoskeletal therapy. *Bioeng. Trans. Med.* 2022;7(2):e10295.
42. Collon K, Gallo MC, Lieberman JR. Musculoskeletal tissue engineering: Regional gene therapy for bone repair. *Biomaterials* 2021;275:120901.
43. Zhang Z, Wang R, Xue H, Knoedler S, Geng Y, Liao Y, et al. Phototherapy techniques for the management of musculoskeletal disorders: Strategies and recent advances. *Biomater. Res.* 2023;27(1):123.
44. Žnidarič M, Kozinc Z, Škrinjar D. Potential of molecular biophysical stimulation therapy in chronic musculoskeletal disorders: A narrative review. *Eur. J. Transl. Myol.* 2023;33(4):11894.

45. Akkawi I. Ozone therapy for musculoskeletal disorders: Current concepts. *Acta. Biomed.* 2020;91(4):e2020191.
46. de Sire A, Agostini F, Lippi L, Mangone M, Marchese S, Cisari C, et al. Oxygen–Ozone therapy in the rehabilitation field: State of the art on mechanisms of action, safety and effectiveness in patients with musculoskeletal disorders. *Biomolecules* 2021;11(3):356.
47. Enayati M, Liu W, Madry H, Neisiany RE, Cucchiarini M. Functionalized hydrogels as smart gene delivery systems to treat musculoskeletal disorders. 2024;331:103232.
48. Park S, Rahaman KA, Kim Y-C, Jeon H, Han H-S. Fostering tissue engineering and regenerative medicine to treat musculoskeletal disorders in bone and muscle. *Bioact. Mater.* 2024;40:345–65.
49. Perna A, Proietti L. Editorial on: Musculoskeletal rehabilitation: Current challenges and new perspectives. *J. Clin. Med.* 2023;12(12):3981.

https://doi.org/10.1142/9789819819645_0002

Chapter 2

The Aging Musculoskeletal Disorder Patient: A Call to Action

Jonathan D. Schwartzman[1], Asif Aziz[1], Luis Jimenez-Chavez[1], Joanne Dore[1], Abdullah Faruk Uyanık[1], Ali Yüce[2], Aadil Mumith[1,3], Melanie J. Coathup[1,*]

[1]*Biionix Cluster, College of Medicine, University of Central Florida, Orlando, FL 32827, United States*
[2]*Prof. Dr. Cemil Tascioglu Training and Research Hospital, Kaptan Paşa, Darülaceze Cd. No: 27, 34384 Şişli/İstanbul, Türkiye*
[3]*Basingstoke and North Hampshire Hospital, Hampshire Hospitals NHS Foundation Trust, Basingstoke, RG24 7AL, UK*

Chapter Outline

* **Corresponding author:** Dr. Melanie Coathup, Biionix Cluster, Department of Medicine, College of Medicine, University of Central Florida, FL 32827, United States. Email: melanie.coathup@ucf.edu

Abstract

Aging is a major cause of impaired musculoskeletal healing. As humans age, the capacity of tissues to regenerate and repair naturally declines due to a series of interlaced and complex changes at the molecular, cellular, material, and structural levels. This natural, age-related decline can result in a plethora of clinical challenges, and understanding this multifaceted interplay is essential for developing effective strategies to prevent and treat age-related musculoskeletal disorders such as sarcopenia, osteoporosis, and osteoarthritis (OA). Advances in medical research, together with more active lifestyles, are lengthening life, and record life expectancy does not appear to be approaching its limit. Evidence confirms that we are living longer; however, it remains unclear whether we are living "better." As the global proportion of the oldest-old (>85 years of age) and the number of centenarians continue to increase, a rise in age-related musculoskeletal degenerative disease and disability is projected. This combined with higher patient expectations for superior health outcomes is calling for a change in the approach to and delivery of health care for the elderly. As such, this shift necessitates urgency in educating clinicians on the fundamental alterations in regenerative capacity for this cohort and subsequently training them to tailor musculoskeletal care accordingly. In this chapter, we highlight the key molecular, cellular, material, and structural factors that drive the aging process within musculoskeletal tissues. We describe the clinical consequences of age-associated decline with a focus on the Star Triad, examine whether humans become too old for total joint replacement, and review the unique and significant impact of cancer therapy on musculoskeletal morbidity in the elderly. Challenges due to osteoporosis, OA, and Achilles tendon rupture are discussed, and finally, we highlight salient critical unmet gaps, both for clinicians and researchers, and propose strategies to bridge them.

1. Aging as a Central Modifier of Musculoskeletal Health

Aging is among the most significant determinants of impaired musculoskeletal healing. With global life expectancy continuing to rise, the proportion of individuals aged 65 and above is projected to continue to increase dramatically, paralleled by a surge in musculoskeletal disease burden. Recent literature estimates that 16% of the world's population will be elderly (≥65 years of age) by 2050, with an increasing proportion aged ≥85 years [1]; this group carries the highest risk of fragility fractures, tendon degeneration, degraded articular cartilage, narrowed intervertebral discs, sarcopenia, and impaired postsurgical recovery [2, 3]. Globally, satisfactory musculoskeletal health is essential to enable mobility and wellness in old age. However, the limited regenerative capacity of these tissues and their inadequate ability to repair mean that achieving clinical success with conventional therapeutic musculoskeletal strategies can be challenging. In this respect, elderly patients often endure frequent complications in care and require protracted hospital stays [4], thereby posing a high burden on healthcare costs [5, 6]. As such, this shift necessitates urgency in educating clinicians on the fundamental alterations in regenerative capacity in this cohort and subsequently training them to tailor musculoskeletal care accordingly. Human aging is a complex, multifunctional process characterized by a time-related and irreversible deterioration of physiological function. The key primary factors involved are highlighted below.

1.1. *Cellular and Molecular Changes in Aging Musculoskeletal Tissue*

As humans age, the fundamental regenerative potential inherent within musculoskeletal tissues diminishes due to a confluence of factors at the cellular and molecular levels. This includes (i) genomic and epigenetic instability and misfolded proteins, (ii) cellular senescence and inflammation, and (iii) oxidative stress.

1.1.1. *Genomic and Epigenetic Instability, and Misfolded Proteins*

Aging is intrinsically associated with the progressive accumulation of nuclear and mitochondrial DNA (mtDNA) damage [7–10], along with a reduction in the efficacy of innate DNA repair mechanisms [11, 12]. Within cells, this manifests as chromosomal aberrations, telomere shortening, and genomic instability, which increase with each cell division cycle, thereby limiting proliferation and differentiation, among other cellular functions. Further, with age, somatic mutations within mtDNA accumulate in mitotic and postmitotic tissue, as well as in stem cell precursors [13, 14]. In the context of osteogenesis, such mtDNA mutations impair osteoblast metabolism and matrix synthesis due to its heavily adenosine triphosphate (ATP)-dependent nature, thereby increasing bone loss [15]. Epigenetic alterations (i.e., DNA methylation, histone modification, and regulation by noncoding RNAs) compound these processes *via* global hypomethylation and specific hypermethylation, which both downregulate the expression of key osteogenic genes, such as Runt-related transcription factor 2 (RUNX2) and Osterix, while also altering the fundamental structure of chromatin [16]. Age-associated epigenetic alterations have also been reported to modulate the expression of receptor activator of nuclear factor kappa-B ligand (RANKL) and osteoprotegerin (OPG) [16]. Notably, the RANKL–OPG signaling pathway serves as a crucial regulator of bone remodeling and plays a vital role in maintaining bone health. In support of this, aged human mesenchymal stem cells (hMSCs) have been reported to significantly downregulate OPG expression and increase RANKL expression, thereby inhibiting bone formation and shifting the cellular balance toward bone resorption [17, 18]. Similarly, altered DNA methylation patterns are associated with age-related changes in tendons, decreasing their elasticity, promoting degeneration, heightening their susceptibility to injury, and reducing their repair capacity [19]. Strong associations have been reported between epigenetic changes and the aging of cartilage tissue contributing to the development of OA [20], as well as the dysfunction of satellite cell proliferation and differentiation, which are linked to the development of sarcopenia [21].

Cells are bestowed with essential systems to ensure that proteins fold correctly and to eliminate any misfolded proteins that cannot be rescued. Genomic instability can trigger a cascade of events that leads to protein misfolding, which can have a significant impact on cellular health [22]. Protein misfolding, a process where proteins fail to fold into their correct three-dimensional (3D) structure, accumulates with aging due to a decline in the cells' ability to maintain protein homeostasis. The accumulation of aggregates of misfolded proteins leads to proteotoxicity [23] and is a hallmark occurrence in many age-related disorders [24, 25]. For example, associations have been reported between protein misfolding and sarcopenia [26], osteoporosis [27], OA [28], aging-associated tendon degeneration [29], and intervertebral disc degeneration [30]. Together with the daily stresses and injuries placed on musculoskeletal tissue, these aging-related genetic and proteomic alterations result in diminished remodeling potential, delayed healing, impaired function, and increased susceptibility to disease.

1.1.2. *Cellular Senescence and Inflammation*

Heightened levels of cellular senescence have been implicated as a major cause of age-related disease. Senescence is characterized by a stable state of growth arrest in which cells are unable to proliferate despite optimal growth conditions and mitogenic stimuli. Cells also develop increased resistance to apoptotic death [31]. While senescence contributes an important physiological role during healthy homeostasis — a role that limits the proliferation of aged or damaged cells — aging-associated senescence is triggered *via* DNA damage, decreased mitophagy, oxidative stress, and genomic instability, among other factors [32]. To this end, recent evidence highlights the high relevance and role of senescence in musculoskeletal disorders [33]. As cells become senescent, their senescence-associated secretory phenotype (SASP) secretome contributes toward sustaining a chronic inflammatory state, thereby disrupting musculoskeletal tissue remodeling processes. For example, various bone marrow cells, osteoblasts, and osteocytes secrete SASP, which increases their expression of interleukin 6 (IL-6), IL-1β, tumor necrosis factor alpha (TNF-α), and RANKL, which contribute toward osteoclastogenesis while impairing mesenchymal stem cell (MSC) differentiation toward osteoblasts [33]. Thus, age-related senescence actively promotes osteoporosis [34], impairs the bone repair response [35], and implant osseointegration [36]. Notably, senescent chondrocytes have been linked to age-related OA [37], senescent satellite cells and myoblasts to sarcopenia [38], senescent tenocytes to impaired tendon repair [29], and senescent cells to intervertebral disc aging and degeneration [39]. These SASP-induced positive feedback proinflammatory cycles are critical in reducing musculoskeletal recovery *via* impaired tissue formation and increased tissue breakdown.

1.1.3. *Oxidative Stress*

As the primary endogenous source of unstable reactive oxygen species (ROS), mitochondrial dysfunction is arguably one of the most important mechanisms that contribute to aging-associated tissue decline [40]. Aging causes a reduction in ATP production, together with a sustained increase in ROS (i.e., oxidative stress). ROS, especially in excess of available antioxidant buffer, induce various destructive processes including impaired matrix production, the apoptosis of osteoblasts and osteocytes, and the activation of osteoclastogenesis *via* Wnt/β-catenin signaling — thus promoting bone resorption, compounding bone loss [41–45], delaying postoperative bone repair following orthopedic surgery [46], and impairing implant osseointegration [47, 48]. Further, *via* oxidative stress, aging can shift the fate of MSCs toward adipogenesis at the expense of osteogenesis, thereby further exacerbating bone loss [49]. Aging-induced sarcopenia is typically characterized by reduced muscle mass, reduced cross-sectional fiber area, alterations in myosin isotype or fiber type, and the loss of organelles, cytoplasm, and total proteins [50–52]. Sarcopenia negatively impacts multiple physiological parameters including respiration, thermoregulation, and metabolic homeostasis [52]. Notably, emerging evidence suggests that oxidative stress and inflammation are the main pathological drivers in the development of sarcopenia. As ROS-mediated mitochondrial dysfunction is likely a gatekeeper for age-related tissue decline, data suggest the potential role of antioxidant and anti-inflammatory strategies for its treatment [52]. Excessive ROS production can directly damage the components of articular cartilage, including chondrocytes, collagen, and proteoglycans, leading to the breakdown of the extracellular matrix (ECM), compromising cartilage integrity and driving OA [53]. Further, oxidative stress is increasingly recognized as a significant factor that hinders tendon repair and contributes to the development and progression of degenerative tendinopathy in older adults [54]. Chronic tendinopathy is characterized by persistent pain, swelling, and the impairment of tendon and adjacent soft tissue function [55]. Patients >70 years of age often present with a significantly higher incidence of rotator cuff tears compared to the younger cohort. Older patients display a regenerative capacity that is substantially and comparatively impaired and present with higher levels of serum oxidative stress [56]. Notably, oxidative stress and rotator cuff degeneration in mice are reported to be associated with a decrease in collagen type I and localized mechanical property degradation, thereby increasing the susceptibility of the tendon to mechanical rupture or injury [57]. Finally, oxidative stress is reported to promote the degeneration of intervertebral disc degeneration (IDD) in the elderly [58]. Although oxidative stress has been shown to negatively impact inflammation, autophagy, and DNA methylation in IDD [59], the specific pathological mechanism through which oxidative stress–induced damage occurs remains to be elucidated. Nevertheless, some antioxidant therapeutic measures for IDD hold excellent future promise.

1.2. *Structural and Material Changes in Aging Musculoskeletal Tissue*

1.2.1. *Bone Mineral and Collagen Composition*

Over time, bone mineral becomes more crystalline, characterized by larger hydroxyapatite crystals, which make aged bone more brittle [60, 61]. This occurs *via* increased crystallinity altering the elastic modulus of bone, as shown by its reduced ability to dissipate energy during mechanical loading. Similarly, the quality of the collagen itself deteriorates over time *via* various processes including nonenzymatic glycation forming advanced glycation end-products (AGEs) [62, 63]. Accumulating in the collagen matrix, AGEs interfere with collagen cross-linking and bind to the receptor for advanced glycation end-products (RAGE) on osteoblasts, promoting nuclear factor kappa-light-chain-enhancer of activated B cell (NF-κB) signaling and osteoclastogenesis. Further microarchitectural degenerative processes have been cited *via* histomorphometric and high-resolution imaging studies, confirming that aging leads to decreased osteocyte lacunar density by up to 30%, increased cortical porosity, trabecular thinning, altered lacunar shape, and thinning of the canalicular network [64, 65]. These structural changes reduce mechanotransduction, impairing the ability of bone to respond to mechanical loads and repair microdamage. Clinically, these principles underscore aged bone as having overall reduced toughness and an increased risk of fracture despite a similar bone density. Standard metrics such as the dual-energy X-ray absorptiometry (DEXA) scan may subsequently underestimate fracture risk in elderly patients.

1.2.2. *Muscle Mass Loss and Fiber Changes*

Aging leads to significant changes in muscle structure, morphology, and material properties. This is primarily characterized by a decline in muscle mass, strength, and power (i.e., sarcopenia) [66]. Muscle atrophy begins during the third and fourth decades of life, with ~10% of muscle lost by age 50 years [67]. Subsequently, an accelerated rate of muscle loss ensues in both sexes, where ~0.7%–0.8% per year of lower limb muscle atrophy typically occurs in the seventh and eighth decades of life [68]. This decline may be further accelerated into very old age unless interventions occur [69]. Sarcopenia is driven primarily *via* the loss of motor units [70] and atrophy of surviving muscle fibers [67]. During aging-associated muscle loss, signaling pathways that regulate muscle size (e.g., transforming growth factor-beta [TGF-β]/Activin/bone morphogenetic protein [BMP], NF-κB, and insulin-like growth factor [IGF-1]/protein kinase B [Akt]/mammalian target of rapamycin [mTOR] signaling [71, 72]) are altered, and the reduction in whole muscle mass typically correlates with a reduced number of myofibers and, to a lesser degree, a reduction in myofiber area [67]. Further, muscle tissue is gradually replaced by noncontractile adipose and connective tissue. This tissue, located within and adjacent to the muscles, can become stiffer and less elastic, and the interaction between muscle and fascia weakens. To this end, depending on the muscle group, ~2% to 5% of noncontractile tissue has been measured in young individuals, while ~8% to 18% was measured in an elderly male cohort [73]. As such, after 50–60 years of age, the accelerated formation of noncontractile tissue within the muscle potentially negatively impacts overall muscle movement and force transmission [74], with a rate of decline in strength measured at ~2%–4% per year [75, 76]. Finally, the central and peripheral nervous systems become less efficient at activating muscle fibers, together with a gradual loss of motoneurons and degeneration of neuromuscular junctions [77]. The denervation of fibers belonging to a fast-twitch single motor unit is followed by reinnervation of slow-twitch fibers, which leads to a gradual conversion of fiber-type grouping [67]. Thus, there is a steady shift toward a higher proportion of slow-twitch (type I) muscle fibers parallel to a decline in fast-twitch (type II) fibers, thereby reducing muscle force, speed, and reaction times. Translated to the clinic, coordination and control of muscle movements are often affected, thereby contributing to balance problems and falls.

1.2.3. *Tendon Loss and Collagen Composition*

Aging significantly impacts tendon structure, composition, and its material properties, leading to reduced strength, elasticity, and stiffness, thereby increasing the risk of injury, including microtraumas [78]. These changes are primarily due to a decline in collagen production, alterations in collagen fibril structure, and a decrease in tenocyte function. Several signaling pathways play a role in the aging of tendon tissue, with the Janus kinase-signal transducer and activator of transcription (JAK-STAT) [79], NF-κB [80], and Wnt [81] pathways being particularly significant. Collagen accounts for ~60%–85% of tendon dry weight and is an essential contributor to the mechanical properties of tendons [82]. To this end, collagen fibrils can be millimeters in length [83], range between ~1 and 300 nm in diameter [84], and are the principal tensile element in tendon [82]. Approximately 95% of collagen is type I, with types III, V, XI, XII, and XIV comprising the remaining 5% [85]. As aging progresses, collagen biosynthesis declines, and its degradation is increased *via* posttranscriptional hydroxylation, glycosylation, and AGE crosslinking, thereby reducing or enlarging collagen fibril size [86, 87]. Further, the presence of fragmented and disorganized collagen fibers is typically reported, and these changes are considered the structural basis for the mechanical differences observed between mature and aged tendons [87, 88]. Further, aged tendons display a reduction in vascularity [89], and the increased presence of non-tendinous tissues such as adipose, cartilaginous, and calcified tissue compromises tendon structure and thereby reduces its biomechanical properties [90–92]. Together, this loss of collagen and alterations in its structure result in stiffer, less elastic tendons that become less able to stretch, recoil, and dissipate forces, making them more susceptible to tears and other injuries, particularly during activities that involve repetitive motions or high impact. As such, tendinitis, tendinopathy, and tendon tears are more common in older individuals due to these age-related changes.

1.2.4. *Cartilage Aging and Altered Collagen Structure*

Aging leads to decreased cartilage thickness, increased stiffness, and an altered tissue composition. These morphological, biochemical, and mechanical changes are due in part to changes that include reduced water content and altered collagen structure, which together contribute to cartilage degeneration and an increased risk of dysfunction, including OA. Articular cartilage and subchondral bone comprise a functional unit that delivers an essential physiological role in distributing load and absorbing shock during ambulation and movement. Cartilage degeneration is attributed to many factors including metabolism, age, and overloading [93]. Age-related structural changes include a reduction in collagen type II expression and in the thickness and strength of the fibers within. Several signaling pathways play crucial roles and include Notch [94], TGF-β/BMP, fibroblast growth factor (FGF), and Wnt [95]. Cartilage decline is accompanied by functional condensation of the underlying subchondral bone, which displays a characteristic disordered arrangement of trabeculae. An increase in thickness and bone mineral density (BMD) and decreased porosity are also reportedly observed in the subchondral plate during aging [96]. In terms of morphology, and in addition to a decrease in cartilage thickness, age-related surface degeneration occurs *via* cartilage defects and fibrillation, which first occur in the superficial zone of articular cartilage [96, 97]. In healthy cartilage, the orientation and organization of the collagen fibril network run parallel to the articular surface. However, during aging, this changes, and the fibrils instead form an arcade-like Benninghoff architecture, suggesting important negative implications for cartilage mechanics and mechanobiology [98]. To this end, the elastic modulus and tensile strength of articular cartilage decrease markedly. Other age-related changes include increased collagen cross-linking *via* AGEs, loss of large proteoglycan aggregates, increased fibril diameter, accumulation of degraded molecules, and decreased water concentration [99, 100]. Ultimately, cartilage becomes stiffer with age, which reduces its ability to deform and absorb shock, thereby increasing its susceptibility to damage from mechanical stress and injury.

1.2.5. *Intervertebral Disc Aging, Flattening, and Material Dysfunction*

As the body ages, the intervertebral discs undergo significant structural changes. Interestingly, intervertebral discs undergo detrimental age-related changes at a younger age compared to other tissues in the body [101, 102]. These changes encompass alterations in the ECM, cellular biology, and overall disc morphology, including *via* NF-κB, mitogen-activated protein kinases (MAPKs), and hypoxia-inducible factor 1-alpha (HIF-1α) signaling pathways [103]. The nucleus pulposus (NP), normally a gelatinous, hydrated tissue, experiences a decrease in water content with age, leading to a more fibrous presentation. This is largely due to an age-related reduction in aggrecan, the primary proteoglycan responsible for the NP's osmotic properties and hydration [104]. This decline in aggrecan leads to a loss of glycosaminoglycans and a reduction in disc height and pressurization [105, 106]. Notably, the slow peroxidation of lipids linked to collagen and matrix proteins allows for the accumulation of lipofuscin, an "age pigment," which transforms the normally clear NP found in youth to a yellow color in older individuals [107]. Such modifications to structural proteins also contribute to the impaired material function of aging disc tissue. Structural disorganization is also apparent in the annulus fibrosus (AF), where the concentric rings of collagen fibers become irregular, bifurcate, and interdigitate, compromising the AF's ability to contain the NP. These changes are associated with an increase in the number and size of tears and fissures, as well as the presence of granular debris within the disc construct [102]. Further, the primary type I collagen fibers within the outer AF, as well as the type II fibers located within the inner AF, undergo proteolytic damage and form nonenzymatic crosslinks, leading to weakened mechanical strength and increased stiffness. The loss of intradiscal pressure from NP aging causes increased shear stresses in the AF when the spine is loaded under compression. Aging also impacts the cartilaginous endplates (CEPs). The CEPs facilitate nutrient diffusion into the disc, and as they thin, ossify, become sclerotic, develop microfractures within subchondral bone, and undergo a drastic reduction in vascular channels with age, this hinders nutrient supply, accumulates waste products, and exacerbates disc dysfunction [108, 109]. Thus, disc aging involves a cascade of biochemical and structural changes that ultimately compromise its ability to withstand dynamic mechanical forces and maintain spinal stability.

2. The Clinical Consequences of Age-Associated Decline

The cellular, molecular, and structural changes in aged bone result in a plethora of clinical challenges, especially in the domains of osteoporosis, fracture healing, implant integration, cartilage degenerative conditions, and tendon and ligament repair.

2.1. *The Star Triad: Sarcopenia, Tendinopathy, and Arthritis*

In 2020, Minetto *et al.* introduced nomenclature to describe a pathological triad of three interrelated disorders, especially prevalent in elderly patients, known as the Star Triad: sarcopenia, tendinopathy, and arthritis [110]. These processes are uniquely shaped by age-associated inflammatory regulation abnormalities, decreased biomechanical integrity, and loss of regenerative capacity. The triad highlights how these conditions can negatively influence each other, accelerating disease progression and impacting an individual's quality of life. As such, a particularly insidious consequence of musculoskeletal aging is the convergence of degenerative disorders that compound each other and collectively reduce independence. By introducing this nomenclature, Minetto *et al.* provide clinicians with a framework that seeks to emphasize the tandem nature of pathological processes that are often uniquely seen and treated in isolation [110]. Specifically, the team explores the mutual reinforcement of muscle wasting, tendon degeneration, and joint deterioration, which lead to rapid and substantial decreases in elderly quality of life. For the aging musculoskeletal disorder patient, clinicians will routinely encounter individuals in a sarcopenic state, clinically defined by progressive loss of skeletal muscle mass and function, which has been shown to affect over 30% of individuals aged 60 and older [111]. As the skeleton loses muscular support, joints and tendons are subjected to proportionally increased force with a higher likelihood of overload and injury. Subsequent tendinopathies and arthritis limit the functional mobility and endurance of these patients, further accelerating muscular atrophy. The result of this vicious cycle is an escalating decline in functional reserve, which often culminates in long-term disability and generalized frailty. Falls are significant in this cohort, with various studies on geriatric patients citing mortality rates upward of 17% within 30 days of a hip fracture and 33% within 1 year [112]. Older age was found to be an independent risk factor in many of these studies, and other risk factors, namely malnutrition, have been found to increase mortality risk by upward of a factor of 4 [113]. Even in successful surgical cases, approximately 40% of patients lose independence and transition to institutional care [114].

While the triad of sarcopenia, tendinopathy, and arthritis represents a unique set of detrimental processes that facilitate the development of each other in aged cohorts, other medical comorbidities and lifestyle attributes remain particularly salient for comprehensive, personalized care plans. Of particular significance, especially as they relate to the musculoskeletal processes discussed in this chapter, are smoking, obesity, and diabetes mellitus.

2.1.1. *Smoking*

Smoking continues to be one of the most detrimental and preventable health issues in the United States. According to the CDC in 2022, roughly 11.6% of the American population reported current cigarette smoking, including 8.3% of those over the age of 65 years [115–117]. Cigarette smoke contains more than 7,000 chemicals, of which 250 are toxic, including ammonia, cyanide, and carbon monoxide [118]. On an individual level, smoking leads to numerous forms of cancer, heart disease, and many other serious health problems [119]. Alongside these chronic illnesses, smoking also negatively impacts the musculoskeletal system.

It is reported to decrease bone healing and increase the incidence of bone fractures [120], periodontitis, alveolar bone loss, and dental implant failure [121] and is particularly detrimental in men and in the elderly [122]. In terms of joint function, smoking is associated with increased rheumatoid disease activity, poor functional outcomes, a poor therapeutic response [121], increased radiographic OA [123], complications following total joint arthroplasty (TJA) [124, 125], and an increased risk of early total hip arthroplasty (THA) failure [126]. Further, studies reveal an association between smoking and lumbar disc herniation [127]; an increase in the incidence of rotator cuff tears, shoulder dysfunction, and shoulder symptoms [128]; higher complication rates following anterior cruciate ligament (ACL) reconstruction surgery [129]; and negative postoperative outcomes — either molecularly, biomechanically, or clinically — in terms of the performance of knee ligaments and articular cartilage [130]. Further, smokers are reported to display lower levels of type I and IIa muscle fibers, indicating oxidative fiber atrophy [131], and in the elderly, smoking results in a significant reduction in grip strength, chair rise speed, and timed walk tests [132], as well as a decrease in knee muscle strength in healthy adults [133]. Regarding recovery following musculoskeletal injury, nicotine is a strong vasoconstrictor and can decrease blood flow by 24% for 90 minutes after smoking one cigarette [120]. Indeed, hypoxia downregulates osteoblast formation and stimulates osteoclastic activity, thereby increasing the likelihood of a nonunion, malunion, and increased postfracture complication rates [118, 134]. Smoking has also been found to decrease calcium and vitamin D absorption *via* impairment of intestinal calcium absorption — two critical components for healthy bone formation [122]. With chronic use, smoking is associated with decreased BMD, as well as delayed healing of small-to-medium rotator cuff tears after repair surgery [135], where the effects are exacerbated with further use [136]. Patients should be educated regarding the effects of cessation and given the resources to strongly discourage them from smoking [120].

2.1.2. *Obesity*

Worldwide, the rates of people living with obesity have been rising significantly. According to the 2025 World Obesity Atlas, a >115% increase in the number of adults living with obesity is forecast between 2010 and 2030, rising from 524 million to 1.13 billion [137]. By the year 2035, the international economic impact of obesity will reach $4.32 trillion annually if current interventions are not improved [137]. In the United States, between 1994 to 2018, the number of adults aged ≥65 years with obesity increased from 22% to 40%, and presently, 2 in every 5 elderly Americans are obese [138]. Obesity impacts older patients more severely than younger individuals by accelerating biological aging and increasing the risk for chronic illnesses, diabetes, cardiovascular disease, and disability, thereby shortening life expectancy. The relationship between obesity and musculoskeletal biology is complex, but many of the associated processes are attributed to chronic inflammation — specifically *via* the increased proportion of white adipose tissue (WAT) found in older obese adults — and the subsequent increase in proinflammatory cytokine secretion such as TNF-α, IL-1β, and IL-6, leading to osteoclastic activation and bone loss [139]. In support of this, studies using aged mice fed a high-fat diet to induce obesity have shown that obesity decreases BMD and impairs bone regeneration due to these proinflammatory processes [140–142]. A study by Halade *et al.* fed 12-month-old female mice a 10% corn-oil diet for 6 months to induce obesity and found that the mice displayed a significant reduction in bone formation due to an overproduction of osteoclastogenesis, as evidenced by enhanced levels of RANKL and peroxisome proliferator-activated receptor-gamma — a crucial promotor of adipogenesis and inhibitor of osteogenesis — together with the decreased expression of RUNX2 and OPG among other factors [140]. The Global Longitudinal Study of Osteoporosis in Women evaluated a total of 60,393 women aged ≥55 years and reported that obese postmenopausal women displayed a greater risk of upper leg and ankle fractures compared to non-obese postmenopausal women [143]. Further, in 5,995 obese men ≥65 years of age, Nielson *et al.* evaluated the fracture incidence in relation to body mass index (BMI). Results showed that obesity was significantly associated with an increased risk of non-vertebral (68%) and hip (62%) fractures in men [144]. This may be attributable to an obesity-related deficit in physical performance, a chronic inflammatory state, vitamin D deficiency, and increased parathyroid hormone activity in obese individuals.

Adjacent to the Star Triad, obesity — particularly visceral fat — has been found to exacerbate the rate of sarcopenia by significantly lowering muscle mass and strength *via* the infiltration of WAT, creating local inflammation between intermuscular adipose tissue spaces [145, 146]. Sarcopenic obesity significantly increases the risk of disability, poor quality of life, and mortality, and its management often involves lifestyle inventions including calorie restriction, protein supplementation, and aerobic resistance exercises [147]. Further, excess weight (BMI >25 kg/m^2) increases the magnitude of joint loading and alters the stress distribution within the joint, leading to clinical implications including OA and tendinopathy of the back, hip, knee, ankle, foot, and shoulder [148–150], as well as IDD and sciatica [151, 152]. The prevalence of these conditions is reported to increase with increasing levels of BMI in adults ≥60 years of age [153]. Obesity also increases the premature need for TJA [154], reduces the health outcomes following TJA, particularly at a BMI >35 kg/m^2 [155], and increases the risk of TJA infection and the need for THA and total knee arthroplasty (TKA) revision surgery [156]. To this end, the functional and structural limitations imposed by the additional loading of the musculoskeletal system in obesity must produce aberrant mechanics and increase local stresses, thereby profoundly increasing the stress and overuse of soft-tissue structures, such as tendon, fascia, and cartilage. However, the mechanisms for this remain poorly described. Nevertheless, obesity increases the likelihood of a patient presenting with foot and ankle tendinitis, plantar fasciitis, and Achilles tendonitis [157, 158]. Rotator cuff tendonitis and shoulder impingement are increased in obese patients between 53 and 77 years of age [159], and obese patients undergoing ACL reconstruction are at greater risk for developing posttraumatic OA [160]. As lifestyle modification remains the cornerstone of tailored, nonoperative medicine, consideration of a patient's BMI and associated counseling remains critical in effectively caring for aging musculoskeletal patients.

2.1.3. *Diabetes Mellitus*

The prevalence of diabetes mellitus (DM) increases with age and affects approximately 29% of adults over the age of 65 years [161]. According to the International Diabetes Federation, by 2045, this number is projected to increase by 50% [162]. Over the last several decades, as the population has progressively become older and more obese, the number of individuals diagnosed with type II DM (T2DM) has continued to escalate. As the human body ages, homeostatic mechanisms that regulate insulin production naturally decline, and when compounded by increasing levels of obesity, both insulin resistance and impaired beta-cell function increase the risk of developing poor glycemic control and dyslipidemia. To this end, while recent studies have estimated heritability as high as 70% for developing T2DM [163, 164], the risk is threefold higher in those with morbid obesity (BMI $\geq$ 40 kg/m^2) compared to normal-weight individuals, and insulin dependence is reported to be five times higher [165].

Aging impairs the homeostatic maintenance mechanisms that regulate insulin and thus contributes to sustained chronic low-grade inflammation (inflammaging), senescence, mitochondrial dysfunction, and increased oxidative stress within cells [40, 166]. As a multisystem disease, DM can lead to various musculoskeletal disorders. These include muscle cramps, muscle infarction, loss of deep tendon reflexes, peripheral neuropathy, neuropathic joints, adhesive capsulitis (frozen shoulder), carpal tunnel syndrome, flexor tenosynovitis (trigger finger), and Dupuytren's contracture [167, 168]. Furthermore, individuals with type 2 DM (T2DM) are more likely to report musculoskeletal pain in the shoulder/neck, knee, or hip that interferes with usual daily activities [169]. Osteoporosis affects ~33% of individuals with T2DM and 36% of those with T1DM [170, 171]. Research has implicated bone turnover, AGEs, and increased marrow adiposity as potential mechanisms for T2DM-induced bone loss [172]. Further, both T1DM and T2DM are strongly associated with an overall increased fracture risk in men and women, with preferential locations at the hip, vertebrae, humerus, and ankle in T1DM, as well as the hip, vertebrae, and likely humerus, distal forearm, and foot in T2DM [173, 174]. Additionally, 47% of elderly T2DM patients develop T2DM-related sarcopenia [175–177], and 39% of all elderly patients who experience a hospitalizing fall are diabetic [178]. It has been suggested that hyperglycemic conditions lead to hormonal changes, oxidative stress, inflammation, and the accumulation of AGEs that alter the collagen matrix, leading to sarcopenia [176, 179]. Notably, Liu *et al.* showed that the pathogenic mechanism of T2DM-induced sarcopenia may differ from traditional sarcopenia and disuse muscle atrophy [177]. The study revealed that T2DM-induced sarcopenia was instead characterized by a reduction in type I muscle fibers, while primary sarcopenia and disuse-induced muscle atrophy primarily affect type II fibers. Thus, the pathological drivers may be different. To this end, it was speculated that T2DM-induced sarcopenia may occur *via* reduced GLUT4 expression in type I fibers, together with an increased rate of protein degradation, likely involving Akt/mTOR/forkhead box O (FOXO) signaling. As such, to advance the development of more effective diagnostic and therapeutic strategies, further research is crucial to better understand the pathogenesis of T2DM-related sarcopenia.

Diabetes also disrupts the interconnecting soft tissues between muscle and bone. For example, adhesive capsulitis is a painful and severely debilitating condition. Patients present with painful and incomplete elevation and external rotation, atrophy of the supraspinatus and infraspinatus muscles within the rotator cuff — muscles crucial for shoulder movement and stability — limitation of active and passive movement, and bone atrophy, among other symptoms and signs [180]. The condition is caused by inflammatory contracture and thickening of the glenohumeral joint capsule, mainly around the coracohumeral ligament, forming a dense collagen matrix consisting of a high degree of cellularity and abnormal, thickened fibrils. A study by Huang *et al.* [181] investigated 78,827 DM subjects, and after adjustment for age, sex, and dyslipidemia, individuals with either T1DM or T2DM were associated with an increased risk of developing a frozen shoulder compared to the non-DM group, which was comprised of 236,481 individuals. To this end, diabetics are reported to have a 20% increased risk of developing frozen shoulder, and this rises to 36% in insulin-dependent diabetics. Further, 42% of patients with bilateral frozen shoulders are diabetic, individuals with diabetes may experience worse clinical outcomes compared to those without diabetes [180, 182, 183], and the incidence of frozen shoulder increases with age [184]. As with all medical comorbidities, especially metabolic disorders, optimizing holistic care with associated endocrinologists and dieticians is essential for mitigating future musculoskeletal injury risk and giving patients the best chances for recovery following injury.

2.2. *Delayed Bone Healing, Nonunion, and Reduced Implant Integration in the Elderly — Fact or Fiction?*

Fracture healing becomes significantly less reliable in patients ≥65 years of age [185]. Some of the molecular, cellular, and structural factors behind this decline are described in Section 1, but in terms of fracture healing, this impaired response is also likely attributed to diminished angiogenesis, decreased expression of cytokines and growth factors during the pivotal healing cascade that ensues, and reduced osteogenic stem cell recruitment [186]. Nevertheless, more research is necessary to develop a cohesive understanding. Given the delayed bone repair response, it is conceivable that elderly patients are at a higher risk of delayed union or nonunion after fracture. While studies do report an increased nonunion risk in the elderly [187], several other studies report no significant correlation specific to this patient cohort. The risk factors for developing a nonunion across all age groups are numerous and include (i) fracture-related factors such as open fractures and infection; (ii) patient-related factors such as T2DM, smoking, and sarcopenia; and (iii) surgeon-related factors including the surgical approach and type of hardware used [188, 189]. Within the general population and following appropriate management, nonunions are relatively uncommon, with evidence from 5,000 individuals demonstrating the overall risk of nonunion per fracture being 1.9% [190]. However, van Wunnik *et al.* [191] and Mills *et al.* [190] both report that while bone quality diminishes in the elderly, the risk of fracture nonunion does not necessarily increase with age or with age-related osteoporotic bone loss. In support of this, a study by Hernandez *et al.* [192] investigated patients aged 65–79 years and reported that they were less likely to undergo fracture healing complications compared to patients aged 18–29 years. It was speculated that this may be due to the type and severity of fracture, with younger patients more likely to experience more traumatic, high-impact injuries that may subsequently challenge an efficient repair process. However, in 2017, Zura *et al.* [193] examined 47,437 Medicare patients and 56,492 fractures to evaluate the relationship between age and the occurrence of bone fracture nonunion. Remarkably, this study reported that patients aged ≥85 years had a nonunion rate of 1.3%, while those aged 55–59 years presented with a rate of 5.5%. Importantly, this study nevertheless also showed that fractures in the elderly were strongly associated with an increased risk of death within 1 year post-fracture, confirming fracture as a major health concern in this older patient cohort. Van Trikt *et al.* investigated whether the treatment of nonunions in the humerus and femur of 45 patients aged ≥75 years resulted in similar osseous union rates and time to union compared to a younger cohort [194]. Results confirmed that using a protocol of debridement, alignment, compression, stable fixation, bone grafting, and early motion, elderly patients can reliably achieve healing when faced with a nonunion. Finally, Zura *et al.* reported that nonunion in the elderly is exacerbated due to smoking, DM, obesity, and nonsteroidal anti-inflammatory drug (NSAID) use, and they speculated that increasing age is a strong risk factor for nonunion in some bones but a weak or nonsignificant risk in certain other bones [195]. As such, while individuals ≥65 years of age are at increased risk of fracture, whether increased age is an independent risk factor for nonunions remains unclear. Given the continuing rise in the aging population, and with more people living to >85 years of age than ever before, the number of elderly patients requiring treatment for nonunion will undoubtedly grow in the future. Therefore, further important research in this area is warranted. The consequences of nonunion are substantial both in terms of healthcare expenditure and patient outcomes. This includes the need for multiple reoperations, prolonged immobilization, and increased risk of medical complications such as infection, deep vein thrombosis, thromboembolism, and chronic pain [196]. Interestingly, a 2024 machine learning computational model trained with ~750 nonunion cases in long bones showed promise in predicting early fracture healing failure, with 70% specificity and 66% specificity [197]. Thus, machine learning research, though still in its infancy in musculoskeletal pathology, may offer a potential pathway toward tailored prevention and intervention.

The success of an orthopedic implant depends upon bone deposition and ingrowth, as well as integration of the implant surface within surrounding and adjacent bone. Due to a decline in the ability of bone to regenerate and repair during physiological aging, coupled with higher rates of comorbid systemic disease (e.g., T2DM, obesity, smoking, and sarcopenia), an additional important question is whether older age negatively impacts implant osseointegration, thereby leading to an increased risk of early mechanical or aseptic failure and periprosthetic fracture when compared to younger recipients. In essence, is there a timepoint when humans become too old for a TJA or spinal fusion procedure, for example? Due to the significant improvement in quality of life that implant-associated surgery delivers, this question is critical; however, there is limited information on whether osseointegration is compromised and early implant failure ensues in elderly patients with diminished bone quality. Importantly, a study by Bertl *et al.* [198] showed that early implant loosening was not more frequent when assessed in 444 elderly patients (≥65 years of age) compared to younger patients (<55 years of age) over an 11.5-year follow-up period. This study reported that early loosening was infrequent and occurred in 0.34%–0.83% of the 1,517 implants investigated. However, patients ≥80 years of age demonstrated a weak association, where early implant loosening increased to 2.25% compared to patients aged 65–79 years. In support of this, Sendyk *et al.* [199] conducted a systematic review and reported no significant differences in dental implant survival when older (≥60 years of age) versus younger (≥54 years of age) patients were compared (94% vs. 95%, respectively). In terms of function and mobility following TKA, da Casa *et al.* [200] showed that in septuagenarian patients and in the oldest-old (≥84 years of age), significant improvements were achieved and concluded that advanced age, in itself, should not be considered a contraindication for TKA. A similar conclusion was described by Maempel *et al.* [201], who assessed functional outcomes and complications following 3,144 primary TKAs and confirmed that elderly patients aged ≥75 years of age stand to gain considerably from TKA, especially in terms of pain relief. Notably, older patients, particularly those ≥80 years of age, show higher complication and mortality rates following surgery compared with younger patients [201, 200]. Some clinical evidence has also shown higher rates of pedicle screw loosening in older and osteoporotic patients [202, 203]. Further, elderly patients with sarcopenia are reported to demonstrate poorer postoperative outcomes, including a greater risk of dislocation following THA [204] and infection following THA and TKA [205]. As such, treatment to reduce the severity of sarcopenia prior to surgery was suggested as an important consideration moving forward. Nevertheless, and overall, aging does not seem to compromise osseointegration — and if so, only slightly at a later stage in life. In surgical cases, developments in hardware surfacing have enabled such materials as bioactive surfaces and porous titanium coatings designed to improve osseointegration. Even anabolic agents such as teriparatide have been found to enhance fusion mass and improve implant stability with perioperative administration, though these approaches to osteoporotic bone remain vastly underutilized [206]. This may be in part due to inconsistent screening for osteoporosis in orthopedic clinics, as well as decreased follow-up in older patients to identify these complications, both of which embody a gap that future protocols must address.

2.3. *Cancer, Chemotherapy, and Radiation*

As the global population continues to age, and as medical advances prolong life expectancy, the incidence of cancer in individuals aged ≥65 years is projected to accelerate [207]. In 2020, 19.3 million new cancer diagnoses were recorded, and due to our aging society, this is projected to increase to 27.5 million diagnoses by 2040 [208]. Age is a well-established risk factor; ~50%–62.3% of cancer cases occur in the elderly [209, 210], and oncologic disease continues to deliver unique, complex, challenging, and substantial morbidity and mortality to elderly patients. As such, this cohort represents a distinct patient population, and key to approaching their management is understanding the distinct biological, physiological, pharmacokinetic, physical, functional, and comorbid differences these patients have compared to younger individuals [209, 211, 212]. A combination of surgical resection, radiotherapy, and chemotherapy is the cornerstone of cancer therapy. While older patients with cancer tend to have lower surgery rates [213], elderly patients constitute the majority of those treated with radiation, and although radiotherapy is a fundamental and necessary tool, it can cause osteoporosis, osteoradionecrosis, delayed healing, decreased BMD, and pathological insufficiency fractures within bone [214–216]. Further, older individuals are more vulnerable to radiation due to factors including fatigue, microsites, xerostomia, dehydration, infections, and cognitive impairment [217]. Vitzthum *et al.* [218] investigated 28,354 patients aged ≥65 years who treated with radiotherapy for pelvic malignancies. The study showed that the 5-year incidence of pelvic fractures was 12.7% compared to non-treated patients and concluded that advanced age was associated with an increased hazard for pelvic fracture. In support of this, Baxter *et al.* [219] investigated 6,428 women aged ≥65 years and, when compared to nonirradiated patients, reported an increased cumulative 5-year pelvic fracture rate of 14% versus 7.5% in women with anal cancer, 8.2% versus 5.9% in women with cervical cancer, and 11.2% versus 8.7% in women with rectal cancer. Chan *et al.* [220] investigated the effect of stereotactic body radiation therapy in treating spinal metastases and the incidence of vertebral compression fractures in patients aged 70 years and older. A total of 252 patients were examined, and results showed that after 24 months of therapy, the cumulative risk of fracture was 12.3%. Notably, the study reported that in patients >86 years of age, this risk increased to 30.3% after 3.4 months, compared to those younger than 86 years (11.2% at 12.8 months post-exposure), suggesting an increased risk of fracture with advancing age. Overall, bone fractures can occur months to years after treatment, and factors such as the dose delivered, its duration, the location, and repeated exposures can strongly influence the likelihood of a patient developing a postradiation fracture [221]. In a systematic review conducted by Salvini *et al.*, increased risk factors include advanced age, female gender, radiation doses >50 Gy, radiation modality, and periosteal stripping [222], as well as both neoadjuvant and adjuvant chemotherapy [223, 224]. Notably, Razavian *et al.* [221] reported that evidence of osteoporosis, postmenopausal state, and a history of DM also significantly correlated with the increased risk of a postradiation pelvic fracture. Further, in terms of the Star Triad, sarcopenia worsens both acute and late radiation-induced toxicity, prognosis, and quality of life [225–227]. This appears to be an important and challenging problem, but an area that is substantially underexplored. Radiation fibrosis syndrome is a common complication that can negatively impact soft tissues, including muscles, viscera, ligaments, nerves, and tendons. Notably, radiation can promote myopathic muscles that are prone to painful spasms, as well as the progressive fibrosis of tendons and ligaments, which leads to loss of elasticity, shortening, and contracture; reduced joint range of motion; and decreased mobility [228, 229]. When identified early and physical therapy is conducted, these disorders can be abated.

Similar to surgical intervention, elderly patients are also less likely to receive chemotherapy treatment compared to their younger counterparts, despite a comparable or even superior survival benefit reported among patients aged ≥65 years [230–232]. Nevertheless, when given, chemotherapy also negatively impacts BMD, increases bone loss, and contributes to the development of fragility fractures [233–235]. Cytotoxic agents, including methotrexate and cisplatin, induce oxidative stress and damage DNA in osteoblasts, which reduces bone formation. Hormonal therapies, including androgen deprivation and aromatase inhibitors, along with chemotherapy-induced hypogonadism, also accelerate bone loss beyond typical age-related rates [236]. A landmark study by Rees-Punia *et al.* investigated a cohort of 92,431 adults with an average age of 69.4 years. The study found that those with an advanced-stage cancer diagnosis had a greater than twofold increased risk of frailty-related fractures, specifically vertebral and pelvic fractures [237]. Indeed, survivors treated with chemotherapy had an ~31% increased fracture risk within 5 years post-diagnosis. Interestingly, a nonsignificant trend was also observed, where physically active cancer survivors displayed a lower risk of fracture, suggesting the potential role of exercise in fracture prevention. Further, patients treated for non-Hodgkin's lymphoma (NHL), breast, and prostate cancer have also been shown to face an elevated risk of fragility fractures throughout their lives. A study by Huang *et al.* [238] reported that among 162 patients with a mean age of 60 years and treated with variations of R-CHOP-like regimens for aggressive B-cell NHL, nearly 28% had pre-existing vertebral or rib fractures, and an additional 10% developed new fractures within 1 year. As such, having a prevalent fracture strongly predicted developing a new fracture after chemotherapy treatment. Similar to radiation, the presence of sarcopenia negatively impacts tolerance to chemotherapy and can itself be induced by chemotherapy [239, 240]. Not only is the quantity of muscle mass reduced by chemotherapy but also its quality. Dependent on the type of cancer and the chemotherapy regimen given, with or without concurrent radiotherapy, chemotherapy is reported to deplete muscle mass by 2.5%–11.0% per 100 days [241, 242]. The mechanisms responsible for this are not fully understood. Given the importance of healthy muscle mass in aging patients and the high risk and severity of sarcopenia measured in some cases post-oncologic therapy, careful monitoring is necessary, particularly in the elderly cohort. More difficult to quantify are the effects of concomitant deleterious processes in these patients, including chemotherapy, cachexia, and treatment-associated neuropathy, which tend to accelerate sarcopenia, thus increasing fall susceptibility and impairing recovery further [243]. Finally, chemotherapy causes soft tissue damage, manifesting as inflammation, necrosis, or impaired healing, complicating regeneration in aging patients [244]. In this respect, chemotherapy has been reported to induce tendonitis and Achilles tendon rupture [245, 246]. Thus, ultimately, the combined effects of aging, systemic cancer therapy, and the increased risk of developing bone-related metastatic lesions place cancer survivors aged ≥65 years at a dramatically increased risk of musculoskeletal injury [247, 248].

3. Osteoporosis: A Central Challenge in Aging Musculoskeletal Care

Osteoporosis is among the most important musculoskeletal pathologic processes for aging populations worldwide. After age 50, it is estimated that 33% of women and 20% of men will suffer from an osteoporotic fracture at some point during their lives [249]. These fractures most commonly occur in the spine, hip, and wrist and have been cited to occur every ~160/100,000 person-years, increasing with advancing age [250]. Lifetime hip fracture risk in women and men has been reported as 15% and 6%, respectively [251]. Due to the substantial risk of osteoporotic fracture, many of which occur *via* low-energy mechanisms such as ground-level falls, assessment tools are critical in identifying at-risk individuals and mitigating potential complications prophylactically. DEXA remains the gold standard for diagnosis in women aged 65 and men aged 70 years; however, new guidelines recommend earlier screening for those with risk factors, including low body weight or a positive family history. Nevertheless, the limitations of DEXA are gaining increasing awareness. This is in light of recent epidemiological studies reporting that 75% of major osteoporotic fractures occur in patients without densitometric osteoporotic bone [252]. Indeed, the presence of fragility fracture alone — regardless of DEXA findings — is sufficient to diagnose osteoporosis.

One method to address this discrepancy in proactive care is for clinicians to adopt the Fracture Risk Assessment Tool (FRAX), which was introduced in 2008 to estimate a 10-year probability of hip and other major osteoporotic fractures [253]. Using clinical risk factors, including age, prior fractures, smoking, steroid use, and family history, FRAX is calculated in conjunction with femoral neck BMD. Based on several studies that have reported improved targeting of high-risk patients, FRAX has now been introduced into over 80 clinical guidelines worldwide [253].

Treatment interventions such as bisphosphonates and denosumab are known to be highly effective and may reduce the risk of fracture by 50% [254]. Newer anabolic agents, including teriparatide and romosozumab, are effective in patients with more severe bone loss, yet care gaps persist in their administration. Research has shown meaningful reductions in major osteoporotic fractures, with a hazard ratio of 0.91, and hip fractures specifically, with a hazard ratio of 0.80 [255, 256]. Current clinical challenges in the diagnosis and management of osteoporosis include insufficient screening leading to underdiagnosis, inconsistent use of newer tools like FRAX, poor adherence to long-term therapy, and improper follow-up following fracture. Studies investigating newer integrated care models that combine BMD, FRAX, and tailored interventions, including fall prevention protocols, alongside pharmacologic therapy, have revealed improved outcomes [257].

4. The Arthritic Burden of Longevity

In the United States alone, approximately 32.5 million adults, or 14% of the population, are affected by OA of the hip or knee [258]. Like osteoporosis, OA disproportionately impacts those over the age of 65 years. On a global scale, OA affects nearly 600 million people, and recent projections estimate that this will nearly double to over 1 billion by 2050 [259]. This is driven in part by demographic aging and rising rates of obesity. The incidence and prevalence of knee OA increase sharply after age 50 years, with upward of 45% of all individuals eventually becoming symptomatic during their lifetimes. Age-standardized rates of hip OA approach 20% in adults over 50 years of age [260]. This creates a substantial burden on healthcare systems around the world, while in the United States specifically, OA-related hospitalizations account for roughly 1 million per year, with aggregate costs of $15 billion, making it among the most expensive medical conditions in these hospitals [261].

TJA is an established, efficacious, and cost-effective surgical procedure for treating severe, end-stage OA of the hip and knee. Due to the substantial improvement in pain, function, and quality of life delivered to patients, TJA is considered among the most successful of orthopedic procedures, and its use continues to increase worldwide [262]. A total of 719,000 TKAs and 332,000 THAs were performed in the United States in 2010. It is estimated that by 2030, this number will grow by 673% to 3.48 million TKAs and by 174% to 572,000 THA surgeries [263–265]. With this significant rise in TKA and THA procedures, revision TKA and THA will also undoubtedly rise. Revision is most often performed for aseptic loosening, infection, fracture, or dislocation (in THA cases) [264]. Importantly, revision arthroplasty is more technically difficult, time-consuming, and costly and carries higher complication rates with decreased patient satisfaction [266]. A 2021 projection study reported that by 2030, the incidence of revision THA is expected to increase by 43%–70% and TKA by 78%–182% in the United States [267]. Further, from 2030 to 2060, revision THA is expected to reach 110,000 (a 219% increase) and revision TKA 253,000 (a 400% increase) in the United States [268]. As the demand for TJAs continues to rise, a disproportionately greater impact is projected toward elderly patients, as they will need surgery to support function, mobility, and wellness into old age. It will thus become a principal focus of arthroplasty surgeons and their teams to optimize the patient's long-term outcomes with primary arthroplasty procedures, as well as address gaps in effective and cost-efficient healthcare paradigms when revision procedures do occur.

4.1. *Case Study: Shoulder Osteoarthritis*

While primary TJA procedures of the hip and knee have been widely discussed and reported, the aging population also presents the clinician with an increasingly new set of OA-related conditions. For one, shoulder OA leading to arthroplasty is becoming increasingly relevant [269]. The demand for primary shoulder arthroplasty procedures in patients older than 55 years of age is forecast to increase by 755.4% by 2030 [270]. It is estimated that one-third of individuals over 60 years of age exhibit radiographic glenohumeral OA, and shoulder arthroplasty continues to rise accordingly. However, with age-related soft tissue degeneration and a decline in the innate soft tissue repair mechanisms, recent literature suggests that approximately 40% of those aged ≥75 years have asymptomatic full-thickness rotator cuff tears [271–273]. Without adequate soft tissue coverage around the shoulder and altered functional motion, glenohumeral degeneration progresses and may require arthroplasty. However, anatomical total shoulder arthroplasty (ATSA) relies upon a functional and intact rotator cuff; otherwise, the phenomenon of the rocking horse occurs, in which the glenoid compartment gradually loosens due to repetitive edge loading [274]. Thus, surgeons are increasingly utilizing the reverse total shoulder arthroplasty (RTSA) procedure, which instead relies on a functional deltoid. In Germany, between 2012 and 2022, a 121% increase in the use of RTSA for primary OA was reported, and it has since become the default preferred choice in the country for treating elderly patients with shoulder OA [275]. Similarly, in the United States, and following Food and Drug Administration approval in 2003, RTSA has become the most performed shoulder arthroplasty procedure. To this end, an epidemiological study reported that between 2016 and 2020, ~49,000 ATSA procedures were used to treat primary shoulder OA compared with ~96,000 RTSA surgeries [276]. Aside from soft tissue–related indications, the clinical outcome for RTSA use in aging patients is favorable, with 5- to 8-year implant survivorship ranging between 93% and 99%, and with patients presenting with stable functional improvement [277]. Indeed, a recent study that assessed 135 shoulders treated with primary RTSA at a minimum 10-year follow-up found that these improvements did not deteriorate over time when most clinical parameters were evaluated [278]. Further, in patients aged ≥85 years, a multicenter study reported that 76% of these patients rated good or excellent outcomes [279] and that patients can expect significant improvement in shoulder function, a significant reduction in pain, and clinical outcomes comparable to a younger population [280].

4.2. *Treatment Approaches and Emerging Therapies*

Conventional OA management relies on a standard pathway of non-pharmacological and pharmacological approaches that focus on pain management and improving joint function. Management includes lifestyle modifications, such as weight loss, physical therapy to strengthen the muscles around the joint, use of NSAIDs, and corticosteroids. As OA progresses in severity, options include eventual surgery, which may include arthroscopy and cartilage transfer procedures (e.g., mosaicplasty for defects <2 cm^2, autologous chondrocyte implantation for defects >2 cm^2, and matrix-induced autologous chondrocyte implantation), or joint replacement. However, there has been recent and extensive interest in the use of osteobiologics as a treatment approach. Osteobiologics represent such interventions as hyaluronic acid, MSCs, platelet-rich plasma (PRP), and gene-based cartilage therapy. Of note, PRP research and utilization have grown substantially over the past decade despite a lack of consistency in the literature regarding its effectiveness. For example, some meta-analyses of randomized controlled trials, which encompass thousands of OA patients, report that PRP, especially when highly concentrated, provides clinically meaningful improvements in function and pain when compared to hyaluronic acid and placebo [281]. However, other studies have reported favorable outcomes in pain, stiffness, and function over a 6-week course of multiple rounds of PRP, but subsequently, all parameters return to baseline as early as 6 weeks following treatment [282]. In addition, studies also report favorable results when PRP and hyaluronic acid are combined, but the positive clinical outcomes of this approach vary substantially [283, 284]. Indeed, there is a major focus on investigating these therapeutic regimens to delay or eliminate the need for surgery, yet there remains a lack of consensus on optimal dosing and standardized protocols. A similar phenomenon has been reported in recent years following the use of MSCs. This has primarily involved the investigation of adipose-derived or bone marrow–derived MSCs that are administered intra-articularly. This approach may offer a regenerative intervention due to their chondrogenic, paracrine, and immunomodulatory properties. A recent systematic review and meta-analysis published in 2024 examined the outcomes of 31 clinical trials encompassing over 1,400 patients. This study found that the administration of autologous-cultured adipose-derived MSCs yielded rapid pain relief in knee OA, delivering substantial long-term benefits in cartilage regeneration and function [285]. However, more thorough research to investigate the consistency of any adverse events, the optimal cell dose, the delivery method, and recommended patient cohorts is still pending longer-term studies. Finally, ongoing research aims to directly modify joint biology *via* gene-based therapies, though none are currently approved for OA. Gene therapy is emerging as a promising approach for treating OA by targeting the underlying mechanisms of the disease. This involves using viral or nonviral vectors to deliver therapeutic genes to the joint either *in vivo* or *ex vivo*, aiming to modulate gene expression and potentially increase cartilage regeneration, thereby modifying the progression and severity of OA. The research currently being undertaken is focused on examining the efficacy of the genes delivered (transcription factors [e.g., RUNX2, HIF-1α], growth factors [e.g., TGFβ, IGF-1, BMP], inflammation-associated cytokines [e.g., TNF-α, IL-1β, IL-6], and noncoding RNAs) and the mode of gene delivery (e.g., direct or indirect delivery) [286, 287]. Other similar vector-based studies include the use of adeno-associated virus systems and aim to deliver anabolic factors, such as FGF, to regenerate cartilage tissue directly and *via* promoting ECM production and chondrocyte proliferation [288]. Overall, gene therapy may lead to more sustained, targeted, site-specific expression of therapeutic proteins in a more physiologically and temporally relevant way. However, further research is needed to improve safety, its cost-effectiveness, delivery, and the gene-editing technologies employed [287].

5. Soft-Tissue Injury

Soft tissue injuries, primarily tears and ruptures, represent an increasingly prevalent clinical concern in the aging population. This is of particular concern to the orthopedic clinician given the difference in common pathologies within this demographic. Well-documented soft tissue injuries, such as to the ACL, remain clinically relevant, yet their incidence is typically less affected by age-related degeneration. For example, ACL injuries requiring reconstructive surgery (ACLR) occur less frequently in patients >50 years of age and exhibit low failure rates of 10.5% over a minimum 10-year postoperative follow-up period. High (91.4%) patient satisfaction was also reported [289]. Post-ACLR, elderly patients have also been shown to exhibit similar functional outcomes to their younger counterparts, though return to activity may be mildly diminished at short- to mid-term follow-up [290]. Damage to tendons can result from acute injuries (e.g., tears or sports injuries) or chronic degeneration (e.g., overuse injuries or degeneration), and the healing capacity varies depending on the extent, duration, and location of the injury. Effective repair of short and intracapsular tendons (e.g., rotator cuff tendons) often depends on tendon–bone integration, whereas effective repair of long and sheathed tendons (e.g., flexor tendons) typically relies on preventing gap formation at the repair site and maintaining tendon glide [291].

5.1. *Case Study: Achilles Tendon Rupture*

Soft-tissue injuries of the Achilles, quadriceps, and patellar tendon pose unique clinical challenges due to their higher prevalence in older patients and, thus, the associated physiological and mechanical degenerative changes inherent in musculoskeletal tissue. Achilles tendon rupture (ATR) accounts for 10.7% of all tendon and ligament injuries [292] and 20% of all large tendon injuries [293]. ATR can cause prolonged muscular deficits and profoundly impact quality of life. However, its incidence and characteristics remain poorly understood [294]. When investigated in 27,702 to 33,160 individuals, the incidence of ATR is estimated to range between 2.1 and 47.0 per 100,000 person-years in North America and Europe [294–297]. While traditional accounts of high-risk patients for ATR typically cite the active middle-aged male, recent literature suggests a bimodal distribution with a second and increasingly prominent peak in individuals over 50–60 years of age [296, 298], in the obese [299], and in those with metabolic disorders including DM [300]. This is likely attributable to various degenerative changes, such as medication-related risk factors with corticosteroids and fluoroquinolones, diminished vascular supply, and decreased collagen integrity, which predispose and substantially decrease the tendon load-to-failure ratio [301]. Indeed, minimal trauma in this cohort may lead to ATR, especially following the development of age-associated bone deformities and the localized presence of osteophytes [302]. This tendency must be reconciled with increased focus on the promotion of musculoskeletal fitness, especially resistance and endurance training, in the aging population given their increased risk of soft-tissue injury. For instance, the recent explosion of pickleball popularity has concurrently led to a rising incidence of Achilles injuries in the elderly. One recent study found significant associations between pickleball-related Achilles injuries and older age at the time of injury, and lower BMI, and those with injury were more likely to undergo surgery [303]. Even following surgery, functional outcomes are typically lower in the elderly cohort, with recovery reported as diminished compared with younger patients [304–306]. Conceivably, and in addition to the reduced regenerative capacity of the tissues, sarcopenia, DM, obesity, and age-associated gait alterations may also negatively impact the Achilles tendon repair response following injury. While functional rehabilitation remains a staple in caring for these injuries — whether nonoperative or operative — gaps remain in tailored delivery, including protocols that overlook age-related comorbidities, failure to assess patient-specific risks, and interventions that integrate functional ability, frailty, and tendon biology.

6. Unmet Needs and Gaps in Care for the Aging Musculoskeletal Patient

Advances in medical research, together with more active lifestyles, among other factors, are lengthening life, and record life expectancy does not appear to be approaching its limit [307, 308]. Data show that we are living longer; however, it remains unclear whether we are living "better." As the global proportion of the oldest-old (>85 years of age) and the number of centenarians continue to increase, as described, a rise in age-related musculoskeletal degenerative disease and disability is projected [309, 310]. This combined with higher patient expectations for superior health outcomes is calling for a change in the approach to and delivery of health care for the elderly. Therefore, it becomes especially important to recognize the ways in which current care systems fall short in detecting risk early,

Table 1. A summary of key unmet needs and future directions for the aging musculoskeletal patient.

Domain	Unmet Need	Proposed Solution	Research Priority
Risk screening	Under-screened frailty and bone loss	Preoperative DEXA/FRAX + frailty tools in clinics	RCTs of screening impact on surgical outcomes
Surgical optimization	Suboptimal bone support in implants/surgeries	FLS + orthogeriatric consult + bone-anabolic therapy	Trials of teriparatide + enhanced implant systems
Rehabilitation	Generic rehabilitation neglects multimorbidity	Tailored multidisciplinary, age-specific rehabilitation protocols	Comparative effectiveness of rehabilitation models
Emerging therapies	Slow adoption of orthobiologics and assistive tech	In-practice pilot programs with registry oversight	Adaptive trials of biologics and tech in elderly cohorts
System integration	Fragmented care silos, poor communication	4Ms age-friendly perioperative pathways	Implementation trials of integrated orthogeriatric pathways

deploying appropriate interventions, and utilizing evidence-based therapies for the tailored care of older patients. In this section, we highlight salient critical gaps, both for clinicians and researchers, and propose strategies to bridge them (**Table 1**).

6.1. *Preoperative and Preventative Care: Missed Opportunities in Early Risk Stratification*

Effectively managing the musculoskeletal health of an elderly patient, particularly those facing surgery, involves a combination of preoperative optimization and preventative strategies. This multifaceted approach aims to ultimately mitigate risks and promote overall well-being and functional independence. Current practices for accurately assessing risk often fall short, leading to missed opportunities for preventative care and improved outcomes. As such, insufficient risk identification remains a substantial problem for the aging population. The elderly experience an increased incidence of perioperative complications due to their age, multimorbidity (e.g., the Star Triad), polypharmacy, functional status changes and fall risk, and cognitive impairment. As a result, musculoskeletal treatment can require prolonged hospital stays and repeated surgeries, with many patients unable to return to their pre-injury or pre-disease level of activity [4, 311], posing a high burden on healthcare costs [5, 6]. At present, age and medical comorbidities are considered the main parameters in the risk-stratifying evaluation of surgical outcomes in older patients [312]. However, these tools often fail to capture the unique physiological decline and decreased resilience to stress that is common in older adults. Focusing on biological and not chronological age, and on factors such as frailty, may provide a more accurate description of a patient's true risk. To this end, the elderly benefit from the use of the Comprehensive Geriatric Assessment (CGA), which facilitates the evaluation of several aspects of elderly life including depression and cognitive disorders, social status, multimorbidity, fall risk, frailty, geriatric syndromes, nutritional status, and polypharmacy [313]. There is growing evidence that preoperative CGA successfully identifies patients at the highest risk of complications and improves postoperative outcomes in older adults [314, 315]. The subject of frailty is of high significance and is often a subject of confusion when it comes to actionable management. Frailty is a complex syndrome characterized by a multisystem physiological decline, as well as increased susceptibility to stress and negative clinical consequences, thereby increasing overall vulnerability to adverse health outcomes. Frailty is highly prevalent in old age and, in the nonsurgical population, is a proven predictor of hospitalization, incidence of falls, disability, morbidity, and death [316]. In the clinical setting, frailty is rarely investigated despite readily available and validated tools including the Modified Frailty Index, Clinical Frailty Scale, FRAIL scale [317, 318], and gait-speed tests [319]. However, at present, there is no agreed-upon and universally recognized frailty screening tool considered most adequate for elderly patients, and a tool that best suits the resources that are located and available within the immediate hospital setting is advised [313].

6.1.1. *Clinical Action*

Despite there being numerous guidelines for managing musculoskeletal conditions, a gap between these guidelines and real-world practice exists [320–322]. Among the simplest ways to act proactively in caring for aging musculoskeletal patients is to integrate regular assessments into routine care. For example, utilizing osteoporosis screening regardless of the apparent relevance of the nature of the patient's chief complaint. Indeed, only ~20%–30% of older adults are screened for osteoporosis or fall risk during routine care, and metrics such as DEXA and FRAX remain under-utilized [323]. The integration of DEXA, FRAX, and frailty screening tools into both preclinic documents and surgical preparation workflows is simple and cost-effective on a large scale. Clinicians may also include specific proactive prehabilitation into their plans, which may involve muscle strength and balance evaluation, tailored resistance training, aerobic activities, nutritional support, hydration, and medication reconciliation, implemented within a tailored care model depending on the patient's functional status and goals, as well as based on the potential medical or surgical interventions.

6.1.2. *Research Action*

Future research should ideally aim to more concretely trial the assessment of structured preclinical and preoperative risk stratification pathways to increase efficiency and effectiveness. Studies may compare standard models versus enhanced models, which may include screening with or without prehabilitation, for outcomes including nonunion and implant longevity. At the inception of many diseases, subtle and seemingly unremarkable biological and physicochemical changes can occur prior to onset and prior to the disease manifesting clinically distinct symptoms. As such, research that identifies and validates more precise biomarkers and early detection markers and systems, aimed at predicting skeletal muscle and bone aging, as well as the likelihood of a patient developing a musculoskeletal disorder, is essential. For example, after discovering a suitable biomarker or multi-biomarker signature, the engineering of new materials and devices and the design of responsive electronic systems able to monitor electrical and/or biochemical on-body or in-body signals, continuously, in real-time, and *via* a closed-loop system, may promote home-based personal medicine avenues over current hospital-based care systems. This may significantly reduce time to diagnosis and healthcare costs [307]. Thus, the continued pursuit of improving digital health technologies, including telemedicine, wearables, and mobile health applications, may revolutionize musculoskeletal care. Furthermore, advances in imaging capabilities, including computed tomography, magnetic resonance imaging, DEXA, and positron emission tomography, continue to significantly improve diagnostic capabilities in patients [324]. Advancements in artificial intelligence (AI) coupled with machine learning (ML) are also likely to play a pivotal role in further improving the earlier detection and more precise imaging and monitoring of musculoskeletal conditions. In this respect, the use of deep learning models has been shown to achieve physician-level accuracy when diagnosing and detecting complex medical pathologies, including cancer [325, 326]. Furthermore, AI-ML home-health monitoring systems, which include computer vision analytics for the deep learning–based and spatiotemporal detection of patient mobilization activities, may transform the monitoring of the elderly in their homes [327, 328]. Through collecting complex streams of data in real time, longitudinally tracking movements, and then analyzing the data, these systems can iteratively learn the expected daily levels of activity, including walking speed, total daily activity, and ability to get out of bed. Using the well-defined criteria outlined in the Index of Independence in Activities of Daily Living [329], the AI-ML systems utilize these proven parameters to monitor the cognitive and physical capabilities of the elderly on a daily basis. Furthermore, using predictive reasoning, the systems can then immediately identify any unusual changes that may suggest the onset of cognitive or functional decline and intervene by sounding an alert or offering behavioral suggestions. Importantly, these systems may detect subtle declines in function, which a human may otherwise miss [330, 331]. This system may therefore not only deliver more comprehensive and personalized data on the dynamic nature of musculoskeletal disease progression and functioning but also potentially facilitate timely access to the appropriate healthcare team to prevent serious injury [332].

6.2. *Treatment-Level Gaps: Optimization of Operative, Nonoperative, and Postoperative Interventions and Rehabilitation*

Optimizing care for musculoskeletal patients requires a multifaceted approach following both surgical and nonsurgical interventions. However, several treatment-level gaps exist that can hinder this development. Inadequate treatment optimization, especially with respect to evolving technologies, leads to inconsistent use of anabolic and antiresorptive agents, for example. This is especially noteworthy in managing postfracture musculoskeletal care, leading to suboptimal osteoporosis treatment protocols. Indeed, research has found that upward of 25% of patients treated for fragility fractures are lost to follow-up following their first hospital or clinical visit [333]. Further, osteoporosis is often not recognized until one or more fractures occur, yet postfracture screening remains uncommon [334]. Notably, Barton *et al.* [334] surveyed 36 orthopedic surgeons and found that many expressed discomfort in prescribing medications for osteoporosis (due to bisphosphonate-induced side effects of atypical fractures and osteonecrosis of the jaw [335]); in addition, 22% of respondents knew what a FRAX score is. The study concluded that a fracture liaison service (FLS), a model that relies on the use of a dedicated healthcare professional to evaluate patients for osteoporosis and/or osteoporotic fracture and to initiate treatment, may offer an optimal level of patient care. It remains to be seen whether osteo-regenerative treatment modalities, including bone scaffolding, teriparatide-aided fusion, and porous-reinforced implants, will become standard of care following the optimization of training barriers, cost, and evidence [336]. Rehabilitation is crucial for avoiding complications such as joint stiffness, muscle atrophy, or scar tissue formation, and as such, it plays an integral component in the successful management of acute and chronic musculoskeletal injuries [337]. Despite the importance of proper rehabilitation protocols in musculoskeletal care, as well as the substantiated benefits of early mobilization [338, 339], many patients continue to experience prolonged immobilization or receive generic physiotherapy plans. As such, poor functional outcomes following musculoskeletal trauma remain a major public health concern. A multidisciplinary team — including specialists in physical and occupational therapy — together with a thorough understanding of a patient's gaps in home support, delirium prevention, and medication management, may assist in creating rehabilitation plans that work with age-specific needs.

6.2.1. *Clinical Action*

Utilizing the FLS and/or integrating orthogeriatric teams into both elective and trauma workflows has been extensively studied and is associated with various benefits, including decreased time to surgery, decreased mortality, a lower risk of fracture and major re-fractures, and improved postoperative functional status [340–342]. Surgical team education on perioperative use of bone anabolic agents and adjunctive implant devices may facilitate more tailored care while decreasing subsequent injuries. Furthermore, malnutrition is very prevalent in geriatric patients with hip fracture, for example, and is significantly associated with increased mortality, hospital-acquired complications, and length of stay [343, 344]. A study by Malafarina *et al.* [343] concluded that nutritional intervention was cost-effective, and early nutritional intervention improves protein and energy intake, thereby improving functional recovery post-fracture. Further, nutritional supplementation is associated with a reduced length of hospital stay, lower risk of complications, and unfavorable outcomes, including death <12 months postfracture [345–348]. Indeed, evidence-based guidelines and care standards recommend offering oral nutritional supplementation to all older adults with hip fracture — not just those already malnourished. Nevertheless, in less than half of elderly patients within 29 hospitals, its implementation was reported to be mainly restricted to cognitively impaired, frail, and terminally ill patients [348]. A structured approach to delivering a nutritional care plan to all older adults is strongly encouraged to reduce complications and improve outcomes following fracture, as well as other musculoskeletal injuries. Further, sleep quality, quantity, and architecture change with increasing age [349]. Sleep plays a vital role in muscle tissue maintenance, and sleep disturbances and insufficient sleep have been shown to reduce muscle mass and strength in the elderly [350], as well as increase musculoskeletal pain [351]. Therefore, proactive methods to improve sleep quantity and quality in elderly patients are also highly encouraged. Developing multidisciplinary care plan teams — including pharmacy, social work, dieticians, physical therapy, and geriatrics — will more comprehensively guide postoperative care, mitigate potential complications, such as falls, and facilitate rehabilitation compliance and adequate follow-up.

6.2.2. *Research Action*

Improving current treatments and exploring novel therapies is the contemporary focus of musculoskeletal research. This includes the discovery and development of more effective pharmacologic therapies (e.g., Navitoclax, a Bcl-2 inhibitor aimed at eliminating senescent cells and reducing the symptoms of OA [352]), advancements in genomics and biotechnology (e.g., adeno-associated virus-mediated cartilage regeneration therapies), which enable the development of more targeted therapeutic approaches, as well as the investigation of biotechnologies such as PRP, bone marrow aspirate, adipose-derived MSCs, amniotic cell therapies [353, 354]. Importantly, research into how the impact and progression of musculoskeletal disorders and their treatment vary between men and women, as well as the specific risk factors associated with sex, is also under widespread scrutiny [355–357]. While still in their infancy, various orthobiologics and implant development technologies show promise and may become widespread in the next decade. Notably, further information on this highly active research area is provided in subsequent chapters of this book. The subjects covered include bioactive scaffolds, grafts, and coatings; smart biomaterials; 3D printing; nanotechnology; gene delivery approaches; robotic-assisted surgery and artificial intelligence; and testing and assessment models of musculoskeletal disease, among others. In terms of their clinical use, the optimal use of osteo-regenerative therapeutics, including best practices regarding dose, timing, cell processing methodology, biomanufacturing, and duration of intervention per patient cohort, needs further investigation. Further, best practices depending on the musculoskeletal procedures to be used remain elusive in some instances. For example, in hip–spine syndrome, evidence is lacking on which surgery to perform first — TJA or spinal fusion surgery [358]. Answers may be achieved *via* multicenter randomized controlled trials, structured to develop validated protocols for evidence-based best use of these novel technologies and surgical approaches. Assistive technologies including wearables, exoskeletons, and sensor-based balancing systems have also been found to have positive results [359, 360] despite their integration into clinical practice remaining primarily anecdotal. Assessment of outcomes based on various types of rehabilitation models, including home-based compared with inpatient facilities, as well as within various cohorts of geriatric patients, is necessary. Studies structured to determine how these interventions impact function, complications, and readmission rates will significantly guide future management.

Finally, to facilitate the efficient translation of new technologies to patients, beginning early during device/biotechnology development, the creation of a multidisciplinary team is essential to ensure a comprehensive perspective is discharged. This includes collaboration between surgeons, nurses, engineers, and data scientists, among others, to ensure the technology is evaluated and implemented with a holistic understanding of its potential impact on patient care, clinical workflow, and ethical considerations. This will lead to improved assessment, planning, informed decisions, safer implementation, and patient outcomes. Further, clinicians may assist in the development and adoption of novel musculoskeletal intervention technologies by enrolling or recommending patients for well-designed trials and registries. Collaboration with partners in bioengineering or occupational therapy teams may also pilot these innovations in clinical practice. Adaptive and robust trials to evaluate biologics and advanced wearable technology, especially for older musculoskeletal patients, will be key in developing evidence-based protocols for safety, dosing, functional gain, and cost-effectiveness.

6.3. *System-Level and Care Coordination Barriers*

Pervasive integration failure between providers and electronic medical records continues to inhibit the optimal care of aging patients, many of whom are especially susceptible to lapses in care and unnecessary testing, given their often complex comorbidity management [361]. These paradigms lead to fragmented and inefficient care [362]. Especially in older, frail adults post-discharge, the growing gap in shared decision-making, medication review, and follow-up presents a critical gap in modern healthcare systems.

6.3.1. *Clinical Action*

Utilization of the 4Ms framework, "What Matters, Medication, Mentation, Mobility," can help structure perioperative care [363]. With this multifaceted approach and coordinated care *via* orthogeriatric pathways, interdepartmental handoff, and multidisciplinary meetings, the aging population will likely be less costly to the healthcare system and achieve superior outcomes. Even at the individual provider level, this framework may yield substantial results by having a standardized framework for investigating and understanding patient-specific factors that may support or impede care. "What Matters" signifies specific treatment goals for each patient, which have been shown to improve adherence, satisfaction, and quality of life [363]. For musculoskeletal patients, this may take the form of tailoring prehabilitation, surgical, and postoperative rehabilitation decisions toward maintaining independence rather than achieving some technical outcome. "Medication" entails a comprehensive medical reconciliation, given the rates of polypharmacy present in up to 50% of older orthopedic patients. When individuals with polypharmacy are then prescribed common postoperative medication regimens, this strongly predicts postoperative delirium and falls [364]. Indeed, studies have shown that incorporating pharmacy teams into preoperative assessment has reduced adverse drug events by nearly 20% in pilot studies [365]. "Mentation" refers to adequate screening for delirium and cognitive impairment preoperatively to enable targeted strategies prior to their onset, which may include delirium-prevention sitters or bundles, which decrease delirium incidence and shorten inpatient length of stay [366]. Finally, "Mobility" refers to early mobilization protocols, which are commonly associated with reduced postoperative complications when integrated into orthogeriatric pathways. Regarding the prevention of common orthogeriatric complications, early mobilization is associated with a decreased incidence of pressure ulcers, stiffness, and loss of independence [367, 368].

In practice, these investments in understanding each patient from a more robust perspective save time and cost by preventing complications and encouraging greater agency from the patient. Large cohort studies of hip fracture patients have demonstrated that such orthogeriatric co-management models, in which geriatricians and orthopedic surgeons collaborate from admission to discharge, shorten length of stay and lower 30-day readmission rates [369]. Importantly, these programs do not necessarily increase clinic or hospital workload when tasks are appropriately distributed across allied health providers and coordinated through standardized care models. This concerted effort makes integration both feasible and sustainable for otherwise busy providers and services.

6.3.2. *Research Action*

The implementation of scientific studies may evaluate quality improvement in caring for older musculoskeletal patients, as well as the development of frameworks for coordinating between providers, electronic medical record (EMR) systems, and pharmacies. For example, quality improvement initiatives that establish and compare benchmark outcomes, including readmissions, return to baseline functions, and complications, across institutions that adopt the 4Ms framework. EMR-based alerts and decision support tools have become increasingly popular in many systems, and studies investigating their utility and associated patient outcomes would be timely. Regarding the musculoskeletal patient, alerts and decision-support tools including automated FRAX scoring, delirium risk calculations, and polypharmacy flags may trigger early intervention without significant provider burden [370]. Exploration of telehealth and remote monitoring, particularly in rural communities or mobility-limited older adults, may adjunct or replace traditional follow-up and expedite the postoperative course. Future studies investigating orthogeriatric pathways compared to traditional treatment approaches, in terms of outcomes, cost-effectiveness, and scalability across diverse healthcare systems, may inform decisions at the hospital, regional, state, and federal levels of healthcare policy.

Early pilot studies for these approaches are both clinically effective and economically favorable. Indeed, FLSs have demonstrated cost savings by preventing complications such as secondary fractures, and EMR-integrated care pathways have reduced redundant testing and medication errors [371]. However, large-scale, multicenter studies specific to the musculoskeletal aging population remain limited, representing a key gap for health services research. Further, the future of system-level care is trending toward integrated, value-based models where musculoskeletal health is managed within a broader framework of aging care. This is likely to be facilitated by innovations in post-acute virtual rehabilitation platforms and smart devices including hardware implants with technology to track post-operative mobilization and bacterial growth, as well as the exponential growth of AI-driven predictive analytics. For clinicians, the trend of targeted use of existing and emerging tools and teams to close critical gaps in the care of older musculoskeletal adults will continue to streamline workflows, reduce provider burden, and improve patient-centered outcomes.

7. Conclusions

To truly elevate musculoskeletal care in the context of an aging global population, system-level transformation is necessary, from proactive risk identification and tailored surgical approaches to breakthrough therapeutics and coordinated rehabilitation. For clinicians, this entails embracing age-centered frameworks and multidisciplinary collaboration. For researchers, it represents a call to action with rigorous, large-scale trials and implementation studies that investigate the unique biophysiological, functional, and social challenges of older patients. Together, these efforts may redefine standards of care internationally and improve outcomes across the musculoskeletal injury population.

References

1. United Nations. World Population Ageing 2020: Highlights: Living arrangements of older persons, *Webpage*, 2020.

2. Curtis EM, Moon RJ, Harvey NC, Cooper C. The impact of fragility fracture and approaches to osteoporosis risk assessment worldwide. *Bone*. Nov. 2017;104:29–38. https://doi.org/10.1016/j.bone.2017.01.024
3. Roberts S, Colombier P, Sowman A, Mennan C, Rölfing JHD, Guicheux J, et al. Ageing in the musculoskeletal system. *Acta Orthop.* Dec. 2016;87(sup363):5–25. https://doi.org/10.1080/17453674.2016.1244750
4. Meinberg EG, Clark D, Miclau KT, Marcucio R, Miclau T. Fracture repair in the elderly: Clinical and experimental considerations. *Injury*. Jun. 2019;50:S62–S65. https://doi.org/10.1016/j.injury.2019.05.005
5. Zhang C, Feng J, Wang S, Gao P, Xu L, Zhu J, et al. Incidence of and trends in hip fracture among adults in urban China: A nationwide retrospective cohort study. *PLOS Med.* Aug. 2020;17(8):e1003180. https://doi.org/10.1371/journal.pmed.1003180
6. Papadimitriou N, Tsilidis KK, Orfanos P, Benetou V, Ntzani EE, Soerjomataram I, et al. Burden of hip fracture using disability-adjusted life-years: A pooled analysis of prospective cohorts in the CHANCES consortium. *Lancet Public Heal.* May 2017;2(5):e239–e246. https://doi.org/10.1016/S2468-2667(17)30046-4
7. Moskalev AA, Shaposhnikov MV, Plyusnina EN, Zhavoronkov A, Budovsky A, Yanai H, et al. The role of DNA damage and repair in aging through the prism of Koch-like criteria. *Ageing Res. Rev.* Mar. 2013;12(2):661–84. https://doi.org/10.1016/j.arr.2012.02.001
8. Forsberg LA, Rasi C, Razzaghian HR, Pakalapati G, Waite L, Thilbeault KS, et al. Age-related somatic structural changes in the nuclear genome of human blood cells. *Am. J. Hum. Genet.* Feb. 2012;90(2):217–28. https://doi.org/10.1016/j.ajhg.2011.12.009
9. Park CB, Larsson N-G. Mitochondrial DNA mutations in disease and aging. *J. Cell Biol.* May 2011;193(5):809–18. https://doi.org/10.1083/jcb.201010024
10. DeBalsi KL, Hoff KE, Copeland WC. Role of the mitochondrial DNA replication machinery in mitochondrial DNA mutagenesis, aging and age-related diseases. *Ageing Res. Rev.* Jan. 2017;33:89–104. https://doi.org/10.1016/j.arr.2016.04.006
11. Wu Z, Zhang W, Song M, Wang W, Wei G, Li W, et al. Differential stem cell aging kinetics in Hutchinson-Gilford progeria syndrome and Werner syndrome. *Protein Cell.* Apr. 2018;9(4):333–50. https://doi.org/10.1007/s13238-018-0517-8

12. Burtner CR, Kennedy BK. Progeria syndromes and ageing: What is the connection? *Nat. Rev. Mol. Cell Biol.* Aug. 2010;11(8):567–78. https://doi.org/10.1038/nrm2944
13. Taylor RW, Turnbull DM. Mitochondrial DNA mutations in human disease. *Nat. Rev. Genet.* May 2005;6(5):389–402. https://doi.org/10.1038/nrg1606
14. Baines HL, Turnbull DM, Greaves LC. Human stem cell aging: Do mitochondrial <scp>DNA</scp> mutations have a causal role? *Aging Cell*. Apr. 2014;13(2):201–05. https://doi.org/10.1111/acel.12199
15. Dobson PF, Dennis EP, Hipps D, Reeve A, Laude A, Bradshaw C, et al. Mitochondrial dysfunction impairs osteogenesis, increases osteoclast activity, and accelerates age related bone loss. *Sci. Rep.* Jul. 2020;10(1):11643. https://doi.org/10.1038/s41598-020-68566-2
16. Xiao W. An overview on epigenetic regulation of bone development. *J. Bone Res.* 2023;11:244. https://doi.org/10.35248/2572-4916.23.11.244
17. Lin T, Gibon E, Loi F, Pajarinen J, Córdova LA, Nabeshima A, et al. Decreased osteogenesis in mesenchymal stem cells derived from the aged mouse is associated with enhanced NF-κB activity. *J. Orthop. Res.* Feb. 2017;35(2):281–88. https://doi.org/10.1002/jor.23270
18. Sanghani-Kerai A, Osagie-Clouard L, Blunn G, Coathup M. The influence of age and osteoporosis on bone marrow stem cells from rats. *Bone Joint Res.* Apr. 2018;7(4):289–97. https://doi.org/10.1302/2046-3758.74.BJR-2017-0302.R1
19. Zhang EY, Blanch TE, Ahmed SB, Jiang X, Dyment NA, Heo SC. Epigenetic regulation and mechanobiological adaptation in tenocytes during maturation. *APL Bioeng.* Jun. 2025;9(2). https://doi.org/10.1063/5.0271050
20. Zhang M, Theleman JL, Lygrisse KA, Wang J. Epigenetic mechanisms underlying the aging of articular cartilage and osteoarthritis. *Gerontology* 2019;65(4):387–96. https://doi.org/10.1159/000496688
21. Liang W, Xu F, Li L, Peng C, Sun H, Qiu J, et al. Epigenetic control of skeletal muscle atrophy. *Cell. Mol. Biol. Lett.* Jul. 2024;29(1):99. https://doi.org/10.1186/s11658-024-00618-1
22. Ainslie A, Huiting W, Barazzuol L, Bergink S. Genome instability and loss of protein homeostasis: Converging paths to neurodegeneration?. *Open Biol.* Apr. 2021;11(4):200296. https://doi.org/10.1098/rsob.200296
23. Aman Y, Schmauck-Medina T, Hansen M, Morimoto RI, Simon AK, Bjedov I, et al. Autophagy in healthy aging and disease. *Nat. Aging*. Aug. 2021;1(8):634–50. https://doi.org/10.1038/s43587-021-00098-4

24. López-Otín C, Blasco MA, Partridge L, Serrano M, Kroemer G. The hallmarks of aging. *Cell.* Jun. 2013;153(6):1194–217. https://doi.org/10.1016/j.cell.2013.05.039
25. Cecarini V, Bonfili L, Cuccioloni M, Mozzicafreddo M, Angeletti M, Keller JN, et al. The fine-tuning of proteolytic pathways in Alzheimer's disease. *Cell. Mol. Life Sci.* 73(18):3433–51. https://doi.org/10.1007/s00018-016-2238-6
26. Altun M, Besche HC, Overkleeft HS, Piccirillo R, Edelmann MJ, Kessler BM, et al. Muscle wasting in aged, sarcopenic rats is associated with enhanced activity of the ubiquitin proteasome pathway. *J. Biol. Chem.* Dec. 2010;285(51):39597–608. https://doi.org/10.1074/jbc.M110.129718
27. Iyer S, Adams DJ. Bone and the unfolded protein response: In sickness and in health. *Calcif. Tissue Int.* May 2023;113(1):96–109. https://doi.org/10.1007/s00223-023-01096-x
28. Hughes A, Oxford A, Tawara K, Jorcyk C, Oxford J. Endoplasmic reticulum stress and unfolded protein response in cartilage pathophysiology; contributing factors to apoptosis and osteoarthritis. *Int. J. Mol. Sci.* Mar. 2017;18(3):665. https://doi.org/10.3390/ijms18030665
29. Kwan KYC, Ng KW, Rao Y, Zhu C, Qi S, Tuan RS, et al. Effect of aging on tendon biology, biomechanics and implications for treatment approaches. *Int. J. Mol. Sci.* Oct. 2023;24(20):15183. https://doi.org/10.3390/ijms242015183
30. Wen T, Xue P, Ying J, Cheng S, Liu Y, Ruan D. The role of unfolded protein response in human intervertebral disc degeneration: Perk and IRE1-α as two potential therapeutic targets. *Oxid. Med. Cell. Longev.* Jan. 2021;2021(1):6492879. https://doi.org/10.1155/2021/6492879
31. Di Micco R, Krizhanovsky V, Baker D, d'Adda di Fagagna F. Cellular senescence in ageing: From mechanisms to therapeutic opportunities. *Nat. Rev. Mol. Cell Biol.* Feb. 2021;22(2):75–95. https://doi.org/10.1038/s41580-020-00314-w
32. McHugh D, Gil J. Senescence and aging: Causes, consequences, and therapeutic avenues. *J. Cell Biol.* Jan. 2018;217(1):65–77. https://doi.org/10.1083/jcb.201708092
33. Wan M, Gray-Gaillard EF, Elisseeff JH. Cellular senescence in musculoskeletal homeostasis, diseases, and regeneration. *Bone Res.* Sep. 2021;9(1):41. https://doi.org/10.1038/s41413-021-00164-y

34. Huo S, Tang X, Chen W, Gan D, Guo H, Yao Q, et al. Epigenetic regulations of cellular senescence in osteoporosis. *Ageing Res. Rev.* Aug. 2024;99: 102235. https://doi.org/10.1016/j.arr.2024.102235
35. Xing X, Huang H, Gao X, Yang J, Tang Q, Xu X, et al. Local elimination of senescent cells promotes bone defect repair during aging. *ACS Appl. Mater. Interfaces*. Jan. 2022;14(3):3885–99. https://doi.org/10.1021/acsami.1c22138
36. Yang N, Nakagawa M, Nishiura A, Yamada M, Morikuni H, Honda Y, et al. Identification of senescent cells in peri-implantitis and prevention of mini-implant loss using senolytics. *Int. J. Mol. Sci.* Jan. 2023;24(3):2507. https://doi.org/10.3390/ijms24032507
37. Loeser RF. Aging and osteoarthritis: The role of chondrocyte senescence and aging changes in the cartilage matrix. *Osteoarthr. Cartil.* Aug. 2009;17(8):971–79. https://doi.org/10.1016/j.joca.2009.03.002
38. Alcalde-Estévez E, Asenjo-Bueno A, Sosa P, Olmos G, Plaza P, Caballero-Mora MÁ, et al. Endothelin-1 induces cellular senescence and fibrosis in cultured myoblasts. A potential mechanism of aging-related sarcopenia. *Aging (Albany. NY).* Jun. 2020;12(12):11200–23. https://doi.org/10.18632/aging.103450
39. Silwal P, Nguyen-Thai AM, Mohammad HA, Wang Y, Robbins PD, Lee JY, et al. Cellular senescence in intervertebral disc aging and degeneration: Molecular mechanisms and potential therapeutic opportunities. *Biomolecules*. Apr. 2023;13(4):686. https://doi.org/10.3390/biom13040686
40. Maldonado E, Morales-Pison S, Urbina F, Solari A. Aging hallmarks and the role of oxidative stress. *Antioxidants*. Mar. 2023;12(3):651. https://doi.org/10.3390/antiox12030651
41. Almeida M, Han L, Martin-Millan M, O'Brien CA, Manolagas SC. Oxidative stress antagonizes Wnt signaling in osteoblast precursors by diverting β-catenin from T cell factor- to forkhead box O-mediated transcription. *J. Biol. Chem.* Sep. 2007;282(37):27298–05. https://doi.org/10.1074/jbc.M702811200
42. Domazetovic V. Oxidative stress in bone remodeling: Role of antioxidants. *Clin. Cases Miner. Bone Metab.* 2017;14(2):209. https://doi.org/10.11138/ccmbm/2017.14.1.209
43. Lean JM, Jagger CJ, Kirstein B, Fuller K, Chambers TJ. Hydrogen peroxide is essential for estrogen-deficiency bone loss and osteoclast formation. *Endocrinology*. Feb. 2005;146(2):728–35: https://doi.org/10.1210/en.2004-1021

44. Huh Y-J, Kim JM, Kim H, Song H, So H, Lee SY, et al. Regulation of osteoclast differentiation by the redox-dependent modulation of nuclear import of transcription factors. *Cell Death Differ.* Jul. 2006;13(7):1138–46. https://doi.org/10.1038/sj.cdd.4401793
45. Agidigbi TS, Kim C. Reactive oxygen species in osteoclast differentiation and possible pharmaceutical targets of ROS-mediated osteoclast diseases. *Int. J. Mol. Sci.* Jul. 2019;20(14):3576. https://doi.org/10.3390/ijms20143576
46. Almeida M, O'Brien CA. Basic biology of skeletal aging: Role of stress response pathways. *J. Gerontol. Ser. A Biol. Sci. Med. Sci.* Oct. 2013;68(10):1197–208. https://doi.org/10.1093/gerona/glt079
47. Zhou Z, Jiang W, Yan J, Liu H, Ren M, Li Y, et al. Trichostatin a enhances the titanium rods osseointegration in osteoporotic rats by the inhibition of oxidative stress through activating the AKT/Nrf2 pathway. *Sci. Rep.* Dec. 2023;13(1):22967. https://doi.org/10.1038/s41598-023-50108-1
48. Huang J, Li R, Yang J, Cai M, Lee Y, Wang A, et al. Bioadaptation of implants to In vitro and In vivo oxidative stress pathological conditions via nanotopography-induced FoxO1 signaling pathways to enhance osteoimmunal regeneration. *Bioact. Mater.* Oct. 2021;6(10):3164–76. https://doi.org/10.1016/j.bioactmat.2021.02.023
49. Kim M, Kim C, Choi YS, Kim M, Park C, Suh Y. Age-related alterations in mesenchymal stem cells related to shift in differentiation from osteogenic to adipogenic potential: Implication to age-associated bone diseases and defects. *Mech. Ageing Dev.* May 2012;133(5):215–25. https://doi.org/10.1016/j.mad.2012.03.014
50. Chemello F, Bean C, Cancellara P, Laveder P, Reggiani C, Lanfranchi G. Microgenomic analysis in skeletal muscle: Expression signatures of individual fast and slow myofibers. *PLoS One*. Feb. 2011;6(2):e16807. https://doi.org/10.1371/journal.pone.0016807
51. Yin Y, Li N, Jia W, Wang N, Liang M, Yang X, et al. Skeletal muscle atrophy: From mechanisms to treatments. *Pharmacol. Res.* Oct. 2021;172:105807. https://doi.org/10.1016/j.phrs.2021.105807
52. Chen M, Wang Y, Deng S, Lian Z, Yu K. Skeletal muscle oxidative stress and inflammation in aging: Focus on antioxidant and anti-inflammatory therapy. *Front. Cell Dev. Biol.* Aug. 2022;10. https://doi.org/10.3389/fcell.2022.964130
53. Zahan, O-M, Serban O, Gherman C, Fodor D. The evaluation of oxidative stress in osteoarthritis. *Med. Pharm. Reports*. Jan. 2020;93(1):12–22. https://doi.org/10.15386/mpr-1422

54. Xia X, Fang Z, Qian Y, Zhou Y, Huang H, Xu F, et al. Role of oxidative stress in the concurrent development of osteoporosis and tendinopathy: Emerging challenges and prospects for treatment modalities. *J. Cell. Mol. Med.* Jul. 2024;28(13). https://doi.org/10.1111/jcmm.18508
55. Kane SF, Olewinski LH, Tamminga KS. Management of chronic tendon injuries. *Am. Fam. Physician.* Aug. 2019;100(3):147–57. [Online]. Available from: http://www.ncbi.nlm.nih.gov/pubmed/31361101
56. Yazar İ, Sarıkaya B, Koyuncu I, Gönel A, Bozkurt C, Sipahioğlu S, et al. Evaluation of oxidative stress in degenerative rotator cuff tears. *J. Shoulder Elb. Surg.* Oct. 2022;31(10):e490–97. https://doi.org/10.1016/j.jse.2022.03.011
57. Morikawa D, Itoigawa Y, Nojiri H, Sano H, Itoi E, Saijo Y, et al. Contribution of oxidative stress to the degeneration of rotator cuff entheses. *J. Shoulder Elb. Surg.* May 2014;23(5):628–35. https://doi.org/10.1016/j.jse.2014.01.041
58. Wen P, Zheng B, Zhang B, Ma T, Hao L, Zhang Y. The role of ageing and oxidative stress in intervertebral disc degeneration. *Front. Mol. Biosci.* Nov. 2022;9. https://doi.org/10.3389/fmolb.2022.1052878
59. Cao G, Yang S, Cao J, Tan Z, Wu L, Dong F, et al. The role of oxidative stress in intervertebral disc degeneration. *Oxid. Med. Cell. Longev.* Jan. 2022;2022(1). https://doi.org/10.1155/2022/2166817
60. Paschalis EP, Betts F, DiCarlo E, Mendelsohn R, Boskey AL. FTIR microspectroscopic analysis of normal human cortical and trabecular bone. *Calcif. Tissue Int.* Dec. 1997;61(6):480–6. https://doi.org/10.1007/s002239900371
61. Paschalis EP, Betts F, DiCarlo E, Mendelsohn R, Boskey AL. FTIR microspectroscopic analysis of human iliac crest biopsies from untreated osteoporotic bone. *Calcif. Tissue Int.* Dec. 1997;61(6):487–92. https://doi.org/10.1007/s002239900372
62. Burr DB. Changes in bone matrix properties with aging. *Bone.* Mar. 2019;120:85–93. https://doi.org/10.1016/j.bone.2018.10.010
63. Karim L, Tang SY, Sroga GE, Vashishth, D. Differences in non-enzymatic glycation and collagen cross-links between human cortical and cancellous bone. *Osteoporos. Int.* Sep. 2013;24(9):2441–7. https://doi.org/10.1007/s00198-013-2319-4
64. Vashishth D, Verborgt O, Divine G, Schaffler MB, Fyhrie DP. Decline in osteocyte lacunar density in human cortical bone is associated with accumulation of microcracks with age. *Bone.* Apr. 2000;26(4):375–80. https://doi.org/10.1016/S8756-3282(00)00236-2

65. Hesse B, Langer M, Varga P, Pacureanu A, Dong P, Schrof S, et al. Alterations of mass density and 3D osteocyte lacunar properties in bisphosphonate-related osteonecrotic human jaw bone, a synchrotron μCT study. *PLoS One*. Feb. 2014;9(2):e88481. https://doi.org/10.1371/journal.pone.0088481
66. Cruz-Jentoft AJ, Baeyens JP, Bauer JM, Boirie Y, Cederholm T, Landi F, et al. Sarcopenia: European consensus on definition and diagnosis. *Age Ageing*. Jul. 2010;39(4):412–23. https://doi.org/10.1093/ageing/afq034
67. Lexell J, Taylor CC, Sjöström M. What is the cause of the ageing atrophy? *J. Neurol. Sci.* Apr. 1988;84(2–3):275–94. https://doi.org/10.1016/0022-510X(88)90132-3
68. Koster A, Ding J, Stenholm S, Caserotti P, Houston DK, Nicklas BJ, et al. Does the amount of fat mass predict age-related loss of lean mass, muscle strength, and muscle quality in older adults? *J. Gerontol. Ser. A Biol. Sci. Med. Sci.* Aug. 201166A(8):888–95. https://doi.org/10.1093/gerona/glr070
69. Power GA, Dalton BH, Rice CL. Human neuromuscular structure and function in old age: A brief review. *J. Sport Heal. Sci.* Dec. 2013;2(4):215–26. https://doi.org/10.1016/j.jshs.2013.07.001
70. Campbell MJ, McComas AJ, Petito F. Physiological changes in ageing muscles. *J. Neurol. Neurosurg. Psychiatry*. Apr. 1973;36(2):174–82. https://doi.org/10.1136/jnnp.36.2.174
71. Vainshtein A, Sandri M. Signaling pathways that control muscle mass. *Int. J. Mol. Sci.* Jul. 2020;21(13):4759. https://doi.org/10.3390/ijms21134759
72. Sartori R, Romanello V, Sandri M. Mechanisms of muscle atrophy and hypertrophy: Implications in health and disease. *Nat. Commun.* Jan. 2021;12(1):330. https://doi.org/10.1038/s41467-020-20123-1
73. Overend TJ, Cunningham DA, Paterson DH, Lefcoe MS. Thigh composition in young and elderly men determined by computed tomography. *Clin. Physiol.* Nov. 1992;12(6):629–40. https://doi.org/10.1111/j.1475-097X.1992.tb00366.x
74. Lindle RS, Metter EJ, Lynch NA, Fleg JV, Fozard JL, Tobin J, et al. Age and gender comparisons of muscle strength in 654 women and men aged 20–93 yr. *J. Appl. Physiol.* Nov. 1997;83(5):1581–87. https://doi.org/10.1152/jappl.1997.83.5.1581
75. Delmonico MJ, Harris TB, Visser M, Park SW, Conroy MB, Velasquez-Mieyer P, et al. Longitudinal study of muscle strength, quality, and adipose tissue infiltration. *Am. J. Clin. Nutr.* Dec. 2009;90(6):1579–85. https://doi.org/10.3945/ajcn.2009.28047

76. Goodpaster BH, Park SW, Harris TB, Kritchevsky SB, Nevitt M, Schwartz AV, et al. The loss of skeletal muscle strength, mass, and quality in older adults: The health, aging and body composition study. *J. Gerontol. Ser. A Biol. Sci. Med. Sci.* Oct. 2006;61(10):1059–64. https://doi.org/10.1093/gerona/61.10.1059
77. Gonzalez-Freire M, de Cabo R, Studenski SA, Ferrucci LA. The neuromuscular junction: Aging at the crossroad between nerves and muscle. *Front. Aging Neurosci.* Aug. 2014;6. https://doi.org/10.3389/fnagi.2014.00208
78. Magnusson SP, Kjaer M. The impact of loading, unloading, ageing and injury on the human tendon. *J. Physiol.* Mar. 2019;597(5):1283–98. https://doi.org/10.1113/JP275450
79. Chen M, Xiao L, Dai G, Lu P, Zhang Y, Li Y, et al. Inhibition of JAK-STAT signaling pathway alleviates age-related phenotypes in tendon stem/progenitor cells. *Front. Cell Dev. Biol.* Mar. 2021;9. https://doi.org/10.3389/fcell.2021.650250
80. Cai Z, Zhang Y, Liu S, Liu X. Celecoxib, beyond anti-inflammation, alleviates tendon-derived stem cell senescence in degenerative rotator cuff tendinopathy. *Am. J. Sports Med.* Jul. 2022;50(9):2488–96. https://doi.org/10.1177/03635465221098133
81. Chen M, Li Y, Xiao L, Dai G, Lu P, Rui Y, Noncanonical Wnt5a signaling regulates tendon stem/progenitor cells senescence. *Stem Cell Res. Ther.* Dec. 2021;12(1):544. https://doi.org/10.1186/s13287-021-02605-1
82. Screen HRC, Berk DE, Kadler KE, Ramirez F, Young MF. Tendon functional extracellular matrix. *J. Orthop. Res.* Jun. 2015;33(6):793–99. https://doi.org/10.1002/jor.22818
83. Craig AS, Birtles MJ, Conway JF, Parry DAD. An estimate of the mean length of collagen fibrils in rat tail-tendon as a function of age. *Connect. Tissue Res.* Jan. 1989;19(1):51–62. https://doi.org/10.3109/03008208909016814
84. Parry DAD, Craig AS. Quantitative electron microscope observations of the collagen fibrils in rat-tail tendon. *Biopolymers.* May 1977;16(5):1015–31. https://doi.org/10.1002/bip.1977.360160506
85. Riley GP, Harrall RL, Constant CR, Chard MD, Cawston TE, Hazleman BL. Tendon degeneration and chronic shoulder pain: Changes in the collagen composition of the human rotator cuff tendons in rotator cuff tendinitis. *Ann. Rheum. Dis.* Jun. 1994;53(6):359–66. https://doi.org/10.1136/ard.53.6.359
86. Hudson DM, Archer M, Rai J, Weis M, Fernandes RJ, Eyre DR. Age-related type I collagen modifications reveal tissue-defining differences

between ligament and tendon. *Matrix Biol. Plus*. Dec. 2021;12:100070. https://doi.org/10.1016/j.mbplus.2021.100070

87. Dunkman AA, Buckley MR, Mienaltowski MJ, Adams SM, Thomas SJ, Satchell L, et al. Decorin expression is important for age-related changes in tendon structure and mechanical properties. *Matrix Biol.* Jan. 2013;32(1):3–13. https://doi.org/10.1016/j.matbio.2012.11.005
88. Frantz C, Stewart KM, Weaver VM. The extracellular matrix at a glance. *J. Cell Sci.* Dec. 2010;123(24):4195–200. https://doi.org/10.1242/jcs.023820
89. Brewer BJ. Aging of the rotator cuff. *Am. J. Sports Med.* Mar. 1979;7(2):102–10. https://doi.org/10.1177/036354657900700206
90. Wood LK, Brooks SV. Ten weeks of treadmill running decreases stiffness and increases collagen turnover in tendons of old mice. *J. Orthop. Res.* Feb. 2016;34(2):346–53. https://doi.org/10.1002/jor.22824
91. Sakellariou G, Iagnocco A, Filippucci E, Ceccarelli F, Di Geso L, Carli L, et al. Ultrasound imaging for the rheumatologist XLVIII. Ultrasound of the shoulders of patients with rheumatoid arthritis. *Clin. Exp. Rheumatol.* 2013;31(6):837–42. [Online]. http://www.ncbi.nlm.nih.gov/pubmed/24373322
92. Lui PPY, Wong CM. Biology of tendon stem cells and tendon in aging. *Front. Genet.* Jan. 2020;10. https://doi.org/10.3389/fgene.2019.01338
93. Lotz M, Loeser RF. Effects of aging on articular cartilage homeostasis. *Bone*. Aug. 2012;51(2):241–48. https://doi.org/10.1016/j.bone.2012.03.023
94. Li Y, Li T, Zhu C, Li H, Fang R, Li R, et al. Stable-dynamic hydrogels mimicking the pericellular matrix for articular cartilage repair. *Adv. Healthc. Mater.* May 2025;14(12). https://doi.org/10.1002/adhm.202405081
95. Mariani E, Pulsatelli L, Facchini A. Signaling pathways in cartilage repair. *Int. J. Mol. Sci.* May 2014;15(5):8667–98. https://doi.org/10.3390/ijms15058667
96. Ren P, Niu H, Gong H, Zhang R, Fan Y. Morphological, biochemical and mechanical properties of articular cartilage and subchondral bone in rat tibial plateau are age related. *J. Anat.* Mar. 2018;232(3):457–71. https://doi.org/10.1111/joa.12756
97. Bae WC, Temple MM, Amiel D, Coutts RD, Niederauer GG, Sah RL. Indentation testing of human cartilage: Sensitivity to articular surface degeneration. *Arthritis Rheum.* Dec. 2003;48(12):3382–94. https://doi.org/10.1002/art.11347
98. van Turnhout M, Haazelager M, Gijsen M, Schipper H, Kranenbarg S, van Leeuwen J. Quantitative description of collagen structure in the articular

cartilage of the young and adult equine distal metacarpus. *Anim. Biol.* 2008;58(4):353–70. https://doi.org/10.1163/157075608X383674

99. Buckwalter JA, Woo SL, Goldberg VM, Hadley EC, Booth F, Oegema TR, et al. Soft-tissue aging and musculoskeletal function. *J. Bone Jt. Surg.* Oct. 1993;75(10):1533–48. https://doi.org/10.2106/00004623-199310000-00015
100. Martin JA, Buckwalter JA. Roles of articular cartilage aging and chondrocyte senescence in the pathogenesis of osteoarthritis. *Iowa Orthop. J.* 2001;21:1–7. [Online]. http://www.ncbi.nlm.nih.gov/pubmed/11813939
101. Miller JA, Schmatz, C, Schultz AB. Lumbar disc degeneration: Correlation with age, sex, and spine level in 600 autopsy specimens. *Spine (Phila. Pa. 1976).* Feb. 1988;13(2):173–8. [Online]. http://www.ncbi.nlm.nih.gov/pubmed/3406837
102. Boos N, Weissbach S, Rohrbach H, Weiler C, Spratt KF, Nerlich AG. Classification of age-related changes in lumbar intervertebral discs. *Spine (Phila. Pa. 1976).* Dec. 2002;27(23):2631–44. https://doi.org/10.1097/00007632-200212010-00002
103. Vo NV, Hartman RA, Patil PR, Risbud MV, Kletsas D, Iatridis JC, et al. Molecular mechanisms of biological aging in intervertebral discs, *J. Orthop. Res.* Aug. 2016;34(8):1289–306. https://doi.org/10.1002/jor.23195
104. Roughley PJ. Biology of intervertebral disc aging and degeneration. *Spine (Phila. Pa. 1976).* Dec. 2004;29(23):2691–99. https://doi.org/10.1097/01.brs.0000146101.53784.b1
105. Kumaresan S, Yoganandan N, Pintar FA, Macias M, Cusick JF. Morphology of young and old cervical spine intervertebral disc tissues. *Biomed. Sci. Instrum.* 2000;36:141–6. [Online]. http://www.ncbi.nlm.nih.gov/pubmed/10834223
106. Prescher A. Anatomy and pathology of the aging spine. *Eur. J. Radiol.* Jul. 1998;27(3):181–95. https://doi.org/10.1016/S0720-048X(97)00165-4
107. Hormel SE, Eyre DR. Collagen in the ageing human intervertebral disc: An increase in covalently bound fluorophores and chromophores. *Biochim. Biophys. Acta — Protein Struct. Mol. Enzymol.* Jun. 1991;1078(2):243–50. https://doi.org/10.1016/0167-4838(91)90565-H
108. Edelson JG, Nathan H. Stages in the natural history of the vertebral end-plates. *Spine (Phila. Pa. 1976).* Jan. 1988;13(1):21–6. https://doi.org/10.1097/00007632-198801000-00006
109. Bibby SRS, Jones DA, Ripley RM, Urban JPG. Metabolism of the intervertebral disc: Effects of low levels of oxygen, glucose, and pH on rates of energy

metabolism of bovine nucleus pulposus cells. *Spine (Phila. Pa. 1976).* Mar. 2005;30(5):487–96. https://doi.org/10.1097/01.brs.0000154619.38122.47

110. Minetto MA, Giannini A, McConnell R, Busso C, Torre G, Massazza G. Common musculoskeletal disorders in the elderly: The star triad. *J. Clin. Med.* Apr. 2020;9(4):1216. https://doi.org/10.3390/jcm9041216
111. Yuan S, Larsson SC. Epidemiology of sarcopenia: Prevalence, risk factors, and consequences. *Metabolism.* Jul. 2023;144:155533. https://doi.org/10.1016/j.metabol.2023.155533
112. Fakler JKM, Pieroh P, Höch A, Roth A, Kleber C, Löffler M, et al. Predictors of long-term mortality in older patients with hip fractures managed by hemiarthroplasty: A 10-year study based on a population registry in Saxony, Germany. *Patient Saf. Surg.* Apr. 2024;18(1):15. https://doi.org/10.1186/s13037-024-00398-9
113. Gonul R, Tasar PT, Tuncer K, Karasahin O, Binici DN, Sevinc C, et al. Mortality-related risk factors in geriatric patients with hip fracture. *Ann. Geriatr. Med. Res.* Jun. 2023;27(2):126–33. https://doi.org/10.4235/agmr.23.0010
114. Li H, Huang H, Zhang X, Wang Y, Ren X, Cui Y, et al. Postoperative long-term independence among the elderly with meningiomas: Function evolution, determinant identification, and prediction model development. *Front. Oncol.* Mar. 2021;11:639259. https://doi.org/10.3389/fonc.2021.639259
115. CDC. *The Burden of Cigarette Smoking.* 2024. https://www.cdc.gov/tobacco/campaign/tips/about/#impact (accessed Jul. 29, 2025).
116. Clark D, Nakamura M, Miclau T, Marcucio R. Effects of aging on fracture healing. *Curr. Osteoporos. Rep.* Dec. 2017;15(6):601–8. https://doi.org/10.1007/s11914-017-0413-9
117. U. S. C. Bureau. Older Population and Aging. https://www.census.gov/topics/population/older-aging.html (accessed Jul. 29, 2025).
118. Tarakji B, Cil A, Butin RE, Bernhardt M. Adverse effects of smoking on musculoskeletal health. *Mo. Med.* 2017;114(4):268–71. [Online]. http://www.ncbi.nlm.nih.gov/pubmed/30228609
119. CDC. *Cigarette Smoking.* https://www.cdc.gov/tobacco/about/index.html (accessed Jul. 29, 2025).
120. Hernigou J, Schuind F. Tobacco and bone fractures. *Bone Joint Res.* Jun. 2019;8(6):255–65. https://doi.org/10.1302/2046-3758.86.BJR-2018-0344.R1
121. AL-Bashaireh AM, Haddad LG, Weaver M, Kelly DL, Chengguo X, Yoon S. The effect of tobacco smoking on musculoskeletal health: A systematic

review. *J. Environ. Public Health.* Jul. 2018;2018:1–106. https://doi.org/10.1155/2018/4184190
122. Ward KD, Klesges RC. A meta-analysis of the effects of cigarette smoking on bone mineral density. *Calcif. Tissue Int.* May 2001;68(5):259–70. https://doi.org/10.1007/BF02390832
123. Zhang Y, Zeng C, Li H, Yang T, Deng ZH, Yang Y, et al. Relationship between cigarette smoking and radiographic knee osteoarthritis in Chinese population: A cross-sectional study. *Rheumatol. Int.* Jul. 2015;35(7):1211–7. https://doi.org/10.1007/s00296-014-3202-0
124. Duchman KR, Gao Y, Pugely AJ, Martin CT, Noiseux NO, Callaghan JJ. The effect of smoking on short-term complications following total hip and knee arthroplasty. *J. Bone Jt. Surg.* Jul. 2015;97(13):1049–58. https://doi.org/10.2106/JBJS.N.01016
125. Kim AH, ElNemer W, Cartagena-Reyes MA, Marrache M, Thompson JM, Aiyer AA. The cost-effectiveness of smoking cessation programs for prevention of wound complications following total ankle arthroplasty: A break-even analysis. *Foot Ankle Orthop.* Jan. 2024;9(1):24730114241239315. https://doi.org/10.1177/24730114241239315
126. Lombardi AV, Berend KR, Adams JB, Jefferson RC, Sneller MA. Smoking may be a harbinger of early failure with ultraporous metal acetabular reconstruction. *Clin. Orthop. Relat. Res.* Feb. 2013;471(2):486–97. https://doi.org/10.1007/s11999-012-2748-y
127. Huang W, Qian Y, Zheng K, Yu L, Yu X. Is smoking a risk factor for lumbar disc herniation?. *Eur. Spine J.* Jan. 2016;25(1):168–76. https://doi.org/10.1007/s00586-015-4103-y
128. Bishop JY, Santiago-Torres JE, Rimmke N, Flanigan DC. Smoking predisposes to rotator cuff pathology and shoulder dysfunction: A systematic review. *Arthrosc. J. Arthrosc. Relat. Surg.* Aug. 2015;31(8):1598–605. https://doi.org/10.1016/j.arthro.2015.01.026
129. Novikov DA, Swensen SJ, Buza JA, Gidumal RH, Strauss EJ. The effect of smoking on ACL reconstruction: A systematic review. *Phys. Sportsmed.* Oct. 2016;44(4):335–41. https://doi.org/10.1080/00913847.2016.1216239
130. Kanneganti P, Harris JD, Brophy RH, Carey JL, Lattermann C, Flanigan DC. The effect of smoking on ligament and cartilage surgery in the knee. *Am. J. Sports Med.* Dec. 2012;40(12):2872–8. https://doi.org/10.1177/0363546512458223
131. Montes de Oca M, Loeb E, Torres SH, De Sanctis J, Hernández N, Tálamo C. Peripheral muscle alterations in non-COPD smokers. *Chest.* Jan. 2008;133(1):13–8. https://doi.org/10.1378/chest.07-1592

132. Rapuri PB, Gallagher JC, Smith LM. Smoking is a risk factor for decreased physical performance in elderly women. *J. Gerontol. Ser. A Biol. Sci. Med. Sci.* Jan. 2007;62(1):93–9. https://doi.org/10.1093/gerona/62.1.93
133. Kok MO, Hoekstra T, Twisk JWR. The longitudinal relation between smoking and muscle strength in healthy adults. *Eur. Addict. Res.* 2012;18(2):70–5. https://doi.org/10.1159/000333600
134. Nåsell H, Ottosson C, Törnqvist H, Lindé J, Ponzer S. The impact of smoking on complications after operatively treated ankle fractures — A follow-up study of 906 patients. *J. Orthop. Trauma.* Dec. 2011;25(12):748–55. https://doi.org/10.1097/BOT.0b013e318213f217
135. Santiago-Torres J, Flanigan DC, Butler RB, Bishop JY. The effect of smoking on rotator cuff and glenoid labrum surgery. *Am. J. Sports Med.* Mar. 2015;43(3):745–51. https://doi.org/10.1177/0363546514533776
136. Tamaki J, Iki M, Fujita Y, Kouda K, Yura A, Kadowaki E, et al. Impact of smoking on bone mineral density and bone metabolism in elderly men: The Fujiwara-kyo Osteoporosis Risk in Men (FORMEN) study. *Osteoporos. Int.* Jan. 2011;22(1):133–41. https://doi.org/10.1007/s00198-010-1238-x
137. W. O. A. 2025 P. Release, World Obesity Federation, *2025*.
138. Bureau PR. Rising Obesity in an aging America, 2022. https://www.prb.org/wp-content/uploads/2022/07/Todays-Research-on-Aging-Obesity-in-America-Final.pdf (accessed Aug. 02, 2025).
139. Shapses SA, Pop LC, Wang Y. Obesity is a concern for bone health with aging. *Nutr. Res.* Mar. 2017;39:1–13. https://doi.org/10.1016/j.nutres.2016.12.010
140. Halade GV, El Jamali A, Williams PJ, Fajardo RJ, Fernandes G. Obesity-mediated inflammatory microenvironment stimulates osteoclastogenesis and bone loss in mice. *Exp. Gerontol.* Jan. 2011;46(1):43–52. https://doi.org/10.1016/j.exger.2010.09.014
141. Tencerova M, Figeac F, Ditzel N, Taipaleenmäki H, Nielsen TK, Kassem M. High-fat diet-induced obesity promotes expansion of bone marrow adipose tissue and impairs skeletal stem cell functions in mice. *J. Bone Miner. Res.* Jun. 2018;33(6):1154–65. https://doi.org/10.1002/jbmr.3408
142. Ambrosi TH, Scialdone A, Graja A, Gohlke S, Jank AM, Bocian C, et al. Adipocyte accumulation in the bone marrow during obesity and aging impairs stem cell-based hematopoietic and bone regeneration. *Cell Stem Cell.* Jun. 2017;20(6):771–84.e6. https://doi.org/10.1016/j.stem.2017.02.009
143. Compston JE, Watts NB, Chapurlat R, Cooper C, Boonen S, Greenspan S, et al. Obesity is not protective against fracture in postmenopausal women:

GLOW. *Am. J. Med.* Nov. 2011;124(11):1043–50. https://doi.org/10.1016/j.amjmed.2011.06.013

144. Nielson CM, Marshall LM, Adams AL, LeBlanc ES, Cawthon PM, Ensrud K, et al. BMI and fracture risk in older men: The osteoporotic fractures in men study (MrOS). *J. Bone Miner. Res.* Mar. 2011;26(3):496–502. https://doi.org/10.1002/jbmr.235
145. Donini LM, Busetto L, Bischoff SC, Cederholm T, Ballesteros-Pomar MD, Batsis JA, et al. Definition and diagnostic criteria for sarcopenic obesity: ESPEN and EASO Consensus Statement. *Obes. Facts*. 2022;15(3):321–35. https://doi.org/10.1159/000521241
146. Axelrod CL, Dantas WS, Kirwan JP. Sarcopenic obesity: Emerging mechanisms and therapeutic potential. *Metabolism.* Sep. 2023;146:155639. https://doi.org/10.1016/j.metabol.2023.155639
147. Batsis JA, Villareal DT. Sarcopenic obesity in older adults: Aetiology, epidemiology and treatment strategies. *Nat. Rev. Endocrinol.* Sep. 2018;14(9):513–37. https://doi.org/10.1038/s41574-018-0062-9
148. Wearing SC, Hennig EM, Byrne NM, Steele JR, Hills AP. Musculoskeletal disorders associated with obesity: A biomechanical perspective. *Obes. Rev.* Aug. 20067(3):239–50. https://doi.org/10.1111/j.1467-789X.2006.00251.x
149. Felson DT, Goggins J, Niu J, Zhang Y, Hunter DJ. The effect of body weight on progression of knee osteoarthritis is dependent on alignment. *Arthritis Rheum.* Dec. 2004;50(12):3904–909. https://doi.org/10.1002/art.20726
150. Lievense AM. Influence of obesity on the development of osteoarthritis of the hip: A systematic review. *Rheumatology*. Oct. 2002;41(10):1155–62. https://doi.org/10.1093/rheumatology/41.10.1155
151. Hangai M, Kaneoka K, Kuno S, Hinotsu S, Sakane M, Mamizuka N, et al. Factors associated with lumbar intervertebral disc degeneration in the elderly. *Spine J.* Sep. 2008;8(5):732–40. https://doi.org/10.1016/j.spinee.2007.07.392
152. Katsevman GA, Daffner SD, Brandmeir NJ, Emery SE, France JC, Sedney CL. Complexities of spine surgery in obese patient populations: A narrative review. *Spine J.* Apr. 2020;20(4):501–11. https://doi.org/10.1016/j.spinee.2019.12.011
153. Andersen RE, Crespo CJ, Bartlett SJ, Bathon JM,Fontaine KR. Relationship between body weight gain and significant knee, hip, and back pain in older Americans. *Obes. Res.* Oct. 2003;11(10):1159–62. https://doi.org/10.1038/oby.2003.159

154. Changulani M, Kalairajah Y, Peel T, Field RE. The relationship between obesity and the age at which hip and knee replacement is undertaken. *J. Bone Joint Surg. Br.* Mar. 2008;90-B(3):360–63. https://doi.org/10.1302/0301-620X.90B3.19782
155. Lübbeke A, Moons KGM, Garavaglia G, Hoffmeyer P. Outcomes of obese and nonobese patients undergoing revision total hip arthroplasty, *Arthritis Care Res. (Hoboken).* May 2008;59(5):738–45. https://doi.org/10.1002/art.23562
156. George J, Klika AK, Navale SM, Newman JM, Barsoum WK, Higuera, CA. Obesity epidemic: Is its impact on total joint arthroplasty underestimated? An analysis of national trends. *Clin. Orthop. Relat. Res.* Jul. 2017;475(7): 1798–806. https://doi.org/10.1007/s11999-016-5222-4
157. Frey C, Zamora J. The effects of obesity on orthopaedic foot and ankle pathology. *Foot Ankle Int.* Sep. 2007;28(9):996–9. https://doi.org/10.3113/FAI.2007.0996
158. Holmes GB, Lin J. Etiologic factors associated with symptomatic achilles tendinopathy. *Foot Ankle Int.* Nov. 2006;27(11):952–9. https://doi.org/10.1177/107110070602701115
159. Wendelboe AM, Hegmann KT, Gren LH, Alder SC, White GL, Lyon JL. Associations between body-mass index and surgery for rotator cuff tendinitis. *J. Bone Jt. Surg. Am. Vol.* Apr. 2004;86(4):743–7. https://doi.org/10.2106/00004623-200404000-00011
160. DiSilvestro KJ, Jauregui JJ, Glazier E, Cherkalin D, Bennett CH, Packer JD, et al. Outcomes of anterior cruciate ligament reconstruction in obese and overweight patients: A systematic review. *Clin. J. Sport Med.* Jul. 2019;29(4):257–61. https://doi.org/10.1097/JSM.0000000000000521
161. Saeedi P, Petersohn I, Salpea P, Malanda B, Karuranga S, Unwin N, et al. Global and regional diabetes prevalence estimates for 2019 and projections for 2030 and 2045: Results from the International Diabetes Federation Diabetes Atlas, 9th edition. *Diabetes Res. Clin. Pract.* Nov. 2019;157:107843. https://doi.org/10.1016/j.diabres.2019.107843
162. Guo J, Huang X, Dou L, Yan M, Shen T, Tang W, et al. Aging and aging-related diseases: From molecular mechanisms to interventions and treatments. *Signal Transduct. Target. Ther.* Dec. 2022;7(1):391. https://doi.org/10.1038/s41392-022-01251-0
163. Suzuki K, Hatzikotoulas K, Southam L, Taylor HJ, Yin X, Lorenz KM, et al. Genetic drivers of heterogeneity in type 2 diabetes pathophysiology. *Nature.* Mar. 2024;627(8003):347–57. https://doi.org/10.1038/s41586-024-07019-6

164. Laakso M, Fernandes Silva L. Genetics of Type 2 diabetes: Past, present, and future. *Nutrients*. Aug. 2022;14(15):3201. https://doi.org/10.3390/nu14153201
165. Gray N, Picone G, Sloan F, Yashkin A. Relation between BMI and diabetes mellitus and its complications among US older adults. *South. Med. J.* Jan. 2015;108(1):29–36. https://doi.org/10.14423/SMJ.0000000000000214
166. Kuhlow D, Florian S, von Figura G, Weimer S, Schulz N, Petzke KJ, et al. Telomerase deficiency impairs glucose metabolism and insulin secretion. *Aging (Albany. NY).* Sep. 2010;2(10):650–8. https://doi.org/10.18632/aging.100200
167. Wyatt LH, Ferrance RJ. The musculoskeletal effects of diabetes mellitus. *J. Can. Chiropr. Assoc.* Mar. 2006;50(1):43–50. [Online]. http://www.ncbi.nlm.nih.gov/pubmed/17549168
168. Sözen T, Çalık Başaran N, Tınazlı M, Özışık L. Musculoskeletal problems in diabetes mellitus. *Eur. J. Rheumatol.* Sep. 2019;5(4):258–65. https://doi.org/10.5152/eurjrheum.2018.18044
169. Carvalho-e-Silva AP, Ferreira ML, Ferreira PH, Harmer AR. Does type 2 diabetes increase the risk of musculoskeletal pain? Cross-sectional and longitudinal analyses of UK biobank data. *Semin. Arthritis Rheum.* Aug. 2020;50(4):728–34. https://doi.org/10.1016/j.semarthrit.2020.05.007
170. Starup-Linde J, Støy J, Grinderslev PB, Langdahl B, Harsløf T. Prevalence and risk factors for osteoporosis in type 1 diabetes — results from an observational study. *Osteoporos. Int.* May 2025;36(5):823–31. https://doi.org/10.1007/s00198-025-07443-y
171. Sharma P, Sharma RK, Gaur K. Understanding the impact of diabetes on bone health: A clinical review. *Metab. Open*. Dec. 2024;24:100330. https://doi.org/10.1016/j.metop.2024.100330
172. Odetti P, Rossi S, Monacelli F, Poggi A, Cirnigliaro M, Federici M, et al. Advanced glycation end products and bone loss during aging. *Ann. N. Y. Acad. Sci.* Jun. 2005;1043(1):710–17. https://doi.org/10.1196/annals.1333.082
173. Janghorbani M, Van Dam RM, Willett WC, Hu FB. Systematic review of Type 1 and Type 2 diabetes mellitus and risk of fracture. *Am. J. Epidemiol.* Jun. 2007;166(5):495–505. https://doi.org/10.1093/aje/kwm106
174. Van Hulten V, Rasmussen N, Driessen JHM, Burden AM, Kvist A, van den Bergh JP. Fracture patterns in Type 1 and Type 2 diabetes mellitus: A narrative review of recent literature. *Curr. Osteoporos. Rep.* Dec. 2021;19(6):644–55. https://doi.org/10.1007/s11914-021-00715-6

175. Takahashi F, Hashimoto Y, Kaji A, Sakai R, Kawate Y, Okamura T, et al. Vitamin intake and loss of muscle mass in older people with Type 2 diabetes: A prospective study of the KAMOGAWA-DM cohort. *Nutrients*. Jul. 2021;13(7):2335. https://doi.org/10.3390/nu13072335
176. Chen H, Huang X, Dong M, Wen S, Zhou L, Yuan X. The association between sarcopenia and diabetes: From pathophysiology mechanism to therapeutic strategy. *Diabetes, Metab. Syndr. Obes.* May 2023;16:1541–54. https://doi.org/10.2147/DMSO.S410834
177. Liu Z, Guo Y, Zheng C. Type 2 diabetes mellitus related sarcopenia: A type of muscle loss distinct from sarcopenia and disuse muscle atrophy. *Front. Endocrinol. (Lausanne).* May 2024;15:1375610. https://doi.org/10.3389/fendo.2024.1375610
178. Tilling LM, Darawil K, Britton M. Falls as a complication of diabetes mellitus in older people. *J. Diabetes Complications*. May 2006;20(3):158–62. https://doi.org/10.1016/j.jdiacomp.2005.06.004
179. Gesing A. The thyroid gland and the process of aging. *Thyroid Res.* 2015;8(Suppl 1):A8. https://doi.org/10.1186/1756-6614-8-S1-A8
180. Bunker T. Frozen shoulder. *Orthop. Trauma*. Feb. 2011;25(1):11–8. https://doi.org/10.1016/j.mporth.2011.01.007
181. Huang Y, Fann CY, Chiu YH, Yen MF, Chen LS, Chen HH, et al. Association of diabetes mellitus with the risk of developing adhesive capsulitis of the shoulder: A longitudinal population-based followup study. *Arthritis Care Res. (Hoboken).* Jul. 2013;65(7):1197–202. https://doi.org/10.1002/acr.21938
182. Dyer BP, Burton C, Rathod-Mistry T, Blagojevic-Bucknall M, van der Windt DA. Diabetes as a prognostic factor in frozen shoulder: A systematic review. *Arch. Rehabil. Res. Clin. Transl.* Sep. 2021;3(3):100141. https://doi.org/10.1016/j.arrct.2021.100141
183. Dyer BP, Rathod-Mistry T, Burton C, van der Windt D, Bucknall M. Diabetes as a risk factor for the onset of frozen shoulder: A systematic review and meta-analysis. *BMJ Open*. Jan. 2023;13(1):e062377. https://doi.org/10.1136/bmjopen-2022-062377
184. Cao W, Chen J, Pu J, Fan Y, Cao Y. Risk factors for the onset of frozen shoulder in middle-aged and elderly subjects within 1 year of discharge from a hospitalization that involved intravenous infusion: A prospective cohort study. *Front. Med.* Jun. 2022;9:911532. https://doi.org/10.3389/fmed.2022.911532

185. Nikolaou VS, Efstathopoulos N, Kontakis G, Kanakaris NK, Giannoudis PV. The influence of osteoporosis in femoral fracture healing time. *Injury*. Jun. 2009;40(6):663–8. https://doi.org/10.1016/j.injury.2008.10.035
186. Gruber R, Koch H, Doll BA, Tegtmeier F, Einhorn TA, Hollinger JH. Fracture healing in the elderly patient. *Exp. Gerontol.* Nov. 2006;41(11):1080–93. https://doi.org/10.1016/j.exger.2006.09.008
187. Foulke BA, Kendal AR, Murray DW, Pandit H. Fracture healing in the elderly: A review. *Maturitas*. Oct. 2016;92:49–55. https://doi.org/10.1016/j.maturitas.2016.07.014
188. Brinker MR, O'Connor DP. The biological basis for nonunions. *JBJS Rev.* Jun. 2016;4(6). https://doi.org/10.2106/JBJS.RVW.15.00078
189. Vander Voort W, Davison J, Hendrickson N, Buckwalter J, Guetschow B, Glass N, et al. Sarcopenia is associated with nonunion of open tibia and ankle fractures. *Iowa Orthop. J.* 2020;40(1):153–58. [Online]. http://www.ncbi.nlm.nih.gov/pubmed/32742224
190. Mills LA, Aitken SA, Simpson AHRW. The risk of non-union per fracture: Current myths and revised figures from a population of over 4 million adults. *Acta Orthop.* Jul. 2017;88(4):434–9. https://doi.org/10.1080/17453674.2017.1321351
191. van Wunnik BPW, Weijers PHE, van Helden SH, Brink PRG, Poeze M. Osteoporosis is not a risk factor for the development of nonunion: A cohort nested case–control study. *Injury*. Dec. 2011;42(12):1491–4. https://doi.org/10.1016/j.injury.2011.08.019
192. Hernandez RK, DoTP, Critchlow CW, Dent RE, Jick SS. Patient-related risk factors for fracture-healing complications in the United Kingdom general practice research database. *Acta Orthop.* Dec. 2012;83(6):653–60. https://doi.org/10.3109/17453674.2012.747054
193. Zura R, Braid-Forbes MJ, Jeray K, Mehta S, Einhorn TA, Watson JT, et al. Bone fracture nonunion rate decreases with increasing age: A prospective inception cohort study. *Bone* Feb. 2017;95:26–32. https://doi.org/10.1016/j.bone.2016.11.006
194. van Trikt CH, Donders JCE, Klinger CE, Wellman DS, Helfet DL, Kloen P. Operative treatment of nonunions in the elderly: Clinical and radiographic outcomes in patients at minimum 75 years of age. *BMC Geriatr.* Dec. 2022;22(1):985. https://doi.org/10.1186/s12877-022-03670-8
195. Zura R, Mehta S, Della Rocca GJ, Steen RG. Biological risk factors for nonunion of bone fracture. *JBJS Rev.* Jan. 2016;4(1):e5. https://doi.org/10.2106/JBJS.RVW.O.00008

196. Vanderkarr MF, Ruppenkamp JW, Vanderkarr M, Holy CE, Blauth M. Risk factors and healthcare costs associated with long bone fracture non-union: A retrospective US claims database analysis. *J. Orthop. Surg. Res.* Oct. 2023;18(1):745. https://doi.org/10.1186/s13018-023-04232-3
197. Donié C, Reumann MK, Hartung T, Braun BJ, Histing T, Endo S, et al. Predictive model development to identify failed healing in patients after non–union fracture surgery, In: *2024 46th Annual International Conference of the IEEE Engineering in Medicine and Biology Society (EMBC)* 2024 Jul. 15 (pp. 1–4). https://doi.org/10.1109/EMBC53108.2024.10782650
198. Bertl K, Ebner M, Knibbe M, Pandis N, Kuchler U, Ulm C, et al. How old is old for implant therapy in terms of early implant losses?. *J. Clin. Periodontol.* Dec. 2019;46(12):1282–93. https://doi.org/10.1111/jcpe.13199
199. Sendyk DI, Rovai ES, Pannuti CM, Deboni MCZ, Sendyk MCZ, Wennerberg A. Dental implant loss in older versus younger patients: A systematic review and meta-analysis of prospective studies. *J. Oral Rehabil.* Mar. 2017;44(3):229–36. https://doi.org/10.1111/joor.12465
200. da Casa C, Fidalgo H, Nieto J, Cano-Lallave E, Blanco JF. Total knee arthroplasty for the oldest old. *Geriatrics*. Aug. 2021;6(3):75. https://doi.org/10.3390/geriatrics6030075
201. Maempel JF, Riddoch F, Calleja N, Brenkel IJ. Longer hospital stay, more complications, and increased mortality but substantially improved function after knee replacement in older patients. *Acta Orthop.* Jul. 2015;86(4):451–6. https://doi.org/10.3109/17453674.2015.1040304
202. Wu J-C, Huang WC, Tsai HW, Ko CC, Wu CL, Tu TH, et al. Pedicle screw loosening in dynamic stabilization: Incidence, risk, and outcome in 126 patients. *Neurosurg. Focus*. Oct. 2011;31(4):E9. https://doi.org/10.3171/2011.7.FOCUS11125
203. Xu F, Zhou S, Zou D, Li W, Sun Z, Jiang S. The relationship between S1 screw loosening and postoperative outcome in patients with degenerative lumbar scoliosis. *BMC Musculoskelet. Disord.* Feb. 2022;23(1):186. https://doi.org/10.1186/s12891-022-05107-0
204. Chang K, Albright JA, Testa EJ, Balboni AB, Daniels AH, Cohen E. Sarcopenia is associated with an increased risk of postoperative complications following total hip arthroplasty for osteoarthritis. *Biology (Basel).* Feb. 2023;12(2):295. https://doi.org/10.3390/biology12020295.
205. Babu JM, Kalagara S, Durand W, Antoci V, Deren ME, Cohen E. Sarcopenia as a risk factor for prosthetic infection after total hip or knee arthroplasty.

J. Arthroplasty. Jan. 2019;34(1):116–22. https://doi.org/10.1016/j.arth.2018.09.037

206. Pan T-Y, Chang C-C, Chen H-T, Tsou H-K, Lin Y-C, Hsu C-H. Effectiveness of teriparatide for spine fusion in osteoporotic patient: A systematic review and meta-analysis of comparative studies. *World Neurosurg*. Nov. 2023;179:8–17. https://doi.org/10.1016/j.wneu.2023.07.056
207. Li L, Shan T, Zhang D, Ma F. Nowcasting and forecasting global aging and cancer burden: Analysis of data from the GLOBOCAN and Global Burden of Disease Study. *J. Natl. Cancer Cent.* Sep. 2024;4(3):223–32. https://doi.org/10.1016/j.jncc.2024.05.002
208. American Cancer Society, No Title.
209. Van Herck Y, Feyaerts A, Alibhai S, Papamichael D, Decoster L, Lambrechts Y, et al. Is cancer biology different in older patients?. *Lancet Heal. Longev.* Oct. 2021;2(10):e663–677. https://doi.org/10.1016/S2666-7568(21)00179-3
210. Kalita M, Saha DMI, Chakrabarti A. Global burden of cancer pattern in 2020 & prediction to 2040 among older adults. *Indian J. Med. Res.* Dec. 2024;160:397. https://doi.org/10.25259/ijmr_1729_23
211. Chang S, Goldstein NE, Dharmarajan KV. Managing an older adult with cancer: Considerations for radiation oncologists. *Biomed Res. Int.* 2017;2017:1–13. https://doi.org/10.1155/2017/1695101
212. Marosi C, Köller M. Challenge of cancer in the elderly. *ESMO Open*. 2016;1(3):e000020. https://doi.org/10.1136/esmoopen-2015-000020
213. Akinoso-Imran AQ, O'Rorke M, Kee F, Jordao H, Walls G, Bannon FJ. Surgical under-treatment of older adult patients with cancer: A systematic review and meta-analysis. *J. Geriatr. Oncol.* May 2022;13(4):398–409. https://doi.org/10.1016/j.jgo.2021.11.004
214. Chatzimavridou-Grigoriadou V, Barraclough LH, Kochhar R, Buckley L, Alam N, Higham CE. Radiotherapy-related insufficiency fractures and bone mineral density: What is the connection? *Endocr. Connect.* Apr. 2023;12(7). https://doi.org/10.1530/EC-22-0328
215. Berk L. The effects of high-dose radiation therapy on bone: A scoping review. *Radiat. Oncol. J.* Jun. 2024;42(2):95–103. https://doi.org/10.3857/roj.2023.00969
216. Kim S, Kim YS. Radiation-induced osteoradionecrosis of the ribs in a patient with breast cancer: A case report. *Radiol. Case Reports*. Aug. 2022;17(8):2894–98. https://doi.org/10.1016/j.radcr.2022.01.067
217. Prathap R, Kirubha S, Rajan AT, Manoharan S, Elumalai K. The increasing prevalence of cancer in the elderly: An investigation of epidemiological

trends. *AGING Med.* Aug. 2024;7(4):516–27, https://doi.org/10.1002/agm2.12347

218. Vitzthum LK, Park H, Zakeri K, Heide ES, Nalawade V, Mundt AJ, et al. Risk of pelvic fracture with radiation therapy in older patients. *Int. J. Radiat. Oncol.* Mar. 2020;106(3):485–92. https://doi.org/10.1016/j.ijrobp.2019.10.006
219. Baxter NN. Risk of pelvic fractures in older women following pelvic irradiation. *JAMA*. Nov. 2005;294(20):2587. https://doi.org/10.1001/jama.294.20.2587
220. Chan AW, Zeng KL, Moore-Palhares D, Atenafu EG, Chen H, Myrehaug S, et al. Spine stereotactic body radiation therapy in geriatric patients: Implications of age and dose on iatrogenic vertebral compression fracture risk. *Int. J. Radiat. Oncol.* Apr. 2025;121(5):1185–93. https://doi.org/10.1016/j.ijrobp.2024.11.082
221. Razavian N, Laucis A, Sun Y, Spratt DE, Owen D, Schonewolf C, et al. Radiation-induced insufficiency fractures after pelvic irradiation for gynecologic malignancies: A systematic review. *Int. J. Radiat. Oncol.* Nov. 2020;108(3):620–34. https://doi.org/10.1016/j.ijrobp.2020.05.013
222. Salvini M, El Motassime A, Cavola F, Ruberto P, Ziranu A, Maccauro G. Recent advances in the surgical management of radiation-induced fractures following soft tissue sarcomas. *J. Clin. Med.* May 2024;13(11), 3126. https://doi.org/10.3390/jcm13113126
223. Bartelstein, MK, Yerramilli D, Christ AB, Kenan S, Ogura K, Fujiwara T, et al. Postradiation fractures after combined modality treatment in extremity soft tissue sarcomas. *Sarcoma*. Mar. 2021;2021:1–11. https://doi.org/10.1155/2021/8877567
224. Bishop AJ, Zagars GK, Allen PK, Moon BS, Lin PP, et al. Treatment-related fractures after combined modality therapy for soft tissue sarcomas of the proximal lower extremity: Can the risk be mitigated?. *Pract. Radiat. Oncol.* May 2016;6(3):194–200. https://doi.org/10.1016/j.prro.2015.09.004
225. Medici F, Rizzo S, Buwenge M, Arcelli A, Ferioli M, Macchia G, et al. Everything you always wanted to know about sarcopenia but were afraid to ask: A quick guide for radiation oncologists (impAct oF saRcopeniA In raDiotherapy: The AFRAID Project). *Curr. Oncol.* Nov. 2022;29(11):8513–28. https://doi.org/10.3390/curroncol29110671
226. Bergamaschi L, Marvaso G, Zaffaroni M, Vincini MG, D'Ecclesiis O, Volpe S, et al. Prognostic impact of sarcopenia's occurrence during radiotherapy in oropharyngeal cancer patients. *Cancers (Basel).* Jan. 2023;15(3):723. https://doi.org/10.3390/cancers15030723

227. Yang J-F, Huang WY, Lo CH, Lee MS, Lin CS, Shen PC, et al. Significant muscle loss after stereotactic body radiotherapy predicts worse survival in patients with hepatocellular carcinoma. *Sci. Rep.* Nov. 2022;12(1):19100. https://doi.org/10.1038/s41598-022-21443-6
228. Hojan K, Milecki P. Opportunities for rehabilitation of patients with radiation fibrosis syndrome. *Reports Pract. Oncol. Radiother.* Jan. 2014;19(1):1–6. https://doi.org/10.1016/j.rpor.2013.07.007
229. Simman R, Bach K, Abbas F, Klomparens K, Brickman BJ. Management of radiation-induced tissue injuries: A review of current treatment strategies. *Plast. Reconstr. Surg. — Glob. Open.* Jun. 2023;11(6):e5043. https://doi.org/10.1097/GOX.0000000000005043
230. Jiang Y, Xie J, Huang W, Chen H, Xi S, Li T, et al. Chemotherapy use and survival among young and middle-aged patients with gastric cancer. *Clin. Transl. Gastroenterol.* Oct. 2020;11(10):e00253. https://doi.org/10.14309/ctg.0000000000000253.
231. Khattak MA, Townsend AR, Beeke C, Karapetis CS, Luke C, Padbury R, et al. Impact of age on choice of chemotherapy and outcome in advanced colorectal cancer. *Eur. J. Cancer.* Jun. 2012;48(9):1293–8. https://doi.org/10.1016/j.ejca.2011.09.029
232. McKibbin T, Frei CR, Greene RE, Kwan P, Simon J, Koeller JM. Disparities in the use of chemotherapy and monoclonal antibody therapy for elderly advanced colorectal cancer patients in the community oncology setting. *Oncologist.* Aug. 2008;13(8):876–85. https://doi.org/10.1634/theoncologist.2008-0061
233. Bruning P, Pit M, de Jong-Bakker M, van den Ende A, Hart A, van Enk A. Bone mineral density after adjuvant chemotherapy for premenopausal breast cancer. *Br. J. Cancer.* Feb. 1990;61(2):308–10. https://doi.org/10.1038/bjc.1990.58
234. Mancuso S, Scaturro D, Santoro M, Di Gaetano G, Vitagliani F, Falco V, et al. Bone damage after chemotherapy for lymphoma: A real-world experience. *BMC Musculoskelet. Disord.* Dec. 2021;22(1):1024. https://doi.org/10.1186/s12891-021-04904-3
235. Nisha Y, Dubashi B, Bobby Z, Sahoo JP, Kayal S, Ananthakrishnan R, et al. Cytotoxic chemotherapy is associated with decreased bone mineral density in postmenopausal women with early and locally advanced breast cancer. *Arch. Osteoporos.* Mar. 2023;18(1):41. https://doi.org/10.1007/s11657-023-01231-z

236. Kourtis E, Zygogiannis K, Fanourgiakis I, Koulalis D, Stathopoulos KD. Understanding and managing fracture risk in patients with cancer: A literature review. *Cureus*. Apr. 2025. https://doi.org/10.7759/cureus.83082
237. Rees-Punia E, Newton CC, Parsons HM, Leach CR, Diver WR, Grant AC, et al. Fracture risk among older cancer survivors compared with older adults without a history of cancer. *JAMA Oncol.* Jan. 2023;9(1):79. https://doi.org/10.1001/jamaoncol.2022.5153
238. Huang L-W, Sun D, Link TM, Lang T, Ai W, Kaplan LD, et al. High incidence of fractures after R-CHOP-like chemotherapy for aggressive B-cell non-Hodgkin lymphomas. *Support. Care Cancer*. Sep. 2021;29(9):5399–408. https://doi.org/10.1007/s00520-021-06120-0
239. Davis MP, Panikkar R. Sarcopenia associated with chemotherapy and targeted agents for cancer therapy. *Ann. Palliat. Med.* Jan. 2019;8(1):86–101. https://doi.org/10.21037/apm.2018.08.02
240. Bozzetti F. Forcing the vicious circle: Sarcopenia increases toxicity, decreases response to chemotherapy and worsens with chemotherapy. *Ann. Oncol.* Sep. 2017;28(9):2107–118. https://doi.org/10.1093/annonc/mdx271
241. Bozzetti F. Chemotherapy-induced sarcopenia. *Curr. Treat. Options Oncol.* Jan. 2020;21(1):7. https://doi.org/10.1007/s11864-019-0691-9
242. Jang MK, Park S, Park C, Doorenbos AZ, Go J, Kim S. Does neoadjuvant chemotherapy regimen affect sarcopenia status in patients with breast cancer?. *The Breast*. Dec. 2022;66:1–7. https://doi.org/10.1016/j.breast.2022.08.009
243. Teissonnière M, Point M, Biver E, Hadji P, Bonnelye E, Ebeling PR, et al. Bone effects of anti-cancer treatments in 2024. *Calcif. Tissue Int.* Mar. 2025;116(1):54. https://doi.org/10.1007/s00223-025-01362-0
244. Fan C, Foster BK, Wallace WH, Xian CJ. Pathobiology and Prevention of cancer chemotherapy-induced bone growth arrest, bone loss, and osteonecrosis. *Curr. Mol. Med.* Mar. 2011;11(2):140–51. https://doi.org/10.2174/156652411794859223
245. Alqahtani A, Sabha M, Abdelfattah T, Srour K, Dhayihi T, Kahaleh B, et al. Tendonitis and tendon rupture after treatment with Rituximab: A case series. *Am. J. Ther.* Sep. 2017;24(5):e592–95. https://doi.org/10.1097/MJT.0000000000000591
246. Kesikburun B. Bilateral spontaneous rupture of the Achilles' tendon during chemotherapy treatment. *Turkish J. Oncol.* 2016. https://doi.org/10.5505/tjo.2016.1323

247. Guise TA. Bone loss and fracture risk associated with cancer therapy. *Oncologist.* Nov. 2006;11(10):1121–31. https://doi.org/10.1634/theoncologist.11-10-1121
248. Hu Z, Yang S, Xu Z, Zhang X, Wang H, Fan G, et al. Prevalence and risk factors of bone metastasis and the development of bone metastatic prognostic classification system: A pan-cancer population study. *Aging* (Albany. NY). Nov. 2023;15(22):13134–49. https://doi.org/10.18632/aging.205224
249. Sözen T, Özışık L, Başaran N. Ç. An overview and management of osteoporosis. *Eur. J. Rheumatol.* Mar. 2017;4(1):46–56. https://doi.org/10.5152/eurjrheum.2016.048
250. Zhu Y, Xing X, Liu S, Chen W, Zhang W, Zhang Y. Epidemiology of low-energy wrist, hip, and spine fractures in Chinese populations 50 years or older. *Medicine (Baltimore).* Jan. 2020;99(5):e18531. https://doi.org/10.1097/MD.0000000000018531
251. Kannus P, Parkkari J, Sievänen H, Heinonen A, Vuori I, Järvinen M. Epidemiology of hip fractures. *Bone.* Jan. 1996;18(1):S57–63. https://doi.org/10.1016/8756-3282(95)00381-9
252. Wainwright SA, Marshall LM, Ensrud KE, Cauley JA, Black DM, Hillier TA, et al. Hip fracture in women without osteoporosis. *J. Clin. Endocrinol. Metab.* May 2005;90(5):2787–93. https://doi.org/10.1210/jc.2004-1568
253. Schini M, Johansson H, Harvey NC, Lorentzon M, Kanis JA, McCloskey EV. An overview of the use of the fracture risk assessment tool (FRAX) in osteoporosis. *J. Endocrinol. Invest.* Oct. 2023;47(3):501–11. https://doi.org/10.1007/s40618-023-02219-9
254. Black DM, Schwartz AV, Ensrud KE, Cauley JA, Levis S, Quandt SA, et al. Effects of continuing or stopping alendronate after 5 Years of treatment. *JAMA.* Dec. 2006;296(24):2927. https://doi.org/10.1001/jama.296.24.2927
255. Khalid S, Calderon-Larrañaga S, Hawley S, Ali MS, Judge A, Arden N, et al. Comparative anti-fracture effectiveness of different oral anti-osteoporosis therapies based on “real-world” data: a meta-analysis of propensity-matched cohort findings from the UK Clinical Practice Research Database and the Catalan SIDIAP Data. *Clin. Epidemiol.* Oct. 2018;10:1417–31. https://doi.org/10.2147/CLEP.S164112
256. Adami G, Biffi A, Porcu G, Ronco R, Alvaro R, Bogini R, et al. A systematic review on the performance of fracture risk assessment tools: FRAX, DeFRA, FRA-HS. *J. Endocrinol. Invest.* Apr. 2023;46(11):2287–97. https://doi.org/10.1007/s40618-023-02082-8

257. Gomez F, Curcio CL, Brennan-Olsen SL, Boersma D, Phu S, Vogrin S, et al. Effects of the falls and fractures clinic as an integrated multidisciplinary model of care in Australia: A pre–post study. *BMJ Open*. Jul. 2019; 9(7):e027013. https://doi.org/10.1136/bmjopen-2018-027013
258. Callahan LF, Cleveland RJ, Allen KD, Golightly Y. Racial/ethnic, socioeconomic, and geographic disparities in the epidemiology of knee and hip osteoarthritis. *Rheum. Dis. Clin. North Am.* Feb. 2021;47(1):1–20. https://doi.org/10.1016/j.rdc.2020.09.001
259. Steinmetz JD, Culbreth GT, Haile LM, Rafferty Q, Lo J, Fukutaki KG, et al. Global, regional, and national burden of osteoarthritis, 1990–2020 and projections to 2050: A systematic analysis for the Global Burden of Disease Study 2021. *Lancet Rheumatol.* Sep. 2023;5(9):e508–22. https://doi.org/10.1016/S2665-9913(23)00163-7
260. Neogi T. The epidemiology and impact of pain in osteoarthritis. *Osteoarthr. Cartil.* Sep. 2013;21(9):1145–53. https://doi.org/10.1016/j.joca.2013.03.018
261. Schepman P, Thakkar S, Robinson RL, Beck CG, Malhotra D, Emir B, et al. A retrospective claims-based study evaluating clinical and economic burden among patients with moderate to severe osteoarthritis pain in the united states. *J. Heal. Econ. Outcomes Res.* Mar. 2022;9(1):58–67. https://doi.org/10.36469/jheor.2022.31895
262. Simpson AHRW. Incidence, complications and novel treatment strategies: Joint arthroplasty. In: *Musculoskeletal Infection*. Cham: Springer International Publishing; 2022. p. 227–82.
263. Kaufman M, Meaike J, Izaddoost S. Orthopedic prosthetic infections: Diagnosis and orthopedic salvage. *Semin. Plast. Surg.* May 2016;30(02):066–072. https://doi.org/10.1055/s-0036-1580730
264. Kurtz S, Ong K, Lau E, Mowat F, Halpern M. Projections of primary and revision hip and knee arthroplasty in the United States from 2005 to 2030. *J. Bone Jt. Surg.* Apr. 2007;89(4):780–85. https://doi.org/10.2106/JBJS.F.00222
265. Caldwell M, Hughes M, Wei F, Ngo C, Pascua R, Pugazhendhi AS, et al. Promising applications of D-amino acids in periprosthetic joint infection. *Bone Res.* Mar. 2023;11(1):14. https://doi.org/10.1038/s41413-023-00254-z
266. Vanhegan IS, Malik AK, Jayakumar P, Ul Islam S, Haddad FS. A financial analysis of revision hip arthroplasty. *J. Bone Joint Surg. Br.* May 2012;94-B(5):619–23. https://doi.org/10.1302/0301-620X.94B5.27073

267. Schwartz AM, Farley KX, Guild GN, Bradbury TL. Projections and epidemiology of revision hip and knee arthroplasty in the United States to 2030. *J. Arthroplasty*. Jun. 2020;35(6):S79–85. https://doi.org/10.1016/j.arth.2020.02.030
268. Sloan M, Sheth N. Projected volume of primary and revision total joint arthroplasty in the United States, 2030–2060. Presented at: *Annual Meeting of the American Academy of Orthopaedic Surgeons*; Mar. 2018. p. 16.
269. Day JS, Lau E, Ong KL, Williams GR, Ramsey ML, Kurtz SM. Prevalence and projections of total shoulder and elbow arthroplasty in the United States to 2015. *J. Shoulder Elb. Surg.* Dec. 2010;19(8):1115–20. https://doi.org//10.1016/j.jse.2010.02.009
270. Padegimas EM, Maltenfort M, Lazarus MD, Ramsey ML, Williams GR, Namdari S. Future patient demand for shoulder arthroplasty by younger patients: National Projections. *Clin. Orthop. Relat. Res.* Jun. 2015;473(6):1860–67. https://doi.org/10.1007/s11999-015-4231-z
271. Kim HM, Teefey SA, Zelig A, Galatz LM, Keener JD, Yamaguchi K. Shoulder strength in asymptomatic individuals with intact compared with torn rotator cuffs. *J. Bone Jt. Surgery-American Vol.* Feb. 2009;91(2):289–96. https://doi.org/10.2106/JBJS.H.00219
272. Milgrom C, Schaffler M, Gilbert S, van Holsbeeck M. Rotator-cuff changes in asymptomatic adults. The effect of age, hand dominance and gender. *J. Bone Joint Surg. Br.* Mar. 1995;77-B(2):296–98. https://doi.org/10.1302/0301-620X.77B2.7706351
273. Meng C, Jiang B, Liu M, Kang F, Kong L, Zhang T, et al. Repair of rotator cuff tears in patients aged 75 years and older: Does it make sense? A systematic review. *Front. Public Heal.* Jan. 2023;10:060700. https://doi.org/10.3389/fpubh.2022.1060700
274. Raval P, Singh H. Shoulder arthroplasty in the elderly. *J. Clin. Orthop. Trauma*. Jun. 2025;65:102976. https://doi.org/10.1016/j.jcot.2025.102976
275. Hochberger F, Herrmann P, Rudert M, List K, Stratos I. Trends in shoulder arthroplasty in germany: A 10-year epidemiological analysis of patients with primary osteoarthritis of the shoulder. *Healthcare*. May 2024;12(9):949. https://doi.org/10.3390/healthcare12090949
276. Mayfield CK, Korber SS, Hwang NM, Bolia IK, Gamradt SC, Weber AE, et al. Volume, indications, and number of surgeons performing reverse total shoulder arthroplasty continue to expand: A nationwide cohort analysis from 2016-2020. *JSES Int.* Sep. 2023;7(5):827–34. https://doi.org/10.1016/j.jseint.2023.05.002

277. Su F, Nuthalapati P, Feeley BT, Lansdown DA. Outcomes of anatomic and reverse total shoulder arthroplasty in patients over the age of 70: A systematic review. *JSES Rev. Reports, Tech.* May 2023;3(2):181–8. https://doi.org/10.1016/j.xrrt.2023.02.003
278. Kriechling P, Calek A-K, Hatziisaak K, Hochreiter B, Bouaicha S, Wieser K. Clinical outcomes do not deteriorate over time following primary reverse total shoulder arthroplasty. *JBJS Open Access.* Jul. 2024;9(3). https://doi.org/10.2106/JBJS.OA.23.00171
279. Gómez Alcaraz J, Pardo García JM, Sevilla Fernández J, Delgado Díaz E, Moreno Beamud JA. Artroplastia total primaria de cadera en pacientes mayores de 85 años: Riesgos, complicaciones y resultados a medio-largo plazo. *Rev. Esp. Cir. Ortop. Traumatol.* Jan. 2021;65(1):13–23. https://doi.org/10.1016/j.recot.2020.05.003
280. Selman F, Moreira B, Perry NPJ, Kriechling P, Gressl M, Wieser K. Reverse total shoulder arthroplasty outcomes in elderly patients. *JSES Int.* May 2025;9(3):815–22. https://doi.org/10.1016/j.jseint.2025.01.006
281. Bensa A, Previtali D, Sangiorgio A, Boffa A, Salerno M, Filardo G. PRP injections for the treatment of knee osteoarthritis: The improvement is clinically significant and influenced by platelet concentration: A meta-analysis of randomized controlled trials. *Am. J. Sports Med.* Mar. 2025;53(3):745–54. https://doi.org/10.1177/03635465241246524
282. Shahid A, Malik A, Bukhari A, Shaikh A, Rutherford J, Barkatali B. Do platelet-rich plasma injections for knee osteoarthritis work? *Cureus.* Feb. 2023. https://doi.org/10.7759/cureus.34533
283. Fossati C, Randelli FM, Sciancalepore F, Maglione D, Pasqualotto S, Ambrogi F, et al. Efficacy of intra-articular injection of combined platelet-rich-plasma (PRP) and hyaluronic acid (HA) in knee degenerative joint disease: A prospective, randomized, double-blind clinical trial. *Arch. Orthop. Trauma Surg.* Oct. 2024;144(11):5039–51. https://doi.org/10.1007/s00402-024-05603-z
284. Du D, Liang Y. A meta-analysis and systematic review of the clinical efficacy and safety of platelet-rich plasma combined with hyaluronic acid (PRP + HA) versus PRP monotherapy for knee osteoarthritis (KOA). *J. Orthop. Surg. Res.* Jan. 2025;20(1):57. https://doi.org/10.1186/s13018-024-05429-w
285. Lee H, Lim Y, Lee S-H. Rapid-acting pain relief in knee osteoarthritis: Autologous-cultured adipose-derived mesenchymal stem cells outperform stromal vascular fraction: A systematic review and meta-analysis. *Stem Cell*

Res. Ther. Nov. 2024;15(1):446. https://doi.org/10.1186/s13287-024-04034-2

286. Evans CH, Ghivizzani SC, Robbins PD. Osteoarthritis gene therapy in 2022. *Curr. Opin. Rheumatol.* Jan. 2023;35(1):37–43. https://doi.org/10.1097/BOR.0000000000000918
287. Li X, Shen L, Deng Z, Huang Z. New treatment for osteoarthritis: Gene therapy. *Precis. Clin. Med.* Jun. 2023;6(2). https://doi.org/10.1093/pcmedi/pbad014
288. Hollander JM, Goraltchouk A, Rawal M, Liu J, Luppino F, Zeng L, et al. Adeno-associated virus-delivered fibroblast growth factor 18 gene therapy promotes cartilage anabolism. *Cartilage.* Dec. 2023;14(4):492–505. https://doi.org/10.1177/19476035231158774
289. Micicoi G, Fairag R, Machado A, Douiri A, Bronsard N, Ernat J, et al. Anterior cruciate ligament reconstruction in patients older than 50 years: A descriptive study with minimum 10-year follow-up. *Orthop. J. Sport. Med.* Dec. 2024;12(12), https://doi.org/10.1177/23259671241292071
290. Saad Berreta R, Knapik DM, Lawand J, Moews L, Villarreal-Espinosa JB, Pallone L, et al. Anterior cruciate ligament reconstruction in patients aged 50 years and older results in improvements in activity and functional outcome measures, whereas reported complication rates vary widely: A systematic review. *Arthrosc. J. Arthrosc. Relat. Surg.* Jun. 2025;41(6):2146–62. https://doi.org/10.1016/j.arthro.2024.08.008
291. Killian ML, Cavinatto L, Galatz LM, Thomopoulos S. The role of mechanobiology in tendon healing. *J. Shoulder Elb. Surg.* Feb. 2012;21(2):228–37. https://doi.org/10.1016/j.jse.2011.11.002
292. Clayton RAE, Court-Brown CM. The epidemiology of musculoskeletal tendinous and ligamentous injuries. *Injury.* Dec. 2008;39(12):1338–44. https://doi.org/10.1016/j.injury.2008.06.021
293. Gillies H, Chalmers J. The management of fresh ruptures of the tendo achillis. *J. Bone Joint Surg. Am.* Mar. 1970;52(2):337–43. [Online]. http://www.ncbi.nlm.nih.gov/pubmed/5440011
294. Briggs-Price S, Mangwani J, Houchen-Wolloff L, Modha G, Fitzpatrick E, Faizi M, et al. Incidence, demographics, characteristics and management of acute Achilles tendon rupture: An epidemiological study. *PLoS One.* Jun. 2024;19(6):e0304197. https://doi.org/10.1371/journal.pone.0304197.
295. Huttunen TT, Kannus P, Rolf C, Felländer-Tsai L, Mattila VM. Acute achilles tendon ruptures. *Am. J. Sports Med.* Oct. 2014;42(10):2419–23. https://doi.org/10.1177/0363546514540599
296. Ganestam A, Kallemose T, Troelsen A, Barfod KW. Increasing incidence of acute Achilles tendon rupture and a noticeable decline in surgical treatment

from 1994 to 2013. A nationwide registry study of 33,160 patients. *Knee Surgery, Sport. Traumatol. Arthrosc.* Dec. 2016;24(12):3730–37. https://doi.org/10.1007/s00167-015-3544-5
297. Sheth U, Wasserstein D, Jenkinson R, Moineddin R, Kreder H, Jaglal SB. The epidemiology and trends in management of acute Achilles tendon ruptures in Ontario, Canada. *Bone Joint J.* Jan. 2017;99-B(1):78–86. https://doi.org/10.1302/0301-620X.99B1.BJJ-2016-0434.R1
298. Park S-H, Lee HS, Young KW, Seo SG. Treatment of acute achilles tendon rupture. *Clin. Orthop. Surg.* 2020;12(1):1. https://doi.org/10.4055/cios.2020.12.1.1
299. Yoon YK, Park JH, Han SH, Lee JW, Park KH. Obesity is an independent risk factor for achilles tendon rupture: A nationwide longitudinal cohort study in South Korea. *Foot Ankle Orthop.* Jan. 2022;7(1). https://doi.org/10.1177/2473011421S00509
300. Cramer A, Jacobsen NC, Hansen MS, Sandholdt H, Hölmich P, Barfod KW. Diabetes and treatment with orally administrated corticosteroids negatively affect treatment outcome at follow-up after acute Achilles tendon rupture. *Knee Surg. Sports Traumatol. Arthrosc.* 2021 May;29(5):1584–92. https://doi.org/10.1007/s00167-020-06371-0
301. Sankova MV, Beeraka NM, Oganesyan MV, Rizaeva NA, Sankov AV, Shelestova OS, et al. Recent developments in Achilles tendon risk-analyzing rupture factors for enhanced injury prevention and clinical guidance: Current implications of regenerative medicine. *J. Orthop. Transl.* Nov. 2024;49:289–307. https://doi.org/10.1016/j.jot.2024.08.024
302. Usman MA, Murtaza B, Winangun PAN, Kennedy D. Chronic rupture of achilles tendon caused by Haglund's deformity: A case report. *Medicina.* Sep. 2022;58(9):1216. https://doi.org/10.3390/medicina58091216
303. McCahon JAS, Miller M, Riebesell S, Pedowitz DI, Parekh SG, Daniel JN. Pickleball and the rising incidence of Achilles tendon injuries in the elderly. *Foot Ankle Spec.* Oct. 2024. https://doi.org/10.1177/19386400241286591
304. Sonohata M, Okamoto T, Uchihashi K, Motooka T, Tanaka H, Kitajima M, et al. Subcutaneous Achilles tendon rupture in an eighty-year-old female with an absence of risk factors. *Orthop. Rev.* Mar. 2010;2(1). https://doi.org/10.4081/or.2010.e11
305. Yang X, Meng H, Quan Q, Peng J, Lu S, Wang A. Management of acute Achilles tendon ruptures. *Bone Joint Res.* Oct. 2018;7(10):561–9. https://doi.org/10.1302/2046-3758.710.BJR-2018-0004.R2
306. Olsson N, Petzold M, Brorsson A, Karlsson J, Eriksson BI, Grävare Silbernagel K. Predictors of clinical outcome after acute Achilles tendon

ruptures. *Am. J. Sports Med.* Jun. 2014;42(6):1448–55. https://doi.org/10.1177/0363546514527409

307. Manero A, Crawford KE, Prock-Gibbs H, Shah N, Gandhi D, Coathup MJ. Improving disease prevention, diagnosis, and treatment using novel bionic technologies. *Bioeng. Transl. Med.* Jan. 2023;8(1):e10359. https://doi.org/10.1002/btm2.10359
308. Oeppen J, Vaupel JW. Broken limits to life expectancy. *Science* May 2002;296(5570):1029–31. https://doi.org/10.1126/science.1069675
309. Engberg H, Oksuzyan A, Jeune B, Vaupel JW, Christensen K. Centenarians — a useful model for healthy aging? A 29-year follow-up of hospitalizations among 40000 Danes born in 1905. *Aging Cell.* May 2009;8(3):270–6. https://doi.org/10.1111/j.1474-9726.2009.00474.x
310. Vaupel JW. Biodemography of human ageing. *Nature* Mar. 2010;464(7288): 536–42. https://doi.org/10.1038/nature08984
311. Chen Y, Zhou Y, Lin J, Zhang S. Challenges to improve bone healing under diabetic conditions. *Front. Endocrinol. (Lausanne).* Mar. 2022;13. https://doi.org/10.3389/fendo.2022.861878
312. Polanczyk CA, Marcantonio E, Goldman L, Rohde LEP, Orav J, Mangione CM, et al. Impact of age on perioperative complications and length of stay in patients undergoing noncardiac surgery. *Ann. Intern. Med.* Apr. 2001; 134(8):637–43. https://doi.org/10.7326/0003-4819-134-8-200104170-00008
313. Schipa C, Luca E, Ripa M, Sollazzi L, Aceto P. Preoperative evaluation of the elderly patient. *Saudi J. Anaesth.* Oct. 2023;17(4):482–90. https://doi.org/10.4103/sja.sja_613_23
314. Chow WB, Rosenthal RA, Merkow RP, Ko CY, Esnaola NF. Optimal preoperative assessment of the geriatric surgical patient: A best practices guideline from the American College of Surgeons National Surgical Quality Improvement Program and the American Geriatrics Society. *J. Am. Coll. Surg.* Oct. 2012;215(4):453–466. https://doi.org/10.1016/j.jamcollsurg.2012.06.017
315. Harari D, Hopper A, Dhesi J, Babic-Illman G, Lockwood L, Martin F. Proactive care of older people undergoing surgery ('POPS'): Designing, embedding, evaluating and funding a comprehensive geriatric assessment service for older elective surgical patients. *Age Ageing* Jan. 2007;36(2):190–6. https://doi.org/10.1093/ageing/afl163
316. Fried LP, Tangen CM, Walston J, Newman AB, Hirsch C, Gottdiener J, et al. Frailty in older adults: Evidence for a phenotype. *J. Gerontol. Ser. A Biol. Sci. Med. Sci.* Mar. 2001;56(3):M146–M157. https://doi.org/10.1093/gerona/56.3.M146

317. Bellamy JL, Runner RP, Vu CCL, Schenker ML, Bradbury TL, Roberson JR. Modified frailty index is an effective risk assessment tool in primary total hip arthroplasty. *J. Arthroplasty* Oct. 2017;32(10):2963–68. https://doi.org/10.1016/j.arth.2017.04.056
318. Bandeen-Roche K, Xue Q-L, Ferrucci L, Walston J, Guralnik JM, Chaves P, et al. Phenotype of frailty: Characterization in the Women's health and aging studies. *J. Gerontol. Ser. A Biol. Sci. Med. Sci.* Mar. 2006;61(3):262–6. https://doi.org/10.1093/gerona/61.3.262
319. Huisman MG, van Leeuwen BL, Ugolini G, Montroni I, Spiliotis J, Stabilini C, et al. 'Timed Up & Go': A screening tool for predicting 30-Day morbidity in onco-geriatric surgical patients? A multicenter cohort study. *PLoS One* Jan. 2014;9(1):e0086863. https://doi.org/10.1371/journal.pone.0086863
320. Hall AM, Scurrey SR, Pike AE, Albury C, Richmond HL, Matthews J, et al. Physician-reported barriers to using evidence-based recommendations for low back pain in clinical practice: A systematic review and synthesis of qualitative studies using the theoretical domains framework. *Implement. Sci.* Dec. 2019; 14(1):49. https://doi.org/10.1186/s13012-019-0884-4
321. Zadro J, O'Keeffe M, Maher. Do physical therapists follow evidence-based guidelines when managing musculoskeletal conditions? Systematic review. *BMJ Open* Oct. 2019;9(10):e032329. https://doi.org/10.1136/bmjopen-2019-032329
322. Suman A, Dikkers MF, Schaafsma FG, van Tulder MW, Anema JR. Effectiveness of multifaceted implementation strategies for the implementation of back and neck pain guidelines in health care: A systematic review. *Implement. Sci.* Dec. 2015;11(1):126. https://doi.org/10.1186/s13012-016-0482-7
323. Camp K, Hartos J, Atanda A. Use of clinical practice guidelines and quality metrics to assess primary care management of osteoporosis. *Gerontol. Geriatr. Med.* Jan. 2023;9. https://doi.org/10.1177/23337214231202152
324. Nguyen A, Lee P, Rodriguez EK, Chahal K, Freedman BR, Nazarian A. Addressing the growing burden of musculoskeletal diseases in the ageing US population: Challenges and innovations. *Lancet Heal. Longev.* May 2025;6(5):100707. https://doi.org/10.1016/j.lanhl.2025.100707
325. Cheng J-Z, Ni D, Chou Y-H, Qin J, Tiu C-M, Chang Y-C, et al. Computer-aided diagnosis with deep learning architecture: Applications to breast lesions in US images and pulmonary nodules in CT scans. *Sci. Rep.* Apr. 2016;6(1):24454. https://doi.org/10.1038/srep24454

326. Kooi T, Litjens G, van Ginneken B, Gubern-Mérida A, Sánchez CI, Mann R, et al. Large scale deep learning for computer aided detection of mammographic lesions. *Med. Image Anal.* Jan. 2017;35:303–12. https://doi.org/10.1016/j.media.2016.07.007
327. Yeung S, Rinaldo F, Jopling J, Liu B, Mehra R, Downing NL, et al. A computer vision system for deep learning-based detection of patient mobilization activities in the ICU. *npj Digit. Med.* Dec. 2019;2(1):11. https://doi.org/10.1038/s41746-019-0087-z
328. Tran D, Bourdev L, Fergus R, Torresani L, Paluri M. Learning spatiotemporal features with 3D convolutional networks. In: *2015 IEEE International Conference on Computer Vision (ICCV)*, Dec. 2015, pp. 4489–97. https://doi.org/10.1109/ICCV.2015.510
329. Katz S, Downs TD, Cash HR, Grotz RC. Progress in development of the index of ADL. *Gerontologist* Mar. 1970;10(1) Part 1:20–30. https://doi.org/10.1093/geront/10.1_Part_1.20
330. Ho A. Are we ready for artificial intelligence health monitoring in elder care? *BMC Geriatr.* Dec. 2020;20(1):358. https://doi.org/10.1186/s12877-020-01764-9
331. Kaye JA, Maxwell SA, Mattek N, Hayes TL, Dodge H, Pavel M, et al. Intelligent systems for assessing aging changes: Home-based, unobtrusive, and continuous assessment of aging. *J. Gerontol. Ser. B Psychol. Sci. Soc. Sci.* July 2011;66B(Supplement 1):i180–i190. https://doi.org/10.1093/geronb/gbq095
332. McMurray J, Strudwick G, Forchuk C, Morse A, Lachance J, Baskaran A, et al. The importance of trust in the adoption and use of intelligent assistive technology by older adults to support aging in place: Scoping review protocol. *JMIR Res. Protoc.* Nov. 2017;6(11):e218. https://doi.org/10.2196/resprot.8772
333. Bennett MJ, Center JR, Perry L. Primary care follow-up of patients after attending a fracture liaison service: An integrative review. *Arch. Osteoporos.* May 2025;20(1):65. https://doi.org/10.1007/s11657-025-01521-8
334. Barton DW, Griffin DC, Carmouche JJ. Orthopedic surgeons' views on the osteoporosis care gap and potential solutions: Survey results. *J. Orthop. Surg. Res.* Dec. 2019;14(1):72. https://doi.org/10.1186/s13018-019-1103-3
335. Bauer DC. Osteoporosis treatment after hip fracture. *JAMA Netw. Open.* July 2018;1(3):e180844. https://doi.org/10.1001/jamanetworkopen.2018.0844
336. Schwartzman JD, McCall M, Ghattas Y, Pugazhendhi AS, Wei F, Ngo C, *et al.* Multifunctional scaffolds for bone repair following age-related

biological decline: Promising prospects for smart biomaterial-driven technologies. *Biomaterials* Dec. 2024;311:122683. https://doi.org/10.1016/j.biomaterials.2024.122683
337. Jain NB, Schneider BJ, Murrell WB, Hettrich CM, Archer KR. What's new in orthopaedic rehabilitation. *J. Bone Jt. Surg.* Nov. 2018;100(22):1993–99. https://doi.org/10.2106/JBJS.18.00828
338. Phillips TD, Shoemaker MJ. Early access to physical therapy and specialty care management for American workers with musculoskeletal injuries. *J. Occup. Environ. Med.* Apr. 2017;59(4):402–11. https://doi.org/10.1097/JOM.0000000000000969
339. You DZ, Leighton JL, Schneider PS. Current concepts in rehabilitation protocols to optimize patient function following musculoskeletal trauma. *Injury* May 2020;51:S5–S9. https://doi.org/10.1016/j.injury.2020.03.047
340. Huntjens KM, van Geel T, van den Bergh JPW, van Helden S, Willems P, Winkens B, et al. Fracture liaison service: Impact on subsequent nonvertebral fracture incidence and mortality. *J. Bone Jt. Surg.* Feb. 2014;96(4):e29. https://doi.org/10.2106/JBJS.L.00223
341. Huntjens KMB, van Geel TCM, Geusens PP, Winkens B, Willems P, van den Bergh J, et al. Impact of guideline implementation by a fracture nurse on subsequent fractures and mortality in patients presenting with nonvertebral fractures. *Injury* Sept. 2011;42:S39–S43. https://doi.org/10.1016/S0020-1383(11)70011-0
342. Nakayama A, Major G, Holliday E, Attia J, Bogduk N. Evidence of effectiveness of a fracture liaison service to reduce the re-fracture rate. *Osteoporos. Int.* Mar. 2016;27(3):873–9. https://doi.org/10.1007/s00198-015-3443-0
343. Malafarina V, Reginster J-Y, Cabrerizo S, Bruyère O, Kanis JA, Martinez A, et al. Nutritional status and nutritional treatment are related to outcomes and mortality in older adults with hip fracture. *Nutrients* Apr. 2018;10(5):555. https://doi.org/10.3390/nu10050555
344. Chiavarini M, Ricciotti GM, Genga A, Faggi MI, Rinaldi A, Toscano OD, et al. Malnutrition-related health outcomes in older adults with hip fractures: A systematic review and meta-analysis. *Nutrients* Apr. 2024;16(7):1069. https://doi.org/10.3390/nu16071069
345. Lai W-Y, Chiu Y-C, Lu K-C, Huang I-T, Tsai P-S, Huang C-J. Beneficial effects of preoperative oral nutrition supplements on postoperative outcomes in geriatric hip fracture patients. *Medicine (Baltimore).* Nov. 2021;100(47):e27755. https://doi.org/10.1097/MD.0000000000027755

346. Arkley J, Dixon J, Wilson F, Charlton K, Ollivere BJ, Eardley W. Assessment of nutrition and supplementation in patients with hip fractures. *Geriatr. Orthop. Surg. Rehabil.* Jan. 2019;10. https://doi.org/10.1177/2151459319879804
347. Tappenden KA, Quatrara B, Parkhurst ML, Malone AM, Fanjiang G, Ziegler TR. Critical role of nutrition in improving quality of care: An interdisciplinary call to action to address adult hospital malnutrition. *J. Acad. Nutr. Diet.* Sep. 2013;113(9):1219–37. https://doi.org/10.1016/j.jand.2013.05.015
348. Bell JJ, Mitchell RJ, Harris IA, Seymour H, Armstrong E, Harris R, et al. Oral nutritional supplementation in older adults with a hip fracture — findings from a Bi-National clinical audit. *Healthcare* Oct. 2024;12(21):2157. https://doi.org/10.3390/healthcare12212157
349. Foley DJ, Monjan AA, Brown SL, Simonsick EM, Wallace RB, Blazer DG. Sleep complaints among elderly persons: An epidemiologic study of three communities. *Sleep* Aug. 1995;18(6):425–32. https://doi.org/10.1093/sleep/18.6.425
350. Buchmann N, Spira D, Norman K, Demuth I, Eckardt R, Steinhagen-Thiessen E. Sleep, muscle mass and muscle function in older people: A cross-sectional analysis based on data from the Berlin aging study II (BASE-II). *Dtsch. Arztebl. Int.* Apr. 2016. https://doi.org/10.3238/arztebl.2016.0253
351. Chun MY, Cho B-J, Yoo SH, Oh B, Kang J-S, Yeon C. Association between sleep duration and musculoskeletal pain. *Medicine (Baltimore).* Dec. 2018;97(50):e13656. https://doi.org/10.1097/MD.0000000000013656
352. Gil T-H, Zheng H, Lee HG, Shin J-W, Hwang SW, Jang K-M, et al. Senolytic drugs relieve pain by reducing peripheral nociceptive signaling without modifying joint tissue damage in spontaneous osteoarthritis. *Aging (Albany. NY).* Aug. 2022;14(15):6006–27. https://doi.org/10.18632/aging.204204
353. Obana KK, Schallmo MS, Hong IS, Ahmad CS, Moorman CT, Trofa DP, et al. Current trends in orthobiologics: An 11-Year review of the orthopaedic literature. *Am. J. Sports Med.* Sep. 2022;50(11):3121–29. https://doi.org/10.1177/03635465211037343
354. Garza JR, Campbell RE, Tjoumakaris FP, Freedman KB, Miller LS, Santa Maria D, et al. Clinical efficacy of intra-articular mesenchymal stromal cells for the treatment of Knee osteoarthritis: A double-blinded prospective

randomized controlled clinical trial. *Am. J. Sports Med.* Mar. 2020;48(3):588–98. https://doi.org/10.1177/0363546519899923
355. Overstreet DS, Strath LJ, Jordan M, Jordan IA, Hobson JM, Owens MA, et al. A brief overview: Sex differences in prevalent chronic musculoskeletal conditions. *Int. J. Environ. Res. Public Health* Mar. 2023;20(5):4521. https://doi.org/10.3390/ijerph20054521
356. Tosi LL, Templeton K, Pennington AM, Reid KA, Boyan BD. Influence of sex and gender on musculoskeletal conditions and how they are reported. *J. Bone Jt. Surg.* Aug. 2024;106(16):1512–19. https://doi.org/10.2106/JBJS.24.00194
357. Hart DA. Sex differences in musculoskeletal injury and disease risks across the lifespan: Are there unique subsets of females at higher risk than males for these conditions at distinct stages of the life cycle? *Front. Physiol.* Apr. 2023;14. https://doi.org/10.3389/fphys.2023.1127689
358. Bala A, Chona D, Amanatullah DF, Hu SS, Wood KB, Alamin TF, et al. Timing of lumbar spinal fusion affects total hip arthroplasty outcomes. *JAAOS Glob. Res. Rev.* Nov. 2019;3(11):e00133. https://doi.org/10.5435/JAAOSGlobal-D-19-00133
359. Manero A, Rivera V, Fu Q, Schwartzman JD, Prock-Gibbs H, Shah N, et al. Emerging medical technologies and their use in bionic repair and human augmentation. *Bioengineering* July 2024;11(7):695. https://doi.org/10.3390/bioengineering11070695
360. Nairn B, Tsakanikas V, Gordon B, Karapintzou E, Kaski D, Fotiadis DI, et al. Smart wearable technologies for balance rehabilitation in older adults at risk of falls: Scoping review and comparative analysis. *JMIR Rehabil. Assist. Technol.* May 2025;12:e69589–e69589. https://doi.org/10.2196/69589
361. Jones CH, Dolsten M. Healthcare on the brink: Navigating the challenges of an aging society in the United States. *npj Aging* Apr. 2024;10(1):22. https://doi.org/10.1038/s41514-024-00148-2
362. Yi Y, Lee Y, Kang S, Kwon YH, Seo YM, Baek JY, et al. Unmet needs and barriers in providing hospital care for older adults: A qualitative study using the age-friendly health system framework. *Clin. Interv. Aging* Aug. 2023;18:1321–32. https://doi.org/10.2147/CIA.S409348
363. Mate K, Fulmer T, Pelton L, Berman A, Bonner A, Huang W, et al. Evidence for the 4Ms: Interactions and outcomes across the care continuum. *J. Aging Health* Aug. 2021;33(7–8):469–81. https://doi.org/10.1177/0898264321991658

364. Lee Y, Liew Y, Sim MH, Sim XLJ. Association of polypharmacy and perioperative outcomes: Systematic review and meta-analysis. *J. Perioper. Pract.* Feb. 2025. https://doi.org/10.1177/17504589251320818
365. Nanji KC, Patel A, Shaikh S, Seger DL, Bates DW. Evaluation of perioperative medication errors and adverse drug events. *Anesthesiology* Jan. 2016;124(1):25–34. https://doi.org/10.1097/ALN.0000000000000904
366. Deeken F, Sánchez A, Rapp MA, Denkinger M, Brefka S, Spank J, et al. Outcomes of a delirium prevention program in older persons after elective surgery. *JAMA Surg.* Feb. 2022;157(2):e216370. https://doi.org/10.1001/jamasurg.2021.6370
367. Nieto-García L, Carpio-Pérez A, Moreiro-Barroso MT, Alonso-Sardón M. Can an early mobilisation programme prevent hospital-acquired pressure injures in an intensive care unit?: A systematic review and meta-analysis. *Int. Wound J.* Apr. 2021;18(2):209–20. https://doi.org/10.1111/iwj.13516
368. Huang J, Shi Z, Duan F-F, Fan M-X, Yan S, Wei Y, et al. Benefits of early ambulation in elderly patients undergoing lumbar decompression and fusion surgery: A prospective cohort study. *Orthop. Surg.* June 2021;13(4):1319–26. https://doi.org/10.1111/os.12953
369. Van Heghe A, Mordant G, Dupont J, Dejaeger M, Laurent MR, Gielen E. Effects of orthogeriatric care models on outcomes of hip fracture patients: A systematic review and meta-analysis. *Calcif. Tissue Int.* Feb. 2022;110(2):162–84. https://doi.org/10.1007/s00223-021-00913-5
370. Jain RK, Polley E, Weiner M, Iwamaye A, Huang E, Vokes T. An electronic health record (EHR)-based risk calculator can predict fractures comparably to FRAX: A proof-of-concept study. *Osteoporos. Int.* Dec. 2024;35(12):2117–26. https://doi.org/10.1007/s00198-024-07221-2
371. Solomon DH, Patrick AR, Schousboe J, Losina E. The potential economic benefits of improved postfracture care: A cost-effectiveness analysis of a fracture liaison service in the US Health-care system. *J. Bone Miner. Res.* July 2014;29(7):1667–74. https://doi.org/10.1002/jbmr.2180

https://doi.org/10.1142/9789819819645_0003

Chapter 3

Molecular Approaches to Bone Repair and Regeneration

Peter Zeblisky[1], Yasmine Ghattas[1], Kyle Smola[1], Kailee Hernandez[1], Matthew Crowley[1], David Rallison[1], Becky Perron[1], Shane Burke[1,2], Thomas J. Kean[1,2], Mehdi Razavi[1,2,*]

[1]*College of Medicine, University of Central Florida, FL 32827, United States*
[2]*Biionix Cluster, Department of Medicine, University of Central Florida College of Medicine, FL 32827, United States*

Chapter Outline

---

* **Corresponding author:** Mehdi Razavi, 6900 Lake Nona Blvd Orlando, FL 32827. Email: Mehdi.Razavi@ucf.edu

Abstract

Bone possesses a remarkable intrinsic capacity for regeneration; however, critical-size defects resulting from trauma, infection, or surgical resection often exceed this capacity and require clinical intervention. Autologous bone grafting remains the gold standard for such cases due to its osteogenic, osteoinductive, and osteoconductive properties, but it is limited by donor site morbidity and graft availability. This chapter explores the molecular and cellular mechanisms underlying bone repair and regeneration, providing a foundation for understanding emerging therapeutic strategies. We examine the sequential phases of fracture healing ranging from inflammation to remodeling and highlight the roles of key signaling molecules, including bone morphogenic proteins (BMPs), fibroblast growth factors (FGFs), platelet-derived growth factor (PDGF), vascular endothelial growth factor (VEGF), and calcium. This chapter further discusses systemic modulators such as parathyroid hormone, estrogen, and growth hormone, as well as the application of progenitor cells derived from bone marrow, adipose tissue, and periosteum. We delve into genetic and ribonucleic acid (RNA)-based therapies, including viral and nonviral gene delivery systems, gene-activated matrices, and interfering RNA (RNAi) technologies, assessing their potential to enhance bone regeneration. Together, these molecular approaches represent a promising frontier in regenerative medicine, aiming to overcome the limitations of current clinical practices and improve outcomes in bone repair.

1. Introduction

Bones intrinsically have the capacity to heal themselves in response to injury. In the clinical setting, bones mostly do not commonly require exogenous stimulation of regeneration following fracture. The vast majority (90%) of fractures heal normally through a coordinated biological process [1]. Endochondral fracture healing can be grouped into four sequential steps: inflammation, cartilage formation, ossification, and remodeling. In certain cases, bone injuries due to trauma, infection, skeletal abnormalities, or tumor resection can impair this healing process, resulting in nonunion or delayed union. In extreme cases, fractures may even exceed a critical size, defined as those bone defects that will not autonomically heal during a patient's lifetime [2]. This chapter explores the molecular mechanisms of fracture healing as a foundation for understanding therapeutic approaches aimed at enhancing bone repair.

The current gold standard for healing critical-size bone defects is autologous bone grafting. This method involves harvesting bone graft from, for example, the iliac crest of the pelvis of the patient and transplanting it to the site of injury. These grafts are so successful due to their three key attributes. They are osteogenic, meaning they contain living cells that can differentiate into osteoblasts. They are osteoinductive, meaning they can stimulate other cells to differentiate into osteoblasts. Finally, they are osteoconductive, meaning they can act as scaffolds to allow new bone material to grow along their surfaces [3]. Although the current clinical approach has shown efficacy, autografting does not come without disadvantages. This is limited by the amount of bone that can be harvested. There are also various complications to the procedure including donor site morbidity, chronic pain, and infection [4, 5]. Given these limitations, scientists have considered other possible treatments. One alternative is using an allograft or cadaveric bone. While allografts eliminate the need for a second surgical site and are more readily available, they often lack the osteogenic potential of autografts, as the bone has been sterilized, killing the cells. These shortcomings have prompted researchers to develop novel approaches to improve bone repair and regenerative processes. Before diving into the details of these approaches, it is necessary to understand the physiologic processes that underlie innate bone repair. Through analysis of this process, we can begin to pinpoint various genes, peptides, cytokines, and other bioactive molecules for therapeutic intervention.

Self-regeneration is a multifaceted and highly regulated process, which is analogous to embryonic skeletal development. Two mechanisms of bone development exist. The first major mechanism is intramembranous ossification, which induces mesenchymal stem cells (MSCs) to undergo differentiation into osteoblasts. Osteoblasts play an integral role in bone formation by inducing extracellular matrix mineralization and regulating bone remodeling [6]. These cells release several bioactive molecules into the environment, which include (1) type I collagen, which is the major component of organic extracellular bone matrix; (2) osteocalcin and osteopontin (OPN), which are highly incorporated into hydroxyapatite and regulate bone mineralization, respectively; and (3) bone sialoprotein, which promotes hydroxyapatite crystal nucleation and osteoblast differentiation [7, 8]. The second major mechanism is endochondral ossification. This pathway is marked by a highly regulated coordination of chondrocyte differentiation, hypertrophy, and apoptosis, which ultimately results in the formation of trabecular or cortical bone [9, 10]. This is the dominant mechanism underlying typical bone healing [11], and the details regarding components of this pathway are discussed below. Bone repair can be broken down into four major phases: inflammation, soft callus formation, hard callus formation, and remodeling. A summary of this process is outlined in **Figure 1**.

2. Inflammation in Bone Repair and Regeneration

Fracture is associated with disruption to the local bone tissue matrix and the vascular network. As bleeding continues, it is contained by the surrounding tissue and forms a hematoma. The degranulation of platelets, macrophages, and several other inflammatory cells (granulocytes, monocytes, and lymphocytes) works to ward off infection, secrete several bioactive molecules to induce a specialized tissue environment, and transform a platelet plug into a fibrin-laden thrombus [13]. Over the course of the next few days, angiogenesis promotes neovascularization of the injured tissue, osteoblasts deposit type I collagen (granulation tissue), and cellular debris is constantly cleared by phagocytic cells [14]. This cellular response is orchestrated by several cytokines and growth factors (GFs) such as bone morphogenic proteins (BMPs), vascular endothelial growth factor (VEGF), platelet-derived growth factor (PDGF), fibroblast growth factors (FGFs), transforming growth factor-β (TGF-β), stromal-derived factor-1alpha

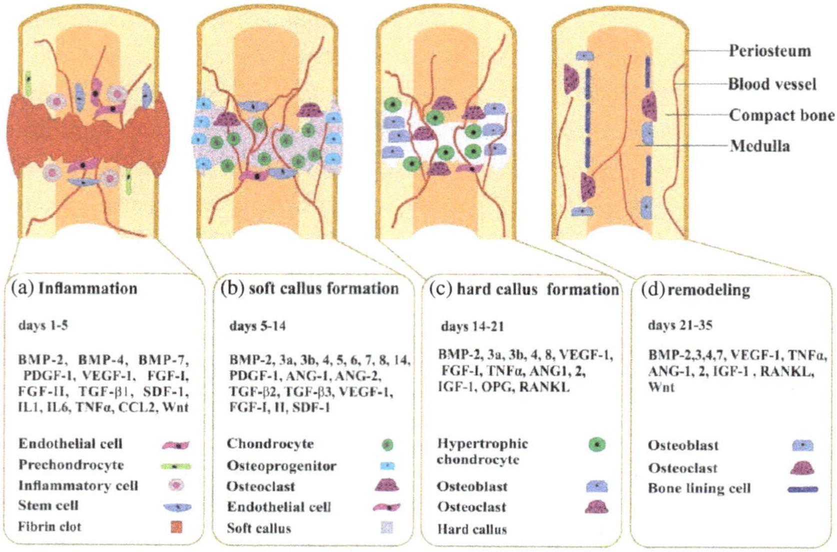

Figure 1. Four stages of bone repair with their respective bioactive molecular and cellular profiles.

Reproduced from Safari *et al.* [12].

(SDF-1α), tumor necrosis factor-alpha (TNF-α), interleukins (ILs), and macrophage colony-stimulating factor (M-CSF) [15, 16]. These factors drive the differentiation of MSCs into osteoblasts, promote inflammatory cell infiltrates, and vascularize the injured tissues.

2.1. *Soft Callus Formation*

This stage is marked by a coordinated effort between chondrocytes and fibroblasts to produce a relatively durable soft callus. Subsequently, this functions as a scaffold to provide mechanical support to the injured area and is a template for bony callus formation. When a fracture occurs, blood fills the wound, and fibrin is formed from fibrinogen through the coagulation cascade. Fibroblasts infiltrate the clot and deposit collagen to stabilize it. Chondrocytes, derived from MSCs, synthesize a cartilaginous matrix that replaces the fibrous granulation tissue. These discrete cartilage and fibrin-rich regions coalesce to become a central fibrocartilaginous plug, thereby splinting the fracture [17]. As this plug is being established, chondrocytes undergo hypertrophy and mineralize the cartilaginous matrix to improve its integrity before undergoing apoptosis. There is increasing evidence that some chondrocytes transdifferentiate into osteoblasts [18]. Fibroblast and chondrocyte proliferation and differentiation are induced through an integrated expression of GFs such as TGF-β2 and TGF-β3, PDGF, FGF-1, and insulin-like growth factor (IGF) [11, 16]. BMPs (2, 4, 5, and 6) mainly drive the maturation of chondrocytes. This allows them to generate high quantities of collagen type II and subsequently type X once they have hypertrophied [19]. Concomitantly, VEGF, angiopoietin I, and angiopoietin II alter vascular morphology, creating larger caliber vessels, capillary ingrowth, and collaterals from existing vessels [20, 21]. These systems are under regulation by CBFA1/runt-related transcription factor 2 (RUNX2), the master bone and cartilage regulatory factor [22]. The expression of this master regulatory factor explains why we see more angiogenesis in the soft callus phase when compared to the inflammatory phase, despite both phases containing VEGF [23].

2.2. *Hard Callus Formation*

This stage is characterized by the formation of a highly mineralized bone matrix due to very high levels of osteoblast activity. The deposition of this mineralized matrix begins in stable areas at the periphery of the soft callus and proceeds toward the center. As soft callus turns over and is replaced by hard callus, there is a concomitant revascularization. The hard callus is similar to healthy bone, with it exhibiting high mechanical strength; however, its matrix is irregular and must undergo remodeling before it is considered a complete restoration of tissue. Two factors are critical for successful hard callus synthesis: the BMP family and the angiogenic family (CBFA1/RUNX2 and VEGF). The BMP family has been directly implicated in driving osteoblast activity and differentiation to create a proteinaceous and mineralized extracellular matrix. In fact, studies have shown that BMPs can induce *de novo* bone formation [24, 25]. Proper vascularization is integral because high oxygen tension within the local environment is necessary for osteoblast differentiation. Healing model systems with increased angiogenic factors showed augmented bone formation and fracture healing [26, 27].

2.3. *Regeneration*

The final stage of bone repair is characterized by high activity of osteoclasts. Osteoclasts originate from hematopoietic stem cells *via* the monocyte/macrophage lineage, sharing a common progenitor with macrophages. They function to resorb bone and remodel the grossly formed hard callus into the original shape of the previously healthy tissue. To execute resorption, osteoclasts first polarize on the bone surface and form a ruffled membrane [28]. The electrogenic proton pump of the osteoclast causes acidification of the microenvironment, which mobilizes the mineral phase of bone and establishes desirable conditions for organic matrix degradation [29]. Two major cytokines are secreted by osteoblasts: M-CSF and receptor activator of nuclear factor κ B (NFκB) ligand (RANKL), which are imperative to induction, differentiation, competency, and survival of osteoclasts. M-CSF is responsible for the initial induction of hematopoietic stem cell differentiation into the osteoclast lineage [30]. RANKL is produced by mature osteoblasts, which binds to macrophages and pre-osteoclasts, directing their transformation into osteoclasts, enabling their ability to resorb bone, and coordinating the appropriate amount of bone formation and resorption, thus proper bone formation within the microenvironment [31]. Another important factor that antagonizes RANKL is osteoprotegerin (OPG), which is also expressed on osteoblasts and competes with RANKL for binding to the receptor, RANK [32]. This regulates the amount of bone resorption, where aberrations in the balance can manifest in joint destruction such as in rheumatoid arthritis [33, 34].

3. Local Enhancement of Bone Repair and Regeneration

3.1. *Bone Morphogenic Proteins and Transforming Growth Factor-β*

BMPs are peptide ligands considered to be part of the TGF-β superfamily. Their signaling effects are enacted through both type I and type II serine-threonine kinase receptors, which activate downstream signaling cascades mediated by both SMAD-dependent and SMAD-independent pathways [35]. Initially discovered in bone extracts, these molecules have been found to be involved in the development and maintenance of organs, including bone, muscle, kidney, and blood vessels. The functions of BMPs and TGF-β are complex, although they have been linked to a vital role in recruiting progenitor cells from the bone marrow, periosteum, and cortical bone [36–41]. During the bone healing process, BMPs and TGF-β are secreted by M2 phenotype macrophages that localized to the fracture site. Alongside other influential GFs such as FGF, PDGF, and IGF, they induce proliferation and subsequently cellular differentiation of MSCs into osteoblasts and, ultimately, the formation of mature bone. This makes them essential during both skeletogenesis and fracture healing, as demonstrated by experiments in which BMP-knockout model organisms were unable to properly form bone [42].

BMP-2 and BMP-7 have been the focus of much research over the past few decades [11, 43]. Some data suggest that BMPs selectively target periosteal stem cell differentiation [44]. Supporting this, Yun *et al.* demonstrated that BMP-2-stimulated periosteal cells promote both chondrogenesis and osteogenesis, and in the marrow space, cells underwent only osteogenesis in response to BMP-2 [41]. Upon histological evaluation, recombinant BMP-7 elicited solely an anabolic impact, facilitating cortical bone repair [45]. While the general contribution of these molecules to bone formation is clearly established, their specific role and the defined pathways through which they enact their effects remain elusive.

Clinical applications of BMPs have been explored, although their efficacy and safety remain controversial. Autografts, considered the gold standard bone grafting material, commonly include BMPs and TGF-β delivered as a mixture of osteoinductive factors [46, 47]. These molecules can be injected or loaded onto a resorbable scaffold including in a patient's own autograft, allowing for their release into the tissue either by diffusion or as the scaffold degrades during the healing process [48–50]. The Food and Drug Administration (FDA) has approved their use in products, such as the INFUSE® collagen sponge (containing BMP-2) and the OP-1® Implant (containing BMP-7). While theoretically sensible, the science confirming the efficacy of BMP and TGF-β has been lacking. BMP-7, for example, was safely used within autografts but was unable to significantly decrease measures, such as pain at the fracture site or radiographical indications of treatment success [51]. BMP-2 was initially thought to lower the risk of secondary interventions in patients with fractures compared to the current standard of care, the intramedullary nail. This included decreased failures of the nail, fewer infections, and faster wound healing [52]. However, deeper analysis failed to unveil significant differences between either treatment modality [53, 54]. Similarly, open tibial fractures were not found to have accelerated healing when the collagen sponge technique was used [55]. Initial laboratory experiments in mouse models showed accelerated repair at the fracture site, but these results have been difficult to replicate outside of the laboratory setting [52].

There are concerns that the use of BMPs may lead to a variety of adverse effects, including heterotopic bone formation, immunologic responses, pseudoarthritis, and increased cancer risk. These seem to be especially true regarding the supraphysiologic doses administered under the current methods of implementation seen today [56–58]. Studies aimed at optimizing the use of BMPs have been published where various biomaterials and loading strategies allowing for the delivery of BMPs were tried. Several strategies have emerged as particularly effective in enhancing both the efficacy and safety of GF delivery systems. For instance, incorporating biomaterials such as heparin, which exhibits high affinity for many cationic GFs, has been shown to stabilize bioactivity and enable sustained release. Advanced delivery architectures, including core–shell microcapsules and nanoparticles-in-scaffolds, allow for controlled, sequential, or on-demand release, more closely mimicking physiological healing processes. In addition, stimuli-responsive systems (e.g., ultrasound- or enzyme-triggered hydrogels) and dual/multi-GF delivery approaches have demonstrated synergistic effects in complex tissue regeneration, offering precise spatiotemporal control and minimizing adverse effects associated with bolus administration [59]. While the potential for BMPs to improve patient outcomes seems evident based on their clearly observed ability to increase bone formation, the success of this research will be necessary to develop clinically useful techniques that can limit the negative effects that have been observed.

3.2. *Fibroblast Growth Factor*

FGF is a protein GF involved in cellular proliferation, migration, differentiation, and survival [41]. FGF acts through tyrosine kinase receptors, influencing the predominant RAS/mitogen-activated protein kinase (MAPK) pathway, the phosphatidylinositol 3-kinase (PI3K)/protein kinase B (AKT) pathway, and the phospholipase C gamma (PLCγ) pathway. The FGF signaling pathway contributes to numerous cellular processes, including angiogenesis, wound healing, and bone formation.

In bone formation, FGF characteristically plays a role in the proliferation of progenitor cells necessary for bone tissue formation and fracture repair [37, 38, 40, 41]. It is secreted by macrophages and fibroblasts at the fracture site in response to damaged blood vessels [42, 60]. FGF is one of the multiple locally secreted mediators capable of recruiting MSCs, which, upon stimulation, proliferate and differentiate into osteoblasts [38, 61, 62]. This process contributes to both intramembranous and endochondral ossification. FGF's stimulatory effect on osteoblast differentiation and inhibitory effect on osteocyte differentiation suggest that the effects of FGF are likely stage-specific [63]. Its effects may also be receptor-specific, an important example is the FGFR3 receptor, which regulates bone density and cortical thickness in differentiated osteoblasts in response to FGF stimulation [64]. FGF is commonly present within autografts. FGF incorporation within gelatin hydrogel/autograft improved fracture union rates in patients with tibial shaft fractures in a clinical trial [65]. Basic FGF also acts as a mitogen for MSCs, causing a higher incorporation of osteocytes into healing bone [66].

Currently, new scaffolding designs are being developed to maximize the delivery and effectiveness of biomolecules such as FGF in autografting. A major challenge in the therapeutic use of GFs, including FGF, is their inherent poor stability, short half-life, and rapid clearance. While various delivery systems, such as slow-release formulations, have been developed to mitigate these issues, fully overcoming them remains an active area of research. Advancements in scaffolding materials, loading strategies, and patient-specific dosing may help overcome these challenges, making them an important focus of current and future studies.

3.3. *Platelet-Derived Growth Factor*

PDGF exists as a dimeric glycoprotein with a vital function in cellular growth and division. Its structure is slightly variable, containing two subunits in combinations of either two alpha (PDGF-$\alpha\alpha$), two beta (PDGF-$\beta\beta$), or one alpha and one beta configurations (PDGF-$\alpha\beta$). PDGF is recognized as a potent mitogen for cells derived from the mesenchymal lineage, including fibroblasts and smooth muscle cells [67, 68]. PDGF, acting on PDGF receptor tyrosine kinases, stimulates the homing and proliferation of cells, including MSCs, and promotes angiogenesis at the wound site [69]. Its activity may be mediated downstream by the PI3K transduction pathway [70].

In bone, PDGF has been shown to activate MSCs to allow for differentiation into osteoblasts. Supporting this, MSC cultures depleted of PDGF tend to have fewer MSCs, although lack of PDGF did not prevent existing cells from undergoing differentiation [71]. Recombinant PDGF is commonly found as an osteoinductive factor within repairing bone [36–41]. This has been translated into a therapeutic, recombinant human PDGF-$\beta\beta$ (rhPDGF-$\beta\beta$) combined with β-tricalcium phosphate (TCP), forming AUGMENT® bone graft, which is used in clinical orthopedic applications [72]. It was shown that PDGF enhances the population of bone marrow MSCs and plays a role in the chemotaxis and activation of macrophages at the fracture site [73]. Clinical trials using rhPDGF-$\beta\beta$ combined with β-TCP (Augment® bone graft) in a hindfoot and ankle arthrodesis have demonstrated comparable fusion rates to autograft, with the added benefit of avoiding donor site morbidity [74]. PDGF in solution can be loaded onto a scaffold that provides a structure for new bone formation. Current research, as with most osteoinductive factors, is aimed at optimizing the use of PDGF to achieve significant improvements in patient outcomes in the clinical setting.

3.4. *Vascular Endothelial Growth Factor*

VEGF is an angiogenic GF considered essential for the growth and proliferation of vascular endothelial cells. It is produced by a variety of cells, including macrophages, platelets, keratinocytes, renal mesangial cells, and many tumor cells [75–80]. Although primarily known for its role in angiogenesis, VEGF also contributes to bone formation, hematopoiesis, wound healing, and general cellular development [81–84]. Vascularization is a key step in the development and formation of new bone. It creates the vessels necessary for the delivery of nutrients, GFs, and MSCs involved in the regenerative process [85]. The specific role of VEGF in fracture healing is multifaceted. VEGF's initial role in bone healing is at the site of the hematoma. In fact, VEGF concentrations within the hematoma have been reported to be up to 15-fold higher than in plasma [86]. The release of VEGF by osteoblastic cells stimulates vascular permeability and new vessel growth in the early stages of healing. TNF-α and IL-1β do not directly promote revascularization but stimulate endothelial activation and indirectly support angiogenesis by upregulating VEGF and other factors. TGF-β1 is released later in the inflammatory phase and helps transition from the proliferative to reparative phases [36, 87, 88]. As healing progresses, VEGF stimulates blood vessels and osteoclasts in the fracture site to initiate skeletal revascularization [89, 90]. Stem cells differentiate into either osteoblasts or chondrocytes and begin forming bone and cartilage, respectively. The consistent, elevated levels of VEGF at this stage induce angiogenesis, which facilitates the recruitment of osteoclast precursors. Thus, the soft bony callus is converted to a hard bony callus during endochondral ossification.

Experiments in which the VEGF gene was knocked out were shown to prevent bone formation, displaying the necessity of this GF in bone tissue development [91]. At this time, the clinical use of VEGF has remained limited to its native presence in autografts and as part of the scaffold matrices that deliver osteoinductive molecules to fracture sites. VEGF has not been found to significantly impact the clinical outcome of patients who receive VEGF as part of their treatment, and the inclusion of VEGF in autografts has been justified mainly by its known role in the healing process [92]. Moving forward, it will be important to evaluate whether VEGF is being translated into clinically meaningful applications in bone regenerative medicine — specifically, those that demonstrate tangible improvements in patient outcomes beyond theoretical or preclinical promise.

3.5. *Mitogen-Activated Protein Kinase Signaling*

During cell proliferation, differentiation, migration, and death, the regulatory MAPK-extracellular signal-regulated kinase (ERK) pathway serves as a key interface between the cell surface and nucleus [93]. Its specific role in bone formation has been unclear, as some studies have suggested a stimulatory role, while others found its effects to be inhibitory [94, 95]. As part of a complex cellular signaling cascade, it is unsurprising that the exact effects of MAPK signaling are variable and difficult to distinguish. The MAPK pathway does appear to be an obligatory transducer for bone healing, as it helps in the transduction of signals from multiple GFs, including FGF, EGF, IGF, and the bioactive compound calcium phosphate [96, 97]. Experiments inhibiting elements of the MAPK pathway revealed an inability of these GFs to enact their effects on regenerating bone [98]. As of now (2025), only the link between the MAPK pathway and various osteoinductive factors has been established. Currently, no bone regeneration treatment strategies directly targeting the MAPK pathway are implemented in the clinical setting.

The involvement of the MAPK pathway in mediating the effects of promising osteoinductive molecules has made it apparent that further characterization of this pathway will be a necessary step in refining their use in bone regenerative medicine. Determining the relationship between the MAPK pathway and specific biomolecules may help improve the clinical applications of these molecules as the field progresses. Treatments that augment the response of the MAPK signaling cascade to a variety of GFs may enhance the effect of these biomolecules to increase their efficacy.

3.6. *Calcium*

Calcium, as a nutrient, is commonly associated with bone formation, as nearly 99% of the body's calcium stores reside in bone in the form of calcium hydroxyapatite ($Ca_{10}[PO_4]6[OH]_2$). The total calcium level in its storage form and in serum is regulated by the parathyroid hormone (PTH)-vitamin D system, which can influence calcium metabolism in the gut, kidneys, and bone itself. Calcium is typically brought into the body through the diet as part of various foods and dietary supplements.

Calcium is deposited into the bone matrix, supplying bone its rigidity and strength. Following the formation of a collagenous matrix, phosphate ions are deposited, initiating the nucleation of hydroxyapatite, a crystalline structure composed of calcium and phosphate. Rather than simply binding to phosphate anions, calcium and phosphate co-precipitate to form this mineral phase, which imparts rigidity to the developing bone. Concurrently, Ca^{2+} is continuously released into the extracellular space by cells involved in bone remodeling, ensuring sufficient availability for osteoblasts and osteoprogenitor cells during the mineralization process [99]. Thus, calcium plays a quintessential role in the formation of the hard bony callus in fracture remodeling. Similarly, calcium also plays an integral regulatory role in both the function and release of previously mentioned GFs. Intracellular Ca^{2+} signaling can modulate GFs including VEGF, BMP2, BMP4, TGF-β, and IGF-1/2, all of which are necessary, especially in the early stages of bone formation [100].

In fracture repair, scaffolds inserted at the fracture site are commonly created with ionic substances including calcium. During the healing process, these resorbable scaffolds break down releasing the added ions, including calcium, into the surrounding space. This increases the local availability of calcium as a regulatory agent as well as a substrate to be used by the body in the bone regenerative process. This technique has been found to be safe in clinical trials, although its ability to improve patient outcomes is still under evaluation [1].

4. Systemic Enhancement of Bone Repair and Regeneration

4.1. *Parathyroid Hormone*

PTH is a polypeptide made of 84 amino acids secreted by the parathyroid glands, with a half-life of less than 5 minutes. It plays an integral role in calcium–phosphate homeostasis and bone remodeling [101]. It is quite a versatile molecule, playing a myriad of roles, including, but not limited to, stimulating bone formation and mineralization, inhibiting osteoblast apoptosis, and stimulating osteoblasts to secrete GFs [29].

4.1.1. *Parathyroid Hormone Regulation*

PTH has an inverse relationship with its major regulatory signal, serum calcium. Thus, by definition, if serum calcium levels are high, then serum PTH levels are low, and *vice versa.* Upregulated calcium release from intracellular stores increases extracellular calcium levels *via* diffusion through cell membranes and channels and, in turn, inhibits PTH secretion from the parathyroid glands. In excess, serum calcium can also bind the Ca^{2+}-sensing receptor (CaSR) and inhibit PTH production at the level of gene transcription..

4.1.2. *Parathyroid Hormone Role*

Many studies have been conducted to pinpoint where exactly PTH expression affects bone healing. PTH plays a critical role in the inflammatory stage of bone formation through stimulation of osteoblasts to secrete GFs. As bone healing progresses, PTH indirectly suppresses osteoclastogenesis by downregulating sclerostin (SOST) and Dickkopf-1 (DKK1), two inhibitors of the Wnt/β-catenin signaling pathway. Enhanced Wnt signaling promotes osteoblast activity and increases OPG expression, which inhibits osteoclast differentiation [102]. This results in an environment that promotes bone formation and mineralization. The effect of PTH is ultimately dependent on its concentration. In response to high levels of PTH, osteoblasts increase the production of RANKL, thereby increasing the binding of RANKL to osteoclast surface receptors and activating the osteoclasts — a step that is critical in the remodeling stage [29]. Therefore, the induction of osteogenesis or resorption is dependent on the amount and length of PTH exposure. Persistent, elevated levels of PTH lead to bone resorption, while intermittent, low doses facilitate bone formation and increase mineral density [1, 103].

4.1.3. *Therapy*

The FDA has approved osteoporotic treatment using PTH derivatives (e.g., PTH1–34 [teriparatide] and PTHrP1–34 [abaloparatide]), taking advantage of daily intermittent low dosages to promote osteoblast activity and bone formation [104, 105]. Both teriparatide and abaloparatide bind to the PTH1 receptor on osteoblasts and stem cells with similar activity to endogenous PTH. Teriparatide therapy improves bone mass and microarchitecture in osteoporotic defects, but unfortunately, its treatment potential is limited due to the appearance of catabolic effects after 2 years of therapy. These catabolic effects are less severe with abaloparatide, a synthetic analog of human recombinant PTH, possibly because it affects RANKL production less than teriparatide [106]. Furthermore, abaloparatide was shown to reduce vertebral and nonvertebral fractures and the number needed to treat for preventing nonvertebral, clinical, and major osteoporotic fractures, compared to teriparatide. Healing of distal radial and pelvic fractures was effectively accelerated in elderly patients supplemented with teriparatide [107]. Currently, preclinical PTH therapy research is investigating the utilization of controlled delivery methods in animal trials that maintain the efficacy of the hormone while avoiding the catabolic effect using scaffolds and prolonged release hydrogels [108, 109].

4.2. *Estrogen*

Estrogen, an endogenous steroidal sex hormone, is vital for the modulation of bone tissue homeostasis and bone mass regulation in both women and men [110, 111]. Thus, reduced bone mineral density, increased risk for osteoporotic fractures, and ultimately bone loss are the distinctive features of estrogen deficiency [112, 12]. Estrogen receptors on bone cells and MSCs bind 17β-estradiol (E2), a potent hormone in the human body. During the repair phase of fracture healing, estrogen upregulates the proliferation and differentiation of osteoblasts, inhibits apoptosis of osteocytes and osteoblasts, and concomitantly induces apoptosis of osteoclasts [113]. Active osteoclast formation is suppressed by the inhibition of RANKL production and the stimulation of osteoblasts and osteocytes to synthesize OPG, the decoy receptor that binds to RANKL in response to estrogen. This competitive interaction of OPG with RANKL decreases osteoclastogenesis in the context of bone remodeling. While estrogen's role in maintaining bone homeostasis is well defined, its specific contributions to fracture repair remain an area of ongoing investigation.

Postmenopausal women at risk of osteoporotic fracture could benefit from the systemic administration of estrogen, but concern remains over nontarget tissue effects such as in the breast, cardiovascular system, and uterus. As a result, adverse effects such as cardiovascular disease, pulmonary embolism, and breast cancer can occur [114]. Controlled delivery for the administration of the lowest effective dose and avoiding systemic side effects is the focus of estrogen-based osteoporotic therapy currently. Animal studies are investigating the efficacy of local estrogen delivery using nanomaterial-based scaffolds and injectable hydrogels [115, 116].

4.3. *Growth Hormone/Insulin-Like Growth Factor-1*

Growth hormone (GH) is a polypeptide hormone secreted by the anterior pituitary gland. GH primarily acts on the liver where it stimulates IGF-1 production. In turn, the IGF signaling pathway induces the proliferation and differentiation of osteoblasts [117]. Childhood GH deficiency has been linked to decreased bone mineral density. If accompanied by low serum IGF-1 levels, the child could be at an increased risk of fractures [118]. Most cells contain transmembrane GH receptors (GHRs) on their surface, which elicit various direct cellular effects when bound to GH. In particular, GHR interactions induce the synthesis of IGF-1 *via* direct or indirect mechanisms. The GHR system classically functions using Janus kinase (JAK) — signal transducer and activator of transcription (STAT) pathway. The activated GHR activates JAK tyrosine kinase and phosphorylates STAT proteins. Upon phosphorylation, STAT proteins translocate to the nucleus, bind specific DNA sequences, and initiate gene transcription.

Both GH and IGF-1 are considered potential anabolic agents due to their major roles in bone mass acquisition and maintenance. IGF-1 supports bone formation by reducing osteoblast apoptosis and promoting osteoblastogenesis, which is crucial for callus formation. In contrast, IGF-1 also indirectly activates osteoclastogenesis through the induction of RANKL synthesis, thus promoting remodeling. In addition, IGF-1 enhances skeletal mineralization by increasing tubular reabsorption of phosphate and upregulating 1 α-hydroxylase activity in the kidney, ultimately leading to elevated serum levels of active vitamin D [119]. This, in turn, contributes to enhanced calcium and phosphate absorption, both of which are essential for mineralization of bone matrix. The administration of GH and IGF-1 can stimulate longitudinal bone growth in humans by acting both directly and indirectly. GH and IGF act independently of one another, but when given together, they exert a synergistic effect. Studies have shown intermittent or continuous treatment of GH in men with idiopathic osteoporosis results in an increase in bone mineral density that is sustained for at least 1 year posttreatment. Although GH may not improve bone density in women with age-related bone loss, it may decrease fracture risk [120, 121].

4.4. *1,25(OH)2 Vitamin D3*

Bone strength, growth, and calcium–phosphorus balance are modulated by vitamin D, a fat-soluble secosteroid [12]. Its metabolically active form, 1α,25-dihydroxyvitamin D_3 (1,25$(OH)_2D_3$), forms a complex with cytoplasmic vitamin D receptors and is transported to the nucleus, where it affects the expression of osteoblastic proteins. Classically, vitamin D also plays an important role in calcium and phosphate reabsorption. This mechanism is vital because if the calcium-to-phosphate ratio is disturbed, bone mineralization fails, ultimately leading to conditions such as rickets in children and osteomalacia in the older population [122]. Inadequate vitamin D concentrations are associated with decreased calcium absorption, causing a compensatory increase in PTH levels, which leads to a lower degree of mineralization and accelerated bone loss due to the mechanisms listed in the PTH section of this chapter [123]. Regarding fracture repair, this issue would most obviously affect mineralization of the callus. In addition, vitamin D is also suspected to upregulate RANKL signaling in osteoblasts. As previously mentioned, this signaling activates osteoclastogenesis, thus facilitating local remodeling and resorption at the fracture site [124]. Current evidence supports vitamin D supplementation for individuals with confirmed deficiency or at high risk of low vitamin D status. Supplementation in these populations may improve physical function and reduce the risk of falls and fractures. However, routine supplementation in the general population is not universally recommended [125].

4.5. *Wnt/β-Catenin Signaling*

Wnt proteins are members of a family of secreted glycoproteins [1, 126]. Osteoblast activation is primarily regulated by Wnt/β-catenin signaling [127]. Wnt signaling plays a critical role in osteoblast commitment, proliferation, differentiation, and the survival of both osteoblasts and osteocytes. Its activation is particularly important during the hard callus phase of fracture healing, facilitating the transition from soft to hard callus and promoting endochondral ossification. Canonical Wnt signaling is initiated when Wnt proteins bind to a receptor complex composed of Frizzled and low-density lipoprotein receptor-related protein 5 or 6 (LRP5/6). This interaction stabilizes cytoplasmic β-catenin, which then translocates to the nucleus to regulate the transcription of osteogenic genes [127]. In osteoblasts, Wnt signaling promotes bone formation, while antagonists such as DKK1 and SOST inhibit this pathway. Loss of these inhibitors results in excessive Wnt activity and increased bone mass, as seen in conditions such as sclerosing bone dysplasia (e.g., van Buchem disease). Conversely, loss-of-function mutations may disrupt the active complex, such as those seen in LRP5, which are associated with insufficient activation of Wnt signaling and reduced bone mass [128].

SOST is the only component of the Wnt pathway exclusively expressed by osteocytes, hence its emergence as a drug target, although successful animal trials antagonizing DKK1 have arisen [127]. Anti-SOST antibody treatment has been shown to enhance bone healing in metaphyseal and proximal tibial defects in rats. A study of postmenopausal women with osteoporosis has shown that anti-SOST antibody (romosozumab) therapy can increase bone mineral density and bone formation compared to placebo and teriparatide [1, 127]. Romosozumab has recently been approved in several countries for the treatment of severe osteoporosis in postmenopausal women at high fracture risk and without a history of heart attack, myocardial infarction, or stroke, due to reports of cardiovascular events [129].

4.6. *Notch signaling*

Notch signaling is categorized as a ligand-receptor signaling pathway marked by high evolutionary conservation [126]. Activation occurs when ligand binding to the Notch receptor triggers two proteolytic cleavages, resulting in the release of the Notch intracellular domain (NICD). The NICD is then translocated into the nucleus, where it activates target genes at the transcriptional level. Studies have shown that signaling through the Notch-2 receptor and Jagged-1 (Jag-1) ligand is involved in MSC differentiation to osteoblasts [126]. The treatment of human MSCs with Jag-1 resulted in an increase in osteoblast-related genes and the induction of osteoblastogenesis [130]. Various animal studies have illustrated that Notch inhibition in bone progenitor cells results in bone marrow–derived MSC pool depletion, leading to age-related bone loss. In 2016, the requirement for Notch and bone marrow–derived MSCs in fracture repair was reported in mouse studies. The study investigated fracture union in mice treated with MSCs and osteoblasts compared to controls, in which MSC knockouts highlighted the importance of Notch signaling in intramembranous ossification of the soft callus. In MSC-specific Notch-knockout mice, the central callus region failed to undergo osteogenic differentiation, remaining as undifferentiated mesenchymal tissue, while peripheral ossification still occurred [131]. In osteoblasts with Notch knockouts, the fracture healed, thus pointing to the importance of Notch in the early stages of callus formation. This data coincides with another study that found Notch overexpression to increase mineralization of the callus and strength of bone while reducing cartilage formation [132]. These findings suggest that intermittent activation of Notch signaling may enhance early osteogenesis and bone strength, making it a promising therapeutic target for bone loss disorders [133].

5. Progenitor Cell Enhancement of Bone Repair and Regeneration

5.1. *Use of Progenitor Cell Lines in Bone Healing*

Multipotent cell lines are a potentially powerful tool for bone healing. Cell-based techniques aid in the healing of delayed union or nonunion fractures by introducing exogenous fibroblastic MSCs capable of differentiating into osteogenic or chondrogenic lineages. These cells function by incorporating themselves into the fracture callus and regenerating bone, as well as influencing the surrounding tissues of the host to promote healing. While the introduction of lineage-committed cell types, such as immature osteoblasts and chondrocytes, has potential for use in cell-based therapy, multipotent stem cells are preferred due to their accessibility for harvesting, easy expandability *in vitro*, renewability, and homogeneity.

The process of cell-based therapy begins with harvesting autologous or allogenic pluripotent cells, which are then clonally expanded *in vitro* to obtain enough cells for fracture healing. Next, the cells are exposed to molecular GFs such as BMP-2, BMP-7, and PDGF to direct their differentiation into bone and cartilage lineages [134]. These cells are allowed to mature and then introduced into the fracture site either by direct injection or by surgical implantation of a biological scaffold seeded with the maturing cells. The most common scaffold materials include allogenic bone grafts, demineralized bone tissue, hydroxyapatite, calcium phosphate, calcium sulfate, and collagen [134]. As these cells continue to develop *in vivo*, they form functional tissue that contributes to the formation of the initial cartilaginous callus and the new mineralized bone. In addition, it has been shown that these cells influence host tissues to accelerate healing and ultimately replace the implanted cells with host cells. The capacity of pluripotent cells to organize the host varies and depends on the progenitor cell type used. The size of the fracture, the type of cells, the GFs used to stimulate the cells, and the type of biomaterial scaffold that is used are various factors that tentatively influence the number of cells required for healing, but fractures may require hundreds of millions of amplified progenitor cells to heal.

Bone marrow stromal cells (BMSCs), adipose-derived MSCs, and periosteum-derived stem cells are the most commonly used cell types for stem cell–based bone repair. These cells are all multipotent and have similar fibroblast-like morphology. In addition to these cells, placenta-derived amniotic epithelial cells and MSCs harvested from the umbilicus have been studied for bone repair. Although both amniotic epithelial cells and umbilical MSCs can differentiate into lineages of all three germ layers, they have been found to have an intermediate level of pluripotency [135,

136]. Umbilical cord mesenchymal cells, in particular, have demonstrated delayed and incomplete differentiation into osteocytes, potentially making them less useful for bone repair therapies.

5.1.1. *Bone Marrow Stromal Cells*

BMSCs were discovered over 50 years ago, originally termed colony-forming unit-fibroblasts, and are the most commonly used progenitor cells. They are a heterogenous population of cells found in the bone marrow stroma with the potential to differentiate into osteogenic, chondrogenic, adipogenic, and hematopoietic-supporting lineages [137]. BMSCs are harvested through bone marrow aspiration from the posterior iliac crest, proximal medial tibia, or proximal humerus, with 200–260 cells per milliliter or 0.001% to 0.01% of nucleated cells in the aspirate, where typically 30–60 mL is taken [138]. These cells adhere to a plastic culture flask surface, which is then washed to separate the BMSCs from the non-adhering cells. After washing, single-cell-derived colonies are cultured and expanded to achieve the necessary population of cells, with a population doubling time averaging 79 hours [134]. Once expanded *in vitro*, BMSCs retain their potential for bone, cartilage, and adipose lineages but exhibit senescent changes after passage 5 [139]. The osteogenic potential is the last lineage lost, causing BMSCs to have more use as an osteogenic agent rather than a chondrogenic or adipogenic agent in stem cell therapy [140]. As implants for bone repair therapy, one of the main effects of BMSCs is to modulate host inflammatory cells and osteoblasts to promote ossification instead of directly forming osteocytes and osteoblasts themselves [141].

5.1.2. *Adipose-Derived Progenitor Cells*

Adipose-derived progenitor cells (ASCs) are another form of MSCs, which are a heterogenous population of cells derived from adipose tissue and are present in subcutaneous, visceral, and organ fat. While their exact location in adipose tissue is unknown, they are typically found in a perivascular niche. Potential ASC lineages include osteogenic, chondrogenic, adipogenic, and myogenic cell types [142]. ASCs are harvested through minimally invasive liposuction with 1 mL of aspirated fat yielding an average of 400,000 cells after enzymatic digestion, with 1%–10% of those cells being ASCs [143]. Like BMSCs, ASCs adhere to a plastic culture flask surface, and they may be separated and expanded by cell culture in a similar fashion. However, ASCs tend to form more colonies than BMSCs, have a shorter population doubling time (60 hours), and are more genetically stable on expansion [134]. The abundance, ease of harvest, and stability of these cells make them an appealing option for stem cell therapies. As with other MSCs, ASCs are immunoprivileged and have been found to have immunosuppressive effects, with studies finding reduced proliferation of allogenic lymphocytes when cultured *in vitro* with ASCs [144]. In addition, a study of rat spinal fusion found that specimens with an implanted ASC containing scaffold showed improved rates of fusion with decreased T cell activation [145]. These qualities may improve the safety and efficacy of stem cell–mediated bone repair by reducing the potential for host rejection of an allogenic stem cell graft. In bone repair experiments, ASCs appear to contribute more directly to new tissue instead of playing an organizing role, with one study using ASC scaffolds in mice reporting an 84%–99% direct contribution of ASCs to the new tissue [146]. However, there has been observed variability in the ability of ASCs to aid in bone repair depending on patient age, gender, and the location from which the ASCs were harvested. While ASCs have a number of attractive qualities, there are also challenges when used in bone repair therapy. For example, ASCs have been found to secrete factors that inhibit chondrocytes and lead to their apoptosis, which could be counterproductive if used in the case of an endochondral fracture [147].

5.1.3. *Periosteum-Derived Progenitor Cells*

Periosteum-derived progenitor cells (PDSCs) are a subset of MSCs found in the cambium layer of the periosteum, adjacent to the bone cortex [148]. Under normal conditions, PDSCs differentiate into osteoblasts and work with osteoclasts to control bone remodeling. In the case of a fracture, PDSCs proliferate and differentiate into both osteogenic and chondrogenic lineages and form the callus around the fracture site. The role of these stem cells as skeletal precursors makes them intriguing subjects for investigation as agents for cell-based bone repair. PDSCs are obtained through periosteal biopsy and, after enzymatic digestion, can be clonally expanded on plastic culture dishes in a similar fashion to BMSCs and ASCs. These colonies display a population doubling time of ~80 hours and may double up to 30 times *in vitro*. PDSCs have low telomerase but remain stable on repeated expansion due to extended telomeres [149]. Interestingly, the use of serum in PDSC culture protocols has been found to give inconsistent results due to the inhibition of cells by the cytokines present, but the expansion potential of PDSCs has been improved by trials using serum-free culture preparation techniques [52]. While further study is required to establish PDSC characteristics and clinical utility, murine studies have shown that PDSCs primed with specific GFs actively contribute to bone regeneration [52].

At the present time, stem cells are not FDA approved for approaches that target bone regeneration, and current studies are phase 1 clinical trials. These studies aim to demonstrate the safety of stem cell–based regeneration techniques, improve methods of cell harvesting and culture, and discover and address potential adverse effects. In addition, further research will aid in determining the viability and feasibility of different types of multipotent cells, such as ASCs and PDSCs, as well as providing additional characterization.

6. Genetic Approaches to Bone Repair and Regeneration

6.1. *Genetic Approaches*

Treating genetic diseases, especially recessive Mendelian diseases, was the driving force for the initial use of genetic therapies [150, 151]. Earlier utilizations included introducing wild-type genes into target cells to compensate for the original genetic defect and maintaining sustained gene expression after incorporation into target cell genomes. There have been some concerns associated with gene therapies, with an emphasis on the safety profiles of the therapies, establishing efficient gene transfer to target cells, avoiding the activation of the body's immune system, and sustaining sufficient gene expression once incorporated into cells [152]. As of 2020, only 14 gene therapies have been approved for clinical use worldwide for various ailments. To help encourage the development of gene research, in 2019, the FDA announced a plan to create pathways in the approval process to expedite certain areas of research, namely those aimed at treating monogenetic defects [153]. Currently, most FDA-approved therapies for conditions needing a specific target protein use the direct application of a protein of interest into the body. For bone regeneration therapies, BMPs are a popular area of interest, especially BMP-2 and BMP-7. The use of recombinant BMP-2 and BMP-7 (rhBMP-2 and rhBMP-7), called INFUSE® and OP-1®, respectively, was approved by the FDA [154]. OP-1® is no longer on the market, but INFUSE® is actively used in the treatment of spinal fusions, dental applications, and acute open tibial fractures. Off-label use of INFUSE® is encouraging, showing bone growth in large defects. INFUSE® is a collagen sponge with rhBMP-2 embedded within it and was approved for use in spinal fusion by the FDA in 2002. During clinical application, INFUSE® encountered challenges due to the rapid diffusion of rhBMP-2 from the collagen sponge after implantation. To compensate, supraphysiologic doses — up to 10^6-fold higher than natural levels — were required, which have been associated with adverse effects such as ectopic bone formation, inflammation, cancer risk, and fertility complications [155]. The use of supraphysiologic protein levels is not an issue unique to INFUSE®. It is one of the main criticisms of direct protein application therapies, which leads to similar adverse effects seen in the use of INFUSE® [155–160]. It is also extremely costly to produce recombinant proteins, limiting the number of people who could afford treatment utilizing direct protein application.

6.2. *Gene Delivery*

Gene therapy has several advantages over the direct application of proteins: (1) It avoids the need to manufacture high levels of the protein since the proteins will be produced *in vivo* [161]. (2) It can induce better localization of osteogenic molecules compared to protein delivery. (3) It is potentially less expensive than recombinant protein [162]. (4) It can produce more active forms of GFs due to synthesis by autologous cells [163]. Gene therapies are a superior method to deliver intracellular-acting products such as transcription factors, signaling molecules, and noncoding species of ribonucleic acid (RNA). Protein insertion into a specific cellular compartment also falls into this category, thus expanding the possible applications of this technology [164]. Even with these advantages, the ideal gene therapy should be delivered off the shelf and applied at the point of care in a single, affordable, and preferably percutaneous procedure. In gene therapy, genes can either be incorporated into target cells in the host, *in vivo*, or be incorporated into autologous or allogeneic cells outside of the body, *ex vivo,* and then implanted into the host. The primary aim of both is to increase the expression of target proteins in the affected cells.

6.2.1. *In Vivo Gene Delivery*

In vivo gene delivery involves introducing genetic material, typically *via* viral or nonviral vectors, directly into the patient's body, where it is taken up by target cells to achieve therapeutic effects [165]. The genes are delivered either locally or systemically [166]. For gene therapies involving bone regeneration, two main approaches have been used: (1) gene vectors are bound to a matrix, known as a gene-activated matrix; or (2) gene vectors are suspended in a solution [152]. Advantages of *in vivo* delivery over *ex vivo* delivery include the following: (1) The simplicity of the process used to introduce the genetic material to host cells; the material is either directly injected at the site of interest or administered intravenously. (2) It avoids the process of needing to harvest, grow, and select cells that will then have to be introduced into the host, vastly lowering the production and storage costs. Disadvantages include low efficiency of gene transfer, requiring a large amount of genetic material and vectors to be used to produce therapeutic effects. This can cause unwanted effects such as inflammatory or immune responses. Vector systems themselves can be potentially toxic, and targeting the cell population of interest is challenging [166, 167].

6.2.2. *Ex Vivo Gene Delivery*

Ex vivo delivery is when genetic material, usually in the form of a vector, is incorporated into target cells outside of the host body, and then those cells are introduced to the site of interest within the host. Often, this approach involves harvesting autologous cells, expanding and genetically modifying these cells outside of the body, followed by insertion into the desired site. In terms of bone regeneration, the desired site is the osseous lesion or bone defect [152]. This approach is often used when damage to the site is extensive and lacks active cells capable of stimulating regeneration [168]. An abbreviated method is possible where suitable tissues, such as fat, muscle, or marrow, are harvested and genetically modified intraoperatively, then reimplanted during the same procedure [169]. In such cases, there is no need to harvest specific cell types, modify them, and then expand them in a laboratory setting using good manufacturing practices, significantly lowering the production cost. Another approach avoids the need to harvest, expand, and then genetically modify host tissues and cells altogether by using an allograft cell line [152]. Advantages of *ex vivo* approaches over *in vivo* approaches include their better safety profile. Genetically modified cells can be monitored for aberrant behavior, and this allows for the cells with the highest gene expression to be individually selected, increasing their protein production efficiency [170]. The number and type of cells modified can be controlled, allowing for the more discriminant selection of modified cells [165]. A low quantity of vectors is vital to achieve desirable therapeutic effects, leading to less immune recognition and lower rates of vector-associated cytotoxicity [171]. Disadvantages include high production costs, impractical clinical application in bone regeneration and storage, and slow production time of the therapeutic dose due to the need to harvest and culture autologous stem cells *in vitro*. While the phase I clinical trial of an *ex vivo* gene therapy for arthritis demonstrated safety and feasibility, it also highlighted the logistical and regulatory complexities that can hinder broader clinical application [172].

6.2.3. *Nonviral Vector Gene Therapies*

The simplest vectors are DNA plasmids (pDNA) which can be reproduced inside of bacteria [152]. Plasmids are extrachromosomal DNA made up of

1,000–20,000 base pairs. They can be picked up by bacteria in the environment or be passed from one bacterium to another in a process called bacterial conjugation. Originally, plasmids contained genes that granted bacterial hosts an advantage against stressors, like antibiotic resistance [173]. Due to the ease of plasmid DNA modification and replication, scientists have made use of them to produce desired proteins to help treat diseases. Once a plasmid is incorporated into a bacterium, it can make endless copies of the plasmid, leading to large amounts of the desired protein being produced. pDNA complexes are used in a variety of nonviral vector methods as well. Most approaches use highly positively charged materials, such as polymers, liposomes, and other polycations, to interact with the negatively charged DNA, forming stable nanoplexes [165]. These complexes have an overall positive charge, enhancing their uptake into the mammalian cell in a process called transfection. Transfection is the nonviral counterpart of the viral process of transduction where genetic material delivered in a nonviral vector is taken up by target cells. Using nonviral vectors has several advantages over viral vectors. They are easier to produce, have less immunogenicity, and do not cause insertional mutations, making them more economical and safer compared to viral vectors [162, 174]. Despite these advantages, their clinical use has been limited due to their relatively low transfection efficiency. This leads to the need to use larger amounts to produce a therapeutic level, which can cause cytotoxicity depending on the vector material used. The efficiency of DNA uptake by target cells is called transfection efficiency, and strategies have been implemented to help increase it, such as chemical methods and physical methods including electroporation and sonoporation [175–177].

6.2.4. *Chemical Nonviral Gene Therapies*

Chemical methods of nonviral vector gene therapies rely mostly on the cationic nature of the vector used in order to attract and bind the anionic pDNA. Examples of cationic vectors include polymers and liposomes. Common polymers used as vectors include polyethylenimine (PEI), chitosan, and polyamidoamine (PAMAM) [178, 179]. Of these, PEI is the most efficient and most commonly studied nonviral gene delivery vector [173]. With the use of a gene-activated matrix, PEI–pDNA nanoplexes were embedded throughout a collagen scaffold to further enhance the overall effectiveness of nonviral approaches [180]. Liposomal vectors have also been shown to be effective in bone regeneration in a pig model using the BMP-2 gene [166]. However, cationic lipids and polymers used as vectors for pDNA have also been shown to cause cytotoxicity when used in the large amounts needed to achieve greater rates of transfection [181]. This poses yet another challenge for researchers to overcome in order to bring these therapeutic approaches to clinical trials [182].

6.2.5. *Physical Nonviral Gene Therapies*

Physical nonviral gene therapies include electroporation and sonoporation. In electroporation, electric pulses open small temporary pores on the cell membrane where DNA can then enter the cytoplasm [163]. Electroporation-induced transfer of BMP-2 and BMP-7 gene-containing plasmids has been shown to induce ectopic bone formation [183]. It has also been used to heal critical bone size defects in a rat model [183]. Sonoporation is an ultrasound-mediated acoustic cavitation that increases cell membrane permeability [163]. It has been shown to be a transient method to deliver genes, creating well-localized gene expression and bone formation *in vivo*, as well as a relatively safe gene delivery method, but has a lower transfection efficiency than electroporation [184]. With the utilization of microbubbles, sonoporation became more efficient for regenerating critical-size bone defects while maintaining its safety in a mouse model [185]. Microbubble-enhanced sonoporation maintained its effectiveness in a clinically relevant mini-pig model and was shown to facilitate uptake of osteogenic plasmids, such as BMP-2-encoding plasmids, and induce ectopic bone formation [176, 186].

Researchers continue to explore strategies to optimize physical gene delivery for bone regeneration. Temporal control has been enhanced using regulated constructs such as doxycycline-inducible systems encoding BMP-2 and BMP-7, which have successfully induced both ectopic and orthotopic bone formation in rat femur models [187]. Spatial control has also been demonstrated using heat-activated and ligand-inducible gene switches, allowing for localized gene expression [188]. To extend the duration of transgene expression, encapsulated cationic microparticles have been employed as sustained-release vehicles [189]. While most studies have focused on BMPs, recent work has shown that low-intensity ultrasound-mediated delivery of basic FGF can also enhance craniofacial bone regeneration [190].

6.2.6. *Viral Vector Gene Therapies*

Gene therapy using viral vectors is the oldest and most well-studied technique [150]. In fact, viral vectors have been used in more than 1,200 human gene therapy trials since 2012 [191]. Since viruses have an innate ability to insert their own genetic material into target cells, they have a higher transduction efficiency than nonviral approaches [152]. Transduction is the viral equivalent of transfection and is the term used to describe the process of genetic material being passed from the viral vector into target cells. Modifications are made to the viral genome to curtail pathogenicity, incorporate genes of interest, and maintain transduction efficiency [165, 192–194]. Pathologic and replication genes are removed to eliminate pathogenicity and create space for desired genes and their regulatory elements to be inserted into the viral vector [152]. There are still concerns about immunogenicity even with these modifications [162]. More than a dozen viral vectors have been studied, but only adenovirus, adeno-associated virus, herpes simplex virus (HSV), retroviruses, and lentivirus have been approved for clinical use [152]. HSV, due to its cytotoxicity, is primarily used in oncolytic applications and is not suitable for bone regeneration and thus will not be discussed further [195].

6.2.7. *Adenoviral Vectors*

Adenovirus is a well-studied viral vector, likely due to its various favorable characteristics. Specifically, it does not integrate with target cell genomes, is straightforward to produce at high viral titers, and has the ability to transduce many different cell types, both dividing and nondividing cells, with high transduction efficiency [196, 197]. Adenoviral vectors containing osteogenic genes, such as BMP-2 and BMP-6, have been used to treat femoral defects, leading to earlier ossification and stronger bony unions compared to untreated defects or control vectors and accelerated ulnar osteotomies and spinal fusions in small animal models [198–201]. Other studies have shown that the timing of vector injection during the bone healing process can significantly influence outcomes, likely due to changes in local cellularity and the ability to retain viral vectors within the lesion at different healing stages [199]. Also of note, adenovirus vectors can provoke both a humoral and a cell-mediated immune response. Consequently, this decreases the number of vectors available to transduce target cells, leading to reduced overall expression rates after 2–4 weeks. Despite this, some studies have shown that enough gene expression occurs to induce irreversible osteogenic responses [152]. While generally safe for localized use in bone lesions, adenoviral vectors have been associated with serious adverse events in systemic applications, including the first reported gene therapy–related death due to an inflammatory response [202].

6.2.8. *Adeno-Associated Viral Vectors*

Adeno-associated viral vectors are gaining popularity due to their safer profiles compared to adenoviral vectors. They still produce a humoral immune response but only trigger a mild cell-mediated response [152]. Genetically modified recombinant adeno-associated viral vectors have a superior safety profile because they are nonpathogenic and immunologically inert, while also inducing a sustained transgene expression [163]. Like adenoviral vectors, they can transduce both nondividing and dividing cells, existing as a concentrated episome [152]. Their small size limits their uses for larger genes; however, this is not an issue for bone regeneration considering the small size of GF genes used. Studies have shown that adeno-associated viral vectors carrying osteogenic genes, such as BMP-2, lead to ectopic and orthotopic bone formation [203, 204]. One study also revealed that administering adeno-associated viral vectors carrying BMP-2 along with adenoviral vectors carrying BMP-2 showed superior bone formation than each separately [203]. Manufacturing is a huge hurdle to bringing their use into a clinical setting due to its complexity and cost. For example, an adeno-associated viral vector–based drug used for spinal muscular atrophy costs $2 million per dose, which significantly limits the number of people able to afford it [205].

6.2.9. *Retroviral Vectors*

Retroviral vectors are straightforward to produce and manipulate and were the first viral vectors developed for human gene therapy [152]. Transduction with retroviral vectors often requires actively dividing cells, which limits their use to mostly *ex vivo* therapies. Retroviral vectors containing genetic information for the LIM mineralization protein (LMP) showed the promotion of bone regeneration in rat femoral defects [206]. Despite successes, the safety of retroviral vectors is a concern for gene therapies treating nonlethal diseases, making clinical acceptance of retrovirus-based therapies challenging. Since retroviruses insert genomes at unpredictable sites in the host, there is the potential for mutagenesis which has been documented in clinical trials [207]. Most bone pathologies are not life-threatening, so even with a small risk of mutagenesis and carcinogenesis, it is not a favorable choice as a vector. These concerns largely restrict retroviral vector use to lethal diseases, such as late-stage cancers and severe immunodeficiency disease.

6.2.10. *Lentiviral Vectors*

Lentiviruses are a subclass of retroviruses, but unlike some retroviruses, they can also transduce nondividing cells, increasing their range of application. Insertional mutagenesis of these retroviruses is still a cause for concern, as there is documented evidence of two participants in an SCID trial using lentiviral vector therapy developing leukemia [208]. An advantage of using lentiviral vectors is that they have long-term gene expression; however, this may not be as important as once believed for bone regeneration [152].

6.3. *Gene-Activated Matrices*

Gene-activated matrices embed genetic material using different kinds of vectors into a scaffold, which is then inserted into the bone lesion or defect. Different additives, drugs, and proteins can be included to help with bone regeneration [209–211]. The scaffolds themselves can be made with different materials, including collagen, hydroxyapatite, β-TCP, glass ceramics, and titanium mesh cages [170]. Generally, scaffolds are required to be both biocompatible and biodegradable [212]. The mechanical properties needed to make an optimal scaffold include adequate pore size, interconnectivity, and integrity to facilitate new cell growth and neovascularization within the scaffold. It is vital to ensure that the rigidity of the scaffold mimics that of bone, because this has been found to influence stem cell differentiation and promote osteogenic differentiation [213]. Scaffolding materials fall under one of two categories: synthetic or natural. Collagen scaffolds are popular due to the number of forms it can take; collagen can be manipulated to make hydrogels, sponges, and three-dimensional (3D)-printed constructs [214–216]. It is a highly biocompatible biopolymer that supports cell growth and has natural degradation. Type I collagen is also the primary protein component of native bone tissue, making it especially useful for bone regeneration research [161]. Another frequently used scaffolding material is calcium phosphate–derived material [217, 218]. TCP, hydroxyapatite, and octacalcium phosphate are all found in bone [219]. Their properties can be manipulated by varying the ratio of calcium and phosphate. Its ability to stimulate MSCs to differentiate into osteogenic cells has been an area of focus in bone tissue engineering [220]. Combining calcium phosphate–derived material and collagen with GFs has further enhanced the regenerative abilities of bone [161]. Other examples of synthetic materials are poly-(L-co-D, L-lactide), while natural materials include chitosan, gelatin, silk, and alginate [212].

Recent studies have begun utilizing more than just passive characteristics to construct scaffolds and have started engineering them to act more like drug and biomolecule delivery systems. Researchers have explored scaffold modifications, including covalent binding, physical entrapment, and micro/nanosphere delivery of osteogenic material to host cells [221, 222]. It was found that even the shape of the delivery vehicle had an impact, with spheres having the most control over the release rate of molecules [212]. As research into gene therapies advanced, researchers started combining gene-based therapies with scaffolds using *ex vivo* and *in vivo* approaches. The *in vivo* approach calls for loading scaffolds with transfection/transduction vectors that will incorporate genetic material into the host cells after implantation *in situ*. This "off-the-shelf" therapy would avoid the cost, labor, and time associated with *ex vivo* culturing and seeding of cells onto scaffolds. The *ex vivo* approach involves seeding already transfected/transduced cells onto the scaffold before implantation. This approach, like other previously mentioned *ex vivo* approaches, has the benefit of being able to select cells with the highest amount of gene expression, making the therapy more effective. Some issues include finding a viable source of cells, establishing cell-handling standards, and transporting and storing live cells [223]. Transfecting/transducing cells on or around scaffolds has been explored using pDNA, viral, nonviral, and RNA-based approaches. In terms of RNA-based approaches, both RNA that promote the upregulation of osteogenic proteins and RNA that downregulates antiosteogenic proteins have been used [161].

6.3.1. *Gene-Activated Matrices with DNA Plasmids and DNA Plasmids Nanoplexes*

As previously stated, pDNA has a relatively low transfection efficiency and needs some kind of vehicle to prevent its degradation *in vivo* [178, 179]. Nonviral vectors are the most commonly used method for delivering pDNA. Most studies using pDNA have it complexed to cationic polymers, such as PEI, chitosan, and PAMAM, to create nanoplexes that go on to transfect cells. Nanoplexes form spontaneously after reaching a specific charge ratio between the cationic molecules and the anionic pDNA molecules. They are then endocytosed, translocated into the nuclei of target cells, and then decomplexed, allowing for the pDNA to induce gene expression. The exact mechanism for decomplexing and nuclear translocation is unknown [224–226]. At larger local concentrations, using these cationic materials has been shown to be cytotoxic [167, 168]. Less commonly, studies have complexed pDNA to calcium phosphate nanoparticles or cell-penetrating peptides. Some studies have found that loading pDNA onto scaffolds that encode for two or more osteogenic proteins can act synergistically, causing greater bone volume regeneration and higher union rates [227, 228]. However, the optimal combination and ratio of osteogenic proteins remain unknown, with some combinations seemingly leading to less bone regeneration than a single type of osteogenic protein alone [229]. Other studies have found that seeding scaffolds with both

BMSCs and pDNA nanoplexes induced greater levels of bone regeneration than scaffolds seeded with BMSCs alone [230]. Instead of exploring different combinations of osteogenic genes and materials to increase the amount of bone regeneration, studies have also looked at modifying other factors that impact bone regeneration, such as the rate of nanoplex release and the body's inflammatory response during recovery and therapeutic treatment. Controlling the release of nanoplexes from scaffolds using enzymatic activity from infiltrating cells has been achieved. Results of these studies have shown better *in vitro* osteogenic differentiation and *in vivo* bone regeneration compared to unmodified gene-activated scaffolds and controls [231]. Another topic of research interest has looked to downregulate the inflammatory response generated by IL-1 by incorporating IL-1 receptor agonists into the scaffold. As a result, IL-1 receptor agonists promoted bone formation *in vivo* and protected seeded BMSC from IL-1's antiosteogenic effects [232–234]. Strategies have been implemented in attempts to eliminate the concern for cytotoxicity associated with cationic polymers by utilizing cell-penetrating peptides, such as glycosaminoglycan binding, to enhance transfection. Results from *in vitro* studies showed that this approach had comparable transfection efficiency to standard reagents with minimal toxicity [235].

Some gene-activated matrices have made it to the clinical trial phase of research. The first clinical trial was an octacalcium phosphate scaffold embedded with naked pDNA-encoding VEGF. It was used to correct alveolar ridge atrophy in 16 participants and jawbone defects in four participants. There were no adverse events reported during the trial or in the 30-month follow-up period. However, no differences were found in bone density within the bone graft zone compared to the control [236].

6.3.2. *Gene-Activated Scaffolds with Other Systems*

Non-nanoplex gene-activated scaffolds have been explored. A study using microvesicles (MVs) coated sequentially with a cationic polymer and then pDNA was used to reduce the cytotoxicity associated with pDNA nanoplexes. These MVs were then loaded onto a demineralized bone matrix scaffold and inserted into bone lesions. They were compared against unloaded scaffolds and PEI-pDNA-loaded scaffolds and showed greater expression of osteocalcin and OPN. Increased bone regeneration and neovascularization *in vivo* compared to PEI–pDNA scaffolds were also found [237]. Utilization of ultrasound-responsive gene-activation techniques, known as sonoporation, has also taken place, with the main goal being to control the transfection of local cells. Ultrasound-sensitive microbubbles, C2C12 cells, and pDNA were introduced into an injectable collagen gel. *In vitro* results showed increased osteogenic differentiation of cells, while *in vivo* results showed ectopic bone formation when injected into murine hind limb muscles [238].

3D printing is an emerging topic of study that utilizes different printing techniques. Inkjet printing prints as a liquid and then hardens into a solid structure. Bioplotting is similar to inkjet printing except continuous filaments of scaffold material are injected out of syringes, forming a solid structure. Stereolithography forms one layer at a time with UV light-activated curing until the desired structure is completed [239, 240]. A study utilizing 3D printing to form its scaffold used an octacalcium phosphate scaffold immersed in a sodium phosphate solution containing pDNA with agitation. This scaffold showed the ability to biodegrade and transfect cells with minimal inflammation while simultaneously integrating and promoting vascularized bone regeneration in bone defects [241].

6.3.3. *Virus-Activated Scaffolds*

The translocation of genetic material into target cell nuclei is more efficient with viral gene therapy methods than nonviral methods [242, 243]. Similar to the nonscaffold-based viral approaches, there are risks of insertional mutation and activation of the host's immune system. Insertional mutations can cause dysfunctional regulation of oncogenes and tumorigenesis [207]. In addition, eliciting an immune response can cause the host to kill viral vectors, prompting the therapy to be less effective or leading to a lethal immune response [244]. Despite these risks, virus applications to scaffolds have resulted in the efficient production of proteins of interest and the enhancement of bone regeneration in numerous *in vivo* studies [161]. Adenoviral vectors in porous scaffolds seeded with

BMSCs using BMP-7, PDGF-β, or a combination of both showed sustained expression of encoded proteins for weeks, normal proliferation of seeded cells, enhanced osteoblastic differentiation, and an increased bone regeneration volume [245, 246]. Furthermore, using two vectors containing different osteogenic proteins simultaneously acted synergistically and resulted in more bone defect regeneration compared to a single vector alone. The type of osteogenic protein expressed affected different aspects of bone regeneration [247]. Studies focused on controlling the release and spatial distribution of viral vectors embedded in scaffolds through physical measures, such as freezing and protein linkages, and *via* chemical means, such as doxycycline-inducible systems, have also been explored [247–250]. BMSCs expressed more protein within the scaffolds compared to nonimmobilized viral vectors, leading to enhanced osteogenic differentiation. Some immobilization methods led to greater transduction in cells local to the bone defect and scaffold, leading to more bone regeneration than the nonimmobilized viral vector scaffolds. In addition, these studies also demonstrated less erroneous bone formation [250]. Other researchers have explored ways to reduce the immune response caused by the use of viral vectors. One such study found that the inflammatory response to scaffold implantation could be reduced by incorporating IL-1 receptor agonists into the scaffold, leading to less scaffold degradation [249]. Regenerating large areas of bone requires a good vascular supply to ensure enough nutrients reach the new tissue to maintain its viability. Thus, bone defect revascularization was shown to be enhanced through the use of hypoxia-inducible factor 1α and VEGF [251, 252].

6.4. *Points to Consider for Future Studies in Bone Repair Gene Therapy*

Numerous studies have revealed findings that should be considered moving forward. Immune responses to materials within bone defects can impair healing and can make gene therapies less effective. Bone regeneration may only require low, transient levels of osteogenic gene expression to promote bone regeneration [176, 253]. Endogenously synthesized osteogenic genes produced by transduced cells were 100 times more effective than recombinant proteins and remained cell-associated with minimal diffusion to distant sites [152]. Finally, cell-to-cell contact is needed for transduced cells expressing osteogenic proteins to cause nontransduced cells to express the same osteogenic proteins, likely due to autocrine and close paracrine mechanisms [152]. Some challenges that need to be tackled to bring viral vectors for bone therapy into the clinical setting include decreasing the number of agents that need to be purified, ensuring vector containment without failure, preventing immune reactions to viral vectors, and preventing transduction of nontarget tissues [163].

6.5. *Cell-Mediated Gene Therapy*

Cell-mediated gene therapy consists of incorporating genetic material into different lines of stem cells. Once the stem cells have the desired genes incorporated, they are then introduced into the bone lesion or defect. Cell-mediated gene therapy can utilize cells that have already demonstrated high transduction efficiency, enabling clinicians to select cell types that are well-suited as delivery vehicles based on their successful genetic modification. It can be safer than *in vivo* delivery of viral vectors by preventing direct contact between vectors and hosts. This minimizes local inflammation and immune responses allowing for multiple cell transplantations [163]. Stem cells have both autocrine and paracrine responses, meaning they can react to osteogenic factors, such as BMPs, and contribute to bone regeneration directly [254]. These are the reasons why cell-mediated gene therapy is considered one of the primary approaches to bone repair and regeneration [197]. Some disadvantages of cell-mediated gene therapy include the high costs associated with harvesting, expanding, genetically modifying, storing, and transporting stem cells, as well as the risks of graft-versus-host disease and immune rejection, all of which present significant barriers to clinical adoption.

6.6. *Considerations for Clinical Applications and Future Studies*

For the majority of gene therapies for bone regeneration, safety remains the main barrier to clinical trials. Most bone defects and lesions are not life-threatening, so the safety profile of the therapies used to treat them needs to be exemplary. Tumorigenicity is an issue when working with stem cells and retroviral vectors [255]. To counteract the possibility of tumor formation, residual stem cells need to be identified and killed once the desired number of cells have differentiated. The introduction of suicide genes or the use of killer antibodies, targeting cell-surface receptors on undifferentiated cells, could be explored [256, 257]. Despite these theoretical concerns, no reports of tumors appearing at sites of cell-mediated gene therapy, specifically for bone regeneration, have occurred. The safer profiles, ease of scalability, and production of nonviral techniques do not overcome their underwhelming performance with low transfection efficiency. This limits their use for *in vivo* bone regeneration.

In terms of gene-activated matrices, more research needs to be performed comparing different gene-activated scaffolds to one another to optimize this therapy. The combination and ratio of different osteogenic genes should be further characterized. These approaches should also aim to compare how they perform to the already accepted protein-based approaches that they are trying to replace. It would be beneficial to know where the gene-based approaches are stronger or weaker than the current protein-based standard. In addition, the sexually dimorphic nature of stem cell behavior, including differences in proliferation, differentiation, and trophic factor expression, has been largely overlooked in the literature despite growing evidence of its importance [258, 259]. As more approaches are being published, it is becoming increasingly difficult to identify the most promising candidates for clinical trials. In addition to identifying the optimal strategy, little to no research has focused on optimizing treatments on a patient-to-patient basis.

7. RNA Approaches to Bone Repair and Regeneration

Bone development and regeneration rely on tightly regulated gene activation and repression in response to a myriad of cell signaling pathways. In recent decades, the use of RNA-based therapies to promote bone repair has substantially increased as our understanding of specific molecular mechanisms has grown [260]. RNA-based therapeutics, along with cells, drugs, or proteins, can be incorporated into scaffolds and delivered to bone defect sites to enhance bone repair. Therapeutic RNAs can be easily synthesized and modified to serve a variety of purposes in bone remodeling. Several RNA therapeutics currently exist, including messenger RNA (mRNA), microRNA (miRNA), and small interfering RNA (siRNA). This section will highlight these three RNA therapeutics, focusing on their mechanisms, molecular targets, and therapeutic applications, as well as the advantages and limitations of current practice.

Although mRNA has been used in various fields of medicine, such as vaccines [261], cancer immunotherapy [49], skin repair [262], and myocardial damage repair [135], its use in bone remodeling was not introduced until 2015 [262]. Since then, numerous advances in the preparation and application of mRNA therapeutics have been developed. mRNA is a single-stranded RNA transcribed from DNA within the cell nucleus and functions as a template for protein synthesis and gene expression. *In vitro* transcription mRNA (IVT mRNA) is a novel drug class used to supplement endogenous mRNA. IVT mRNA is synthesized using a DNA template containing a bacteriophage promoter (such as T7), 5′ and 3′ untranslated regions (UTRs), an open reading frame (ORF), and a poly(A) tail or poly(A/T) sequence [263]. Unlike endogenous mRNA, IVT mRNA does not require nuclear entry for expression, allowing it to bypass the nuclear membrane and be directly translated in the cytoplasm, making it more effective in nonmitotic cells [45, 263]. These advantages over endogenous mRNA provide IVT mRNA with greater therapeutic application for bone remodeling. Before the delivery of mRNA to bone defect sites, modification is necessary to prevent the body's natural immune response from attacking and inhibiting mRNA uptake [264]. Various modifications are currently used, including adding methyl or adenyl groups to nucleotides, introducing additional nucleotides, or deleting ORFs, and several studies have shown efficacious bone remodeling with these modifications [262, 265, 266]. Once modified, mRNA can be delivered into the cytoplasm of cells *via* physical or chemical methods, with the latter being more common. Among the chemical methods, cationic polymers such as poly-L-lysine and PEI [265] and lipoplex nanoparticles [267] are among the most widely used. These methods promote the assembly of positively charged vector carriers with negatively charged mRNA to allow for absorption into the cell. For the IVT mRNA to successfully drive protein synthesis and promote bone remodeling, its stability and sustained release must be tightly regulated. This process depends on specific parameters of the scaffold used to deliver IVT mRNA to bone defect sites, namely the scaffold's biodegradability, chemical composition, and pore size [260]. The two prototypical mRNA-based scaffolds are constructed from fibrin gel and collagen. Depending on the type used and additional modifications, studies have demonstrated sustained protein production and bone remodeling ranging from 11 days to 8 weeks [266, 268].

7.1. *Micro Ribonucleic Acid*

Endogenous miRNA is a short, noncoding RNA that combines with the RNA-induced silencing complex (RISC) to form the miRISC complex [269]. This complex may then bind to specific regions of the 3′ or 5′ UTR of endogenous mRNA, effectively silencing gene expression. Therapeutic applications take advantage of this process to either upregulate osteogenic-related genes or downregulate adverse genes to promote bone remodeling. To upregulate target genes, antisense strands of miRNAs (anti-miRNA, also called antagomirs or miRNA inhibitors) are created that bind with miRNAs and prevent their normal action [135]. To downregulate target genes, molecules identical to endogenous miRNAs are created (miR-mimics) to inhibit translation of mRNAs [260]. The primary targets of miRNAs in bone remodeling are the BMP and Wnt/β-catenin signaling pathways involved in osteogenic differentiation of MSCs. In the BMP signaling pathway, the noggin protein gene (NOG) suppresses osteogenesis by preventing the binding and activation of BMP with its receptor. Various miR-mimics target this pathway, including miR-148b, which promotes osteogenesis by silencing NOG [270, 271]. Inhibition of miR-146a (e.g., using anti-miR-146a) has been shown to enhance bone regeneration in both *in vitro* and *in vivo* models [96, 272]. In the Wnt/β-catenin signaling pathway, RUNX2 can regulate the BMP signaling pathway to affect bone remodeling. miR mimics, such as miR-23a [260], miR-204 [273], miR-103a [135], and miR-467g [274], target RUNX2 to suppress osteogenesis, while miR-135 [275] targets HOXA2, an inhibitor of RUNX2, to enhance osteogenesis. Numerous other miR-mimics have been reported in the literature, and others are currently being investigated for their therapeutic use. Once specific signaling pathways are identified and miR-mimics are created, delivery into the cytoplasm of cells is often accomplished using PEI cationic polymers, similar to mRNA delivery. Scaffolds composed of hydrogel, hyaluronic acid, or collagen are the preferred delivery systems, as they exhibit greater stability and more sustained release of RNA particles compared to nanoparticle-based scaffolds [260]. Similar to mRNA-based therapeutics, collagen is frequently used, as it is the major organic component of bone extracellular matrix. With recent advances in 3D printing technology, specific parameters of the collagen scaffold, such as its mechanical properties, pore size, and microstructure, can be precisely modified for specific bone defect sites [266, 276]. Hyaluronic acid is frequently incorporated with collagen or hydrogel scaffolds to provide additional mechanical support [161, 260].

7.2. *Small Interfering Ribonucleic Acid*

siRNA is a short, double-stranded RNA that regulates genetic expression and protein synthesis. Similar to miR-mimics, siRNA combines with the RISC to degrade endogenous mRNA and silence gene expression. Like miRNA, it functions to downregulate gene expression [260]. siRNA is highly specific to its target mRNA due to the requirement for near-perfect sequence complementarity, and unlike miRNAs, it typically regulates only a single mRNA target. Numerous siRNAs have been discovered that silence genes inhibiting osteocyte formation or promoting osteoclast formation. For example, using siRNAs to silence S1000A4 [277] or guanine nucleotide-binding protein alpha subunit 1 (GNAS1) [278] has been shown to upregulate osteoblast formation and differentiation. Other siRNAs have been designed to silence genes involved in bone degeneration, including tumor necrosis factor-α (TNF-α) [279], RANK [280], and soluble VEGF receptor 1 (sFlt-1) [135]. Lipid-based vectors are efficacious in carrying siRNA to cells, with the most commonly used being FuGENE 6 [281] and biodegradable PEI [272]. Local delivery of siRNA to bone defect sites is commonly achieved through scaffolds made of hydrogel, collagen, or chitosan. These materials have demonstrated necessary mechanical stability to provide siRNA with sustained release and a sufficient duration of action [260]. In addition to their use in remodeling bone defect sites, siRNAs are frequently administered systemically to treat osteoporosis. For this purpose, siRNAs are combined with materials such as bisphosphonate [282], Asp oligopeptide [94], or CH6 aptamer [283], with a high affinity for hydroxyapatite and delivery to osteoporotic bone surfaces.

Although considerable progress has been made since the first use of RNA therapeutics in bone remodeling, there are several areas for discovery and improvement. First, co-delivery of RNAs would allow for simultaneous expression of desired proteins and inhibition of unwanted proteins. The effectiveness of this technique is constrained by differences in molecular weights among mRNAs, miRNAs, and siRNAs [283], as well as the relative concentrations of each RNA subtype. Second, the mechanical stability of scaffolds is a major determinant in the duration of action and efficacy of RNA therapies. Although existing research has demonstrated prolonged release of RNA and extended periods of bone remodeling *in vitro* [268, 284], limited efficacy has been demonstrated *in vivo*. Continued advances in 3D printing technology will hopefully facilitate the development of tissue and site-specific scaffolds with prolonged release of RNA products. Third, bone repair and remodeling are intricate processes with many biochemical mediators and cell signaling pathways. A greater understanding of the interactions between these genetic components will enable researchers to design targeted RNA therapies to promote bone remodeling.

7.3. *RNA Transcript-Activated Scaffolds*

RNA transcript-activated scaffolds use mRNA encoding for osteogenic GFs to enhance bone regeneration at injury sites [285]. mRNA alone is relatively unstable and is rapidly degraded. Stability and transduction efficiency of mRNA can be increased by chemically modifying the bases [286, 287]. By incorporating pseudouridine in place of uridine, transfection efficiency can be increased. Immunogenicity has been shown to decrease with modification of interferon-alpha mRNA [212]. To further enhance stability, a 5′ cap was added to the mRNA strands to decrease degradation within the cytosol [288–290]. Using mRNA over pDNA in scaffolds has some advantages. High levels of desired protein expression are achievable in nondividing or slowly dividing cells due to mRNA's ability to be translated in the cytosol of cells. This also avoids the need to be translocated into cell nuclei, which is the rate-limiting step in pDNA protein expression [285]. Some studies have also shown that mRNA transcript-activated scaffolds have superior effects on bone regeneration compared to pDNA-based scaffolds [212, 291]. One major disadvantage is the cost to chemically modify mRNA is significantly higher than those associated with the production of pDNA.

7.4. *Interfering Ribonucleic Acid-Activated Scaffolds*

These scaffolds contain interfering RNA (RNAi) that are designed to downregulate proteins at the level of posttranscriptional regulation that inhibits bone regeneration [178, 285, 292]. Some common types include miRNA, siRNA, short hairpin RNA (shRNA), and inhibitory nucleotide antagonists (antagomiRs) [293]. shRNA and siRNA target specific RNA for degradation, miRNAs affect the expression of more than one gene through various mechanisms that are dependent on cell type, and antagomiRs are complementary to miRNAs, targeting them for degradation [285, 293–295]. Proteins, such as glycogen synthase kinase-3β, that have been identified to have a negative impact on bone regeneration are targets for downregulation. A study using miRNA microspheres to inhibit this protein revealed improved bone mass and density when compared to scaffolds without miRNA. It also noted that the release speed of the microspheres affected the amount of bone regeneration that occurred, with slow-releasing scaffolds yielding superior results versus fast-releasing scaffolds. The miRNA, itself, was also found to have osteogenic effects [296]. Other studies revealed that scaffolds incorporating miRNAs that promote osteogenic differentiation vastly outperformed scaffolds using noncoding miRNA for controls [297–299]. Osteogenic differentiation was induced in *in vitro* studies, and bone regeneration was shown in *in vivo* studies within the bone defects. Targeting endogenous miRNAs that interfere with bone regeneration is another way to use inhibitory miRNAs to help promote bone formation. Studies have shown that scaffolds containing the antisense miRNA of known endogenous antiosteogenic miRNA enhance bone production and osteogenesis [300–305].

8. Conclusion

Molecular therapeutics have offered us a variety of different approaches to revolutionize bone repair. While some of the methodologies discussed earlier have been translated into clinical medicine and can be accessed today, most of these approaches have just begun to undergo investigation and will take time to optimize their methodologies. As science continues to advance, and we gain a better understanding of the molecular pathology involved in bone repair, we can expect to see new and improved therapeutic interventions to augment bone healing.

References

1. Einhorn TA, Gerstenfeld LC. Fracture healing: Mechanisms and interventions. *Nat. Rev. Rheumatol.* 2015 Jan;11:45–54.
2. Roddy E, DeBaun MR, Daoud-Gray A, Yang YP, Gardner MJ. Treatment of critical-sized bone defects: Clinical and tissue engineering perspectives. *Eur. J. Orthop. Surg. Traumatol.* 2018 Apr;28(3):351–62. https://doi.org/10.1007/s00590-017-2063-0
3. Lichte P, Pape HC, Pufe T, Kobbe P, Fischer H. Scaffolds for bone healing: Concepts, materials and evidence. *Injury.* 2011 Jun;42(6):569–73. https://doi.org/https://doi.org/10.1016/j.injury.2011.03.033
4. Migliorini F, Cuozzo F, Torsiello E, Spiezia F, Oliva F, Maffulli N. Autologous bone grafting in trauma and orthopaedic surgery: An evidence-based narrative review. *J. Clin. Med.* 2021 Sep 24;10(19):4347. https://doi.org/10.3390/jcm10194347
5. Kinaci A, Neuhaus V, Ring DC. Trends in bone graft use in the United States. *Orthopedics.* 2014 Sep;37(9):e783–8.
6. Neve A, Corrado A, Cantatore FP. Osteoblast physiology in normal and pathological conditions. *Cell Tissue Res.* 2011 Feb;343(2):289–302.

7. Ishijima M, Tsuji K, Rittling SR, Yamashita T, Kurosawa H, Denhardt DT, Nifuji A, et al. Osteopontin is required for mechanical stress-dependent signals to bone marrow cells. *J. Endocrinol.* 2007 May;193(2):235–43.
8. Gordon JAR, Tye CE, Sampaio AV, Underhill TM, Hunter GK, Goldberg HA. Bone sialoprotein expression enhances osteoblast differentiation and matrix mineralization in vitro. *Bone.* 2007 Sep;41(3):462–73.
9. Blair HC, Zaidi M, Schlesinger PH. Mechanisms balancing skeletal matrix synthesis and degradation. *Biochem. J.* 2002 Jun 1;364(Pt 2):329–41.
10. Karsenty G, Wagner EF. Reaching a genetic and molecular understanding of skeletal development. *Dev. Cell.* 2002 Apr;2(4):389–406.
11. Gerstenfeld LC, Cullinane DM, Barnes GL, Graves DT, Einhorn TA. Fracture healing as a post-natal developmental process: molecular, spatial, and temporal aspects of its regulation. *J. Cell. Biochem.* 2003 Apr 1;88(5): 873–84.
12. Safari B, Davaran S, Aghanejad A. Osteogenic potential of the growth factors and bioactive molecules in bone regeneration. *Int. J. Biol. Macromol.* 2021;175:544–557.
13. Ai-Aql ZS, Alagl AS, Graves DT, Gerstenfeld LC, Einhorn TA. Molecular mechanisms controlling bone formation during fracture healing and distraction osteogenesis. *J. Dent. Res.*2008 Feb;87(2):107–18.
14. Lin X, Patil S, Gao Y-G, Qian A. The bone extracellular matrix in bone formation and regeneration. *Front. Pharmacol.* 2020 May 26;11:757.
15. Bolander ME. Regulation of fracture repair by growth factors. *Proc. Soc. Exp. Biol. Med.* 1992 Jun;200(2):165–70.
16. Einhorn TA. The cell and molecular biology of fracture healing. *Clin. Orthop. Relat. Res.* 1998 Oct;(355 Suppl):S7–S21.
17. Schindeler, A., McDonald, M. M., Bokko, P. & Little, D. G. in *Semin. Cell Dev. Biol.* 459–466 (Elsevier).
18. Aghajanian P, Mohan S. The art of building bone: Emerging role of chondrocyte-to-osteoblast transdifferentiation in endochondral ossification. *Bone Res.* 2018;6:19. https://doi.org/10.1038/s41413-018-0021-z
19. von der Mark K, Kirsch T, Nerlich A, Kuss A, Weseloh G, Glückert K, Stöss H. Type X collagen synthesis in human osteoarthritic cartilage. Indication of chondrocyte hypertrophy. *Arthritis Rheum.* 35, 806–811.
20. Deckers MML, van Bezooijen RL, van der Horst G, Hoogendam J, van der Bent C, Papapoulos SE, et al. Bone morphogenetic proteins stimulate angiogenesis through osteoblast-derived vascular endothelial growth factor A. *Endocrinology* 2002 Apr;143(4):1545–53.

21. Kalfas IH. Principles of bone healing. *Neurosurg. Focus* 2001 Apr 15;10(4):E1.
22. Zelzer E, Glotzer DJ, Hartmann C, Thomas D, Fukai N, Soker S, et al. Tissue specific regulation of VEGF expression during bone development requires Cbfa1/Runx2. *Mech. Dev.* 2001 Aug;106(1–2):97–106.
23. Pufe T, Wildemann B, Petersen W, Mentlein R, Raschke M, Schmidmaier G. Quantitative measurement of the splice variants 120 and 164 of the angiogenic peptide vascular endothelial growth factor in the time flow of fracture healing: A study in the rat. *Cell Tissue Res.* 2002 Sep;309(3): 387–92.
24. Chen D, Zhao M, Mundy GR. Bone morphogenetic proteins. *Growth Factors.* 2004 Dec;22(4):233–41.
25. Nakase T, Yoshikawa H. Potential roles of bone morphogenetic proteins (BMPs) in skeletal repair and regeneration. *J. Bone Miner. Metab.* 2006;24(6):425–33.
26. Peng H, Usas A, Olshanski A, Ho AM, Gearhart B, Cooper GM, et al. VEGF improves, whereas sFlt1 inhibits, BMP2-induced bone formation and bone healing through modulation of angiogenesis. *J. Bone Miner. Res.* 2005 Nov;20(11):2017–27.
27. Tarkka T, Sipola A, Jämsä T, Soini Y, Ylä-Herttuala S, Tuukkanen J, et al. Adenoviral VEGF-A gene transfer induces angiogenesis and promotes bone formation in healing osseous tissues. *J. Gene Med.* 2003 Jul;5(7):560–6.
28. Väänänen HK, Horton M. The osteoclast clear zone is a specialized cell-extracellular matrix adhesion structure. *J. Cell Sci.* 1995 Aug;108(Pt 8): 2729–32.
29. Teitelbaum SL. Bone resorption by osteoclasts. *Science.* 2000 Sep 1;289(5484):1504–8.
30. Fan X, Biskobing DM, Fan D, Hofstetter W, Rubin J. Macrophage colony stimulating factor down-regulates MCSF-receptor expression and entry of progenitors into the osteoclast lineage. *J. Bone Miner. Res.* 1997 Sep;12(9): 1387–95.
31. Kong YY, Yoshida H, Sarosi I, Tan HL, Timms E, Capparelli C. et al. OPGL is a key regulator of osteoclastogenesis, lymphocyte development and lymph-node organogenesis. *Nature.* 1999 Jan 28;397(6717):315–23.
32. Blair JM, Zhou H, Seibel MJ, Dunstan CR. Mechanisms of disease: Roles of OPG, RANKL and RANK in the pathophysiology of skeletal metastasis. *Nat. Clin. Pract. Oncol.* 2006 Jan;3(1):41–49.

33. Geusens PP, Landewé RBM, Garnero P, Chen D, Dunstan CR, Lems WF, et al. The ratio of circulating osteoprotegerin to RANKL in early rheumatoid arthritis predicts later joint destruction. *Arthritis Rheum.* 2006 Jun;54(6):1772–7.
34. Tanaka S. Regulation of bone destruction in rheumatoid arthritis through RANKL-RANK pathways. *World J Orthop.* 2013 Jan 18;4(1):1–6.
35. Katagiri T, Watabe T. Bone morphogenetic proteins. *Cold Spring Harb. Perspect. Biol.* 2016 Jun 1;8(6):a021899. https://doi.org/10.1101/cshperspect.a021899
36. Schlundt C, El Khassawna T, Serra A, Dienelt A, Wendler S, Schell H, et al. Macrophages in bone fracture healing: Their essential role in endochondral ossification. *Bone.* 2018 Jan;106:78–89. https://doi.org/10.1016/j.bone.2015.10.019
37. Ai-Aql ZS, Alagl AS, Graves DT, Gerstenfeld LC, Einhorn TA. Molecular mechanisms controlling bone formation during fracture healing and distraction osteogenesis. *J. Dent. Res.* 2008 Feb;87:107–18. https://doi.org/10.1177/154405910808700215
38. Barnes GL, Kostenuik PJ, Gerstenfeld LC, Einhorn TA. Growth factor regulation of fracture repair. *J. Bone Miner. Res.* 1999 Nov;14:1805–15.
39. Gerstenfeld LC, Cho TJ, Kon T, Aizawa T, Cruceta J, Graves BD, et al. Impaired intramembranous bone formation during bone repair in the absence of tumor necrosis factor-alpha signaling. *Cells Tiss. Organs.* 2001;169(3):285–94. https://doi.org/10.1159/000047893
40. Schmid GJ, Kobayashi C, Sandell LJ, Ornitz DM. Fibroblast growth factor expression during skeletal fracture healing in mice. *Dev Dyn.* 2009 Mar;238(3):766–74. https://doi.org/https://doi.org/10.1002/dvdy.21882
41. Yun Y-R, Won JE, Jeon E, Lee S, Kang W, Jo H, et al. Fibroblast growth factors: biology, function, and application for tissue regeneration. *J. Tissue. Eng.* 2010 Nov 7;2010;218142.
42. Grimaud E, Heymann D, Rédini F. Recent advances in TGF-β effects on chondrocyte metabolism: Potential therapeutic roles of TGF-beta in cartilage disorders. *Cytokine Growth Factor Rev.* 2002 Jun;13(3):241–57. https://doi.org/https://doi.org/10.1016/S1359-6101(02)00004-7
43. Santo VE, Gomes ME, Mano JF, Reis RL. Controlled release strategies for bone, cartilage, and osteochondral engineering--Part II: Challenges on the evolution from single to multiple bioactive factor delivery. *Tissue Eng Part B Rev.* 2013 Aug;19(4);327–52. https://doi.org/10.1089/ten.teb.2012.0727

44. Melief SM, Schrama E, Brugman MH, Tiemessen MM, Hoogduijn MJ, Fibbe WE, et al. Multipotent stromal cells induce human regulatory T cells through a novel pathway involving skewing of monocytes toward anti-inflammatory macrophages. *Stem Cells.* 2013 Sep;31:1980–91. https://doi.org/10.1002/stem.1432
45. Zou S, Scarfo K, Nantz MH, Hecker JG. Lipid-mediated delivery of RNA is more efficient than delivery of DNA in non-dividing cells. *Int. J. Pharm.* 2010 Apr 15;389(1–2):232–43. https://doi.org/10.1016/j.ijpharm.2010.01.019
46. Bauer TW, Muschler GF. Bone graft materials: An overview of the basic science. *Clin. Orthop. Relat. Res.* 2000 Feb 371, 10–27.
47. Parikh SN. Bone graft substitutes: Past, present, future. *J. Postgrad. Med.* 2002;48, 142–8.
48. Pasanen K, Ekola T, Vasankari T, Kannus P, Heinonen A, Kujala UM, Parkkari J, et al. High ankle injury rate in adolescent basketball: A 3-year prospective follow-up study. *Scand. J. Med. Sci. Sports* 2017;27(6); 643–649. https://doi.org/10.1111/sms.12818
49. Zhou M, Geng YM, Li SY, Yang XB, Che YJ, Pathak J, Wu G, et al. Nanocrystalline Hydroxyapatite-Based Scaffold Adsorbs and Gives Sustained Release of Osteoinductive Growth Factor and Facilitates Bone Regeneration in Mice Ectopic Model. *J. Nanomater.* 2019;2019(1)1202159. https://doi.org/10.1155/2019/1202159
50. Ruan H, Yu Y, Guo X, Jiang Q, Luo Y. The possibility of healing alveolar bone defects with simvastatin thermosensitive gel: in vitro/in vivo evaluation. *Drug Des. Dev. Ther.* 2018;12:1997–2003. https://doi.org/10.2147/DDDT.S163986
51. March L, Smith EUR, Hoy DG, Cross MJ, Sanchez-Riera L, Blyth F, et al. Burden of disability due to musculoskeletal (MSK) disorders. *Best Pract. Res. Clin. Rheumatol.* 2014;28(3):353–66. https://doi.org/10.1016/j.berh.2014.08.002
52. Bolander J, Ji W, Leijten J, Moreira Teixeira L, Bloemen V, Lambrechts D, et al. healing of a large long-bone defect through serum-free in vitro priming of human periosteum-derived cells. *Stem Cell Rep.* 2017;8(3):758–72. https://doi.org/10.1016/j.stemcr.2017.01.005
53. Govender S, Csimma C, Genant HK, Valentin-Opran A, Amit Y, Arbel R, et al. Recombinant human bone morphogenetic protein-2 for treatment of open tibial fractures: A prospective, controlled, randomized study of four hundred and fifty patients. *J. Bone Miner. Metab.* 2002;84(12):2123–34.

54. Lyon T, Scheele W, Bhandari M, Koval KJ, Sanchez EG, Christensen J, et al. Efficacy and safety of recombinant human bone morphogenetic protein-2/calcium phosphate matrix for closed tibial diaphyseal fracture: A double-blind, randomized, controlled phase-II/III trial. *J. Bone Joint Surg.Am.* 2013;95(23):2088–96.
55. Aro HT, Govender S, Patel AD, Hernigou P, Gregorio AP, Popescu GI, et al. Recombinant human bone morphogenetic protein-2: A randomized trial in open tibial fractures treated with reamed nail fixation. *J. Bone Joint Surg.Am.* 2011;93(9):801–8.
56. Carragee EJ, Chu G, Rohatgi R, Hurwitz EL, Weiner BK, Yoon ST, Comer G, et al. Cancer risk after use of recombinant bone morphogenetic protein-2 for spinal arthrodesis. *J. Bone Joint Surg.Am.* 2013;95(17):1537–45.
57. Golish SR. Pivotal trials of orthopedic surgical devices in the United States: predominance of two-arm non-inferiority designs. *Trials* 2017;18(1):348.
58. Zara JN, Siu RK, Zhang X, Shen J, Ngo R, Lee M, et al. High doses of bone morphogenetic protein 2 induce structurally abnormal bone and inflammation in vivo. *Tissue Eng. Part A* 2011;17(9–10):1389–99. https://doi.org/10.1089/ten.TEA.2010.0555
59. Subbiah R, Guldberg RE. Materials science and design principles of growth factor delivery systems in tissue engineering and regenerative medicine. *Adv. Healthc. Mater.* 2019;8(1):e1801000.
60. Lieberman JR, Daluiski A, Einhorn TA. The role of growth factors in the repair of bone: Biology and clinical applications. *J. Bone Joint. Surg. Am.* 2002;84(6):1032–44.
61. Dimitriou R, Tsiridis E, Giannoudis PV. Current concepts of molecular aspects of bone healing. *Injury* 2005;36(12):1392–404.
62. Mountziaris PM, Mikos AG. Modulation of the inflammatory response for enhanced bone tissue regeneration. *Tissue Eng. Part B Rev.* 2008;14(2):179–86.
63. Coutu DL, Galipeau J. Roles of FGF signaling in stem cell self-renewal, senescence and aging. *Aging (Albany NY)* 2011;3(10):920–33.
64. Arvidson K, Abdallah BM, Applegate LA, Baldini N, Cenni E, Gomez-Barrena E, et al. Bone regeneration and stem cells. *J. Cell Mol. Med.* 2011;15(4):718–46. https://doi.org/10.1111/j.1582-4934.2010.01224.x
65. Kawaguchi H, Oka H, Jingushi S, Izumi T, Fukunaga M, Sato K, et al. A local application of recombinant human fibroblast growth factor 2 for tibial shaft fractures: A randomized, placebo-controlled trial. *J. Bone Miner. Res.* 2010;25(12):2735–43.

66. Kawaguchi H, Kurokawa T, Hanada K, Hiyama Y, Tamura M, Ogata E, et al. Stimulation of fracture repair by recombinant human basic fibroblast growth factor in normal and streptozotocin-diabetic rats. *Endocrinology* 1994;135(2):774–81.
67. Hannink M, Donoghue DJ. Structure and function of platelet-derived growth factor (PDGF) and related proteins. *Biochim. Biophy. Acta* 1989; 989(1):1–10.
68. Heldin CH. Structural and functional studies on platelet-derived growth factor. *EMBO J* 1992;11(12):4251–9.
69. Ozaki Y, Nishimura M, Sekiya K, Suehiro F, Kanawa M, Nikawa H, et al. Comprehensive analysis of chemotactic factors for bone marrow mesenchymal stem cells. *Stem Cells Dev.* 2007;16(1):119–29. https://doi.org/10.1089/scd.2006.0032
70. Blažević T, Schwaiberger AV, Schreiner CE, Schachner D, Schaible AM, Grojer CG, et al. 12/15-lipoxygenase contributes to platelet-derived growth factor-induced activation of signal transducer and activator of transcription 3. *J. Biol. Chem.* 2013;288(49):35592–603.
71. Kaigler D, Avila G, Wisner-Lynch L, Nevins ML, Nevins M, Rasperini G, et al. Platelet-derived growth factor applications in periodontal and peri-implant bone regeneration. *Expert Opin. Biol. Ther.* 2011;11(3):375–85.
72. Su N, Du X, Chen L. FGF signaling: Its role in bone development and human skeleton diseases. *Front Biosci.* 2008;13:2842–65.
73. Shah P, Keppler L, Rutkowski J. A review of platelet derived growth factor playing pivotal role in bone regeneration. *J. Oral Implantol.* 2014;40(3): 330–40.
74. DiGiovanni CW, Lin SS, Baumhauer JF, Daniels T, Younger A, Glazebrook M, et al. Recombinant human platelet-derived growth factor-BB and beta-tricalcium phosphate (rhPDGF-BB/β-TCP): An alternative to autogenous bone graft. *J. Bone Joint Surg. Am.* 2013;95(13):1184–92.
75. Boocock CA, Charnock-Jones DS, Sharkey AM, McLaren J, Barker PJ, Wright KA, et al. Expression of vascular endothelial growt factor and its receptors fit and KDR in ovarian carcinoma. *J. Natl. Cancer Inst.* 1995;87(7):506–16.
76. Itakura J, Ishiwata T, Shen B, Kornmann M, Korc M. Concomitant over-expression of vascular endothelial growth factor and its receptors in pancreatic cancer. *Int. J. cancer* 2000;85(1):27–34.
77. Sunderkötter C, Steinbrink K, Goebeler M, Bhardwaj R, Sorg C. Macrophages and angiogenesis. *J. Leukoc. Biol.* 1994;55(3):410–22.

78. Verheul HM, Hoekman K, Luykx-de Bakker S, Eekman CA, Folman CC, Broxterman HJ, et al. Platelet: Transporter of vascular endothelial growth factor. *Clin. Cancer Res.* 1997;3(12 Pt 1):2187–90.
79. Frank S, Hübner G, Breier G, Longaker MT, Greenhalgh DG, Werner S. Regulation of vascular endothelial growth factor expression in cultured keratinocytes: Implications for normal and impaired wound healing. *J. Biol. Chem.* 1995;270:12607–13.
80. Iijima K, Yoshikawa N, Connolly DT, Nakamura H. Human mesangial cells and peripheral blood mononuclear cells produce vascular permeability factor. *Kidney Int.* 1993;44(5):959–66.
81. Gerber HP, Vu TH, Ryan AM, Kowalski J, Werb Z, Ferrara N. VEGF couples hypertrophic cartilage remodeling, ossification and angiogenesis during endochondral bone formation. *Nat. Med.* 5(6):623–8.
82. Ferrara N, Carver-Moore K, Chen H, Dowd M, Lu L, O'Shea KS, et al. Heterozygous embryonic lethality induced by targeted inactivation of the VEGF gene. *Nature* 1996;380(6573):439–42.
83. Chintalgattu V, Nair DM, Katwa LC. Cardiac myofibroblasts: a novel source of vascular endothelial growth factor (VEGF) and its receptors Flt-1 and KDR. *J. Mol. Cell. Cardiol.* 2003;35(3):277–86.
84. Reichardt LF, Tomaselli KJ. Extracellular matrix molecules and their receptors: functions in neural development. *Annu. Rev. Neurosci.* 1991;14: 531–70.
85. Eğri S, Eczacıoğlu N. Sequential VEGF and BMP-2 releasing PLA-PEG-PLA scaffolds for bone tissue engineering: I. Design and in vitro tests. *Artif. cells Nanomed. Biotechnol.* 45(2):321–9.
86. Street J, Winter D, Wang JH, Wakai A, McGuinness A, Redmond HP. Is human fracture hematoma inherently angiogenic? *Clin. Orthop. Relat. Res.* 224–37. https://doi.org/10.1097/00003086-200009000-00033
87. Ukai, T., Shiraishi, C., Moriyama, H., Yoshimoto, M. & Hara, Y. in *Bone.* S155–S155 (ELSEVIER SCIENCE INC 360 PARK AVE SOUTH, NEW YORK, NY 10010-1710 USA).
88. Brancato SK, Albina JE. Wound macrophages as key regulators of repair: Origin, phenotype, and function. *Am. J. Pathol.* 2011;178(1):19–25. https://doi.org/10.1016/j.ajpath.2010.08.003
89. Zelzer E, McLean W, Ng YS, Fukai N, Reginato AM, Lovejoy S, et al. Skeletal defects in VEGF(120/120) mice reveal multiple roles for VEGF in skeletogenesis. *Development* 2002;129(8):1893–904. https://doi.org/10.1242/dev.129.8.1893

90. Maes C, Kobayashi T, Selig MK, Torrekens S, Roth SI, Mackem S, et al. Osteoblast precursors, but not mature osteoblasts, move into developing and fractured bones along with invading blood vessels. *Dev. Cell* 2010;19: 329–44. https://doi.org/10.1016/j.devcel.2010.07.010
91. Street J, Winter D, Wang JH, Wakai A, McGuinness A, Redmond HP. Is human fracture hematoma inherently angiogenic? *Clin. Orthop. Relat. Res.* 2000;378:224–37.
92. Pérez-Gutiérrez L, Ferrara N. Biology and therapeutic targeting of vascular endothelial growth factor A. *Nat. Rev. Mol. Cell Biol.* 2023;24(11):816–34. Epub 20230725. https://doi.org/10.1038/s41580-023-00631-w. PubMed PMID: 37491579
93. Daigang L, Jining Q, Jinlai L, Pengfei W, Chuan S, Liangku H, et al. LPS-stimulated inflammation inhibits BMP-9-induced osteoblastic differentiation through crosstalk between BMP/MAPK and Smad signaling. *Exp. Cell Res.* 2016;341(1):54–60. https://doi.org/https://doi.org/10.1016/j.yexcr.2016.01.009
94. Wang D, Miller SC, Shlyakhtenko LS, Portillo AM, Liu X-M, Papangkorn K, et al. Osteotropic Peptide that differentiates functional domains of the skeleton. *Bioconjug. Chem.* 2007;18(5):1375–8. https://doi.org/10.1021/bc7002132
95. Schindeler A, Little DG. Ras-MAPK signaling in osteogenic differentiation: friend or foe? *J Bone Miner. Res.* 2006;21(9):1331–8. https://doi.org/10.1359/jbmr.060603
96. Zhang Y, Xu J, Ruan YC, Yu MK, O'Laughlin M, Wise H, et al. Implant-derived magnesium induces local neuronal production of CGRP to improve bone-fracture healing in rats. *Nat. Med.* 2016;22(10):1160–9. https://doi.org/10.1038/nm.4162
97. Matsui T, Amano M, Yamamoto T, Chihara K, Nakafuku M, Ito M, et al. Rho-associated kinase, a novel serine/threonine kinase, as a putative target for small GTP binding protein Rho. *EMBO J.* 1996;15(9):2208–16. https://doi.org/https://doi.org/10.1002/j.1460-2075.1996.tb00574.x
98. Gong Y, Liu Y-R, Ji P, Hu X, Shao Z-M. Impact of molecular subtypes on metastatic breast cancer patients: A SEER population-based study. *Sci. rep.* 2017;**7**:45411. https://doi.org/10.1038/srep45411
99. Barradas AMC, Yuan H, van Blitterswijk CA, Habibovic P. Osteoinductive biomaterials: current knowledge of properties, experimental models and biological mechanisms. *Eur. Cell Mater.* 2011;21:407–29; discussion 429. https://doi.org/10.22203/ecm.v021a31

100. Oh B-C. Phosphoinositides and intracellular calcium signaling: Novel insights into phosphoinositides and calcium coupling as negative regulators of cellular signaling. *Exp. Mol. Med.* 2023;55(8):1702–12. Epub 20230801. https://doi.org/10.1038/s12276-023-01067-0. PubMed PMID: 37524877; PMCID: PMC10474053.
101. Shaker JL, Deftos L. Calcium and phosphate homeostasis. *Endotext +Internet]*. 2018.
102. Zhu S, Chen W, Masson A, Li Y-P. Cell signaling and transcriptional regulation of osteoblast lineage commitment, differentiation, bone formation, and homeostasis. *Cell Discov.* 2024;10(1):71. Epub 20240702. https://doi.org/10.1038/s41421-024-00689-6. PubMed PMID: 38956429; PMCID: PMC11219878.
103. Silva BC, Costa AG, Cusano NE, Kousteni S, Bilezikian JP. Catabolic and anabolic actions of parathyroid hormone on the skeleton. *J. Endocrinol. Invest.* 2011;34(10):801–10Epub 20110923. https://doi.org/10.3275/7925. PubMed PMID: 21946081; PMCID: PMC4315330.
104. Capriani C, Irani D, Bilezikian JP. Safety of osteoanabolic therapy: A decade of experience. *J. Bone Miner. Res.* 2012;27(12):2419–28.
105. Makino A, Takagi H, Takahashi Y, Hase N, Sugiyama H, Yamana K, et al. Abaloparatide exerts bone anabolic effects with less stimulation of bone resorption-related factors: A comparison with teriparatide. *Calcif. Tissue Int.* 2018;103:289–97.
106. Ricarte FR, Le Henaff C, Kolupaeva VG, Gardella TJ, Partridge NC. Parathyroid hormone (1–34) and its analogs differentially modulate osteoblastic Rankl expression via PKA/SIK2/SIK3 and PP1/PP2A-CRTC3 signaling. *J. Biol. Chem.* 2018;293(52):20200–13.
107. Aspenberg P, Genant HK, Johansson T, Nino AJ, See K, Krohn K, et al. Teriparatide for acceleration of fracture repair in humans: A prospective, randomized, double-blind study of 102 postmenopausal women with distal radial fractures. *J. Bone Miner. Res.* 2010;25(2):404–14.
108. Huang J, Lin D, Wei Z, Li Q, Zheng J, Zheng Q, et al. Parathyroid hormone derivative with reduced osteoclastic activity promoted bone regeneration via synergistic bone remodeling and angiogenesis. *Small* 2020;16(6):e1905876.
109. Ning Z, Tan B, Chen B, Lau DS, Wong TM, Sun T, et al. Precisely controlled delivery of abaloparatide through injectable hydrogel to promote bone regeneration. *Macromol. Biosci.* 2019;19(6):e1900020.
110. Smy L, Straseski JA. Measuring estrogens in women, men, and children: Recent advances 2012–2017. *Clin. Biochem.* 2018;62:11–23. Epub 20180522.

https://doi.org/10.1016/j.clinbiochem.2018.05.014. PubMed PMID: 29800559.

111. Cauley JA. Estrogen and bone health in men and women. *Steroids.* 2015;99(Pt A):11–5. Epub 20141230. https://doi.org/10.1016/j.steroids.2014.12.010. PubMed PMID: 25555470.
112. Ji M-X, Yu Q. Primary osteoporosis in postmenopausal women. *Chronic dis. Transl. Med.* 2015;1(1):9–13.
113. Kim H-N, Ponte F, Nookaew I, Ucer Ozgurel S, Marques-Carvalho A, Iyer S, et al. Estrogens decrease osteoclast number by attenuating mitochondria oxidative phosphorylation and ATP production in early osteoclast precursors. *Sci. Rep.* 2020;10(1):11933. Epub 20200720. https://doi.org/10.1038/s41598-020-68890-7. PubMed PMID: 32686739; PMCID: PMC7371870.
114. Foessl I, Dimai HP, Obermayer-Pietsch B. Long-term and sequential treatment for osteoporosis. *Nat. Rev. Endocrinol.* 2023;19(9):520–33. Epub 20230718. https://doi.org/10.1038/s41574-023-00866-9. PubMed PMID: 37464088.
115. Chen X, Zhu X, Hu Y, Yuan W, Qiu X, Jiang T, et al. EDTA-modified 17β-estradiol-laden upconversion nanocomposite for bone-targeted hormone replacement therapy for osteoporosis. *Theranostics* 2020;10(7): 3281–92.
116. Segredo-Morales E, Reyes R, Arnau MR, Delgado A, Évora C. In situ gel-forming system for dual BMP-2 and 17β-estradiol controlled release for bone regeneration in osteoporotic rats. *Drug deliv. Transl. Res.* 2018;8(5): 1103–1113.
117. Guntur AR, Rosen CJ. IGF-1 regulation of key signaling pathways in bone. *Bonekey rep.* 2013;2:437.
118. Locatelli V, Bianchi VE. Effect of GH/IGF-1 on bone metabolism and osteoporsosis. *Int. J. Endocrinol.* 2014;2014:235060.
119. Serna J, Bergwitz C. Importance of dietary phosphorus for bone metabolism and healthy aging. *Nutrients* 2020;12(10):3001.
120. Barake M, Arabi A, Nakhoul N, El-Hajj Fuleihan G, El Ghandour S, Klibanski A, et al. Effects of growth hormone therapy on bone density and fracture risk in age-related osteoporosis in the absence of growth hormone deficiency: A systematic review and meta-analysis. *Endocrine* 2018; 59(1):39–49.
121. Gillberg P, Mallmin H, Petrén-Mallmin M, Ljunghall S, Nilsson AG. Two years of treatment with recombinant human growth hormone increases

bone mineral density in men with idiopathic osteoporosis. *J. Clin. Endocrinol. Metab.* 2002;87(11):4900–6.
122. Underwood JL, DeLuca HF. Vitamin D is not directly necessary for bone growth and mineralization. *Am. J. Physiol.* 1984;246(6):E493–8 (1984). https://doi.org/10.1152/ajpendo.1984.246.6.E493
123. van den Bergh JPW, Bours SPG, van Geel TACM,Geusens PP. Optimal use of vitamin D when treating osteoporosis. *Curr. Osteoporos. Rep.* 2011;9(1): 36–42.
124. Suda T, Ueno Y, Fujii K, Shinki T. Vitamin D and bone. *J. Cell Biochem.* 2003;88(2):259–66. https://doi.org/10.1002/jcb.10331
125. Bouillon R, Manousaki D, Rosen C, Trajanoska K, Rivadeneira F, Richards JB. The health effects of vitamin D supplementation: Evidence from human studies. *Nat. Rev. Endocrinol.* 2022;18(2):96–110. Epub 20211123. https://doi.org/10.1038/s41574-021-00593-z. PubMed PMID: 34815552; PMCID: PMC8609267.
126. Majidinia M, Sadeghpour A, Yousefi B. The roles of signaling pathways in bone repair and regeneration. *J. Cell. Physiol.* 2018;233(4):2937–48.
127. Rossini M, Gatti D, Adami S. Involvement of WNT/β-catenin signaling in the treatment of osteoporosis. *Calcif. Tissue Int.* 2013;93(2):121–32.
128. Diegel CR, Kramer I, Moes C, Foxa GE, McDonald MJ, Madaj ZB, et al. Inhibiting WNT secretion reduces high bone mass caused by Sost loss-of-function or gain-of-function mutations in Lrp5. *Bone Res.* 2023;11(1):47. Epub 20230824. https://doi.org/10.1038/s41413-023-00278-5. PubMed PMID: 37612291; PMCID: PMC10447437.
129. Fabre S, Funck-Brentano T, Cohen-Solal M. Anti-sclerostin antibodies in osteoporosis and other bone diseases. *J. clin. med.* 2020;9(11):3439.
130. Zhu F, Sweetwyne MT, Hankenson KD. PKCδ is required for Jagged-1 induction of human mesenchymal stem cell osteogenic differentiation. *Stem Cells* 2013;31(6):1181–92.
131. Wang C, Inzana JA, Mirando AJ, Ren Y, Liu Z, Shen J, et al. NOTCH signaling in skeletal progenitors is critical for fracture repair. *J. Clin. Invest.* 2016;126(4):1471–81.
132. Novak S, Roeder E, Sinder BP, Adams DJ, Siebel CW, Grcevic D, et al. Modulation of Notch1 signaling regulates bone fracture healing. *J. Orthop. Res.* 38(11):2350–61. https://doi.org/10.1002/jor.24650
133. Ji Y, Ke Y, Gao S. Intermittent activation of notch signaling promotes bone formation. *Am. J. Transl. Res.* 2017;9(6):2933–2944.

134. Ho-Shui-Ling A, Bolander J, Rustom LE, Wagoner Johnson A, Luyten FP, Picart C. Bone regeneration strategies: Engineered scaffolds, bioactive molecules and stem cells current stage and future perspectives. *Biomaterials* 2018;180:143–62. https://doi.org/10.1016/j.biomaterials.2018.07.017
135. Zuo B, Zhu J, Li J, Wang C, Zhao X, Cai G, et al. microRNA-103a functions as a mechanosensitive microRNA to inhibit bone formation through targeting Runx2. *J Bone Miner Res.* 2015;30:330–345. https://doi.org/10.1002/jbmr.2352
136. Greco SJ, Liu K, Rameshwar P. Functional similarities among genes regulated by OCT4 in human mesenchymal and embryonic stem cells. *Stem Cells* 2007;25(12):3143–54. https://doi.org/10.1634/stemcells.2007-0351
137. Krebsbach PH, Kuznetsov SA, Bianco P, Robey PG. Bone marrow stromal cells: characterization and clinical application. *Crit. Rev. Oral Biol. Med.* 1999;10:165–81. https://doi.org/10.1177/10454411990100020401
138. Jeyaraman M, Bingi SK, Muthu S, Jeyaraman N, Packkyarathinam RP, Ranjan R, et al. Impact of the process variables on the yield of mesenchymal stromal cells from bone marrow aspirate concentrate. *Bioeng.* 2022;9(2):57. Epub 20220129. https://doi.org/10.3390/bioengineering9020057. PubMed PMID: 35200410; PMCID: PMC8869489.
139. Weng Z, Wang Y, Ouchi T, Liu H, Qiao X, Wu C, et al. Mesenchymal stem/stromal cell senescence: Hallmarks, mechanisms, and combating strategies. *Stem Cells Transl. Med.* 2022;11(4):356–71. https://doi.org/10.1093/stcltm/szac004. PubMed PMID: 35485439; PMCID: PMC9052415.
140. Minieri V, Saviozzi S, Gambarotta G, Lo Iacono M, Accomasso L, Cibrario Rocchietti E, et al. Persistent DNA damage-induced premature senescence alters the functional features of human bone marrow mesenchymal stem cells. *J. Cell Mol. Med.* 2015;19(4):734–43. https://doi.org/10.1111/jcmm.12387
141. Colnot C, Huang S, Helms J. Analyzing the cellular contribution of bone marrow to fracture healing using bone marrow transplantation in mice. *Biochem. Biophys. Res. Commun.* 2006;350(3):557–61. https://doi.org/10.1016/j.bbrc.2006.09.079
142. Tsuji W, Rubin JP, Marra KG. Adipose-derived stem cells: Implications in tissue regeneration. *World J. Stem Cells* 2014;6(3):312–21. https://doi.org/10.4252/wjsc.v6.i3.312
143. Aust L, Devlin B, Foster SJ, Halvorsen YDC, Hicok K, du Laney T, et al. Yield of human adipose-derived adult stem cells from liposuction aspirates. *Cytotherapy* 2004;6(1):7–14. https://doi.org/10.1080/14653240310004539

144. Cui L, Yin S, Liu W, Li N, Zhang W, Cao Y. Expanded adipose-derived stem cells suppress mixed lymphocyte reaction by secretion of prostaglandin E2. *Tissue Eng.* 2007;13(6):1185–95. https://doi.org/10.1089/ten.2006.0315
145. McIntosh KR, Lopez MJ, Borneman JN, Spencer ND, Anderson PA, Gimble JM. Immunogenicity of allogeneic adipose-derived stem cells in a rat spinal fusion model. *Tissue Eng. Part A* 2009;15(9):2677–86. https://doi.org/10.1089/ten.TEA.2008.0566
146. Cowan CM, Shi YY, Aalami OO, Chou YF, Mari C, Thomas R, et al. Adipose-derived adult stromal cells heal critical-size mouse calvarial defects. *Nat. Biotechnol.* 2004;22(5):560–67. https://doi.org/10.1038/nbt958
147. Lee CS, Burnsed OA, Raghuram V, Kalisvaart J, Boyan BD, Schwartz Z. Adipose stem cells can secrete angiogenic factors that inhibit hyaline cartilage regeneration. *Stem Cell Res. Ther.* 2012;3(4):35. https://doi.org/10.1186/scrt126
148. Melis S, Trompet D, Chagin AS, Maes C. Skeletal stem and progenitor cells in bone physiology, ageing and disease. *Nat. Rev. Endocrinol.* 2025;21(3):135–53. Epub 20241008. https://doi.org/10.1038/s41574-024-01039-y. PubMed PMID: 39379711.
149. De Bari C, Dell'Accio F, Vanlauwe J, Eyckmans J, Khan IM, Archer CW, et al. Mesenchymal multipotency of adult human periosteal cells demonstrated by single-cell lineage analysis. *Arthritis Rheum* 54(4):1209–21. https://doi.org/10.1002/art.21753
150. Friedmann T. A brief history of gene therapy. *Nat. Genet.* 1992;2(2):93–8 (1992).
151. Friedmann T, Roblin R. Gene therapy for human genetic disease? Proposals for genetic manipulation in humans raise difficult scientific and ethical problems. *Science* 1972;175(4025):949–55.
152. De la Vega RE, Atasoy-Zeybek A, Panos JA, Van Griensven M, Evans CH, Balmayor ER. Gene therapy for bone healing: Lessons learned and new approaches. *Transl. Res.* 2021;236:1–16. https://doi.org/10.1016/j.trsl.2021.04.009
153. Gottlieb S, M.D. (ed Food and Drug Administration). U.S. Food and Drug Administration, 2019.
154. Sampath TK, Vukicevic S. Biology of bone morphogenetic protein in bone repair and regeneration: A role for autologous blood coagulum as carrier. *Bone* 2020;141:115602. https://doi.org/10.1016/j.bone.2020.115602

155. James AW, LaChaud G, Shen J, Asatrian G, Nguyen V, Zhang X, et al. A review of the clinical side effects of bone morphogenetic protein-2. *Tissue Eng. Part B Rev* 2016;22(4):284–97.
156. Tannoury CA, An HS. Complications with the use of bone morphogenetic protein 2 (BMP-2) in spine surgery. *Spine J.* 2014;14(3):552–9.
157. Woo EJ. Adverse events reported after the use of recombinant human bone morphogenetic protein 2. *J. Oral Maxillofac. Surg.* 2012;70(4):765–7.
158. Carragee EJ, Hurwitz EL, Weiner BK. A critical review of recombinant human bone morphogenetic protein-2 trials in spinal surgery: Emerging safety concerns and lessons learned. *Spine J.* 2011;11(6):471–91.
159. Mroz TE, Wang JC, Hashimoto R, Norvell DC. Complications related to osteobiologics use in spine surgery: A systematic review. *Spine* 2010;35(9 Suppl):S86–104.
160. Zara JN, Siu RK, Zhang X, Shen J, Ngo R, Lee M, et al. High doses of bone morphogenetic protein 2 induce structurally abnormal bone and inflammation in vivo. *Tissue Eng Part A* 2011;17(9–10):1389–99.
161. Laird NZ, Acri TM, Tingle K, Salem AK. Gene- and RNAi-activated scaffolds for bone tissue engineering: Current progress and future directions. *Adv. Drug Deliv. Rev.* 2021;174:613–27. https://doi.org/10.1016/j.addr.2021.05.009
162. Evans C. Gene therapy for the regeneration of bone. *Injury* 2011;42(6):599–604.
163. Ishihara A, Bertone AL. Cell-mediated and direct gene therapy for bone regeneration. *Expert Opin. Biol. Ther.* 2012;12(4):411–23.
164. Evans CH, Huard J. Gene therapy approaches to regenerating the musculoskeletal system. *Nat. Rev. Rheumatol* 2015;11(4):234–42.
165. Elangovan S, Gajendrareddy P, Ravindran S, Salem AK. Emerging local delivery strategies to enhance bone regeneration. *Biomed. Mater.* 2020;15(6):062001.
166. Park J, Lutz R, Felszeghy E, Wiltfang J, Nkenke E, Neukam FW, et al. The effect on bone regeneration of a liposomal vector to deliver BMP-2 gene to bone grafts in peri-implant bone defects. *Biomaterials* 2007;28(17):2772–82.
167. Moghimi SM, Symonds P, Murray JC, Hunter AC, Debska G, Szewczyk A. A two-stage poly(ethylenimine)-mediated cytotoxicity: Implications for gene transfer/therapy. *Mol. Ther.* 2005;11(6):990–95.
168. Fischer J, Kolk A, Wolfart S, Pautke C, Warnke PH, Plank C, et al. Future of local bone regeneration-protein versus gene therapy. *J. Craniomaxillofac. Surg.* 2011;39(1):54–64.

169. Evans CH, Liu FJ, Glatt V, Hoyland JA, Kirker-Head C, Walsh A, et al. Use of genetically modified muscle and fat grafts to repair defects in bone and cartilage. *Eur. Cell Mater.* 2009;18:96–111.
170. Dimitriou R, Jones E, McGonagle D, Giannoudis PV. Bone regeneration: Current concepts and future directions. *BMC Med.* 2011;9:66. https://doi.org/10.1186/1741-7015-9-66
171. Park S-Y, Kim K-H, Kim S, Lee Y-M, Seol Y-J. BMP-2 gene delivery-based bone regeneration in dentistry. *Pharmaceutics* 2019;11(8):393. https://doi.org/10.3390/pharmaceutics11080393
172. Evans CH, Robbins PD, Ghivizzani SC, Wasko MC, Tomaino MM, Kang R, et al. Gene transfer to human joints: Progress toward a gene therapy of arthritis. *Proc. Natl. Acad. Sci. USA.* 2005;102(24):8698–703.
173. Lungwitz U, Breunig M, Blunk T, Göpferich A. Polyethylenimine-based non-viral gene delivery systems. *Eur. J. Pharm. Biopharm.* 2005;60(2):247–66. https://doi.org/10.1016/j.ejpb.2004.11.011
174. Shapiro G, Lieber R, Gazit D, Pelled G. Recent advances and future of gene therapy for bone regeneration. *Curr. Osteoporos. Rep.* 2018;16(4): 504–11.
175. Kimelman-Bleich N, Pelled G, Zilberman Y, Kallai I, Mizrahi O, Tawackoli W, et al. Targeted gene-and-host progenitor cell therapy for nonunion bone fracture repair. *Mol. Ther.* 2011;19(1):53–9.
176. Bez M, Sheyn D, Tawackoli W, Avalos P, Shapiro G, Giaconi JC, et al. In situ bone tissue engineering via ultrasound-mediated gene delivery to endogenous progenitor cells in mini-pigs. *Sci. Transl. Med.* 2017;9(390): eaal3128.
177. Patil S, Gao Y-G, Lin X, Li Y, Dang K, Tian Y, et al. The development of functional non-viral vectors for gene delivery. *Int. J. Mol. Sci.* 2019;20(21): 5491.
178. Yin H, Kanasty RL, Eltoukhy AA, Vegas AJ, Dorkin JR, Anderson DG. Non-viral vectors for gene-based therapy. *Nat. Rev. Genet.* 2014;15(8): 541–55.
179. Hall A, Lächelt U, Bartek J, Wagner E, Moghimi SM. Polyplex evolution: Understanding biology, optimizing performance. *Mol. Ther.* 2017;25(7): 1476–90.
180. Tierney EG, Duffy GP, Hibbitts AJ, Cryan S-A, O'Brien FJ. The development of non-viral gene-activated matrices for bone regeneration using polyethyleneimine (PEI) and collagen-based scaffolds. *J. Control Release* 2012;158(2):304–11.

181. Shtykalova S, Deviatkin D, Freund S, Egorova A, Kiselev A. Non-viral carriers for nucleic acids delivery: Fundamentals and current applications. *Life.* 2023;13(4):903. Epub 20230329. https://doi.org/10.3390/life13040903. PubMed PMID: 37109432; PMCID: PMC10142071.
182. Lv H, Zhang S, Wang B, Cui S, Yan J. Toxicity of cationic lipids and cationic polymers in gene delivery. *J Control Release* 2006;114(1):100–9.
183. Kawai M, Bessho K, Maruyama H, Miyazaki JI, Yamamoto T. Human BMP-2 gene transfer using transcutaneous in vivo electroporation induced both intramembranous and endochondral ossification. *Anat. Rec. A. Discov. Mol. Cell Evol. Biol.* 2005;287(2):1264–71.
184. Sheyn D, Kimelman-Bleich N, Pelled G, Zilberman Y, Gazit D, Gazit Z. Ultrasound-based nonviral gene delivery induces bone formation in vivo. *Gene. Ther.* 2008;15(4):257–66.
185. Shapiro G, Wong AW, Bez M, Yang F, Tam S, Even L., et al. Multiparameter evaluation of in vivo gene delivery using ultrasound-guided, microbubble-enhanced sonoporation. *J. Control Release* 2016;223:157–64.
186. Osawa K, Okubo Y, Nakao K, Koyama N, Bessho K. Osteoinduction by microbubble-enhanced transcutaneous sonoporation of human bone morphogenetic protein-2. *J. Gene. Med.* 2009;11(7):633–41.
187. Feichtinger GA, Hofmann AT, Slezak P, Schuetzenberger S, Kaipel M, Schwartz E, et al. Sonoporation increases therapeutic efficacy of inducible and constitutive BMP2/7 in vivo gene delivery. *Hum. Gene. Ther. Methods* 2014;25(1):57–71.
188. Wilson CG, Martín-Saavedra FM, Padilla F, Fabiilli ML, Zhang M, Baez AM, et al. Patterning expression of regenerative growth factors using high intensity focused ultrasound. *Tissue Eng. Part C Methods* 2014;20(10): 769–79.
189. Qiao C, Zhang K, Jin H, Miao L, Shi C, Liu X, et al. Using poly(lactic-co-glycolic acid) microspheres to encapsulate plasmid of bone morphogenetic protein 2/polyethylenimine nanoparticles to promote bone formation in vitro and in vivo. *Int. J. Nanomedicine* 2013;8:2985–95.
190. Kaur H, Uludağ H, El-Bialy T. Effect of nonviral plasmid delivered basic fibroblast growth factor and low intensity pulsed ultrasound on mandibular condylar growth: A preliminary study. *Biomed. Res. Int.* 2014;2014:426710.
191. Ginn SL, Alexander IE, Edelstein ML, Abedi MR, Wixon J. Gene therapy clinical trials worldwide to 2012-an update. *J. Gene. Med.* 2013;15(2): 65–77. https://doi.org/10.1002/jgm.2698

192. Flotte T. Gene therapy progress and prospects: Recombinant adeno-associated virus (rAAV) vectors. *Gene. Ther.* 2004;11(10):805–10.
193. Montini E, Cesana D, Schmidt M, Sanvito F, Ponzoni M, Bartholomae C, et al. Hematopoietic stem cell gene transfer in a tumor-prone mouse model uncovers low genotoxicity of lentiviral vector integration. *Nat. Biotechnol* 2006;24(6):687–96.
194. Guan M, Rodriguez-Madoz JR, Alzuguren P, Gomar C, Kramer MG, Kochanek S, et al. Increased efficacy and safety in the treatment of experimental liver cancer with a novel adenovirus-alphavirus hybrid vector. *Cancer Res.* 2006;66(3):1620–29.
195. Pol J, Kroemer G, Galluzzi L. First oncolytic virus approved for melanoma immunotherapy. *Oncoimmunology* 2016;5(1):e1115641.
196. Crystal RG. Adenovirus: The first effective in vivo gene delivery vector. *Hum. Gene. Ther.* 2014;25(1):3–11.
197. Kimelman N, Pelled G, Helm GA, Huard J, Schwarz EM, Gazit D. Gene- and stem cell–based therapeutics for bone regeneration and repair. *Tissue Eng.* 2007;13(6):1135–50.
198. Baltzer AW, Lattermann C, Whalen JD, Wooley P, Weiss K, Grimm M, et al. Genetic enhancement of fracture repair: Healing of an experimental segmental defect by adenoviral transfer of the BMP-2 gene. *Gene. Ther.* 2000;7(9):734–9.
199. Betz OB, Betz VM, Nazarian A, Egermann M, Gerstenfeld LC, Einhorn TA, et al. Delayed administration of adenoviral BMP-2 vector improves the formation of bone in osseous defects. *Gene. Ther.* 2007;14(13):1039–44.
200. Southwood LL, Frisbie DD, Kawcak CE, Ghivizzani SC, Evans CH, McIlwraith CW. Evaluation of Ad-BMP-2 for enhancing fracture healing in an infected defect fracture rabbit model. *J. Orthop. Res.* 2004;22(1):66–72.
201. Laurent JJ, Webb KM, Beres EJ, McGee K, Li J, van Rietbergen B, et al. The use of bone morphogenetic protein-6 gene therapy for percutaneous spinal fusion in rabbits. *J. Neurosurg. Spine* 2004;1(1):90–4.
202. Raper SE, Chirmule N, Lee FS, Wivel NA, Bagg A, Gao G-P, et al. Fatal systemic inflammatory response syndrome in a ornithine transcarbamylase deficient patient following adenoviral gene transfer. *Mol. Genet. Metab.* 2003;80(1–2):148–58.
203. Chen Y, Luk DK, Cheung KM, Lu WW, An XM, Ng SS, et al. Combination of adeno-associated virus and adenovirus vectors expressing bone

morphogenetic protein-2 produces enhanced osteogenic activity in immunocompetent rats. *Biochem. Biophys. Res. Commun.* 2004;317(3):675–81.
204. Gafni Y, Pelled G, Zilberman Y, Turgeman G, Apparailly F, Yotvat H, et al. Gene therapy platform for bone regeneration using an exogenously regulated, AAV-2-based gene expression system. *Mol. Ther.* 2004;9(4):587–95.
205. Dyer O. Covid-19: Remdesivir has little or no impact on survival, WHO trial shows. *BMJ* 2020;371:m4057.
206. Strohbach CA, Rundle CH, Wergedal JE, Chen ST, Linkhart TA, Lau K-HW, et al. LMP-1 retroviral gene therapy influences osteoblast differentiation and fracture repair: A preliminary study. *Calcif. Tissue Int.* 2008; 83(3):202–11.
207. Hacein-Bey-Abina S, Garrigue A, Wang GP, Soulier J, Lim A, Morillon E., et al. Insertional oncogenesis in 4 patients after retrovirus-mediated gene therapy of SCID-X1. *J. Clin. Invest.* 2008;118(9):3132–42.
208. Bushman FD. Retroviral insertional mutagenesis in humans: Evidence for four genetic mechanisms promoting expansion of cell clones. *Mol. Ther.* 2020;28(2):352–56. https://doi.org/10.1016/j.ymthe.2019.12.009
209. Ferreira AM, Gentile P, Chiono V, Ciardelli G. Collagen for bone tissue regeneration. *Acta. Biomater.* 2012;8(9):3191–200.
210. Dong C, Lv Y. Application of collagen scaffold in tissue engineering: Recent advances and new perspectives. *Polymers* 2016;8(2):42.
211. Li Z, Du T, Ruan C, Niu X. Bioinspired mineralized collagen scaffolds for bone tissue engineering. *Bioact. Mater.* 2021;6(5):1491–511.
212. Elangovan S, Khorsand B, Do AV, Hong L, Dewerth A, Kormann M, et al. Chemically modified RNA activated matrices enhance bone regeneration. *J. Control Release* 2015;218:22–8.
213. Engler AJ, Sen S, Sweeney HL, Discher DE. Matrix elasticity directs stem cell lineage specification. *Cell* 2006;126(4):677–89.
214. Elangovan S, D'Mello SR, Hong L, Ross RD, Allamargot C, Dawson DV, et al. The enhancement of bone regeneration by gene activated matrix encoding for platelet derived growth factor. *Biomaterials* 2014;35(2):737–47.
215. Heo DN, Hospodiuk M, Ozbolat IT. Synergistic interplay between human MSCs and HUVECs in 3D spheroids laden in collagen/fibrin hydrogels for bone tissue engineering. *Acta. Biomater* 2019;95:348–56.
216. Shrestha A, Allen BN, Wiley LA, Tucker BA, Worthington KS. Development of high-resolution three-dimensional-printed extracellular matrix scaffolds and their compatibility with pluripotent stem cells and early retinal cells. *J. Ocul. Pharmacol. Ther.* 2020;36(1):42–55.

217. Acri TM, Laird NZ, Jaidev LR, Meyerholz DK, Salem AK, Shin K. Nonviral gene delivery embedded in biomimetically mineralized matrices for bone tissue engineering. *Tissue Eng. Part A* 2021;27(15–16): 1074–83.
218. Akkineni AR, Luo Y, Schumacher M, Nies B, Lode A, Gelinsky M. 3D plotting of growth factor loaded calcium phosphate cement scaffolds. *Acta. Biomater.* 2015;27:264–74.
219. Levingstone TJ, Herbaj S, Dunne NJ. Calcium phosphate nanoparticles for therapeutic applications in bone regeneration. *Nanomaterials* 2019;9(11): 1570.
220. Shih Y-RV, Hwang Y, Phadke A, Kang H, Hwang NS, Caro EJ, et al. Calcium phosphate-bearing matrices induce osteogenic differentiation of stem cells through adenosine signaling. *Proc. Natl. Acad. Sci. USA* 2014; 111(3):990–5.
221. De Witte T-M, Fratila-Apachitei LE, Zadpoor AA, Peppas NA. Bone tissue engineering via growth factor delivery: From scaffolds to complex matrices. *Regen. Biomater.* 2018;5(4):197–211.
222. Mouriño V, Boccaccini AR. Bone tissue engineering therapeutics: Controlled drug delivery in three-dimensional scaffolds. *J. R. Soc. Interface* 2010;7(43):209–27.
223. Ahrlund-Richter L, De Luca M, Marshak DR, Munsie M, Veiga A, Rao M. Isolation and production of cells suitable for human therapy: Challenges ahead. *Cell Stem Cell* 2009;4(1):20–6.
224. Benjaminsen RV, Mattebjerg MA, Henriksen JR, Moghimi SM, Andresen TL. The possible "proton sponge" effect of polyethylenimine (PEI) does not include change in lysosomal pH. *Mol. Ther.* 2013;21(1):149–57.
225. Cohen RN, van der Aa MAEM, Macaraeg N, Lee AP, Szoka FC Jr. Quantification of plasmid DNA copies in the nucleus after lipoplex and polyplex transfection. *J. Control Release* 2009;135(2):166–74.
226. Grandinetti G, Reineke TM. Exploring the mechanism of plasmid DNA nuclear internalization with polymer-based vehicles. *Mol. Pharm.* 2012;9(8):2256–67.
227. Khorsand B, Nicholson N, Do AV, Femino JE, Martin JA, Petersen E, et al. Regeneration of bone using nanoplex delivery of FGF-2 and BMP-2 genes in diaphyseal long bone radial defects in a diabetic rabbit model. *J. Control Release* 2017;248:53–59.
228. Raftery RM, Castaño IM, Chen G, Cavanagh B, Quinn B, Curtin CM, et al. Translating the role of osteogenic-angiogenic coupling in bone

formation: Highly efficient chitosan-pDNA activated scaffolds can accelerate bone regeneration in critical-sized bone defects. *Biomaterials* 2017;149: 116–27.

229. D'Mello SR, Elangovan S, Hong L, Ross RD, Sumner DR, Salem AK. A pilot study evaluating combinatorial and simultaneous delivery of polyethylenimine-plasmid DNA complexes encoding for VEGF and PDGF for bone regeneration in calvarial bone defects. *Curr. Pharm. Biotechnol* 2015;16(7):655–60.
230. D'Mello S, Elangovan S, Salem AK. FGF2 gene activated matrices promote proliferation of bone marrow stromal cells. *Arch. Oral. Biol.* 2015; 60(12):1742–9.
231. Malek-Khatabi A, Javar HA, Dashtimoghadam E, Ansari S, Hasani-Sadrabadi MM, Moshaverinia A. In situ bone tissue engineering using gene delivery nanocomplexes. *Acta. Biomater* 2020;108:326–36.
232. Martino MM, Maruyama K, Kuhn GA, Satoh T, Takeuchi O, Müller R, et al. Inhibition of IL-1R1/MyD88 signalling promotes mesenchymal stem cell-driven tissue regeneration. *Nat. Commun.* 2016;7:11051.
233. Sun G, Wang Y, Ti Y, Wang J, Zhao J, Qian H. Regulatory B cell is critical in bone union process through suppressing proinflammatory cytokines and stimulating Foxp3 in Treg cells. *Clin. Exp. Pharmacol. Physiol.* 2017; 44(4):455–62.
234. Claes L, Recknagel S, Ignatius A. Fracture healing under healthy and inflammatory conditions. *Nat. Rev. Rheumatol.* 2012;8(3):133–43.
235. Raftery RM, Walsh DP, Ferreras LB, Castaño IM, Chen G, LeMoine M, et al. Highly versatile cell-penetrating peptide loaded scaffold for efficient and localised gene delivery to multiple cell types: From development to application in tissue engineering. *Biomaterials* 2019;216:119277.
236. Bozo IY, Drobyshev AY, Redko NA, Komlev VS, Isaev AA, Deev RV. Bringing a gene-activated bone substitute into clinical practice: From bench to bedside. *Front. Bioeng. Biotechnol.* 2021;9:599300. https://doi.org/10.3389/fbioe.2021.599300
237. Liang Z, Luo Y, Lv Y. Mesenchymal stem cell-derived microvesicles mediate BMP2 gene delivery and enhance bone regeneration. *J. Mater. Chem. B* 2020;8(30):6378–89.
238. Nomikou N, Feichtinger GA, Saha S, Nuernberger S, Heimel P, Redl H, et al. Ultrasound-responsive gene-activated matrices for osteogenic gene therapy using matrix-assisted sonoporation. *J Tissue Eng. Regen. Med.* 2018;12(1):e250–60.

239. Arealis G, Nikolaou VS. Bone printing: New frontiers in the treatment of bone defects. *Injury* 2015;46(Suppl 8):S20–2.
240. Campos DFD, Blaeser A, Buellesbach K, Sen KS, Xun W, Tillmann W, et al. Bioprinting organotypic hydrogels with improved mesenchymal stem cell remodeling and mineralization properties for bone tissue engineering. *Adv. Healthc. Mater.* 2016;5(11):1336–45.
241. Bozo IY, Deev RV, Smirnov IV, Fedotov AY, Popov VK, Mironov AV, et al. 3D printed gene-activated octacalcium phosphate implants for large bone defects engineering. *Int. J. Bioprint.* 2020;6(3):275.
242. Robinson M, Schor S, Barouch-Bentov R, Einav S. Viral journeys on the intracellular highways. *Cell Mol. Life Sci.* 2018;75(20):3693–714.
243. Medina-Kauwe LK, Xie J, Hamm-Alvarez S. Intracellular trafficking of nonviral vectors. *Gene. Ther.* 2005;12(24):1734–51.
244. Mingozzi F, High KA. Immune responses to AAV vectors: Overcoming barriers to successful gene therapy. *Blood* 2013;122(1):23–36.
245. Zhang Y, Ma Y, Wu C, Miron RJ, Cheng X. Platelet-derived growth factor BB gene-released scaffolds: Biosynthesis and characterization. *J. Tissue Eng. Regen. Med.* 2016;10(10):E372–81.
246. Zhang Y, Wu C, Luo T, Li S, Cheng X, Miron RJ. Synthesis and inflammatory response of a novel silk fibroin scaffold containing BMP7 adenovirus for bone regeneration. *Bone* 2012;51(4):704–13.
247. Zhang Y, Miron RJ, Li S, Shi B, Sculean A, Cheng X. Novel mesoporous bioglass/silk scaffold containing adPDGF-B and adBMP7 for the repair of periodontal defects in beagle dogs. *J. Clin. Periodontol.* 2015;42(3): 262–71.
248. Xue J, Lin H, Bean A, Tang Y, Tan J, Tuan RS, et al. One-step fabrication of bone morphogenetic protein-2 gene-activated porous poly-L-lactide scaffold for bone induction. *Mol. Ther. Methods Clin. Dev.* 2017;**7**:50–9.
249. Rowland CR, Glass KA, Ettyreddy AR, Gloss CC, Matthews JRL, Huynh NPT, et al. Regulation of decellularized tissue remodeling via scaffold-mediated lentiviral delivery in anatomically-shaped osteochondral constructs. *Biomaterials* 2018;177:161–75.
250. Hu WW, Wang Z, Krebsbach PH. Virus immobilization on biomaterial scaffolds through biotin--avidin interaction for improving bone regeneration. *J. Tissue Eng. Regen. Med.* 2016;10(2):E63–72.
251. Zhang Y, Huang J, Wang C, Zhang Y, Hu C, Li G, et al. Application of HIF-1α by gene therapy enhances angiogenesis and osteogenesis in alveolar bone defect regeneration. *J. Gene. Med.* 2016;18(4–6):57–64.

252. Koç A, Finkenzeller G, Elçin AE, Stark GB, Elçin YM. Evaluation of adenoviral vascular endothelial growth factor-activated chitosan/hydroxyapatite scaffold for engineering vascularized bone tissue using human osteoblasts: In vitro and in vivo studies. *J. Biomater. Appl.* 2014; 29(5):748–60.
253. Logeart-Avramoglou D, Bourguignon M, Oudina K, Ten Dijke P, Petite H. An assay for the determination of biologically active bone morphogenetic proteins using cells transfected with an inhibitor of differentiation promoter-luciferase construct. *Anal Biochem* 2006;349(1):78–86.
254. Turgeman G, Pittman DD, Müller R, Kurkalli BG, Zhou S, Pelled G, et al. Engineered human mesenchymal stem cells: A novel platform for skeletal cell mediated gene therapy. *J. Gene. Med.* 2001;3(3):240–51.
255. Wang Y, Huso DL, Harrington J, Kellner J, Jeong DK, Turney J, et al. Outgrowth of a transformed cell population derived from normal human BM mesenchymal stem cell culture. *Cytotherapy* 2005;7(6):509–19.
256. Schuldiner M, Itskovitz-Eldor J, Benvenisty N. Selective ablation of human embryonic stem cells expressing a “suicide” gene. *Stem Cells* 2003;21(3): 257–65.
257. Choo AB, Tan HL, Ang SN, Fong WJ, Chin A, Lo J, et al. Selection against undifferentiated human embryonic stem cells by a cytotoxic antibody recognizing podocalyxin-like protein-1. *Stem Cells* 2008;26(6):1454–63.
258. Seebach C, Henrich D, Tewksbury R, Wilhelm K, Marzi I. Number and proliferative capacity of human mesenchymal stem cells are modulated positively in multiple trauma patients and negatively in atrophic nonunions. *Calcif. Tissue Int.* 2007;80(4):294–300.
259. Siegel G, Kluba T, Hermanutz-Klein U, Bieback K, Northoff H, Schäfer R. Phenotype, donor age and gender affect function of human bone marrow-derived mesenchymal stromal cells. *BMC Med.* 2013;11:146.
260. Leng Q, Chen L, Lv Y. RNA-based scaffolds for bone regeneration: Application and mechanisms of mRNA, miRNA and siRNA. *Theranostics* 2020;10(7):3190–205. https://doi.org/10.7150/thno.42640
261. Petsch B, Schnee M, Vogel AB, Lange E, Hoffmann B, Voss D, et al. Protective efficacy of in vitro synthesized, specific mRNA vaccines against influenza A virus infection. *Nat. Biotechnol.* 2012;30(12):1210–6. https://doi.org/10.1038/nbt.2436
262. Elangovan S, Khorsand B, Do AV, Hong L, Dewerth A, Kormann M, et al. Chemically modified RNA activated matrices enhance bone regeneration. *J. Control. Release* 2015;218:22–8. https://doi.org/10.1016/j.jconrel.2015.09.050

263. Yamamoto A, Kormann M, Rosenecker J, Rudolph C. Current prospects for mRNA gene delivery. *Eur. J. Pharm. Biopharm.* 2009;71(3):484–9. https://doi.org/10.1016/j.ejpb.2008.09.016
264. Awasthi S, Hook LM, Pardi N, Wang F, Myles A, Cancro MP, et al. Nucleoside-modified mRNA encoding HSV-2 glycoproteins C, D, and E prevents clinical and subclinical genital herpes. *Sci. Immunol* 2019;4(39): eaaw7083. https://doi.org/10.1126/sciimmunol.aaw7083
265. Khorsand B, Elangovan S, Hong L, Dewerth A, Kormann MSD, Salem AK. A comparative study of the bone regenerative effect of chemically modified RNA encoding BMP-2 or BMP-9. *AAPS J* 2017;19(2):438–46. https://doi.org/10.1208/s12248-016-0034-8
266. Zhang W, De La Vega RE, Coenen MJ, Müller SA, Peniche Silva CJ, Aneja MK. An improved, chemically modified RNA encoding BMP-2 enhances osteogenesis in vitro and in vivo. *Tissue Eng. Part A* 2019;25(1–2):131–44. https://doi.org/10.1089/ten.TEA.2018.0112
267. Kaczmarek JC, Patel AK, Kauffman KJ, Fenton OS, Webber MJ, Heartlein MW, et al. Polymer-lipid nanoparticles for systemic delivery of mRNA to the lungs. *Angew. Chem. Int. Ed. Engl.* 2016;55(44):13808–12. https://doi.org/10.1002/anie.201608450
268. Badieyan ZS, Berezhanskyy T, Utzinger M, Aneja MK, Emrich D, Erben R, et al. Transcript-activated collagen matrix as sustained mRNA delivery system for bone regeneration. *J. Control. Release* 2016;239:137–48. https://doi.org/10.1016/j.jconrel.2016.08.037
269. Curtin CM, Castaño IM, O'Brien FJ. Scaffold-based microRNA therapies in regenerative medicine and cancer. *Adv. Healthc. Mater.* 2018;7(1):1700695. https://doi.org/10.1002/adhm.201700695
270. Liao Y-H, Chang Y-H, Sung L-Y, Li K-C, Yeh C-L, Yen T-C, et al. Osteogenic differentiation of adipose-derived stem cells and calvarial defect repair using baculovirus-mediated co-expression of BMP-2 and miR-148b. *Biomaterials* 2014;35(18):4901–10. https://doi.org/10.1016/j.biomaterials.2014.02.055
271. Xie Q, Ma A, Jiang J, Cheng Z, Song D, Yuan YC, et al. Stress corrosion cracking behavior of fine-grained AZ61 magnesium alloys processed by equal-channel angular pressing. *Metals* 2017;7(9):343.
272. Xie Q, Wei W, Ruan J, Ding Y, Zhuang A, Bi X, et al. Effects of miR-146a on the osteogenesis of adipose-derived mesenchymal stem cells and bone regeneration. *Sci. Rep.* 2017;7(1):42840. https://doi.org/10.1038/srep42840
273. Huang S, Wang S, Bian C, Yang Z, Zhou H, Zeng Y, et al. Upregulation of miR-22 promotes osteogenic differentiation and inhibits adipogenic

differentiation of human adipose tissue-derived mesenchymal stem cells by repressing HDAC6 protein expression. *Stem Cells Dev.* 2012;21(13): 2531–40. https://doi.org/10.1089/scd.2012.0014

274. Kureel J, John AA, Dixit M, Singh D. MicroRNA-467g inhibits new bone regeneration by targeting Ihh/Runx-2 signaling. *Int. J. Biochem. Cell Biol* 2017;85:35–43. https://doi.org/10.1016/j.biocel.2017.01.018
275. Xie Q, Wang Z, Zhou H, Yu Z, Huang Y, Sun H, et al. The role of miR-135-modified adipose-derived mesenchymal stem cells in bone regeneration. *Biomaterials.* 2016;75:279–94. Epub 20151021. https://doi.org/10.1016/j.biomaterials.2015.10.042. PubMed PMID: 26513420.
276. Aldaadaa A, Owji N, Knowles J. Three-dimensional printing in maxillofacial surgery: Hype versus reality. *J. Tissue Eng.* 2018;9:2041731418770909. https://doi.org/10.1177/2041731418770909
277. Kato C, Kojima T, Komaki M, Mimori K, Duarte WR, Takenaga K, et al. S100A4 inhibition by RNAi up-regulates osteoblast related genes in periodontal ligament cells. *Biochem. Biophys. Res. Commun.* 2005;326(1):147–53. https://doi.org/10.1016/j.bbrc.2004.11.010
278. Cheema SK, Chen E, Shea LD, Mathur AB. Regulation and guidance of cell behavior for tissue regeneration via the siRNA mechanism. *Wound Repair Regen.* 2007;15(3):286–95. https://doi.org/10.1111/j.1524-475X.2007.00228.x
279. Guo HH, Yu CC, Sun SX, Ma XJ, Yang XC, Sun KN, et al. Adenovirus-mediated siRNA targeting TNF-α and overexpression of bone morphogenetic protein-2 promotes early osteoblast differentiation on a cell model of Ti particle-induced inflammatory response in vitro. *Braz. J. Med. Biol. Res.* 2013;46(10):831–8. https://doi.org/10.1590/1414-431x20133092
280. Sezlev Bilecen D, Uludag H, Hasirci V. Development of PEI-RANK siRNA complex loaded PLGA nanocapsules for the treatment of osteoporosis. *Tissue Eng. Part A.* 2019;25(1–2):34–43. https://doi.org/10.1089/ten.TEA.2017.0476
281. Selinger CI, Day CJ, Morrison NA. Optimized transfection of diced siRNA into mature primary human osteoclasts: Inhibition of cathepsin K mediated bone resorption by siRNA. *J. Cell Biochem.* 2005;96(5):996–1002. https://doi.org/10.1002/jcb.20575
282. Giger EV, Castagner B, Räikkönen J, Mönkkönen J, Leroux J-C. siRNA transfection with calcium phosphate nanoparticles stabilized with PEGylated chelators. *Adv. Healthc. Mater.* 2013;2(1):134–44. https://doi.org/10.1002/adhm.201200088

283. Liang C, Guo B, Wu H, Shao N, Li D, Liu J, et al. Aptamer-functionalized lipid nanoparticles targeting osteoblasts as a novel RNA interference-based bone anabolic strategy. *Nat. Med.* 2015;21(3):288–94. https://doi.org/10.1038/nm.3791
284. Wang Y, Tran KK, Shen H, Grainger DW. Selective local delivery of RANK siRNA to bone phagocytes using bone augmentation biomaterials. *Biomaterials.* 2012;33(33):8540–7. https://doi.org/10.1016/j.biomaterials.2012.07.039
285. Leng Q, Chen L, Lv Y. RNA-based scaffolds for bone regeneration: Application and mechanisms of mRNA, miRNA and siRNA. *Theranostics.* 2020; 10(7):3190–205.
286. Karikó K, Buckstein M, Ni H, Weissman D. Suppression of RNA recognition by Toll-like receptors: The impact of nucleoside modification and the evolutionary origin of RNA. *Immunity* 2005;23(2):165–75.
287. Kormann MSD, Hasenpusch G, Aneja MK, Nica G, Flemmer AW, Herber-Jonat S, et al. Expression of therapeutic proteins after delivery of chemically modified mRNA in mice. *Nat. Biotechnol.* 2011;29(2):154–7.
288. Stepinski J, Waddell C, Stolarski R, Darzynkiewicz E, Rhoads RE. Synthesis and properties of mRNAs containing the novel "anti-reverse" cap analogs 7-methyl (3′-O-methyl) GpppG and 7-methyl (3′-deoxy) GpppG. *RNA.* 2001;7(10):1486–95.
289. Vaidyanathan S, Azizian KT, Haque AKMA, Henderson JM, Hendel A, Shore S, et al. Uridine depletion and chemical modification increase Cas9 mRNA activity and reduce immunogenicity without HPLC purification. *Mol. Ther. Nucleic. Acids.* 2018;12:530–42.
290. Guo P, Moss B. Interaction and mutual stabilization of the two subunits of vaccinia virus mRNA capping enzyme coexpressed in Escherichia coli. *Proc. Natl. Acad. Sci. USA.* 1990;87(11):4023–7.
291. Khorsand B, Elangovan S, Hong L, Kormann MSD, Salem AK. A bioactive collagen membrane that enhances bone regeneration. *J. Biomed. Mater. Res. Part B Appl. Biomater.* 2019;107(6):1824–32.
292. Curtin CM, Castaño IM, O'Brien FJ. Scaffold-based microRNA therapies in regenerative medicine and cancer. *Adv. Healthc. Mater.* 2018;7(1): 1700695.
293. Setten RL, Rossi JJ, Han S-P. The current state and future directions of RNAi-based therapeutics. *Nat. Rev. Drug Discov.* 2019;18(6):421–46.
294. Pritchard CC, Cheng HH, Tewari M. MicroRNA profiling: Approaches and considerations. *Nat. Rev. Genet.* 2012;13(5):358–69.

295. Krützfeldt J, Rajewsky N, Braich R, Rajeev KG, Tuschl T, Manoharan M, et al. Silencing of microRNAs in vivo with 'antagomirs'. *Nature.* 2005;438(7068):685–9.
296. Zhang X, Li Y, Chen YE, Chen J, Ma PX. Cell-free 3D scaffold with two-stage delivery of miRNA-26a to regenerate critical-sized bone defects. *Nat. Commun.* 2016;7:10376.
297. Mei Y, Bian C, Li J, Du Z, Zhou H, Yang Z, et al. miR-21 modulates the ERK--MAPK signaling pathway by regulating SPRY2 expression during human mesenchymal stem cell differentiation. *J. Cell Biochem.* 2013; 114(6):1374–84.
298. Meng Y, Liu C, Zhao J, Li X, Li Z, Wang J, et al. An injectable miRNA-activated matrix for effective bone regeneration: In vivo. *J Mater Chem B.* 2016;4:6942–54.
299. Meng Y-B, Li X, Li Z-Y, Zhao J, Yuan X-B, Ren Y, et al. microRNA-21 promotes osteogenic differentiation of mesenchymal stem cells by the PI3K/β-catenin pathway. *J. Orthop. Res.* 2015;33(7):957–64.
300. James EN, Van Doren E, Li C, Kaplan DL. Silk biomaterials-mediated miRNA functionalized orthopedic devices. *Tissue Eng. Part A.* 2019; 25(1–2):12–23.
301. Liu J, Li D, Dang L, Liang C, Guo B, Lu, et al. Osteoclastic miR-214 targets TRAF3 to contribute to osteolytic bone metastasis of breast cancer. *Sci Rep.* 2017;7:40487.
302. Wang X, Guo B, Li Q, Peng J, Yang Z, Wang A, et al. miR-214 targets ATF4 to inhibit bone formation. *Nat Med.* 2013;19(1):93–100.
303. Liao XB, Zhang ZY, Yuan K, Liu Y, Feng X, Cui RR, et al. MiR-133a modulates osteogenic differentiation of vascular smooth muscle cells. *Endocrinology* 2013;154(9):3344–52.
304. Li Z, Hassan MQ, Volinia S, van Wijnen AJ, Stein JL, Croce CM, et al. A microRNA signature for a BMP2-induced osteoblast lineage commitment program. *Proc. Natl. Acad. Sci. USA.* 2008;105(37):13906–11.
305. Mencía Castaño I, Curtin CM, Duffy GP, O'Brien FJ. Next generation bone tissue engineering: Non-viral miR-133a inhibition using collagen-nanohydroxyapatite scaffolds rapidly enhances osteogenesis. *Sci. Rep.* 2016;6:27941.
306. Hanratty BM, Ryaby JT, Pan X-H, Li G. Thrombin related peptide TP508 promoted fracture repair in a mouse high energy fracture model. *J. Orthop. Surg. Res.*2009;4:1.

307. Cakarer S, Olgac V, Aksakalli N, Tang A, Keskin C. Acceleration of consolidation period by thrombin peptide 508 in tibial distraction osteogenesis in rats. *Br. J. Oral Maxillofac. Surg.* 2010;48(8):633–6.
308. Hedberg EL, Kroese-Deutman HC, Shih CK, Crowther RS, Carney DH, Mikos AG, et al. Effect of varied release kinetics of the osteogenic thrombin peptide TP508 from biodegradable, polymeric scaffolds on bone formation in vivo. *J. Biomed. Mater. Res. A* 2005;72(4):343–53.
309. Leskelä H, Risteli J, Niskanen S, Koivunen J, Ivaska KK, Lehenkari P. Osteoblast recruitment from stem cells does not decrease by age at late adulthood. *Biochem. Biophys. Res. Commun.* 2003;311(4):1008–13.
310. Golombek S, Pilz M, Steinle H, Kochba E, Levin Y, Lunter D, et al. Intradermal delivery of synthetic mRNA using hollow microneedles for efficient and rapid production of exogenous proteins in skin. *Mol. Ther. Nucleic. Acids* 2018;11:382–92. https://doi.org/10.1016/j.omtn.2018.03.005
311. Zhao D, Huang S, Lu F, Wang B, Yang L, Qin L, et al. Vascularized bone grafting fixed by biodegradable magnesium screw for treating osteonecrosis of the femoral head. *Biomaterials* 2016;81:84–92. https://doi.org/10.1016/j.biomaterials.2015.11.038

https://doi.org/10.1142/9789819819645_0004

Chapter 4

Scaffolds, Grafts, and Coatings

Maryam Tajabadi[1,*], Hamideh Barghamadi[2], Zahra Pakdaman Lahiji[2], Elnaz Momeninasab[2]

[1]*School of Metallurgy and Materials Engineering, Iran University of Science and Technology (IUST), Narmak, Tehran 16844, Iran*
[2]*Department of Medical Engineering, South Tehran Branch, Islamic Azad University, Tehran 15847/43311, Iran*

Chapter Outline

* **Corresponding author:** School of Metallurgy and Materials Engineering, Iran University of Science and Technology (IUST), Narmak, Tehran 16844, Iran. E-mail: mtajabadi@iust.ac.ir

Abstract

Physiological functions, such as controlling calcium levels, and mechanical support provided by bone make it an essential connective tissue. Collagen is the principal structural component of bone, whereas calcium-containing minerals, such as hydroxyapatite, further mechanically support the bone matrix. The blood vessels create a three-dimensional network by vertically infiltrating the dense layers of bone *via* Haversian systems. Natural bone regeneration occurs in minor fractures, but not in severely injured ones. Healing is influenced by injury site size and angiogenesis, which determine the repaired tissue properties. Messenger factors, including cytokines, morphogens, growth factors, and angiogenic factors, are present during the process of bone tissue repair. Present methods in this important area of reconstructive surgery make use of biomaterials, autografts, allografts, or xenografts. Each approach has its own set of pros and cons. Bone autograft containing natural blood vessels, for instance, is the gold standard for fixing bone abnormalities, but recent synthetic-based scaffolds may speed up the healing process and even restore missing tissue. Scaffold materials, including metal, ceramic, polymer, and biofunctionalized materials, are crucial for cell and tissue development, nutrient penetration, and transport. The surface properties of these materials significantly impact cell interaction, affecting cell adhesion, growth, proliferation, and differentiation. The three-dimensional structure also significantly influences the quality of the newly created tissue. In light of the above, this chapter begins with a brief overview of the several grafts used in bone regeneration before moving on to describe the many scaffolds used in bone tissue engineering and weighing in on the pros and cons of each. Following this, and since the surface features of the materials have a significant impact on cellular activity, is a discussion of the various methods and kinds of coatings used for scaffolding surfaces.

Graphical Abstract

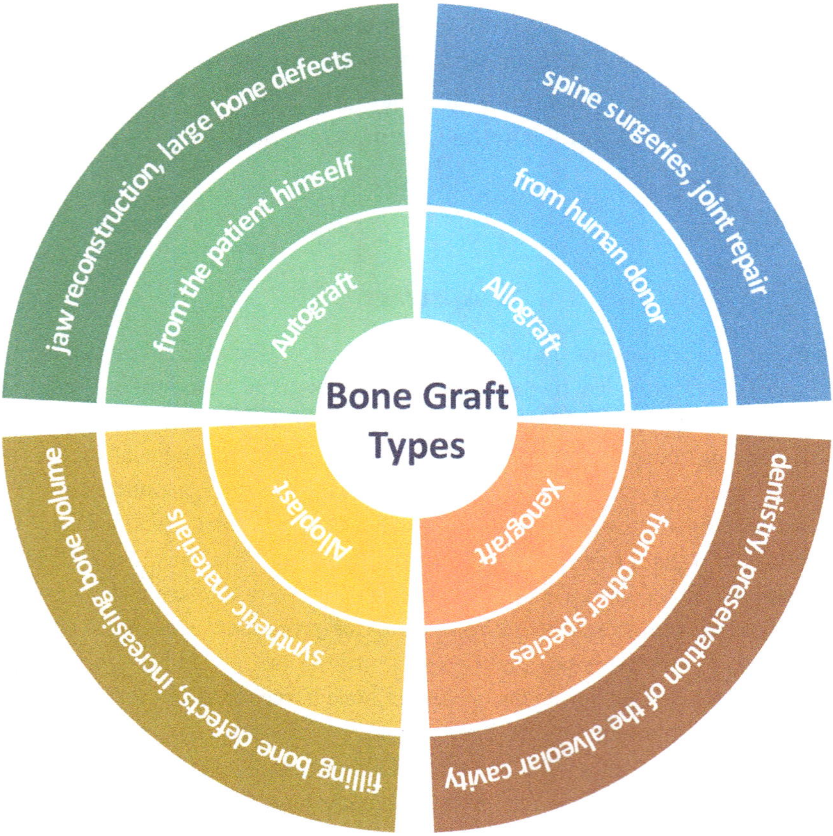

1. Introduction

Osseous tissue is a connective tissue that plays a crucial role in various bodily functions, including locomotion, support for soft tissues, and storage of important minerals such as calcium and phosphate. It also serves as a reservoir for bone marrow. Biomechanically, the nanoscale arrangement of the components that make up bone — collagen type I (30%) and hydroxyapatite (HA) (70%) — makes it a very strong material. Bone production involves two phases: (i) osteoblasts synthesize and secrete unmineralized osteoid, followed by (ii) mineralization of the osteoid matrix, incorporation of calcium and phosphate ions to produce HA crystals, and stiffening of the bone tissue. The mechanical qualities of trabecular and cortical bone are in part, determined by the degree of biomineralization [1, 2]. With the frequency of orthopedic-related injuries and diseases on the rise, there is an increasing demand for appropriate surgical rehabilitation. For more than a century, medical professionals have been using bone grafting to encourage the formation of new bone in regions that have suffered damage and the creation of defects. In significant injury cases, and presently, more than 2.2 million grafts are required annually to regenerate bone tissue [3]. Bone grafting is a surgical treatment approach that involves transferring bone fragments or synthetic bone substitute materials into a recipient site, promoting regeneration at the injury site. It supports the integration of the patient's osseous cells with the transplanted material and can be made from the patient's own bone (autogenic), donor bone (allogeneic or xenogenic), or through the use of synthetic biomaterials (alloplastic scaffolds) [4]. Bone grafts are used to treat many bone injuries, including fractures (caused by traumatic accidents, falls, or gunshot wounds), fracture nonunions, arthritis, bone infections, and congenital diseases (such as rickets). The role of a bone graft during treatment is to provide a scaffold onto which new bone grows, thereby regenerating, strengthening, and protecting the damaged bone structure [5]. An autograft, allograft, xenograft, or alloplastic scaffold should ideally possess osteoinductive properties (directly facilitating osteogenesis), osteoconductive characteristics, and promote osteointegration within the native bone tissue architecture [6]. Its mechanical strength, pore size, porosity, and chemical composition are among the variables that affect the success rate of a grafted material. The choice of grafting method depends on the patient's condition and the type of injury [7].

Limitations in graft supply, an adverse immune response, and the requirement for an additional procedure to source autograft are some disadvantages of this traditional treatment. Potential new avenues for repairing fractured bone include tissue engineering and regenerative medicine approaches. Bone tissue engineering (BTE) is an innovative method that uses scaffolds, which aim to provide an ideal three-dimensional environment to promote cell proliferation and differentiation, to repair bone tissue by augmenting osteogenesis and boosting angiogenesis, thereby mimicking the natural bone environment. The capacity to support loads, and an optimal surface topology, pore size, and rigidity are all desirable qualities in a scaffold [8, 9]. Using a porous scaffold allows for cell-to-cell communication, cell movement, new cell growth, vascularization-mediated nutrient and oxygen exchange, and waste product removal. In the field of tissue engineering, two predominant methodologies have emerged for the creation of scaffolds. The first involves the use of synthetic scaffolds, which are constructed from various biomaterials. The second approach utilizes biological scaffolds, which are derived from tissues obtained from either allogenic or xenogeneic sources.

Cellular–molecular interactions with scaffolds are of paramount importance in the processes of tissue regeneration and repair. Scholarly research has shown that the use of bioactive compounds and nanostructured materials has promise for enhancing the recruitment and differentiation of osteoprogenitor cells. This intervention has the potential to provide therapeutic benefits in both laboratory and animal research contexts. Within this specific field, it is conventional to employ scaffolds in conjunction with growth factors (GFs) and stem cells (SCs). Regulatory signals, such as peptide motifs, play a crucial role in the preservation of tissue shape and function. By meticulous manipulation of these signals, scientists can gain control over certain medicinal treatments or regeneration processes. Another potential strategy for augmenting cellular interactions with scaffolds is the use of nanofillers. Nanofillers, such as silver or HA nanoparticles, can increase the mechanical strength and stability of scaffolds by increasing their surface area, which in turn improves cellular adhesion, proliferation, and differentiation, leading to improved results [10, 11]. In a nutshell, materials that replicate the natural environment and functionality of human bone are the most suitable for producing bone scaffolds. The selection of fabrication methods, such as additive manufacturing, can significantly influence the response of cells to scaffolds [12]. To comprehensively cover these topics, the following sections will discuss bone grafts, scaffolds, and coatings from the perspective of material type, modification, and fabrication methods.

2. Bone Grafts

2.1. *Autologous Bone Graft*

A patient's own bone graft, *autograft*, when implanted into a bony defect, either alone or in conjunction with other biomaterials, can promote bone repair. Autograft is the preferred type of bone graft in orthopedic and dental medicine due to its ability to stimulate bone growth, its compatibility with the body's natural processes, and its effectiveness in repairing larger defects [13]. In the United States, over 200,000 autologous bone grafts are performed annually. In China, autologous bone grafting is the most common surgical technique in orthopedics. The quantity and quality of cortical, cancellous, and corticocancellous bone tissue may be restored *via* several bone-graft choices, including vascularized and non-vascularized varieties, which are further divided into categories based on the applicable bone type [14]. Contrary to the structural support provided by cortical grafts, the use of cancellous grafts is largely limited to compressive resistance [15]. Cancellous grafts are excellent because they promote and stimulate bone growth, whereas corticocancellous grafts strike a satisfactory compromise between bioactivity and mechanical strength. Larger defects or areas with poor blood flow need vascularized grafts. Furthermore, autografts are much more successful when used in composite form for certain procedures, such as ligament replacement and joint repair [16]. For a bone graft to incorporate, a robust osteogenic response is required from the locally situated osteoprogenitor cells, GFs, and connective tissue matrix, together with a scaffold that possesses osteoinductive and/or osteoconductive properties. As mentioned, autograft is crucial for bone regeneration, as living cells, such as osteoblasts and osteoprogenitor cells, are present and can aid in the process of new bone production, that is, its osteogenic ability determines its efficacy [17, 18]. Besides, autograft acts as a physical template for the development of new bone during regeneration due to its osteoconductive properties [19]. Furthermore, autograft has bone-inducing properties that contain GFs such as bone morphogenetic proteins (BMPs) that can stimulate the differentiation of progenitor cells into osteoblasts and further strengthen bone formation [18, 20]. The autograft, with its living cells and blood vessels, promotes vascularization and can effortlessly incorporate into the surrounding tissue, minimizing the risk of immune system rejection and other complications [21].

When selecting an area of bone to serve as a graft donor, clinicians consider the bone defect location, patient position during surgery, and the required amount of graft material. Autografts collected from different anatomical locations can be used for reconstruction of the skull vault, the lower jaw, and other orthopedic applications. The most common donor sites used are the dorsal crest of the ilium, the proximal humerus, and the proximal tibia. These sections can serve as templates to guide surgery, shape implants, or produce the grafted bone stock [22]. In dentistry, and due to the limited amount of bone available, and thus the need to use additional techniques, this treatment method is only used in special cases such as in jaw reconstruction and to repair congenital bone defects, tumors, and bone fracture repair [23]. As mentioned earlier, autologous cancellous grafts are considered optimal for use in bone transplantation and in filling osseous defects where mechanical support is not required. They contain osteoblasts, mesenchymal stem cells (MSCs), BMPs, and GFs, providing an excellent scaffold for vascular ingrowth and infiltration of osteoblastic cells, making them often used as a supplementary treatment. The structure can reach strengths similar to cortical bone graft after 6 months to 1-year post-implantation [24].

The induced membrane (Masquelet) method is a surgical technique that uses cancellous autograft chips to treat necrotic or infected bone tissue defects, where it reduces graft resorption and promotes local bone revascularization and corticalization. The harvesting process includes creating a small incision, drilling a hole, and using a bone curette to remove the graft. Ensuring a proper match between the size of the curette and the drill with the donor bone is crucial to avoid any potential complications at the donor site. It is important to promptly pack the harvested graft into the recipient site, although it can be temporarily stored in a blood-soaked sponge if needed. Alternatively, frozen cancellous allograft can be used, which has demonstrated successful outcomes and is readily accessible on the market [25]. Free vascularized fibular bone grafts (FVFGs) are microsurgical procedures that replace dead bone with healthy, structurally robust bone from a patient's fibula. Their efficacy is remarkable in the treatment of larger defects (>6 cm) that have proven difficult for other grafts to bridge. FVFGs provide a practical solution for repairing segmental diaphyseal defect lesions caused by primary or metastatic disease, thereby avoiding the need for amputation and the associated life-threatening risks involved when undergoing surgery [26]. FVFGs are also used to manage avascular necrosis of the femoral head, unsuccessful spinal fusions, and complex arthrodesis. Due to a robust blood supply, FVFGs are highly effective, even in cases where the recipient site has poor vascularity. With over 600 publications available on PubMed (2025), FVFGs are one of the most widely utilized types of bone transplants due to their unique anatomical characteristics, dependability, and flexibility [27].

The skeleton is a complicated organ containing nerve fibers that communicate with skeletal cells. The peripheral nerve terminals, which release neurogenic factors and detect skeletal signals, mediate bone metabolism and skeletal pain [28]. The effects of the neurological system on bone healing have recently been the center of attention in bone regeneration studies. These studies have demonstrated that both material-driven approaches and the use of biologically enhanced neurogenic repair signals can stimulate effective bone regeneration and nerve regeneration [29–31]. New insights into the role of the central nervous system in regulating bone homeostasis and skeletal interoception provide promising avenues for biomaterial advancement. Autograft donor sites often include sensory nerves (SNs), which enhance the above-mentioned features [32]. However, a complex and technically challenging surgical technique is required to repair motor and mixed nerves. Achieving appropriate alignment and orientation of the autograft is essential to ensure optimal reconstruction, as misalignment can lead to poor functional outcomes [33]. Also, to fill the nerve gap, the autograft must have sufficient length and diameter and provide a suitable environment for axon regeneration. In addition, scar tissue and a lack of vascularization at the repair site may prevent nerve regeneration when using autograft [33, 34].

As a result of their improved osteogenic, osteoinductive, and osteoconductive qualities, autografts continue to be the preferred option for spinal arthrodesis; however, there are some drawbacks. Acute and chronic donor-site pain is a major issue, affecting a substantial number of patients, especially those undergoing iliac crest bone grafts. Alternative sources such as rib and fibula transplants have specific concerns, including subsequent muscular weakness and respiratory complications. The donor site selected must be customized to the patient's specific needs, weighing the advantages of autograft against the risk of donor-site complications. Innovative reconstruction strategies, such as infusing an allograft cancellous expander into the osseous cavity, backfilling the harvest site with coralline HA, and integrating absorbable mesh with bone cement to encourage bone remodeling, along with the introduction of osteoinductive materials like BMP, have the potential to reduce reliance on traditional grafting techniques [16]. Moreover, although autologous grafts are histocompatible, provide structural support, and have no risk of disease transmission, due to limited supply, autograft material must be harvested during surgery, which adds time to the procedure and increases the risk of infection. Complication rates in bone graft harvesting procedures are high, with 8.6% of cases involving major and 20.6% involving minor complications [14]. Additional restrictions include the need for general anesthesia and the potential for significant blood loss and embolism. Recently, autologous bone grafts may be harvested from the intramedullary canal of the femur or tibia using a new technique, the Reamer-Irrigator-Aspirator (RIA), which allows for substantial amounts of cancellous bone to be obtained [35]. The RIA technique reduces pulmonary bone marrow embolism during nailing of the femur and when extracting bone and marrow from the femoral canal. Maximizing autologous bone graft harvest, minimizing complications, and improving the healing of long bone defects are all goals of the RIA surgical approach. Additionally, this technique is reported to reduce postoperative discomfort at the donor site. Despite potential biomechanical compromise, only 2% of cases involve fracture or cortical perforation [36].

In addition to the above-mentioned items, clinical guidelines for indications, techniques, and complications when using an autologous bone grafting approach are lacking. To address the highlighted concerns, further evaluations are required to establish the correct horizon in bone grafts. Various models, including *in vivo*, *ex vivo*, and *in vitro* approaches, are utilized to investigate each formulated treatment strategy. Researchers commonly use *ex vivo* and *in vitro* bone models to study bone metabolism and fracture healing. However, these models are not fully reliable since cell-specific normalization is so difficult to achieve. In addition, there are certain limitations to consider, including species-specific differences and ethical considerations for *in vivo* evaluation [37]. Biomedical research aims to translate experimental results to clinical settings, and researchers must draw justifiable conclusions based on data from appropriate animal models. Animal testing is performed on various species, including mice, dogs, and non-human primates. In dentistry, minipigs are preferred for evaluating the efficacy of bone products, while dogs are used for studies when investigating compromised oral conditions. Mice are useful for studying the osteoconductive characteristics of bone graft materials, particularly for assessing regeneration in calvaria and long bone defects. The use of rabbit models is declining, and mouse models are also typically used for genetic-based studies. Over the past decade, scientific advances and government guidelines have led to the replacement, reduction, and refinement of animal models in bone regeneration research, thereby focusing on *in vitro* or *in silico* biomaterial approaches to bone regeneration [38–40].

2.2. *Allogeneic Bone Graft*

When it comes to orthopedic surgery, treating large bone defects is a challenge. As mentioned above, to restore stability and stimulate regeneration, bone graft replacements are often used. Allografts are harvested from donors of an identical species, meticulously chosen and prepared following extensive evaluation, and preserved in bone repositories [41]. Allografts offer advantages such as containing GFs and conferring osteoconductive properties, which aids tissue growth in three dimensions. These grafts are advantageous since they are simple to apply, safe, and readily available. Of course, there is a shortage of allogeneic bone graft donors due to the rising demand for procedures such as spinal fusion, joint fusion, and arthroplasty [42]. Allografts are the most commercially successful bone grafts used to date and account for 57% of the current bone graft market [43]. Allogeneic bone integration is similar to non-vascularized autologous bone grafts, but the size of the allograft influences the incorporation time due to a lack of cells in the donated region to promote bone healing and beneficial immune reactions. Cancellous allograft is commonly used to treat partial bone defects, particularly in revision arthroplasty [44]. Allografts, made from live donors or cadaveric bone material, can be of a cortical, cancellous, or cortico-cancellous nature and are available in various sizes and shapes [45, 46]. Organizations known as "bone banks" supply safe and efficacious bone tissue for surgical applications, guaranteeing sterility, low immunogenicity, and maintenance of the physical integrity of the graft as well as the presence of inherent inductive proteins. The American Association of Tissue Banks and the Food and Drug Administration (FDA) oversee the procurement, handling, and application of allografts, and under federal law, the FDA is also in charge of overseeing human cells, tissues, and cellular-based products. Prior to use, allograft material that is suitable for distribution and implantation requires meticulous attention to detail. Assessing a donor's medical and social history for illnesses or diseases that might make tissue donation contraindicated is known as donor screening. Notifying relevant personnel of a potential donor's death, establishing initial donor eligibility, getting permission from family members or caregivers, sending a recovery team, obtaining tissue within 12 hours of death for non-refrigerated cadavers, conducting autopsies, and transporting harvested donor tissue, blood samples, and pertinent medical records to the tissue processing center are all part of the procurement of human bone allografts. Tissue banks have strong exclusionary criteria, and FDA requirements mandate allograft monitoring for recall reports [47].

The term "allograft" can refer to a variety of different kinds of bone transplants, such as mineralized bone allograft (MBA), fresh-frozen bone allograft (FFB), freeze-dried bone allograft (FDBA), mineralized freeze-dried bone allograft (MFDBA), decalcified freeze-dried bone allograft (DFDBA), autolyzed antigen-extracted allogeneic bone (AAA bone), demineralized bone matrix (DBM), and decellularized extracellular matrix (dECM), as summarized in **Figure 1**. Due to concerns over disease transmission and the host immunogenic response, fresh allografts are rarely used, despite their improved qualities compared to processed bone. Because of their short shelf life, unprocessed allografts are often stored by freezing or *via* freeze-drying. Total structural strength is also improved when using frozen cortical allografts. Lyophilization may damage collagen fibers, potentially affecting their mechanical qualities. Reducing the mineral content of bone increases the availability of extracellular matrix

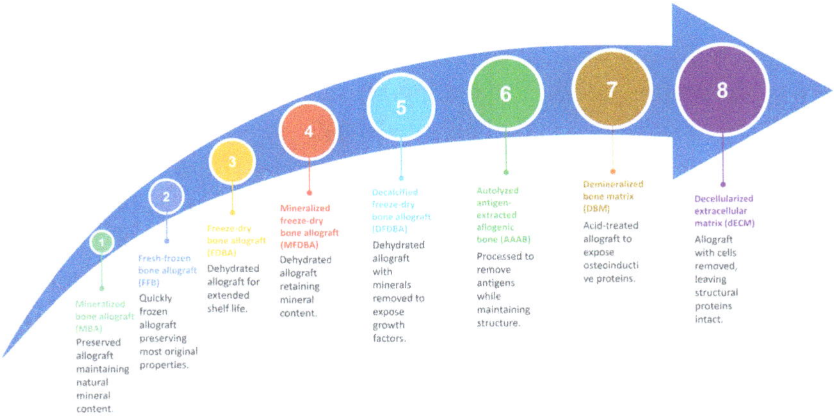

Figure 1. An overview of the different types of allografts and their key applications.

(ECM), thereby increasing osteoinductivity. BMPs and non-collagenous proteins (NCPs) are potential causes of osteoinductivity. To achieve osteoinductivity, however, certain minerals could be useful, including copper, zinc, and magnesium. Because DBM has a lower mineralized matrix content, it is more accessible to biological agents that promote bone formation. Despite its lack of structural strength, DBM has outstanding osteoinductive properties [44]. In neutral phosphate-buffered solutions, a DBM is incubated to produce AAA bone. The degree to which AAA bone is demineralized determines its structural strength. Physical, chemical, and enzymatic treatments are used to prepare the dECM by removing cellular components without compromising the structure of the ECM. Decellularized ECM can be tissue-derived or cell-derived. Tissue-derived bone dECM retains tissue-specific memory, including natural architecture and bioactive components, and promotes cell differentiation. Additionally, immunomodulatory cytokines are preserved. Matricellular proteins, fibronectin, laminin, elastin, and collagen are some of the extracellular macromolecules that make up dECM biomaterials [48]. dECM materials improve oxygen delivery and have received FDA approval for musculoskeletal repair. They are versatile and can be utilized in various forms such as powders, hydrogels, and bioinks for 3D printing applications [49].

The infection risks posed from viruses and other agents exist, but there have been very few documented cases of HIV in allografts. Other infections, such as bacterial infections and hepatitis B and C, cannot be entirely eliminated [44, 50]. To remove harmful substances and deliver a more biocompatible product, the allograft should be sterilized and disinfected using techniques including ethylene oxide gas sterilization, cold physical plasma, antibiotic disinfection, gamma-ray and electron beam irradiation, and peracetic acid treatment, achieving a sterility assurance level of 10^{-6}. dECM may be cross-linked, laser beam modified, solvent cast, or electrospun to improve its mechanical characteristics and stability. To enhance its osteogenic capacity, sterile bone dECM may be recellularized using MSCs. Although MSCs from younger donors have shown a more robust differentiation ability, bone tissue obtained from older donors are more efficient at sustaining the osteogenic differentiation of SCs [44, 46, 51].

For structural, oncological limb salvage surgeries, allograft bone is essential; however, after 10 years, failure rates may approach 60%. This is because different biological processes influence the functional capability and integration of the graft. A 50% reduction in bone strength at 10 years post-surgery was reported in a study of 13 unsuccessful human allograft retrievals, and this loss was linked to a rise in the frequency of microfractures and a decline in bone mineral density. This implies that tissue deterioration might be a contributing factor in the functional failure of allograft limb salvage surgeries [52]. Recent years have seen the development of various methods to improve the effectiveness of allografts, including cell seeding, co-transplantation, and determining the optimal sterilization method. Techniques such as pharmacological immunosuppression, decalcification, irradiation, and cryopreservation have also been employed to enhance the efficiency of allografts. The following text will delve into some of these aspects.

Composite allotransplantation (CAT) represents a promising advancement in the field of transplantation, particularly in addressing the challenges associated with organ rejection and the adverse effects of long-term immunosuppressive therapy. While CAT has demonstrated potential in preventing severe acute rejection through innovative approaches like donor-derived bone co-transplantation, practical limitations in vascularized bone transplants remain a significant hurdle. The ongoing necessity for systemic immunosuppression in vascularized composite allotransplantation (VCA) highlights the need for improved strategies to mitigate rejection while minimizing the associated risks of immunosuppressive agents. Emerging technologies such as genomic editing offer a hopeful avenue for reducing reliance on these toxic regimens, potentially enhancing the success and safety of future transplantations. Continued research and development in this area are essential to optimize outcomes and expand the applicability of CAT and VCA in clinical practice [53]. Studying bone fragment co-transplantation with bone marrow (BF-BM) aspirate infusion revealed that the co-transplanted bone fragments were viable for 6 months after transplantation but thereafter shrunk and degraded 10 months later. Additionally, dendritic cells, T helper cells, and regulatory T cells were influenced by BF-BM in a regulatory manner. During the 5-year follow-up period, no complications were encountered by any participant, regardless of whether they received BF-BM or not. Researchers found that BF-BM safeguards the kidneys and controls the immunological response, making it a safe and useful treatment option for patients [54]. A preclinical *in vivo* study reported that a commercially produced porcine enamel matrix derivative (EMD) can enhance bone formation when combined with a DFDBA and investigated in a nude mouse calf muscle model. EMD is considered osteopromotive rather than osteoinductive, meaning it supports bone growth but does not directly contribute to *de novo* bone growth [55]. To treat serious musculoskeletal injuries, researchers investigated the osteogenic capacity of decellularized bone allografts cellularized using bone marrow-derived MSCs (BMSCs). According to the research, BMSCs attached themselves to the allograft surface within 2 hours of application and continued to grow for 14 days. More potential was seen when these *in vitro* osteogenic results were compared to those that investigated the use of a beta-tricalcium phosphate (β-TCP) scaffold. Assays for *in vivo* transplantation in immunodeficient mice validated the ability of the allograft to stimulate bone growth. The findings imply that allografts may provide structural support for BMSC adherence, create a favorable microenvironment for cell survival and development, and promote new bone formation [56].

As the sterilization method is a decisive step in the preparation of allografts, a study compared the success of three different sterilization methods of human bone allografts: cryopreservation, gamma (γ) irradiation combined with cryopreservation, and solvent dehydration combined with γ irradiation (TPB). The human-derived MSCs (hMSCs) seeding effectiveness was determined to be equal between all three allografts; variations were seen in cell metabolism, osteoblastic gene expression, and *in vivo* bone production. *In vivo*, new bone formation was more common with frozen allografts (89%), but optimum hMSC survival, osteoblastic differentiation, and bone formation were possible with TPB allografts (72%). From this data, it was concluded the optimal sterilization techniques were TPB and cryopreservation, as in both of these cases, 100% of the grafts developed bone *in vivo* and after hMSC osteoinduction, but only 61% of γ-irradiated allografts did the same [57]. Further, to investigate their ability to induce new bone, studies were conducted on commercially available DFDBA. The results revealed that different preparations of the DFDBA, even when samples were obtained from the same bone bank, differed in their ability to induce new bone. This indicates inherent differences in the quality of the material and that this tissue is affected by the preparation processes and even the age of the donor [58, 59]. Smoking and age are two of the many variables that affect the success rate of osteointegrated bone transplants. Cigarette smoking, a common habit, significantly impairs graft efficiency, particularly in dental procedures. The habit contributes to oral health issues such as plaque buildup, gingivitis, and periodontitis, which hinder wound healing and can compromise the success of bone grafts and dental implants. The harmful substances in cigarette smoke, including nicotine and carbon monoxide, elevate the risk of infections and increase the failure rates of implants. To this end, research indicates that smokers experience a notable reduction in dental implant success rates and higher instances of crestal bone loss around grafts, regardless of the loading timing. Furthermore, the graft's position can influence the rate of marginal bone loss [60, 61]. Aging has a profound effect on graft efficiency, particularly in bone regeneration following trauma or surgical procedures. As individuals age, the balance of bone remodeling is disrupted due to altered activity of key cells like osteocytes, osteoclasts, and osteoblasts, which are essential for bone maintenance. This disruption affects the integration of bone grafts, influenced by factors such as graft selection and the mechanical properties of implants, which are critical for osteogenesis. In older adults, MSCs show reduced responsiveness, impairing their ability to migrate and attach to implants. Furthermore, systemic issues, such as medications and health conditions, can weaken the bone-graft interface. Osteoporosis, common in the elderly and particularly among women, worsens bone loss due to hormonal changes and other factors. The decline in metabolic rate with age leads to abnormalities that further compromise bone health. Recent research indicates that restoring levels of nicotinamide adenine dinucleotide may improve health and longevity. Age-related changes in movement and loading conditions also affect the mechanical strains on bone, impacting the integration potential of MSCs and macrophages at the graft interface. Overall, aging introduces numerous challenges to graft efficiency, highlighting the need for tailored strategies to enhance outcomes in older patients undergoing bone surgery who might experience inflammation. Contemporary osteogenesis procedures that promote bone formation within implants aim to tackle these challenges. Proposed solutions include addressing inflammation, inhibiting microbial adhesion, and augmenting osteoinductive and osteoconductive characteristics to enhance grafting results [62, 63]. Finally, and in conclusion, the union rates of allogeneic grafts are now equivalent to those of autologous grafts, and this may largely be due to the protocols that regulate the use of nonionic detergents, hydrogen peroxide, and denatured alcohol. This has greatly improved the safety profile of the transplants [64].

2.3. *Xenogenic Bone Graft*

Xenograft refers to the transfer of bone tissue from one species to another, typically from coral exoskeletons, eggshells, cows, pigs, and horses. Dentists have commonly used xenografts due to their non-resorbable nature, unlike allografts, which are susceptible to resorption over time. Their disadvantage is caused by moral, religious, and health issues, including the possibility of contracting diseases [65, 66]. The history of bone xenotransplantation dates back to the 17th century, with the first bone transplantation performed in 1668. However, the first report of bovine bone transplantation dates back to 1957 [67]. Xenografts, particularly porcine and bovine types, have been explored as alternatives to autologous bone grafts in orthopedic and dental surgeries due to their cost-effectiveness and abundant availability [68]. Over the past 30 years, studies have demonstrated their effectiveness, such as in a two-stage lateral window sinus lift procedure where both porcine xenografts and autologous bone grafts resulted in significant bone growth without infection or inflammation [69]. Follow-up after 3 years indicated comparable outcomes in implant durability and patient satisfaction between the two materials [70]. In another study involving tooth extraction, two bovine xenografts, Bio-Oss® and a new product, Osseus®, were evaluated for their ability to maintain alveolar cavity integrity over a 24-week recovery period. Results showed no significant differences in the effectiveness of the two grafts, confirming both as suitable for implantation [71]. A meta-analysis of 25 trials revealed considerable variability in the characteristics of xenograft bone replacements, including factors like porosity, crystallinity, calcium-to-phosphorus ratio, and osteogenesis. The graft sizes varied significantly (1,000 μm to 5 mm), and pore sizes ranged widely (1.3–1,000 μm). The results revealed that comparing different xenografts and determining the optimal product is complicated, as the selection of biomaterials and the assessment of outcomes need to be considered independently. This complexity is primarily attributed to the critical role of porosity and pore interconnectivity in the process of bone regeneration [72].

Unfortunately, the majority of clinical studies that have investigated the transplantation of bovine bone to humans have had negative outcomes. This includes graft rejection, poor local tissue reactivity, and the inability of the graft to integrate with the host bone [73]. Regrettably, inadequate material preparation has generated protein residues that have led to transplant rejection. The alpha-Gal epitope, which is expressed on glycolipids and glycoproteins in non-primate animals and New World monkeys, is the biggest clinical obstacle to bone xenotransplantation. This antibody may cause acute rejection of tissues with vascular beds, complement activation, and clotting. It makes up 1% of all circulating antibodies in humans. Xenografts go through decellularization, which lowers epitope levels and builds a scaffold of biologic tissue, to stop host rejection caused by alpha-Gal [68]. Further, the pain and suffering of animals used for xenotransplantation raises ethical questions. Animals have a right to life, and utilizing their transplanted organs for medical purposes is considered immoral by some critics. There are serious concerns over the conditions in which these animals are raised, as well as the potential for harsh treatment [74]. The possibility of disease transmission from animals to humans is also a significant ethical factor. There are also fears that xenotransplantation could lead to the emergence of new zoonotic diseases that could have devastating public health consequences. To prevent the spread of diseases, severe safeguards must be used, yet doing so raises challenging ethical issues. The advancement of xenotransplantation technologies necessitates the resolution of these issues [74, 75].

Contemporary investigations have also aimed to comprehend the inflammatory cascade that results after xenograft implantation. According to a novel theory, the response at the implantation site may cause either the graft to degrade and then cause *de novo* bone creation, or it might cause an inflammatory response to a foreign substance. Thus, the physicochemical properties of the used graft may dictate the kind of response [76]. A study conducted on CD1 mice investigated the reaction of host tissue to a xenogeneic bone substitute called Bio-Oss™. The study found that within the first 15 days of implantation, Bio-Oss™ induced high vascularization and the formation of multinucleated giant cells. This phenomenon is dependent on the composition of the bone substitute materials, which control their stability. The slow degradation of Bio-Oss™ helps maintain the stability of the biomaterial over time in the implantation bed. The presence of multinucleated giant cells at the implantation site, believed to be responsible for degrading bone substitute materials, varies depending on the biomaterial's physicochemical structure. These cells help blood vessels to grow by releasing vascular endothelial growth factor (VEGF) and other chemokines and through generating acid phosphatases and osteoclast-specific cell markers. The concentration and type of these chemicals show how biodegradable a biomaterial is [77].

In the last few years, the number of commercial brands that offer xeno and xeno-synthetic bone transplants has increased. Collagen and other proteins have supplemented certain bone-based scaffolds to enhance their regenerative capacity and inhibit migration and aggregation, particularly of any scaffold particles. In this regard, research examined the biocompatibility of three distinct bone xenograft formulations: InterOss®, InterOss® Collagen, and a control formulation called InterCollagen®. The findings demonstrated that none of the three materials displayed any detrimental effects on the development and growth of cells. The materials degraded in distinct ways after implantation. Minor surface alterations, increased cellular activity, and minimal degradation were all signs of material reabsorption in InterOss®. Hydrolytic degradation of InterOss® Collagen, leading to the separation of apatite particles from collagen fibers, occurred after fibrous capsule formation surrounding the implant. The research revealed a significant presence of blood vessels, a factor crucial for tissue regeneration. However, the study findings point to the biocompatibility and regenerative potential of these bone xenograft formulations having different degradation mechanisms and speeds depending on their modifications with collagen [78]. More recently, the first effective clinical use of a xenograft–allograft combination (cerabone® plus mixed with maxgraft®) for alveolar ridge augmentation before dental implantation has been introduced. The defect was repaired utilizing a novel xenogeneic bone replacement comprising hyaluronate coupled with allogeneic bone granules. The new xenograft provided volume stability and strong structural support and retained the alveolar ridge contour. After 3 years of follow-up, the dental implant remained stable and showed no symptoms of infection [79]. In recent years, there has been a significant focus on the production of bone grafts, which has helped to overcome the challenges previously mentioned. The sections that follow will cover some recent developments in bone grafts, as shown in **Figure 2**.

2.4. *Recent Advances in Bone Graft Technology*

2.4.1. *Surface-Modified Bone Grafts*

Bone grafts have been subjected to various surface modification techniques to improve their biological and mechanical performance. A physicochemical coating is obtained by applying different coatings, such as bioactive glass (BG), calcium phosphate, or GFs, to the graft surface, resulting in accelerated callus resolution and increased bone volume [80]. Surface modification is carried out with the aim of improving biocompatibility, bone induction, and bone conduction *via* physical, chemical, and biological alterations. Surface modification techniques are performed through physicochemical coating, radiation bonding, and biochemical

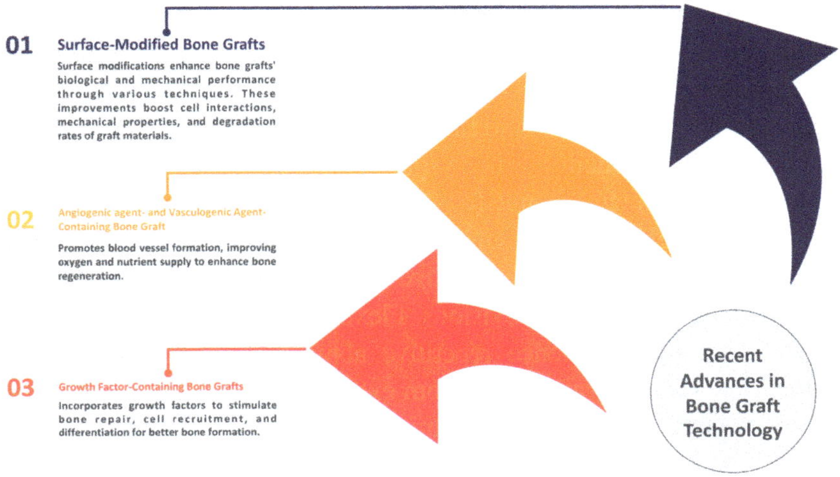

Figure 2. The innovative advances in bone graft technology have been significant. Each of these methods, from surface modifications to enhance tissue interactions to the use of angiogenic factors and growth factor-containing allografts, has helped to improve the repair and regeneration processes. These advances may offer new perspectives in developing novel medical treatments.

immobilization. Radiation bonding is performed by using radiation to bond polymers or functional groups onto the bonding surface, while biochemical immobilization is carried out by attaching biological molecules such as proteins or peptides to the graft surface [81, 82]. Acid etching and collagen coating are two methods that may improve the characteristics of bone grafts, including demineralized tooth matrix. These alterations cause the pores to enlarge and the surfaces to become rougher, which improves cell integration and keeps the calcium-to-phosphorus (Ca/P) molar ratio constant at 1.67, which is representative of the HA mineral phase inherent in natural bone [82]. Recent advancements in the development of injectable bone grafts have been achieved through a modified graft that employs a co-stabilization method using surfactants and HA nanoparticles. This innovative approach addresses issues faced by traditional emulsion-templated foams, such as small pore sizes and inadequate cell attachment. The inclusion of HA nanoparticles as stabilizers enhances the viability of hMSCs [83]. The modified surface causes faster and more effective bone regeneration as it increases progenitor cell attachment, proliferation, and differentiation, and surface changes can also improve the mechanical properties and the degradation rate of bone grafting materials. Surface-modified grafts are used in various dental and orthopedic procedures, such as bone defect repair, and in spinal implant and fusion procedures, and it has been shown that compared to unmodified bone grafts, it improves integrity [81, 84]. Crush injuries, which account for 30% of all hand injuries, frequently cause severe tendon damage and necessitate tendon grafting. However, tendon grafting can result in restrictive adhesions and poor digit motion, leading to multiple surgical revisions. Flexor tendons, classified as intrasynovial tendons, experience repetitive abrasion during hand motion. Standard tendon autografts come from extrasynovial tendon sources, but these have been associated with diminished function. A chemical compound, carbodiimide-derivatized hyaluronic acid combined with lubricin, has been used to modify the tendon graft surface, increasing gliding ability and surface durability against abrasion. Findings indicated that the intrasynovial allogeneic graft group exhibited superior digit function, reduced adhesion formation, improved flexion, and enhanced graft gliding compared to the extrasynovial autologous grafts group. However, the intrasynovial allogeneic graft group experienced diminished healing at the distal tendon-bone junction. This procedure provides a promising avenue for expanding the selection of donor graft sites [85].

Polydopamine (PDA) coatings are increasingly being utilized for surface functionalization purposes due to their strong adsorption capabilities, ability to bind bioactive drugs, and compatibility with various materials. These coatings play a significant role in regulating the bone repair environment, enhancing shear strength, and exhibiting slow degradation under physiological conditions. Despite their advantages, existing literature primarily addresses the physical and chemical properties of PDA coatings, lacking detailed insights into the mechanisms by which PDA promotes bone regeneration [86]. Bone grafts modified with PDA become more suitable for repairing bone abnormalities by enhancing important qualities. To improve graft performance as a bone substitute, this surface modification promotes cell adhesion, proliferation, osteodifferentiation, and mineralization. Besides, the adhesive properties of dopamine allow it to form strong bonds with metal ions, enabling the creation of a nano-coating that improves tissue fixation while maintaining the graft's porous structure [87]. As described previously, the decellularization of biological tissues removes immunogenic components, resulting in mineralized collagen that possesses desirable mechanical properties. One significant modification of this technique involves coating small porcine intestinal submucosa with PDA, which creates a periosteal-like film with strong potential for bone regeneration. This approach uses dopamine to regulate collagen mineralization in hard tissues, specifically improving calcium phosphate incorporation on decellularized collagen membranes. The process allows for the controlled diffusion of calcium and phosphate ions, promoting mineral supersaturation over a period of 1–14 days. The resulting PDA-collagen complex features low crystallinity polycrystals on its surface and within collagen fibers, thereby significantly enhancing its biocompatibility. Notably, the PDA-mineralized-collagen membrane demonstrates excellent cellular activity [88]. One notable approach in the modification of allografts involves the incorporation of PDA into decellularized live hyaline cartilage grafts. This modification utilizes a macromolecule backbone to prevent the rigid crosslinking often seen with smaller dopamine molecules. The results indicated that PDA-modified grafts exhibited improved adhesive strength with surrounding tissue after chelating with ferric ions [89].

2.4.2. *Angiogenic Agent- and Vasculogenic Agent-Containing Bone Graft*

The orthopedic field faces challenges in regenerating bone in large segmental defects due to blood supply issues, thereby requiring angiogenesis and vasculogenesis for successful transplantation. Angiogenesis is the formation of new blood vessels from preexisting capillaries; it happens in a variety of contexts, including health, injury, and illness. In contrast, vasculogenesis works to improve the grafted tissue's oxygen and nutritional supply by encouraging the development of new blood vessels inside the bone graft, resulting in improved integration of the graft within the surrounding native bone. The establishment of the appropriate milieu for effective bone integration is greatly aided by including pro-angiogenic characteristics within the graft material. The early angiogenesis phase, which begins in the first few weeks after grafting and lasts for several months, is crucial for achieving targeted bone repair. By facilitating vasculogenesis and the development of new blood vessels, angiogenesis might be further improved [90–92]. Autografts, the current gold standard, have significant angiogenic potential, forming arteries and increasing blood supply at transplant sites. However, without revascularization, their rejuvenation and remodeling capabilities are limited, leading to complications. The challenge lies in achieving sufficient blood vessel formation in larger bone defects due to the restricted longitudinal growth of blood vessels from the host tissue to the center of the graft. Recent breakthroughs in bone healing mechanisms have unveiled fresh opportunities for treating bony defects, including the utilization of synthetic materials, GFs, and cells. The key to a triumph lies in the vascularization, bridging, and remodeling of bone, which requires new blood vessels for bone formation, migration, differentiation, and cell survival [93, 94]. A study examined three xenogeneic bone grafting materials, including two equine and porcine: Gen-Os and anorganic Bio-Oss, respectively. The materials were all made of calcium oxide phosphate, which was not very crystalline; however, Bio-Oss contained larger particles and a carbonated phase, while both Gen-Os were composed of collagen. The angiogenic potential of Gen-Oss materials was higher than that of the Bio-Oss material. Periodontal bone defect-associated cells increase VEGF synthesis, endothelial cell proliferation, and stimulate angiogenesis. Results indicated that collagen was responsible for the clinical success of both Gen-Os materials [95]. VEGF is crucial for angiogenesis and is significantly involved in bone development and healing. Modulating VEGF levels can potentially improve bone repair mechanisms. It plays a vital role in the different stages of bone healing, such as inflammation, endochondral ossification, and intramembranous ossification. Furthermore, VEGF is important in distraction osteogenesis and is essential for repair and regeneration within scaffolds, as well as in the function and activity of skeletal SCs and the release of GFs [96]. Several bone grafting materials have shown significant angiogenic potential, as evidenced by research indicating enhanced VEGF and fibroblast growth factor-2 (FGF-2) release by fibroblasts after direct and indirect exposure to various types of grafts. The results were dependent on their size and concentration [97]. A recent study explored the use of catecholic amino acid 3,4-dihydroxyphenylalanine (DOPA) to create a PDA coating on allogeneic bone, which was then chelated with VEGF. Results indicated that the DOPA-coated allogeneic bone mimicked the characteristics of natural bone, and VEGF-loaded grafts demonstrated excellent biocompatibility while promoting osteogenic signals *in vitro*. After 12 weeks, the VEGF-loaded allografts successfully healed the bone defect and showed a continuous and intact bone cortex [98].

When bone grafts are implanted, they initially lack sufficient blood vessels and blood supply, and this condition creates hypoxia and causes cell death and graft failure. The oxygen needed to maintain bone tissue survival can be provided by scaffolds or biological materials that carry oxygen and allow the graft to mature. A sufficient oxygen supply is necessary for osteogenesis and bone repair because it facilitates the oxygen-consuming reactions that support bone cell proliferation and differentiation [99, 100]. Electric fields (EFs) can cause SCs to undergo differentiation by generating reactive oxygen species (ROS) and activating crucial signaling pathways [101]. Furthermore, the differentiation of SCs can be influenced by the activation and expression of NADPH-oxidase, as ROS is predominantly generated by this enzyme in SCs. The regulated generation of ROS can trigger signaling molecules related to cellular differentiation. Some studies have described the activation of mitogen-activated protein kinase (MAPK) pathways followed by the extracellular signal-regulated kinase 1,2 (ERK1, 2), c-Jun N-terminal kinase (JNK), and p38 signaling cascade as an example [102]. It is widely agreed that ROS can regulate the growth and specialization of MSCs and pluripotent SCs [103]. Collectively, it is theorized that elevated levels of intracellular ROS caused by EF exposure may function as a signaling molecule to potentially trigger different differentiation processes.

2.4.3. *Growth Factor-Containing Bone Grafts*

As previously mentioned, GFs are critical in the structure and function of bone and are incorporated or released from bone graft materials to enhance the bone regeneration process [104, 105]. GFs are signaling molecules that play an important role in stimulating and strengthening the natural mechanisms of bone repair and regeneration [106]. They play a crucial role in bone repair by binding to specific receptors on target cells.

This triggers a series of signals within the cells, regulating the processes involved in bone healing [107–109]. These GFs work together to promote the recruitment, differentiation, and proliferation of bone-forming cells and MSCs, which are vital for the formation of new bone. When GFs are present in bone grafts, they have several benefits and can enhance the quality of newly formed bone, increase angiogenesis, enhance blood flow, and support bone regeneration [110, 111]. It is not always sufficient to rely solely on GFs. Guided bone regeneration (GBR) is a technique that selectively directs tissue healing by utilizing different cytotypes of growth turnover. It does this by utilizing semipermeable membranes that allow gases and nutrients to exchange while preventing the penetration and proliferation of unwanted cells. A graft is utilized to stabilize the clot and promote undisturbed tissue healing. GFs are often used with this biomaterial to enhance tissue healing [112]. In an implantology study, researchers looked at how well a combination of concentrated growth factors (CGF) and deproteinized bovine bone mineral (DBBM) grafts preserved alveolar ridges. A total of 38 participants, 19 from each group, participated in the research. Although there was no significant difference in the development of a new bone contour between the two groups, results showed that the CGF group delivered an improved wound healing index, a greater gray value of alveolar bone volume, and less postoperative pain [111]. A series of GFs, including platelet-derived growth factors (PDGF), VEGF, BMPs, and FGF, are involved in bone regeneration. VEGF-A is a master regulator of angiogenesis. Its overexpression by genetically modified human osteoprogenitor cells induces bone loss through excessive osteoclast recruitment. Since during bone growth, angiogenesis and osteogenesis are physiologically associated with the expression of VEGF, a study investigated the potential effectiveness of VEGF delivery on its physiological function. The results showed that the homogeneous distribution of VEGF protein is associated with the matrix, the physiological pair of angiogenesis, and maintains osteogenesis, providing an attractive and clinically applicable strategy for vascular bone engineering [113]. Today, PDGF-containing grafts have the desired integration rates and fewer side effects, whereas BMP-7 is no longer accessible. BMP-2 may cause tumor development and inflammatory side effects [114]. Recent research has focused on introducing a new form of BMP called “Recombinant BMP” (rhBMP) as a replacement for traditional BMP. The advantage of rhBMP is that it is easier to synthesize and more readily available for clinical use. However, there are still some challenges to overcome. One issue is that rhBMP has a lower bone-inducing activity compared to purified BMP. Quantitative analysis has shown that the bone-inducing activity of rhBMP is less than one-tenth of that of purified BMP. Another challenge is that rhBMPs are soluble in the body and disperse shortly after implantation, so they do not induce bone formation in large quantities without a carrier. Thus, to allow sufficient bone induction *in vivo*, a carrier capable of acting as a slow-delivery system is required [115]. In a study involving 11 patients with missing teeth, researchers discovered that combining rhBMP-2 with a xenogenic bone substitute mineral called Bio-Oss® can greatly enhance GBR therapy. The study focused on 34 Brånemark implants placed in different areas of the same jaw, which required lateral ridge augmentation. By applying rhBMP-2 to the xenogenic bone substitute through a lyophilization process, the researchers observed a significant decrease in defect height after 6 months. Histomorphometric analysis revealed an average area density of 37% newly formed bone at test sites and 30% at control sites [116]. One potent healing factor that encourages the development of both hard and soft tissues is PDGF. For fibroblasts, cementoblasts, and osteoblasts in the gingiva and periodontal ligaments, PDGF is an effective chemotactic and mitogenic agent. Incorporation of rhPDGF with biological or synthetic grafts represents an innovative approach for bone grafting, particularly in periodontal tissue regeneration. This GF has been synthesized to enhance the healing process by actively recruiting cells to repair damaged tissues. Approved by the FDA for various applications, including periodontal and orthopedic bone defects, rhPDGF has shown promising results in preclinical and clinical studies [117]. A systematic review of 63 clinical studies, with an average follow-up of 10.7 months, highlighted the efficacy and safety of rhPDGF in promoting alveolar bone and soft tissue regeneration. The review found no serious adverse effects, aside from common postoperative complications. The results indicated that rhPDGF is particularly beneficial when used in combination with allografts and xenografts, for treating periodontal defects and gingival recession. Furthermore, rhPDGF has shown positive outcomes in GBR and alveolar ridge preservation when paired with allografts or xenografts [118].

New trends, however, tend to produce completely biodegradable materials with the above-mentioned characteristics capable of synchronizing its degradation rate with osseous tissue, *i.e.,* an alloplastic scaffold.

3. Alloplastic Scaffolds in Bone Regeneration

Scaffolds, or alloplastic bone grafts, are synthetic materials designed to complement and replace natural bone tissue. The primary component of bone, HA, is a naturally occurring mineral that is often incorporated into these scaffolds. These artificial grafts can facilitate the proliferation of the patient's own cells, enabling the growth of new bone as they integrate with the material. Available in various sizes and shapes, alloplastic grafts serve multiple purposes, including soft tissue support and bone replacement. As osteoconductive substitutes for natural bone grafts, they are regarded as economical options [119, 120]. Scaffolds can prevent donor site complications and reduce the risk of disease transmission compared to autologous or allogeneic bone grafts, resulting in fewer side effects [121]. The FDA and the Japanese Ministry of Health, Labor, and Welfare (PMDA) regulate alloplastic bone graft products in the United States and Japan, respectively. In the United States, between 1996 and December 2020, 87 alloplastic bone graft scaffold products have been approved. In Japan, HA and β-TCP make up 80% of all alloplastic bone graft products. The available forms of scaffold materials are mainly particles in the United States, Japan, and Korea. However, only four alloplastic bone graft products are approved by both the PMDA and the FDA: Cytrans® Granules (GC), OSferion Dental (Olympus Terumobiomaterial), Cerasorb® M (Zimmer Biomet Dental G.K.), and Arrow Bone-β (Brain Base Corporation). The lack of standardization in indication descriptions leads to ambiguity and inconsistency among products [121]. Researchers have made considerable progress in producing novel scaffold materials, which might lead to safer, standardized replacements in the future. Unlike allogeneic bone grafts, which promote the development of new attachments, scaffolds assist in bone repair and regeneration.

Architecture has a significant impact on cell behavior, particularly in tissue engineering and wound healing. The surface topography, pore size, and shape of biomaterials may modulate the immune response, which impacts macrophage activation. To perform diverse roles in the healing process, macrophages may take on two different phenotypes: M1 and M2. Angiogenic and osteogenic processes are inhibited by M1, while M2 inhibits inflammation and enhances tissue development. More efficient healing may be achieved by deliberately designing biomaterials that promote sequential activation of M1 and M2 macrophages. Evidence suggests that seeded macrophages on rough surfaces take on an M2-like phenotype, which is advantageous for BTE since it suppresses immunological processes while boosting angiogenesis, ECM synthesis, and tissue regeneration [122]. Dimensions, geometric arrangement, and pore connectivity are critical aspects to optimizing bone ingrowth within a scaffold [123]. To avoid challenges including stress shielding and implant-related osteopenia, stiffness is an important biomechanical component of bone engineering scaffolds. By interacting with tension-bearing actin structures, scaffolds influence key cellular behaviors, including focal adhesion formation, motility, proliferation, and differentiation. Cell adhesion and osteogenic gene expression are both enhanced by more robust matrices. According to research, human MSCs differentiate most effectively into osteogenic cells when exposed to the stiffest substrate group (25–40 kPa). However, the ideal scaffold stiffness range for BTE in terms of maximizing a scaffold's pro-osteogenic effect needs further investigation. Further, load-bearing capacity is crucial for scaffold design, as cyclic loading promotes cell proliferation, mineralization, osteogenic differentiation, and bone formation. Additionally, a scaffold's topographic properties encompass its surface characteristics, including roughness and texture. The presence of these features can improve cellular activity, such as protein adsorption, cell adhesion and proliferation, and bone formation. Surface modifications, such as sandblasting or acid-etching, can further enhance these effects [8, 124].

There is evidence that interconnected porous scaffolds with a minimum 100 μm pore diameter promote optimum bone growth. This is because while pores larger than 100 μm facilitate angiogenesis, pores smaller than this size might hinder it. Pore diameters ranging between 200 and 400 μm are considered optimal for the development and regeneration of bone tissue. Osteogenic differentiation, cell-seeding efficiency, and cell dispersion are all affected by the variance in pore diameters [125]. For resorbable scaffold materials used in BTE to promote tissue stability and development, their degradation rate must coincide with that of bone formation. For efficient optimization of materials in bone defect regeneration, it is necessary to focus not only on enhancing mechanical qualities but also on optimizing the synthesis of the ECM and gaining a thorough knowledge of the scaffold degradation process. The degradation of scaffolds in the human body is influenced by factors such as age, nutritional condition, and lifestyle. On the other hand, and from a materials perspective, factors including material composition, the local physiological environment, the method of fabrication, scaffold structure, and surface characteristics play a role in affecting scaffold degradation [125, 126].

Researchers report that by modifying the composition of the alloplastic bone graft, tailorable bone growth might be caused [127]. This property may be employed *via* cell transplantation with GFs, offering better handling and manipulated resorption rates. GFs can be released in a controlled manner during decomposition of specific components, resulting in accelerated new bone formation [127]. Another method for improving the scaffold's biological response is to modify them using natural polymers and the content of the osseous ECM. A preclinical trial explored the effectiveness of different biphasic calcium phosphate formulations combined with an HA-collagen membrane for treating localized alveolar ridge defects. The study, involving six female foxhounds, reported successful healing of grafted sites without complications, indicating good integration of graft particles within the bone. Additionally, new bone formation was noted around and within the graft particles, which were surrounded by dense connective tissue and marrow spaces [128]. According to the theory behind personalized medicine, each person has distinct traits on several levels, necessitating individualized approaches to health problems. New tools for imaging, proteomics, DNA sequencing, and wireless health monitoring have shown substantial inter-individual diversity in disease processes, lending credence to this notion [129]. In line with the principles of personalized medicine, state-of-the-art computer-aided design and manufacturing (CAD/CAM) software enables the creation of unique scaffolds using xenogenic or alloplastic blocks that are derived from computed tomography-generated images of bone defects. These scaffolds offer an alternative to traditional bone augmentation procedures. In a clinical study, grafting bilateral horizontal lesions using HA/TCP versus xenogenic custom-made scaffolds were assessed for their implant-bone recovery response. Results showed that xenogenic grafts achieved 17.8% new bone growth, while alloplastic scaffolds reached 19.9%, with both types demonstrating similar horizontal gains. Despite the positive outcomes and a 1-year survival rate for scaffolds and implants, further research with an extended follow-up is necessary to validate this bone augmentation technique [130]. As alloplastic scaffolds offer advantages such as the absence of infectious disease transmission and ethical or religious controversies, future studies are expected to aim to enhance the use of alloplastic materials in terms of cell migration and angiogenesis, creating appropriate space without inhibiting wound healing while maintaining stable blood clot formation and a suitable resorption rate [127].

3.1. *Metal-Based Scaffolds*

Metals have historically been the primary materials employed to fabricate orthopedic devices, largely due to their superior mechanical properties and structural integrity, making them appealing biomaterials for bone implant technologies. Nonetheless, the application of metals as scaffolds presents certain challenges. One significant issue is that metal implants typically exhibit a higher Young's modulus compared to natural bone, which can result in stress shielding, where the presence of the implant diminishes the mechanical load carried by the bone, leading to bone resorption. Furthermore, the limited degradability of metals poses another significant concern, as it may impede the ability of host cells to generate new bone tissue and could potentially lead to chronic complications such as corrosion and inflammation [12]. Improvements in the biodegradability and multifunctionality of metallic scaffolds have been a focus of recent research in BTE. For improved clinical applications, researchers aim to increase their biocompatibility, stimulate bone formation, and regulate metal ion release. The release of bioactive metal ions by these metal scaffolds may promote blood vessel creation, limit bone resorption, and even display antimicrobial capabilities [131, 132]. Titanium and magnesium, along with their respective alloys, are frequently employed in the field of BTE due to their exceptional mechanical properties. Iron (Fe), zinc (Zn), and magnesium (Mg) are the most frequently employed biodegradable metals in scaffold production [133].

Zinc demonstrates an appropriate corrosion rate for BTE applications. Zinc alloys frequently exhibit satisfactory mechanical characteristics for load-bearing constructions, although they are associated with concerns over toxicity. When compared to other biodegradable metals, zinc alloys offer superior mechanical characteristics and a reduced degradation rate [134]. Magnesium scaffolds have demonstrated encouraging outcomes in enhancing osteogenic activity and facilitating bone formation. A daily intake of 350 mg of magnesium can result in a 25 mg deposition within bone. Magnesium has a comparable elastic modulus to bone, which makes it an appropriate material for scaffolds. Magnesium alloys have biodegradable properties and are favorable in terms of biocompatibility and mechanical characteristics. It plays an important role in enhancing the osteogenic effect by facilitating fibronectin adsorption, activating integrins, and influencing the osteogenic activities of bone MSCs. This ultimately promotes their differentiation into osteogenic lineages, as well as having an impact on macrophage polarization [135, 136]. The use of hierarchical porous scaffolds has the potential to increase bone regeneration by increasing angiogenesis *via* the release of proangiogenic ions and the enhancement of cell adhesion. While an ideal scenario has not yet been established, the structural characteristics and topology of porous structures significantly influence angiogenesis and ossification, since they contribute to tissue development, cell migration, waste clearance, and nutrition supply [137, 138]. In one experiment, researchers constructed a porous scaffold, changed its surface using a polymer, and then covered it with PDA mixed with magnesium. Bone development, cell proliferation, and adhesion were all improved by this altered scaffold, according to the *in vitro* studies reported. The study found that the release of Mg^{2+} ions stimulated angiogenesis, and when implanted into a rabbit's thigh, blood vessel formation and osteogenesis were significantly increased. The study suggests that magnesium incorporation positively influences bone cell growth and proliferation, facilitates angiogenesis by enhancing blood vessel growth, improves endothelial cell cultures, and promotes substantial vascular development, as confirmed *via* the chorioallantoic membrane assay [139, 140].

Iron is a crucial element present in hemoglobin, playing a vital role in oxygen transport and cellular development in humans. The daily requirement for iron in individuals ranges from 8 to 27 mg [141]. In recent years, iron-based implants have garnered significant interest among researchers due to their remarkable mechanical characteristics. While these implants exhibit favorable plasticity, strength, and high biocompatibility, understanding their degradation procedure needs more attention. A study on degradable iron-based alloys for bone regeneration has shown encouraging results. In the trial, implants of two different densities and a control group were implanted into the proximal tibia of Merino sheep and demonstrated high biocompatibility. However, for clinical usage, the rate of degradation would need to be greatly enhanced, and biocompatibility would need to be re-evaluated. The research indicated that the degraded alloy particles surrounded the implants, but no inflammatory response was seen. Although the iron-based porous bone replacement implants exhibited acceptable biocompatibility, further analysis is required to establish their potential for clinical applications [142]. Recently, iron-bioceramic composites have been developed as biodegradable implant materials with customized degradation behavior and bioactive properties. Research employing a sheep animal model and the surgical implantation of five sets of samples (Fe-HA, Fe-TCP, Fe-BCP composites, and pure-Fe and SS316L as controls) into the proximal area of the radial bone found that the composites exhibited minimal tissue response during wound healing. Real-time ultrasound analysis demonstrated a diminished echo pattern within the peri-implant biodegradation region, while peripheral whole blood indicators showed typical dynamic changes. Histological investigation revealed a decreased inflammatory giant cell population and a larger degradation layer on the composites compared to pure Fe, which means that the corrosion of pure iron was less pronounced than that of the iron bio-ceramic composite implants; also, pure iron exhibited lower bioactivity [143].

The incorporation of noble metals, particularly gold, into the iron scaffold enhances its characteristics. The introduction of a minor quantity of gold into the iron scaffold creates a galvanic couple, which accelerates the degradation rate relative to pure iron. Additionally, this process facilitates the increased formation of HA onto the scaffold surface, thereby promoting demineralization and ultimately enhancing biological activity [144]. The incorporation of magnesium into iron enhances its corrosion rate while simultaneously improving its plasticity and mechanical properties [145]. Additionally, Fe–Mn–10Cu was implanted into the femur of New Zealand white rabbits for 90 days, and this resulted in enhanced osteogenesis and new bone formation, which correlated with the addition of copper. Degradation of the Fe–Mn–Cu samples commenced 3 months post-implantation through galvanic corrosion. Furthermore, Fe–35Mn–1Ag was implanted into the shoulder and thigh regions of Sprague–Dawley rats, where a heightened tissue inflammatory response was noted at 4 weeks, subsequently decreasing as the degradation rate diminished. Notably, the presence of silver increased the corrosion rate, bringing the corrosion rate of Fe–35Mn–1Ag in line with that of WE43 [141]. The incorporation of cobalt into iron scaffolds increases overall magnetization, whereas the presence of vanadium, chromium, and manganese leads to a reduction in saturation magnetic flux density [146]. The study findings suggest that incorporation of iron-based superparamagnetic nanoparticles into a scaffold could be used as an internal magnetic source and exhibited positive biosafety characteristics. The enhanced magnetic field activates receptors on the cell surface, initiating signaling pathways that help restore damaged bones. By manipulating human umbilical cord-derived MSCs within the magnetic scaffold, researchers observed an increase in gene expression. *In vivo* experiments showed accelerated bone regeneration, along with higher bone mineral density and a larger proportion of new bone area. The superparamagnetic scaffold also exhibited positive biosafety characteristics [147].

Various clinical applications have employed titanium and its alloys in the fabrication of scaffolds over the past several years. Clinical trials have shown that cylindrical titanium bone scaffolds are effective for successful bone defect reconstruction and complete functional recovery [148]. Because of their biocompatibility and resistance to corrosion, titanium and titanium alloys are essential materials for use in orthopedics. Unfortunately, problems have arisen during practical application due to issues such as a greater Young's modulus and a limited osteogenic induction capacity. Researchers have investigated a wide range of modification techniques, including coating, surface functionalization, 3D structure transformation, altering alloy compositions, and surface structure transformation. Implications for clinical practice have been enhanced by recent advancements in materials science research, which have led to improved bone tissue manufacturing [149]. 3D-printed porous titanium scaffolds were used in a study to resolve bone problems in both dogs and people. The supports were placed on 20 dogs and 3 human patients. The supports assisted with bone growth. After 18 months, the scaffolding led to full repair in all cases following implantation in dogs. Three people with neoplasms in the maxilla who underwent oral and maxillofacial surgery were given a custom-designed porous titanium scaffold made using 3D printing technology. After 3 years, the first patient's eating and sleeping habits had improved, and the second patient's scaffold had successfully integrated within the surrounding bone, and joint conditions were normal. The third patient's tumor growth did not return, and the scaffold appeared similar to normal spongy bone [150]. Although implants that look like bone tissue have been made with metallic scaffolding, they can leach harmful ions and cause inflammation and allergic reactions, which can impede biocompatibility and lead to tissue loss. Surface modifications could be introduced to incorporate cell-recognizable ligands and signaling GFs, as well as improve cell adhesion and proliferation. In this regard, bio-ceramics and biopolymers are being investigated, as they display promising potential [151]. The sections on advanced scaffolds and coatings will delve deeper into this topic.

3.2. *Ceramic-Based Scaffolds*

Bioceramics represent a category of ceramic material utilized for the repair or replacement of impaired bone or muscle tissues within the human skeletal framework [152]. The interaction between bioceramics and tissues varies depending on the specific material used for bone restoration. Implants made of nontoxic ceramics may kill tissues; bioinert materials can create fibrous membranes; bioactive materials can build interfacial connections; or tissue can replace bioresorbable ceramics. Bioinert ceramics exhibit no interaction with biological tissues. In contrast, bioactive ceramics, including HA and TCP, may mimic the chemical and crystallographic properties of natural bone apatite by creating a physiologically active hydroxyl-carbonated apatite layer on the implant [149, 153]. In healing environments, the bioceramics used to fill osseous defects degrade through simple physicochemical dissolution and/or cell-mediated, primarily osteoclastic, resorption. Factors affecting the dissolution rate include the calcium-to-phosphate ratio, crystallization purity, surface area-to-volume ratio, pore architecture, local acidity, fluid convection, and temperature [154]. It usually takes 3–6 months for a scaffold to resorb entirely. However, slow resorption rates are necessary for situations such as GBR and sinus lift, where robust space creation and primary implant stability are needed [121]. There are two main types of ceramic scaffolds: solid scaffolds that provide fixed shapes and injectable scaffolds that allow for shape adjustments. Alumina and zirconia are examples of bioinert ceramics utilized for solid structural purposes, while calcium phosphates are examples of bioactive ceramics used for BTE in both solid and injectable forms [155–157].

Osteoconductivity, an essential property for bone healing, is determined by the physicochemical characteristics of biomaterials, such as their chemical composition, surface properties, and architectural geometry. According to previous studies and because of their structural and chemical similarities to native bone minerals, bioceramics based on calcium phosphate, such as HA, TCP, biphasic calcium phosphate, octa calcium phosphate (OCP), and coralline HA, are used for osteoinduction. The first publication that described the use of calcium phosphates in bone healing was reported by Albee and Morrison in 1920. Some calcium phosphate ceramics, like OCP, are relatively stable, while others, like TCP, are very soluble, due to differences in chemical composition and Ca/P ratio. The incorporation of ions and GFs into the HA structure may boost its biological activities, resulting in a rise in bone density and osteoblast proliferation. Furthermore, osteoconductive materials, such as bioglass, enable mineral deposition due to their ability to bind noncollagenous matrix proteins [158, 159]. The ideal pore size and porosity of the scaffold are critical for effective bone substitute materials, as they permit bone ingrowth and neovascularization. Porous calcium phosphate scaffolds facilitate bone formation through three mechanisms: first, invasion of newly formed bone tissue onto the surface of the material through the network of interconnected pores; second, macrophage activity before invasion or penetration of bone marrow; and third, the material itself creates the microenvironment necessary to locally induce osteogenic differentiation of the osteoprogenitor cells contained within the hematopoietic bone marrow [160]. The modified framework enhances vascularization and self-resorption, which speeds up bone regeneration and improves osteogenic differentiation. Bone mineralization, total volume, bone quality, and tissue necrosis may all be severely impacted by infection-induced inflammation, which in turn slows down the healing process. To address critical-sized bone lesions, researchers have created a porous antibiotic-treated HA scaffold that may replace the gold standard treatment, that is, bone autografts. A group of 24 New Zealand white rabbits underwent surgery to create a defect in the femur. The defects were then treated with either the HA scaffold or a pulverized autograft. Results revealed the bone autograft underperformed when in the presence of an infection. However, the HA scaffolds treated with an antibiotic successfully encouraged bone repair and reduced the bacterial load [161]. Moreover, when coatings of deferoxamine and konjac glucomannan were applied to HA scaffolds, an improved bone repair response was measured, as reported by Zhao *et al.* [162].

Additionally, BG, invented in the 1960s, is a versatile ceramic material that can bond with bone, stimulate bone and blood vessel growth, and dissolve at different rates and sizes. It is used in various medical applications, including orthopedic surgery, cranial and teeth replacement, tissue engineering scaffolds, and metal implant coatings, making it a versatile option [163]. Bioglasses form a unique layer called hydroxyl-carbonated apatite, which induces a cellular response. Scientists are investigating the causes of this phenomenon, which involves proteins and osteoprogenitor cells migrating to the bone surface to produce ECM. To maximize ECM formation, the precise concentration of Si and Ca ions is critical, and the ionic dissolution products of the BG control the proliferation and differentiation of osteoprogenitors [164, 165]. A review of BG scaffolds for bone engineering suggests that their mechanical strength is not a limiting factor. Some existing scaffolds can resist compression pressures, much like original bones; however, they also have drawbacks, including low mechanical reliability and fracture toughness. New research that improves the composition, processing, and sintering conditions has made it possible to make BG scaffolds with predetermined pore topologies and strength levels that are similar to human trabecular and cortical bones. The scientific community has reported brittleness as a limiting issue. Researchers must use state-of-the-art manufacturing processes to develop robust BG scaffolds and then test their effectiveness in animal models [166]. The incorporation of trace metals like Zn, Mg, and strontium (Sr) may boost the biological effects of BG, which promote cell interactions. For example, strontium ranelate is used to treat osteoporosis owing to its antiresorptive and anabolic properties. Sr-containing BGs have been produced in research and integrated into composite scaffolds based on chitosan (CS) and alginate to increase mechanical strength and biological behavior. Based on the investigation, scaffolds with a modest concentration of BG have been discovered to be more suited for repairing significant levels of bone damage. These scaffolds demonstrate improved mechanical strength, cell differentiation efficiency, and biomineralization [165, 167]. Also, research revealed that BTE using injectable collagen gel containing BG may provide a novel treatment option, according to research. The gel improves mineralization, neovascularization, and cell infiltration within 14 days [168].

Ceramic scaffolds, especially HA scaffolds, have recently seen developmental efforts aimed at optimizing their physiological and biochemical characteristics. Bioactive compounds such as BMP-2 or peptides linked to BMP-2 have been integrated into the scaffolds as one method. These compounds help cells adhere to one another, reproduce, and differentiate into osteogenic tissues, all of which contribute to osteoinduction [169]. Another approach is to enhance cell incorporation and differentiation within the scaffold using SCs, such as human adipose-derived SCs or hypoxia-preconditioned BM-MSCs. Scientists reported that adding hypoxia-preconditioned BM-MSCs improved angiogenesis, and combining doped-HA with BM-MSCs improved osteogenesis by employing the doped element [170]. Researchers have been exploring the use of drug carriers such as CS and poly (lactide-co-glycolide) on the surface of HA scaffolds for drug delivery and antibacterial purposes. They have also successfully immobilized drug carriers and biomolecules onto the scaffold surface using a polymeric coating. Additionally, antimicrobial HA scaffolds containing silver ions have recently been created [171]. The utilization of magnetic nanoparticles (MNPs) is another way that HA scaffolds have been shown to improve bone regeneration. MNPs are reported to alter the protein corona, which boosted the production of proteins involved in cell proliferation. The administration of MNPs expedited bone regeneration and stimulated osteoblast growth [172, 173].

3.3. *Polymer-Based Scaffolds*

Polymeric scaffolds represent a promising avenue in BTE and are categorized into two primary types: natural and synthetic polymers. The ideal biocompatible polymers for use in BTE scaffolds are those that provide regulated degradation and easy excretion *via* metabolic processes. Among synthetic polymers, the most prevalent include polycaprolactone (PCL), polyglycolic acid (PGA), poly lactic-glycolic acid (PLGA), and polyurethane. The most frequently utilized natural polymers consist of polysaccharides such as starch, alginate, chitin/CS, and derivatives of hyaluronic acid, as well as proteins such as soy, collagen, fibrin gels, and silk. Notably, protein-based polymeric scaffolds exhibit superior cell adhesion properties compared to polysaccharides, which is attributed to the presence of amino acids that serve as fundamental components in facilitating this adhesion. Researchers discovered that i-Factor™ Bone Graft, a unique composite material consisting of a P-15 collagen fragment, provides superior results compared to local autograft bone in single-level anterior cervical discectomy and fusion procedures. The study followed patients for 2 years after their surgery and compared those who received autograft with those who received i-Factor™ in a cortical ring allograft. Results showed a higher fusion rate and neurological success in i-Factor™ subjects, and no allergic reactions were associated with this scaffold [174]. Although materials produced from natural sources may offer some benefits, such as biological recognition, they also carry the risk of being immunogenic or containing harmful contaminants. The regulated characteristics and repeatable large-scale manufacture of synthetic polymers have made them attractive for use as scaffolds in tissue engineering and cell transplantation [175, 176]. Upon implantation, polymer scaffolds elicit an inflammatory response within the body, triggering biochemical signaling pathways. This response attracts various immune cells, including monocytes, which adhere to the scaffold and differentiate into macrophages in response to these signals. The characteristics of the scaffold significantly influence macrophage activity, thereby impacting the immune response and, consequently, the repair and regeneration of damaged tissues [177]. The extracellular microenvironment could be imitated by porous scaffolds, which sustain tissue structure while facilitating cell adhesion, migration, growth, and survival. Their capacity to promote bone growth in living organisms is dependent on the size of their pores and the strength of the connections between them. Porous scaffolds (such as foam or sponge scaffolds), fibrous scaffolds, microsphere-based scaffolds, and hydrogels are the four geometric types of polymer scaffolds [178]. Many methods exist for controlling the porosity of the scaffolds used in BTE, including rapid prototyping (RP), laser sintering, freeze-drying, leaching, and supercritical CO_2 foaming. Electrospinning is effective for producing nanometer-sized fibers with high surface-area-to-volume ratios, and in promoting cell adhesion, but it can lead to small pore sizes that hinder cell infiltration. This may be overcome using direct melt electrowriting and other modified collector methods to generate macroporous scaffolds with bigger and more ordered pore sizes. This in turn allows cells to penetrate more easily [179]. RP technologies are revolutionizing BTE by providing innovative solutions for the reconstruction of bone defects. Traditional scaffold fabrication methods often fall short in terms of mechanical strength and pore geometry, which are crucial for effective bone regeneration. RP techniques, including stereolithography (SLA), selective laser sintering (SLS), and fused deposition modeling (FDM), allow for the creation of precise 3D structures, thereby enhancing the regenerative capabilities of scaffolds. The global market for 3D printing in medical applications has experienced significant growth, reflecting the increasing adoption of these technologies. SLA offers high resolution but struggles with biocompatible materials, while SLS is particularly effective for bone applications. FDM is popular due to its cost-effectiveness and ability to produce porous scaffolds, although it has limitations regarding material diversity and build time. Additionally, 3D printing shares principles with SLS but typically results in lower biomechanical strength. Despite advancements in biomaterials and manufacturing technologies, challenges persist in optimizing scaffolds, improving material innovation, and effectively incorporating biologically active factors. Continued research in RP for bone regenerative medicine aims to address these issues, ultimately enhancing the effectiveness of BTE [180].

Hydrogels are hydrophilic polymer networks that can be engineered to replicate the biochemical and physical characteristics of the ECM, making them suitable for cell loading and tissue repair. Their high water retention capacity allows them to mimic the softness and hydration of ECM, and their mechanical properties can be tailored for various tissue types through adjustments in monomer concentration, crosslink density, and other factors. Pore size in hydrogels is a critical factor that influences molecular and cell behavior, including nutrient diffusion, cell morphology, and molecular expression [181]. Despite their potential, conventional hydrogels face limitations due to their nanoscale pore sizes, which hinder nutrient and oxygen supply, waste removal, and effective cell seeding. These challenges restrict their clinical application in tissue engineering. To overcome these issues, researchers are developing structured macroporous hydrogels, although obstacles remain, including factors that affect cell survival, the need for injectable forms, control over cell behavior, and enhancement of the mechanical properties to better mimic natural tissue topology [182]. Possible explanations for the variations in the ideal pore diameter include changes in stiffness and the subsequent mechanosensitive cellular responses. Cellular interactions are improved in hydrogels with larger macroporous (~120 μm) in contrast to smaller holes (~5 nm). In addition, various cell types and tissues have distinct pore size requirements; for example, a 100 μm pore size is optimal for superficial cartilage differentiation, whereas a pore size of 200 μm is ideal for intermediate cartilage and endothelial cell activities. The optimal size of macroporous hydrogels reported to enhance the differentiation of endothelial progenitor cells was 200 μm when investigated *in vitro*; however, *in vivo*, a pore size of 300 μm was found to be the optimal size required to enhance vascular invasion [183, 184]. The application of polymer scaffolds has notably decreased the need for bone grafts. However, polymers are characterized by limited bonding capabilities and suboptimal mechanical properties. The elastic modulus of these materials is ~7 GPa for elastic variants and 4 GPa for stiff types, both of which fall short of the elastic modulus observed in cortical and trabecular bone. Furthermore, polymers are susceptible to a deformation phenomenon known as creep, necessitating reinforcement with additional materials; thus, they are often employed in composite forms [178].

3.4. *Composite-Based Scaffolds*

Composite scaffolds in BTE, which combine organic polymers and inorganic phases, have shown promising progress in improving bone regeneration. They are essential for bone healing due to their biocompatibility, biodegradability, bioactivity, and mechanical stability. By combining osteoconductive and osteoinductive elements, composite scaffolds improve bioactivity, encouraging cell attachment and development. They can be engineered to exhibit a range of pore sizes to encourage vascular invasion and angiogenesis, as well as possess interconnected pores for nutrient transport and cell migration. The mechanical characteristics must align with the host tissue being replaced to ensure successful cell mechanoregulation and structural integrity [185, 186]. Composite scaffolds containing ceramic or metal nanoparticles (e.g., HA, BG, magnetic bioceramics, silver, gold, or iron) and polymers (e.g., silk, CS, alginate, or synthetic polymers such as pHEMA, PLGA, etc.) may be used in tissue engineering. Nano- and microfibrous scaffolds are fabricated using processes such as electrospinning, solvent casting, and 3D printing. While solvent casting is easy to use, inexpensive, and creates networks of connected pores, it is not ideal for regulating the shape of the pores. Although electrospinning may mimic the original ECM architecture, it is not always successful in creating porous materials with three dimensions. With the help of CAD software, 3D printing can produce complex 3D objects, including implants customized to each patient. Applying a uniform coating of nanoparticles is challenging, but self-assembly offers spontaneous formation of well-defined structures [187]. Research has focused on creating multifunctional scaffolds that deliver bioactive molecules and provide physicochemical support to various cells. Primary cells or SCs are chosen for their remarkable proliferation and differentiation capabilities, and as such are preferred due to their ability to administer various biomolecules and support diverse cell types [188, 189]. A three-component composite foam scaffold consisting of PCL as the matrix, HA as the whiskers, and L-lysine as the filler component was the subject of a recent study. When compared to the PCL/HA system, the PCL/HA/Lys scaffold demonstrated superior wettability and a higher Young's modulus. The cytokine release profiles of IL-1β, IL-6, and tumor necrosis factor-α from osteoblasts (human fetal osteoblast, hFOB1.19 cells) suggested that the inclusion of HA and L-lysine in PCL scaffolds greatly enhanced the proliferation of pre-osteoblasts when cultured on this material [187]. To accelerate the healing process for bone abnormalities, the researchers created a composite scaffold aimed to encourage bone development and blood vessel production. The researchers combined mesoporous bioactive glass (MBG-NH_2) with silk fibroin (SF). The above-mentioned material incorporated insulin-like GF-1 and VEGF. The scaffold was mechanically strong enough, had a high porosity level and appropriate nanoscale morphology, and during long-term healing, it maintained adequate GF release. MSCs isolated from bone marrow were exposed to the scaffold and showed higher levels of osteogenic marker gene and protein expression, as well as increased angiogenesis marker gene expression and CD31 protein expression. An *in vivo* study conducted in mice with a skull abnormality demonstrated that the scaffold facilitated the development of blood vessels and accelerated healing of the damaged bone [190]. Given the current progress in composites and BTE, which primarily targets complex scenarios, the next section will provide detailed explanations of key advanced techniques designed to produce sophisticated bone-generating structures, including stimuli-responsive scaffolds, ferrogels, biological moiety-containing scaffolds, photobiomodulation (PBM), and low-intensity pulsed ultrasound (LIPUS).

3.5. *Advanced and Biofunctional Scaffolds*

In the realm of scaffold BTE, the intricate interplay of biological processes is crucial for effective bone healing. As has been stated so far, bone repair involves several biological processes such as the regulation of inflammation, angiogenesis, and the formation of new bone tissue. Key cellular players such as endothelial cells, immune cells, osteoclasts, and MSCs contribute to the healing process through proliferation, differentiation, and ECM production [191–193]. Biomaterial-based scaffolds are crucial for managing bone tissue repair processes. These scaffolds can integrate bioactive molecules and SCs and stimulate the Wnt/β-catenin signaling pathway, among others. This activation has been shown to enhance MSC migration and initiate osteogenic pathways, leading to increased cell proliferation and bone formation. The Wnt/β-catenin pathway is essential for fostering osteogenesis and angiogenesis while inhibiting osteoclastogenesis [194]. The process of bone regeneration with the help of these smart materials can occur through three primary mechanisms: (1) the manipulation of surface nanotopography, (2) the incorporation of bioactive molecules, and (3) the seeding of SCs onto scaffolds [195]. Natural polymers, such as silk and Arg-Gly-Asp, are highly useful due to their biological responsiveness, nontoxicity, and biodegradability. They can be used to interact with bioactive agents, including cytokines, GFs, extracellular vesicles, small molecules, or peptides [196]. Some of these scaffolds serve as a matrix enriched with bone peptides that enhance ossification and facilitate bone regeneration by enabling the sustained release of peptides and the activation of signaling pathways [197]. To control cellular recognition of the scaffold, adhesive molecules such as fibronectin may modulate integrin signaling. During the late phase of the osteogenic differentiation process, the NCP osteocalcin is believed to have a crucial role in promoting biomineralization. BMPs, critical proteins used in bone and cartilage tissue engineering, enable the transformation of MSCs and pre-osteoblasts into osteogenic and chondrogenic cells, respectively. Collagen is an appealing material for multifunctional scaffolds because it increases ectopic bone formation and osteogenic differentiation while also providing mechanical support. Controlling the distribution of one or multiple GFs is feasible *via* the use of multifunctional porous or nanoparticulate materials while prolonging the release of the mentioned active agents [198]. Various techniques, such as physical adsorption and covalent binding, are employed to immobilize these bioactive molecules onto the scaffold surface. However, physical connections often result in transient interactions, while covalent binding may diminish the efficacy of the molecules. Furthermore, existing surface modification strategies predominantly emphasize osteoinduction and the differentiation of osteoblasts, with insufficient attention given to osteoclastogenesis, which is crucial for effective bone repair [194]. Biofunctional scaffolds promote osteogenesis, angiogenesis, and osteoclastogenesis, but they face challenges including immune reactions, regulatory hurdles, and long-term stability. Further challenges include cytotoxicity, high costs, and rapid deactivation, necessitating the need for innovative strategies to combat this [194].

Drug delivery systems, pH-sensitive scaffolds, and piezoelectric materials are all categories of smart biomaterials that facilitate bone tissue repair. These approaches have the potential to treat infections, regulate biofilms, transport medications, bioactive substances, and SCs. Knowing the location of the lesion, the patient's activity, and any functional deficiencies, are critical for successful bone regeneration. Other factors that affect performance include age and health [199]. As described in a recent review article, the authors proposed a novel way to categorize smart biomaterials. Biomaterials may be either *inert, active, responsive, or autonomous*, depending on how much they interact with their surroundings and the biological reactions that ensue. Modern smart biomaterials are those that are autonomous, responsive, and active. Distinguishing between "smart biomaterials" and otherwise "intelligent biomaterials" is essential. Smart refers to the acquired ability to apply prior knowledge, while intelligent refers to the innate ability to acquire knowledge. Smart biomaterials cannot exhibit intelligent functions such as self-calibration or self-diagnosis, while intelligent biomaterials cannot be smart [200]. Inert biomaterials are considered biocompatible and relatively harmless, but they can lack certain health benefits. For example, active biomaterials, on the other hand, can provide one-way bioactive properties, which in turn promote tissue regeneration, regulate drug release, as well as facilitate the delivery of antioxidant, anticancer, and antibacterial therapies, among others. To achieve synergistic or additive effects, multifunctional active biomaterials integrate many active ingredients into a single biomaterial. Responsive biomaterials sense and respond to stimuli, subsequently releasing specific therapeutic agents for the delivery of precision medications and other tissue engineering technologies. They can be triggered by internal or external stimuli, allowing for targeted therapeutic delivery to specific cells or processes. Autonomous biomaterials, in contrast, are completely self-contained and can alter their therapeutic effects and environmental characteristics in response to external stimuli and internal biological mechanisms. Although none yet exist, theoretically, these biomaterials aim to detect diseases at an early stage, convey their existence externally, and then treat the disease before damage occurs *via* a closed-loop system. The ability of autonomous biomaterials to mimic the behavior of a living, programmable, and reconfigurable organism without human intervention is comparable to that of a miniature computer system [200]. A study recently described the development of a chemical framework that can transport hydrogels and precisely degrade them based on environmental cues, allowing for reactions to follow user-programmed Boolean logic. The molecular structure and binding of stimuli-responsive segments within the material cross-links were analyzed to show the ability to selectively control gel dissolution and therapeutic release. To show how flexible this approach was, the authors created 17 different stimuli-sensitive materials. These materials produced every possible logical YES/OR/AND result as directed using input combinations *via* an enzyme, a reductant, and light. These hydrogels were used to show the consecutive and environmentally triggered growth of various cell types in specific combinations using one material [201].

In tissue engineering, stimuli-responsive biomaterials that serve as multifunctional scaffolds and imitate ECM properties are essential for facilitating cell-based, genetic, and immunological therapies [202]. The stimuli-responsive scaffolds can react to physical, chemical, and enzyme stimuli. These materials can deliver medications in a time-regulated manner and aid in the promotion of bone repair following tissue loss [203]. The ease of synthesizing photoresponsive functional nanosystems and components has led to their widespread use in antibacterial and anticancer therapies. Brought about by the photophysical effects of radiation, increased adenosine triphosphate (ATP) production and cellular metabolism may result following alterations in intracellular activity and the respiratory chain. This may aid both angiogenesis and bone repair. For their multifunctional properties, several photothermal agents have been researched and produced, including organic nanoparticles, carbon-based nanoparticles, graphene, MXenes, single-elemental nanosheets, gold nanostructures, and transition metal sulfides and oxides. Different stimuli-responsive scaffold compositions might lead to the predominance of certain bone regeneration pathways. Depending on the kind and efficacy of the scaffold, osteogenesis may be greatly enhanced by upregulating heat shock protein expression, making holes in polymeric coatings or shells releasing metallic ions, tumor ablation, and inactivating the BMP-2/Smad signaling pathway [204].

PBM is a modern noninvasive tissue regeneration method that uses a biocompatible range of radiation, in the visible and infrared range, to interact with chromophores within cells, enhancing mitochondrial function and facilitating cell differentiation [205]. In contrast to photodynamic or photothermal therapy, PBM treatment does not need the use of external mediators. This technique has the potential to revolutionize BTE by targeting cytochrome *c* oxidase and influencing osteogenic gene expression, collagen maturation, and mineralization, thereby enhancing molecular secretions and cellular functioning through the production of ATP. Combined with SC populations, bioactive compounds, nanoparticles, or biomaterial scaffolds, PBM tremendously enhances tissue regeneration [206, 207]. Specifically, PBM at wavelengths of 655 nm and 808 nm has been shown to elevate osteogenic gene expression by inducing the production of intracellular ROS, ATP, and nitric oxide, thereby facilitating osteogenesis [208]. However, the application of PBM in BTE is not perfect, and this includes reports of the incomplete repair of extensive bone defects and difficulties in differentiating newly formed bone tissue due to isoradiographic density variations [209].

A recent work aimed to examine a thermo-responsive nanocomposite system using poly(organophosphazene)-based materials and GFs as a bioink. The mechanical characteristics of the thermo-responsive bioink were controlled by adjusting the temperature within the range of 15°C–30°C, and with the highest level of stiffness measured at 37°C. The bioink was combined with BMP-2 and transforming growth factor-beta 1 (TGF-β1) to formulate a scaffold for the restoration of skull abnormalities in mice. A notable enhancement in bone regeneration was measured [210]. CS is a naturally occurring biopolymer that is very useful as a grafting material in the development of thermosensitive and pH-sensitive injectable hydrogels. The formulation of injectable hydrogels based on CS has many advantages, including excellent water absorption, low invasiveness, porous networks, and the capability to be completely shaped into irregular defects. CS hydrogels generated from the protonation/deprotonation of primary amine groups (NH_2) have pH-responsive efficiency that is influenced by the pH of the surrounding environment. At lower pH, the protonation of the -NH_2 group of CS induces electrostatic repulsion, allowing polymer chains to expand and interact with water molecules. This phenomenon efficiently enhances the solubility of the polymer in water. Elevated pH values above the pKa cause the -NH_2 group in CS to deprotonate, resulting in the absence of any net charge. Moreover, this group collapses the globular shape of CS and increases its water-insoluble nature. Hence, the pH-responsive water solubility of CS is contingent upon its pKa value. As a result, the expansion and contraction characteristics of a hydrogel composed of CS are determined by its external and ambient pH [211]. A thermosensitive CS hydrogel with graphene oxide was developed to improve the porous architecture, swelling, protein adsorption, degradation rate, and biomineralization properties. The hydrogel was biocompatible when tested with MSCs, their metabolic activity was maintained, and the hydrogel promoted osteogenic differentiation [212]. Moreover, an investigation into the viability, proliferation, and growth of mouse fibroblasts enclosed in a pH-responsive CS-HA/sodium bicarbonate ($NaHCO_3$) hydrogel over a 7-day duration also yielded encouraging findings [213].

Tissues, such as bone, are dynamically reshaped and remodeled *via* multiple signaling pathways according to their operational needs. These signals are transmitted through chemical and electrical events and modulated by the extracellular network and cells. Notwithstanding the therapeutic advantages of designed scaffolds, their inflexibility in signaling disrupts normal signaling pathways. Hence, it is imperative to develop intelligent biomaterials capable of efficiently generating and transmitting bioelectrical signals that closely resemble those of the native tissue, and tailored for suitable physiological applications. Piezoelectric scaffolds are capable of serving as highly responsive mechanical–electrical guiding systems. Bone inherently functions as a piezoelectric material, and the charges and potentials produced in response to mechanical stimulation may stimulate bone formation. The ability of piezoelectric materials to imitate the physiological microenvironment is crucial in promoting bone regeneration and repair. The intrinsic piezoelectric characteristics and prolonged release of Mg^{2+} from Whitlockite (WH), a naturally occurring calcium phosphate-containing magnesium, have garnered significant interest in the field of bone development. A 3D-printed composite scaffold consisting of piezoelectric Whitlockite (PWH) and PCL was developed to satisfy the physiological criteria for neurovascular bone tissue regeneration. This scaffold aimed to generate an endogenous EF at the site of bone tissue damage. The continuous release of Mg^{2+} from the PWH scaffold exhibited several biological functions and demonstrated a potent synergistic impact coupled with piezoelectricity that suppressed osteoclast activity, facilitated neural differentiation, angiogenesis, and the osteogenic differentiation of BMSCs. Using a rat skull defect model, this PWH scaffold demonstrated exceptional efficacy in promoting neo-bone development by stimulating neurogenic expression and angiogenesis [214].

Wolff's law and the mechanistic theory describe how mechanical loads may enhance or reduce bone mass and shape according to the physical demands of its external environment. The approach known as LIPUS is designed to enhance cell survival and promote tissue regeneration within scaffolds. The impact of this noninvasive method, which uses low-intensity pulse waves on bone to encourage intramembrane ossification healing, has not been well established [215]. However, LIPUS mechanical stimulation activates the integrin/phosphatidylinositol-3-OH kinase/Akt pathway, leading to osteogenic protein upregulation. *In vitro* and *in vivo* studies that investigated the effect of LIPUS on cell behavior within 3D titanium, ceramic, and hydrogel scaffolds revealed that LIPUS promoted bone formation, increased mineral deposition, and improved cell ingrowth. In addition, it improved 3D hydrogel encapsulation, GF delivery, and scaffold modification. Further investigation is required to refine the ultrasonic parameters and assess the impact of LIPUS on other scaffold materials and cell types [216]. A recent study examined the effects of LIPUS and autologous bone on the process of repairing critical-size bone lesions within rat calvaria. The findings indicated that both LIPUS and autologous bone stimulated osteogenesis, resulting in almost full closure of the lesion. After 30 days, the autologous bone group displayed the greatest bone volume, slightly more than that obtained in the LIPUS group. At 7 and 15 days, the LIPUS group exhibited the greatest levels of COX-2 and Osterix (OSX) expression, indicating that LIPUS may serve as a feasible substitute for autologous bone transplants in the healing of intramembranous ossified bone defects [217]. Another study also reported that this technique improved scaffold ossification by promoting proteins involved in bone formation, including COX-2 and OSX, in mitigating apoptosis, and also through fostering dendritic network development [218].

Ferrogels are a category of scaffold material that include MNPs and have exceptional biological properties important for tissue engineering purposes. These materials enable precise manipulation and an instantaneous response to magnetic fields [219]. As often a self-healing substance, ferrogels enhance the properties of tissue engineering scaffolds by imparting dynamic properties [220]. Ferrogel fabrication methods involve creating a porous ferrogel and magnetoactive composite, which can be used in biomedical engineering and microfluidic applications to create deformable scaffolds. These materials currently play a vital role in tissue engineering, particularly in cell culture, drug delivery, biosensing technologies, and wearable electronics [221]. Ferrogels are often produced by integrating iron oxide MNPs into polyacrylamide gels, which has a substantial impact on cellular biological functions. The use of the distinctive characteristics of MNPs has led to the emergence of ferrogels as versatile frameworks in the realm of tissue engineering [222]. It was reported that a gradual increase in the concentration of maghemite nanoparticles within a polyacrylamide gel network led to a significant increase in the Young's modulus, effective viscosity, negative electric potential value, as well as the adhesion index for human skin fibroblasts and human peripheral blood leukocytes. Therefore, in terms of its biomedical application, the inclusion of a small amount of maghemite nanoparticles into the polymer network significantly increased the mechanical and electrical properties of ferrogels and improved the biocompatibility of these systems [223]. Traditional ferrogels often face challenges related to wear and magnetic sensitivity. Recent advancements have incorporated carbon nanotubes (CNTs) into the hydrogel, significantly enhancing its properties. CNTs firmly embedded in the hydrogel network created potential focal adhesion sites for encapsulated fibroblasts and significantly enhanced cell migration, resulting in tissue regeneration and wound healing. In contrast, insufficient migration was reported in the empty matrix [224]. The addition of CNTs to the ferrogel led to an 85% increase in the magnetic moment saturation due to improved grain refinement and magnetization mechanisms. Furthermore, the wear rate of the ferrogel decreased by approximately

40%, which was attributed to the lubricating properties of the CNTs and their synergistic interaction with the MNPs. These improvements position CNT-enhanced ferrogels as a superior polymer composite for application in magnetic sensors and in drug delivery [225]. Another way to modify scaffolds and produce more efficient properties is to incorporate biological elements such as cells, proteins, GFs, or genes, or manipulate the material features to induce neural or vascular regeneration, as depicted in **Figure 3**.

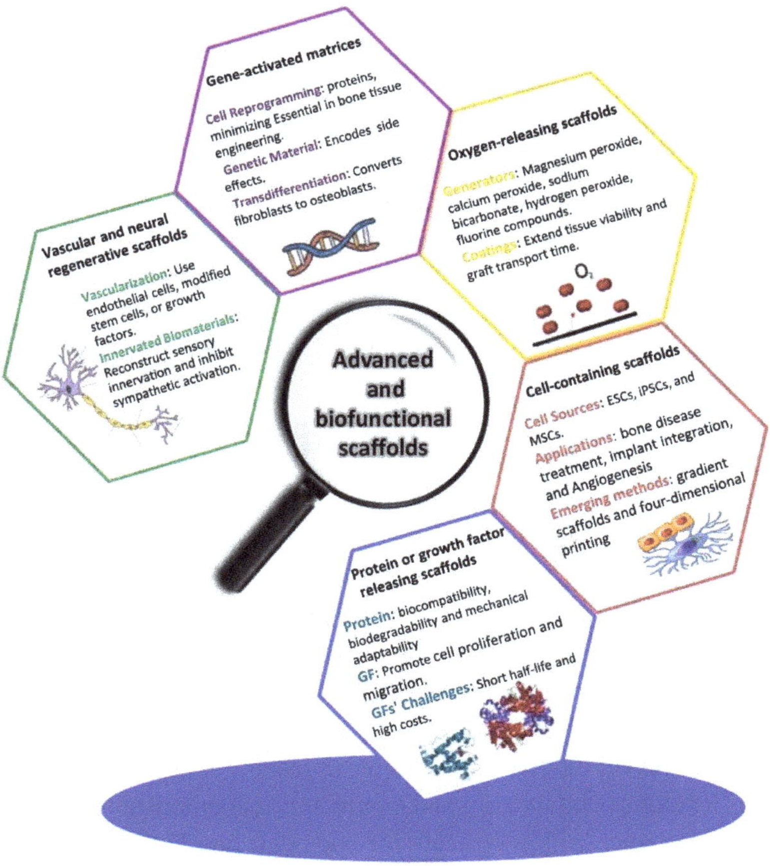

Figure 3. Oxygen-releasing, growth factor-releasing, gene-activated, neurovascular-regenerating, and functionalized cell-containing scaffolds, illustrating their key participants and their applications.

3.5.1. *Cell-Containing Scaffolds*

Bone regeneration is inherently a multifaceted process characterized by diverse biological responses and cellular interactions. The adhesion and proliferation of critical cell types, including macrophages, endothelial cells, and BMSCs, are fostered *via* augmented interactions between cells and the scaffold material [226]. These biofunctionalized scaffolds have several benefits when used, including modulating immune responses, accelerating tissue healing, delivering antimicrobial properties, and stimulating angiogenesis and osteogenesis [227]. Bone scaffolds are created using composites of biopolymers, synthetic polymers, and ceramics with the aim of supporting the growth of MSCs [228]. MSCs have been investigated as a treatment strategy for bone diseases, where traditional surgical procedures and pharmacological approaches have failed. BMSCs are effective in regenerating bone and are reported to be more efficient at differentiating into osteoblasts than adipose-derived MSCs. However, limitations in cell yield, expansion requirements, reduced regenerative ability, and increased patient morbidity and risk necessitate further research into alternative MSC harvest sites [229]. Unfortunately, MSCs cannot be extracted from individuals suffering from systemic disorders, and their small quantity requires further cultivation after separation [230]. Alternatively, other SCs, sourced as embryonic SCs or induced pluripotent stem cells (iPSCs), may be used in future BTE clinical trials. Endothelial cells are also being investigated for potential use in promoting angiogenesis and vascularization [231, 232]. Research has investigated the possibility of using iPSCs to restore bone in animals with critical-size bone defects. The authors reported that scaffolds loaded with either iPSCs or decellularized scaffolds that contained ECM from iPSCs could differentiate these cells into osteoblasts. Grafting iPSCs onto a PLGA/CaP osteoconductive scaffold induced osteogenic differentiation, resulting in an increased bone volume 9 weeks after implantation, compared to using the scaffold alone. Both *in vitro* and *in vivo* studies demonstrated enhanced bone repair in mice within critical-size bone defects [233].

Understanding how cells interact with scaffolds is crucial for effective regenerative medicine. Manufacturing processes often fail to account for important interfacial interactions, which can lead to rejection and diminished outcomes. Personalized scaffolds with an optimal pore structure and signaling to encourage cell adhesion are essential. Surface properties, the incorporation of nano-dimensional materials and nanoparticles, and biomineralization significantly impact cell activity and differentiation [234]. Tissue engineering makes extensive use of biological 3D printing technology owing to its easy operation and controlled precision. This technology aims to produce synthetic tissues that closely resemble human tissues, thereby advancing the field of individualized biomedicine. In BTE, 3D-printed scaffolds can enhance biomineralization and osteoblast adhesion. However, traditional 3D printing has limitations in controlling structure and shape due to high temperatures or specific material treatments. Bioprinting technology overcomes these limitations by incorporating living cells and GFs into scaffolds, mimicking the structure and properties of native bone. There are three main methods of bioprinting: inkjet, extrusion, and laser-assisted bioprinting. Bioink refers to an ink formulation that might include biological components and biomaterials. It has to be biocompatible, bioactive, biodegradable, viscous, and have the appropriate mechanical qualities to be used in a bioprinting process. However, the challenge remains in fabricating scaffolds that meet the structural, mechanical, and osteoconductive/osteoinductive requirements. Emerging approaches in this field include gradient scaffolds and four-dimensional printing technology *via* smart materials, organoids, and cell aggregates/spheroids, allowing for the printing of high cell-density structures [235, 236]. Researchers have developed a device called a "scaffold-on-a-chip" to assist in the assessment of 3D-printed scaffolds engineered for bone regeneration. This device aims to replicate the microenvironment that transplanted bone scaffolds encounter. It consists of a circular space for inserts and a microfluidic channel that surrounds the space. This design enables the monitoring of cell behavior at the interface between the scaffold and blood [237]. By creating 3D-printed biomimetic scaffolds that combine β-TCP with BMSCs, research aims to enhance the healing of alveolar clefts. Hybrid scaffolds made from a mixture of gelatin methacrylate (GelMA) and β-TCP have shown favorable mechanical characteristics and biocompatibility. Bone marrow SCs were shown to adhere to the scaffold surface, where they multiplied, survived, differentiated, and where osteogenesis was promoted [238]. A recent study successfully developed a mineralized bone model using 3D bioprinting techniques. The researchers used a combination of cell-laden alginate–gelatin–graphene oxide hydrogels and cultured them under dynamic loading conditions. They utilized hMSCs and primary human osteoblasts obtained from surgical waste material. The study aimed to compare the effects of two different cell printing densities: a previously reported optimal density of 5 $\times$ 10^6 cells/mL of bioink and a higher physiological density of 10 $\times$ 10^6 cells/mL. The results showed that both bioink cell densities resulted in high cell viability post printing and following 2 weeks of daily mechanical loading. However, bioprinting at the higher cell density resulted in faster mineral formation rates, higher mineral densities, and a 10-fold increase in stiffness. The study also found that physiological cell bioprinting densities positively impacted cell spreading and dendritic interconnections. This technology could be applied to study individual phenotypes of bone disorders, such as osteogenesis imperfecta, and aid clinical decision-making [239]. Despite the promise of bioprinting, challenges remain, particularly concerning cell survival during the printing process, which can inflict physical damage due to shear forces. To mitigate this issue, researchers have utilized microfluidic technology to create cell microcapsules that encapsulate SCs, improving their viability. As described previously, the scaffold's porous structure plays a vital role in promoting cell adhesion and proliferation, with optimal porosity and pore connectivity facilitating 3D growth and enhancing the development of vascular and nerve networks [240].

3.5.2. *Protein- or Growth Factor-Releasing Scaffolds*

Another highly promising strategy in BTE involves the biofunctionalization of scaffolds through the incorporation of proteins and GFs. This process entails the loading of scaffolds with bioactive molecules that enhance the process of bone formation. Essential proteins such as collagen, gelatin, and serum albumin are recognized for their biocompatibility, biodegradability, and mechanical adaptability [241]. In addition to biomaterials and cellular components, GFs are critical for influencing cell proliferation, morphological changes, and migration toward the scaffold surface. By guiding progenitor and inflammatory cells to the transplantation site, GFs initiate the tissue repair process [242]. There are several issues with using GFs in tissue engineering, including their short half-life, immunogenicity, manufacturing challenges, and high prices, although they are crucial for modulating cell activity. BMPs are known for their ability to promote osteoprogenitor cell proliferation and differentiation, making them popular in BTE and grafting strategies. However, BMPs have drawbacks, such as high costs and potential adverse effects like heterotopic bone formation, pseudoarthrosis, and local inflammation. Alternative approaches to BMPs include using small osteoinductive chemicals, which are easy and inexpensive to manufacture, non-immunogenic, and stable in physiological conditions. Moreover, integrins are essential in BTE, regulating cell behavior and facilitating interactions between cells and the ECM. They are classified into three groups: β1-integrins, which enhance cell adhesion to ECM components; β2-integrins, involved in various biological processes; and αv-integrins, which bind ECM proteins through the Arg-Gly-Asp (RGD) motif. In bone, integrins interact with key ECM proteins such as collagen and fibronectin, influencing tissue organization and cell behavior. Recent advancements in biomaterials use integrin interactions to improve tissue engineering outcomes, including surface nanopatterning and the addition of GFs like BMP-2. This highlights the importance of integrins in both natural bone development and engineered tissue constructs [243]. Hydrogels, with their 3D structures, transport bioactive substances, facilitating sustained release for angiogenesis and neural pathway formation. They could promote cellular activities, including neurite development, by enhancing β1-integrin expression. In bone repair, timely delivery of bioactive factors is crucial for bone generation. Sequential release systems based on nanoparticles improve drug delivery efficiency and tissue targeting [244].

Biomaterials may be functionalized as a novel approach for tissue development using biomimetic peptides, which are generated from active regions of soluble or ECM proteins, soluble factors, or naturally occurring substances. These short peptides can be easily designed and cost-effectively synthesized *in vitro* (e.g., cRGD-DWIVA and cRGD-cDWIVA {[*(cyclic(Arg-Gly-Asp-D-Phe-Glu)-Ahx-Ahx)(cyclic(Asp-Trp-Ile-Val-Ala-Glu)-Ahx-Ahx)]-Lys-βAla-Cys-*NH_2}), opening up new opportunities for cheaper and more effective scaffolds. These peptides mediate cell adhesion and induce osteogenic differentiation, as well as angiogenesis [245]. Hybrid scaffolds were created through a biomimetic process of intrafibrillar collagen mineralization and were then coated with an antimicrobial peptide to promote bone/dental tissue growth and to prevent bacterial infection. Highly hydrophilic inorganic collagen scaffolds were the perfect surface for creating a thick and secure layer of antimicrobial peptides. The created structures eliminated Gram-negative *Escherichia coli* and Gram-positive *Streptococcus gordonii* and were also suitable for human BMSCs [246]. A scaffold was created using electrospun PCL fibers combined with bioactive self-assembling peptides (SAPs) P11-4 (Ac-QQRFEWEFEQQ-Am) or P11-8 (Ac-QQRFOWOFEQQ-Am). Both scaffolds containing SAPs were suitable for mouse fibroblasts and induced the formation of apatite minerals *in vitro* (in simulated body fluid; SBF). Scaffolds showed the capacity to regulate the release of bioactive self-assembly peptides, making them appealing for treating pre-critical bone defects [247].

3.5.3. *Gene-Activated Matrices*

Gene-activated scaffolds, developed in the late 1990s, are biocompatible, degradable, and effective in transferring DNA while minimizing toxicity. They enhance cell proliferation, differentiation, and bone repair by delivering targeted genes to specific sites, promoting DNA transcription and translation post-implantation, supplying vital osteogenic factors for bone repair, and aiding the development of MSCs without relying on grafts or prosthetics [248]. Unlike traditional methods that utilize protein-based GFs, which can cause off-target effects due to the high doses needed, gene-based therapies leverage genetic material to encode the desired proteins, minimizing the risk of adverse effects. Gene- and RNA interference-activated scaffolds are tissue engineering devices loaded with nucleic acids aimed at promoting local tissue repair, which may take advantage of the therapeutic activity of proteins without administering supraphysiological doses. Various approaches to formulating these scaffolds have been explored, including activation with plasmid DNA (pDNA), viruses, RNA transcripts, or interfering RNAs [249]. There are two primary types of gene therapy: viral and nonviral. Viral gene therapy utilizes attenuated viruses to deliver desired proteins but poses risks such as immune reactions and insertional mutagenesis, limiting its clinical application. In contrast, nonviral gene therapy employs alternative vectors and cell-penetrating methods, though it often results in lower transgene expression. The integration of gene therapies with scaffolds can involve loading them with transfection vectors or pre-seeding cells, creating a potentially ready-to-use therapeutic solution that simplifies clinical application by reducing the need for extensive cell manipulation [250].

Cell reprogramming, particularly through direct cell reprogramming or transdifferentiation, has gained attention for its potential in bone tissue regeneration and disease modeling. This innovative technique enables the conversion of readily available cells in the body into specific cell types necessary for repairing damaged bone tissue. By utilizing methods such as the overexpression of transcription factors *via* viral vectors, small molecules, and CRISPR/Cas9 technology, researchers can effectively induce these transformations. The resulting transdifferentiated cells have demonstrated the ability to replicate essential functions and support tissue regeneration in live models, particularly in mice. Although clinical applications are still in development, the ability to generate localized transdifferentiated cells *in situ* could allow treatments without invasive surgery [251]. A recent study focused on reprogramming human fibroblasts into chemically induced osteogenic cells (ciOG) holds potential for applications in bone repair and treatment of bone-related diseases. Unlike their original fibroblast counterparts, the ciOG cells demonstrated the ability to form mineralized tissue when implanted into immunodeficient mice. The study also highlighted the influence of engineered culture substrates on osteogenic reprogramming, revealing that ciOG, generated on a nanofiber substrate, accelerated bone matrix formation in a calvarial defect [252]. Recent advancements in direct reprogramming technologies have enabled researchers to convert human fibroblasts into osteoblasts, a significant breakthrough in bone regeneration therapies. This innovative approach allows for the phenotypic transformation of somatic cells into osteoblasts without reverting to a pluripotent state. By introducing specific genes, that is, Runx2, OSX, Oct3/4, and L-Myc, researchers can efficiently generate directly converted osteoblasts (dOBs). Notably, using just three of these genes (OSX, Oct3/4, and L-Myc) also yields effective results. This procedure can prepare large numbers of autologous osteoblasts with high bone-forming ability [253]. The study developed a novel nanogel tectonic material for artificial 3D scaffolding in BTE. dOBs were used, and the gel was highly porous, allowing efficient cell adhesion and substantial bone matrix production. The combination of nanogel and dOBs promoted bone regeneration *in vivo*, suggesting a feasible therapeutic modality for the treatment of bone defects [254].

A novel approach for BTE is the microfluidic-assisted synthesis of pDNA-based nanocomplexes (NCs) that deliver genetic material encoding human BMP-2. The NCs were formed by combining pDNA with CS using a micromixer platform. These NCs were then immobilized onto a nanofibrous PCL scaffold that was functionalized with a metalloprotease-sensitive peptide, allowing for localized and environmentally responsive gene delivery. The osteogenic differentiation of BM-MSCs demonstrated the effectiveness of this gene-activated scaffold, highlighting the potential of this methodology for *in situ* BTE and its applicability in regenerative nanomedicine [255]. By co-delivering pDNA encoding FGF-2 and BMP-2, researchers aimed to leverage the synergistic effects of these GFs and improve bone healing in individuals with diabetes, who frequently face challenges in fracture recovery. In a leporine model of diabetes, scaffolds embedded with PEI-(pBMP-2+pFGF-2) demonstrated significantly improved bone regeneration compared to scaffolds containing only PEI-pBMP-2. This indicated that co-gene-activated scaffolds could be a promising strategy for enhancing bone repair in diabetic patients [256]. IL-1β is a key inflammatory mediator in the fracture process, but its prolonged presence can hinder healing. To address complications in fracture healing such as delayed healing or non-union, a recent study aimed to develop a gene-based therapy that beneficially targets IL-1β while providing a supportive structure for bone regeneration. A collagen-HA scaffold was utilized to deliver nanoparticles containing pDNA encoding for the IL-1 receptor antagonist (IL-1Ra), using PEI as a nonviral gene delivery vector. The research demonstrated that PEI-pDNA nanoparticles effectively transfected into rat BM-MSCs, leading to transient gene expression. While initial viability was affected, the BM-MSCs recovered after 10 days. Importantly, transfection using PEI-pIL-1Ra nanoparticles resulted in the production of functional IL-1Ra, which successfully counteracted the negative effects of IL-1β on BM-MSC osteogenesis. The study found that IL-1Ra gene-activated scaffolds facilitated mineral deposition by BM-MSCs, even under chronic inflammatory conditions, indicating their potential for therapeutic applications *in vivo* for enhancing bone healing [257].

3.5.4. *Vascular- and/or Neural-Regenerating Scaffolds*

BTE involves integrating vascularization and innervation to create functionally superior scaffolds. This approach goes beyond replicating native bone structural features and allows for multifunctional scaffolds that restore bone function and participate in restoring the musculoskeletal system. Incorporating innervation into engineered bone tissue could accelerate the healing process and its response to mechanical stimuli and enhance biological compatibility with host organisms. Biomaterials such as hydrogels, which have a 3D network structure similar to the ECM, can enhance vascularization and innervation and act as a direct carrier for cells, cytokines, and small molecules. Sequential release systems based on nanoparticle technology have been developed to improve drug delivery, efficiency, and tissue targeting [258]. Multiple methods exist to improve vascularization, such as a two-step process, growing angiogenic cells, adding GFs, biological materials, and applying endothelial cells to the surface of the scaffold, or encapsulating these components inside the scaffold itself. A two-stage procedure begins with implanting the scaffold in hypervascular tissue (e.g., muscle) and then transferring it to the injured area after it has completely vascularized. Unfortunately, this treatment is not very applicable since it requires two surgical operations [259, 260]. The second approach involves cultivating endothelial cells and other angiogenic cells on the scaffold prior to its surgical implantation into the injured region. Research has shown that by co-culturing bone scaffolds with human smooth muscle cells and umbilical vein endothelial cells, it is possible to achieve *in vitro* vascularization of the bone scaffold. By using this method, both synthetic and natural scaffolds may be used to build vascular tissue with lumen architecture and the upregulation of appropriate gene expressions [261]. As previously mentioned, the third method involves either encapsulating GFs, biological materials, and endothelial cells inside the scaffold or altering its surface. This makes the scaffold more permeable to blood flow after implantation.

GFs are responsible for promoting the regeneration of bone tissue by stimulating various biological processes, for example, osteogenesis and angiogenesis. Osteogenesis, the bone formation process, relies on the presence of GFs such as PDGF, TGF-β, FGF, IGF, and BMPs. These factors are involved in the creation of the ECM, the differentiation and proliferation of osteogenic cells, and other important steps during bone formation. Conversely, GFs such as PDGF, IGF, FGF, and VEGF can promote the migration and proliferation of endothelial cells, thereby controlling angiogenesis and the formation of new blood vessels without preexisting vascular components. Some of the mentioned GFs have a synergistic effect, establishing a connection between angiogenesis and osteogenesis. For example, PDGF not only promotes osteoblast development but also upregulates VEGF expression. Researchers have found that BMPs may also promote angiogenesis by increasing p38 phosphorylation and activating the Smad signaling pathway, resulting in vessel tube formation [262]. A study conducted *in vivo* used a biodegradable scaffold made of poly (L-lactic acid and glycolide) (PLGA) to deliver VEGF to the irradiated osseous lesions. Radiation treatment frequently damages tissues and impairs their ability to regenerate. A decrease in tissue perfusion and blood flow primarily causes this injury. In comparison to the PLGA scaffolds, the VEGF scaffolds greatly enhanced blood vessel development and function, as well as bone coverage and mineral density. These results point to the potential function of VEGF in improving tissue regeneration in radiation-induced hypovascular conditions [263]. The final strategy utilizes modified SCs and angiogenesis-related genes. This approach aims to improve bone tissue healing by increasing the ability of the SC to generate new bone and vascular structures. However, the lengthy angiogenesis process and the difficulties in controlling the biological components are two obstacles that this method must overcome. Every patient is unique, and their requirements will determine which of these approaches works best [259]. In addition to the mentioned techniques, researchers have investigated how certain ions affect bone regeneration by covering an alginate biopolymer with silicate ions. This method improved bone defect repair and also caused endothelial cells to upregulate angiogenic protein expression (VEGF, KDR, eNOS, bFGF, and HIF1-α). The data revealed that the sustained release of silicate ions facilitated rapid acellular mineral production and increased blood vessel formation [264].

Synthetic biomaterials show promise for treating bone defects but need improvement due to low osteoinductivity, poor integration with host bone, and lack of regeneration of vascular and neural networks. This has led to an increased research interest in neuro-osteology. Sensory Neurons play a crucial role in bone healing, improving osteogenic differentiation and vascular network reconstruction. This has often been overlooked in bone biomaterial design, but SN regeneration represents a new direction in bone regeneration [29]. However, norepinephrine released by adrenergic nerves inhibits bone formation. Recent focus on improving bone regeneration involves the development of innervated biomaterials to reconstruct sensory innervation and inhibit sympathetic nerve activation [265]. Neurons within bone also play an irreplaceable role in bone regeneration and repair after fracture. Signaling molecules mainly contain neurotransmitters, neuropeptides, GFs, and neuronal guidance factors, which work as bridges between the bone and nervous systems. Calcitonin gene-related peptide (CGRP), substance P, norepinephrine, neuropeptide Y, acetylcholine, nerve GF, brain-derived neurotrophic factor, and Semaphorin 3A are all involved in bone regeneration and repair. However, their high cost limits their wide application and short half-life makes it difficult to exert a long-term effect [31, 266]. CGRP, a common neuropeptide, is widely distributed in bone tissue, particularly in the metabolically active metaphysis. It is linked to bone metabolism, osteogenesis, and remodeling, and acts as a bridge between the nervous system and skeletal muscle. CGRP promotes osteogenesis, inhibits bone resorption, promotes vascular growth, and regulates the immune microenvironment [267]. A study explored the therapeutic effect of CGRP-modified BM-MSCs combined with autogenous bone grafting for the treatment of osteonecrosis of the femoral head (ONFH) in rabbits. The researchers found that CGRP-modified BM-MSCs accelerated osteogenic differentiation, improved osteogenesis efficiency, and promoted bone tissue repair and reconstruction, significantly improving the success rate of ONFH treatment [268]. On the other hand, Schwann cells (ScCs) regulate the surrounding microenvironment, and recent research has focused on the function of Schwann cell-derived exosomes (ScC-exos) in promoting bone regeneration. ScC-exos facilitated the proliferation and differentiation of BM-MSCs, enhanced osteogenesis by modulating the TGF-β signaling pathway, and improved the migration and tube formation of endothelial progenitor cells, thus improving vascularization [269]. The researchers developed a 3D-printed scaffold that mimicked the microenvironment of the ossification center, aiming to replicate the bone development process, enhance neural innervation, and ultimately promote bone regeneration. As stated before, 3D bioprinting technology has become a popular tool in BTE, allowing for the assembly of high-density living cells, biomaterials, and bioactive substances. These structures create an optimal microenvironment for cells, enabling personalized structures and communication between cells and the microenvironment. To enhance the regulatory effects of nerves in bone repair, ScC-exos and BM-MSCs were loaded into a bioink to stimulate nerve-bone crosstalk, improve the microenvironment, and promote bone regeneration. A hybrid hydrogel system was used, with thermosensitive GelMA as the base and silk methacrylate (SilMA) added to improve exosome release. The bioprinted constructs promoted osteogenic differentiation of BM-MSCs and stimulated neurovascular network formation, ultimately improving neurovascularized bone repair [270].

The activation of the intraosseous sympathetic nervous system has significant implications for bone defect repair. In mice, the removal of the sympathetic nervous system significantly diminished the bone repair capability and inflammatory response, impeding autologous bone repair. However, in a mouse model of post-traumatic stress disorder (PTSD), mice with PTSD exhibited significantly lower bone repair efficacy compared to those without PTSD. Traumatic stress disorder can enhance sympathetic nerve activation and modulate osteoclast behavior through specific signaling pathways. Research indicates that bone defects often trigger PTSD, prompting the protein TrkA to activate the sympathetic nervous system, leading to an increase in local catecholamine concentration. Catecholamines, such as dopamine, norepinephrine, epinephrine, and their derivatives, can bind to β-adrenoceptors on cell surfaces, causing cellular damage and inhibiting new bone formation. They also promote the expression of the nuclear factor κB receptor RANKL, an osteoclast differentiation factor, which stimulates bone resorption while inhibiting osteoblast formation and osteoclast differentiation, ultimately impairing bone defect repair [271, 272]. A 3D-printed scaffold loaded with the calcium channel blocker, nifedipine, was investigated to reduce the concentration of catecholamine within bone defects and accelerate bone healing. The scaffold was prepared by adding nifedipine-loaded ethosome and laponite into a solution containing sodium alginate, methacrylated gelatin, and BM-MSCs. The released nifedipine closed nerve cell calcium channels, blocking sympathetic activation and inhibiting catecholamine release. This promoted osteogenic differentiation, the migration of BM-MSCs, inhibited osteoclastogenesis, and improved bone regeneration in a rat critical-size calvarial defect model. Sustained release of nifedipine from the scaffold was shown to effectively block sympathetic nervous system activation, thereby offering a promising strategy for future bone defect treatment [273].

3.5.5. *Oxygen-Releasing Scaffolds*

Ensuring cell survival and proliferation is of the utmost importance in tissue engineering. Scaffolds that provide nutrients, growth hormones, and an adequate supply of oxygen are key components in this process. Thus, in regenerative engineering, angiogenesis plays a key role by creating new blood vessels within transplanted tissues to keep oxygen flowing during the integration of the graft. Matrix-based healing of large-scale bone lesions is common, but SCs may not receive enough oxygen, which causes hypoxia-induced necrosis in critical areas. Hypoxia, often resulting from vascular dysfunction, significantly impedes fracture healing in large segmental defects. Insufficient oxygen levels can lead to cellular apoptosis, tissue necrosis, and protracted tissue recovery [274]. To ensure sustainability and best performance, all cells must be located within 200 μm of a blood vessel. It usually takes around 6 weeks for the host's capillaries and arteries to integrate with the implant post-implantation. This time gap in terms of angiogenesis requires a deliberate strategy. Cells inside the implanted construct may be supported by sustainable oxygen release before the onset of angiogenesis, which usually happens within 1–2 weeks. Direct oxygen administration, using perfluorocarbon-based devices that release oxygen, or indirect oxygen administration, using a biomaterial carrier, has been the subject of research and has shown promising results in bone and muscle tissue development. However, there is still a lot of uncharted territory when it comes to the inclusion of agents that release oxygen [275, 276, 99]. Through metabolic programming, oxygen tension influences tissue regeneration. The rapid oxygen release from oxygen-releasing scaffolds raises concerns about their propensity to induce cell death and cytotoxicity, as well as their unpredictable temporal and spatial release, which may threaten their structural integrity [277]. Among the various oxygen generators, magnesium peroxide (MgO_2), calcium peroxide (CaO_2), $NaHCO_3$, hydrogen peroxide (H_2O_2), and fluorine-containing compounds are notable examples. The interaction of these oxygen-generating materials with water can yield oxygen [278]. Due to their enhanced stability, CaO_2 and MgO_2 are typically preferred for sustained oxygen production. Composite biomaterials that combine the advantages of traditional scaffolds with drug-encapsulated microspheres may be created by incorporating oxygen-releasing microspheres into tissue engineering scaffolds. They can also be used as a drug to deliver oxygen to areas following a stroke and where oxygen supply is inadequate. To achieve biocompatibility and tunable biodegradability, a variety of polymers are mixed with oxygen sources. These include polyvinylpyrrolidone, poly(N-isopropylacrylamide), PCL, PLGA, and polyurethane. Oxygel is a novel biomaterial composed of hyaluronic acid and perfluorocarbon and is able to carry oxygen and release it gradually over 90 hours [279, 280]. The decomposition and reduction of H_2O_2 into oxygen and water, aided by the enzyme catalase, is the fundamental mechanism of oxygen release. This method enables a prolonged flow of oxygen that may persist for at least up to 48 hours [281, 282]. These microsystems can provide temporary oxygen to injured regions and require careful material selection. Choosing the correct materials, manufacturing conditions, and implementation techniques are all part of the design process for tailoring the degradation and release time of an oxygen release system. Stimuli-responsive biomaterials could control oxygen production using environmental or internal stimuli [101, 204]. The microsystem has to be programmed to release oxygen precisely when and where it needs to, without accidentally releasing it in the incorrect location [283]. Researchers have improved oxygen diffusion in tissue-engineered scaffolds for transplanted cells by using hollow, hyperbarically loaded microtanks as reservoirs. Biodegradable microtanks were embedded into 3D-printed porous PCL and were shown to enhance bone tissue regeneration, promote osteopontin coverage and mineral deposition, and enhance human adipose-derived SC-mediated bone tissue regeneration [284]. Another study developed an oxygen-releasing scaffold composed of PCL and CaO_2 nanocuboids. The findings indicated that this scaffold facilitated oxygen release for 14 days, supported cell proliferation, and protected pre-osteoblasts from hypoxia-induced cell death. These scaffolds exhibit significant potential for applications in bone regeneration, particularly in enhancing the osseous concentration within bone defect sites [285]. Scientists created a hydrogel/particle scaffold composed of a gradient of microparticles that released oxygen. The hydrogel was formed using oxidized pectin and SF, and the microparticles used were composed of polylactic acid and CaO_2. The mechanical characteristics of the scaffold were found to be enhanced as the microparticle concentration increased. The oxygen-releasing composite was safe for use with MSCs generated from human adipose tissue. When compared with its non-oxygen-releasing analog, it increased cell density and vitality. A low microparticle content promoted chondrogenesis, while a high microparticle concentration favored osteogenesis [286]. Further, oxygen-releasing coatings can enhance tissue preservation in organ transplantation protocols. These coatings, made by encapsulating calcium or urea peroxide microparticles between octadiene plasma polymer films, generate oxygen when exposed to aqueous solutions while limiting toxic ROS, according to a study. When tested under hypoxic conditions, cell viability increased threefold. These coatings have the potential to be applied to a variety of surfaces, thereby extending tissue viability and graft transport time [287]. As these coatings could be considered a valuable modification for orthopedic scaffolds and implants, an extensive overview of coatings and related subjects is presented in the section that follows.

4. Coatings

When a biomaterial is in contact with the biological environment, such as soft tissue, hard tissue, body fluids, or saliva, the interaction between these biological environments and the biomaterial occurs on the surface. Therefore, the biological response to the implanted biomaterial depends on its surface properties, such as surface chemical composition, morphology, surface energy, hydrophilicity or hydrophobicity, and corrosion resistance [288]. The design of biomaterials for implants with optimal surface and mechanical properties is crucial. Therefore, the main properties required are suitable bulk, surface, and biological features. Rarely does one come upon a material that has all the necessary biological, surface, and bulk properties. Surface modification is a cost-effective way to improve a biomaterial's mechanical, tribological, and biocompatibility aspects. To do this, an appropriate coating or surface treatment is applied, which in turn affects surface properties such as electrical, biological, porosity, wear, corrosion, and roughness [289]. What the cell touches plays an essential role in terms of its function. Many cellular activities, including protein absorption, adhesion, proliferation, differentiation, and growth, may be affected by surface modification mechanisms. For a given application, these modifications may be accomplished by altering the surface chemistry, topography, or wettability [290]. Through the manipulation of surface charge or the incorporation of anti-thrombogenic coatings, surface modification methods have the potential to enhance or decrease the probability of blood clot formation in biomedical devices [291, 292].

The influence of surface chemistry on biomaterial design and fabrication cannot be underestimated. It has a significant impact on the material's biological function, affecting its ability to interact with proteins and cells. The way cells and surfaces interact with each other can have a significant impact on various changes that occur during various biological processes. These changes can either activate or inhibit biological events, such as the conversion of the zymogen in the coagulation cascade to an active enzyme, or alter the structural integrity of proteins [293]. Coatings can be applied to implant or scaffold surfaces to improve their osteointegration. One fascinating example of how biological behavior can be altered is the use of a titanium oxide coating on titanium, when combined with elements such as calcium, phosphorus, and sulfur. The thickness of a coating affects the ion current and, by extension, the oxidation rate, which in turn determines how quickly the coating promotes bone formation [394]. Furthermore, the application of a calcium phosphate coating has been shown to promote faster bone growth by strengthening the bond between the implant and the surrounding bone tissue [295]. The surface topography of the implantable material is another one of the main factors that affects cell morphology, growth direction, and proliferation [296]. The surface topography of a biomaterial is important because it enhances the bond between the implanted material and the tissues. When engineering topography, it is necessary to create 3D designs that include features such as micro- and nano-porosity, columns, grooves, and holes. The penetration of cells, diffusion of nutrients, and ingrowth of bone cells are all dependent on porosity. Pore structure, shape, cross-linking, and pore size distribution are some of the macro-parameters that assist intraosseous growth. The substrate architecture can also impact cell division and bone gene expression [297]. Surface charge, the difference in potential between the internal and external surface, influences the biomaterial's biological properties. The charge has been shown to influence protein absorption and cell adhesion, with positively charged surfaces attracting negatively charged cell membranes [298]. Negatively charged surfaces, on the other hand, tend to decrease cellular adhesion. This negative charge would repel the negatively charged cell membrane, generating weaker cell-surface interactions [299]. In addition, surface charge density is also an important parameter. Certain materials, including titanium, zirconium, and aluminum oxides, carry a positive charge. Interestingly, it has been shown that due to the variation in surface charge density, the amount of protein adhesion increased from titanium oxide to aluminum oxide, resulting in varying levels of cell attachment [300].

All matter is composed of atoms, and these atoms provide energy to prevent disintegration, with bulk atoms being more influenced by this energy. Making new surfaces in matter requires surface energy. Surface atoms aim to lower a system's free energy by bonding with water and air atoms, resulting in a surface that is chemically distinct from its inside. Since implanted materials often decrease surface energy when they come into contact with the biological environment, this concept also affects their response when inserted into the body. At the atomic scale, the atoms on the surface reduce the free energy of the system and form bonds with air and water atoms. This occurs in most cases because the chemical composition of the surface is different from the chemical composition inside the substance (e.g., the formation of an oxide layer on the surface of most metals). This issue also applies inside the body, in the sense that when the material is implanted, it tends to reduce its surface energy in contact with the biological conditions of the body. A study investigated how surface charge and wettability affected bone cell mineralization, adhesion, and proliferation on the HA surface. According to the experimental findings, a surface charge may be adjusted without changing the material's volume. With the increasing surface charge, the wettability and energy on an HA surface also increased. Human fetal osteoblasts were used to investigate cell–material interactions. The findings from the *in vitro* experiments that were conducted demonstrated that balancing the combined effects of charge polarity and wettability on the HA surface, as well as the binding of various inorganic ions (e.g., Ca^{2+}, Cl^{-}, Na^{+}, HCO^{3-}) and organic cell adhesion proteins (e.g., fibronectin, vitronectin), led to either reduced or accelerated cell adhesion, proliferation, and mineralization on the polarized HA surface [301].

4.1. *Coating Methods*

Biomaterial coating methods are divided into six categories: chemical methods, thermochemical methods, electrochemical methods, physical methods, electrophysical methods, and 3D printing (**Figure 4**) [302].

4.1.1. *Chemical Methods*

4.1.1.1. Sol-Gel

The sol-gel method is usually used to synthesize oxide materials and sometimes hydrogels and aerogels. This method has several steps. First, the precursor solution, or deposition sol, is formed on the substrate, and then it turns into a gel *via* heat treatment. This method is simple and affordable, and it is possible to adjust the thickness of the coating. Because of their poor adherence to a metal substrate, these coatings are sintered at temperatures higher than 1000°C to enhance their density and adhesion. The final cracking of the coating due to shrinkage is one of this method's drawbacks [303].

4.1.1.2. Biomimetic Coatings

The biomimetic method is a technique that aims to create a bone-like layer on an implant material, thereby improving the bond between the implant and body tissue. This method can be used on ceramics, metals, and

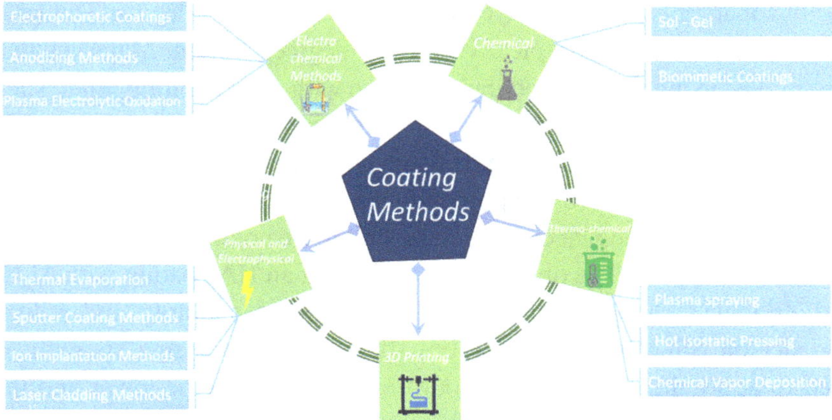

Figure 4. Some of the important coating methods used for bioactive coatings on various implant surfaces.

polymers. The bone-like apatite layer is formed in a solution that mimics the physiological environment, and has a similar pH and ion concentration to blood plasma. Two factors are crucial for apatite deposition, increasing the supersaturated concentration of ions and the presence of functional groups on the surface. Functional groups including Si-OH, Ti-OH, Nb-OH, Ta-OH, Co-OH, and PO_4H_2, are suitable for stimulating apatite deposition. Heat treating the substrate in an aqueous NaOH solution at 60°C for 24 hours is one common method for producing functional groups on a titanium alloy surface, which is a surface modification prior to subsequent HA deposition. Following this, the alloy is heat treated to temperatures ranging from 500°C–800°C [304].

4.1.2. *Thermochemical Methods*

4.1.2.1. Plasma Spraying

Of the thermal spraying processes available, the plasma method is one of the most commonly used techniques for creating a coating. In this process, the plasma environment lies between two electrodes, and spraying takes place in the presence of gases such as argon/hydrogen or argon/helium.

Various materials can be sprayed to create differing sub-layers. The temperature of the flame is typically ~20,000 degrees Kelvin. Materials that are sprayed using this method include those with a low melting point, such as polymers, as well as materials with a high melting point, such as tungsten, oxide ceramics, and so on. If the vacuum environment (low vacuum plasma spraying) is used to apply the coating, greater adhesion strength, less porosity, a homogeneous structure, and more control over the amount of residual stress will be obtained. Heat treating an HA coating with Al_2O_3 and ZrO_2 was shown to significantly improve crystallinity and reduce porosity on SS-316L surfaces [305]. If low-energy plasma spraying is used to apply the coating, the impurities will typically be lower and the density higher. Demnati *et al.* [306] used a low-energy plasma spraying mini-gun to coat HA onto a titanium surface. No cracks were observed within the coating, and the results showed that the HA coatings demonstrated higher crystallinity than coatings prepared using conventional plasma systems, where the degradation rate was reported to be reduced. Other studies related to the spraying of new apatitic powder compositions and *in vivo* evaluation of these coatings are necessary.

4.1.2.2. Hydrothermal Crystallization

The hydrothermal crystallization technique involves depositing a coating onto a metal base when immersed in a solution within a hydrothermal reactor at various temperatures, pH levels, and high pressure. Researchers have used this method to coat Mg-based alloys with calcium phosphate to enhance their corrosion resistance [307] and to deposit HA onto Ti alloy surfaces [308]. In a recent study, the effects of temperature and time of hydrothermal treatment on the subsequent alterations to the surface characteristics and bioactivity of a micro-arc oxidation (MAO) coating on a Ti-6Al-4V alloy surface were systematically investigated. The results showed that with increasing temperature and time of treatment, the amount of HA formation on an MAO coating gradually increases. However, excessive temperature and time caused HA to pulverize on the MAO coating and cover its pores, which will be detrimental to facilitating bone integration. It was found that when the hydrothermal treatment temperature and time were 200°C and 24 h, respectively, the formed HA could not be powdered, but it could completely cover the MAO coating and maintain its porous structure. Further bioactivity tests in SBF showed that the hydrothermally treated MAO coating produced more HA crystal structures and covered a larger area than the sample without hydrothermal treatment.

4.1.2.3. Chemical Vapor Deposition

Chemical vapor deposition is a widely used method to create high-quality coatings on the surface of objects in a reaction chamber. This technique involves using chemical reactions of one or more volatile precursors with heated substrates to coat a thin film. The energy required for this process comes from a variety of sources, such as laser, photon, or heat [302], and it can provide coatings with different structures (e.g., amorphous, polycrystalline) [309] and different levels of purity [302]. The initial connection and subsequent proliferation of osteoblasts, as well as their ability to form bone, are some of the most important factors affecting the success of a bone implant. A study investigated the positive effect of a titanium dioxide (TiO_2) nanostructured coating that was deposited using a metal-organic chemical vapor deposition (MOCVD) method. The bone response in terms of histomorphometry, ultrastructure, and the microhardness at the peri-implant bone interface was evaluated. Microhardness is used to indicate the properties of several microstructural parameters of bone, including the degree of calcification, the arrangement and number of collagen fibers, the ratio between collagen fibers and the matrix, and the amount of mineral per unit volume. The higher the bone hardness value, the higher the level of mineralization and bone maturity. Surface profile measurements showed that the surface of treated implants did not differ from untreated implants in terms of average roughness. However, the maximum roughness height and the average space between the peaks showed that the treated implants presented a surface with a maximum peak height and the lowest density of peaks, thus presenting a surface with more valleys than peaks. According to the histomorphometric analysis, a TiO_2 nanostructured coating demonstrated a positive effect on the metabolism and healing ability of the surrounding bone. Scanning electron microscopy investigations confirmed and highlighted increased bone integration of the treated implants in the cortical bone and, at the same time, demonstrated the osseointegration of the treated implants in the cancellous bone. MOCVD techniques allow control of film quality, which is strongly related to the control of parameters in the deposition chamber, such as temperature, gas feed composition, chamber pressure, and gas flow rate. Due to the technical features of MOCVD, high-quality bone growth (heteroepitaxial growth) was assumed on oriented TiO_2 substrates due to the improved space matching between the growing bone (HA) and the oriented TiO_2 implant coating. TiO_2 coatings obtained by MOCVD stimulated artificial activity of human osteoblast-like cells (MG-63) and increased alkaline phosphatase production and increased osteocalcin on days 7 and 14, resulting in continuous improvement in osteoblast activity and differentiation [310]. According to the literature, low surface roughness reduces cell proliferation and increases cellular synthetic activity, as well as improves bone-implant contact [311].

4.1.3. *Electrochemical Methods*

4.1.3.1. Electrophoretic Coatings

Electrodeposition methods such as electrophoretic and electrochemical deposition are straightforward methods to form homogeneous and multifunctional coatings in conductive and complex geometries. In addition, electrochemistry induces the deposition of nanomaterials and the introduction of biomolecules and polymers, by which various properties such as antibacterial activity, cell proliferation, and osseointegration can be delivered to the surface of the implant. The electrophoretic coating method is a wet process that can control the thickness and morphology of the deposited coating by adjusting the concentration and electrical conditions. In this method, the charged powder particles are dispersed or suspended in a liquid medium and are moved toward the conductive substrate with the opposite charge. This method is used in a variety of applications, including the production of wear-resistant coatings [312], antioxidant ceramic coatings [313], nanostructured materials [314], and bioactive coatings in medical applications [315].

4.1.3.2. Anodizing Methods

Anodizing is an electrochemical process that increases the thickness of the oxide layer that naturally forms on metal surfaces. This process is used on metals such as Ti, Zn, Tn, and especially Al, but it is not suitable for iron and carbon steel because these metals flake during anodization. Anodization changes the microscopic texture of the surface and the crystal structure of the metal near the surface. Anodic layers are generally harder and more adhesive than all kinds of paints and metal coatings; they are also more resistant to corrosion and wear. This technique is performed in an electrochemical cell, which consists of three parts: a cathode, an anode, and an electrolyte solution. In this method, the desired metal of a very high purity percentage is used as the anode, and another metal such as Al, Ti, Pt, Ni, Tn, is used as the cathode. The nature of electrolysis also changes depending on the type of oxide layer and its characteristics (such as the diameter of the holes and the distance between the holes). The anodized metal oxide layer grows as direct current passes through the electrolyte solution. The electric current releases hydrogen in the cathode and oxygen in the anode, causing the oxide layer to grow. In general, the anodizing process produces two types of oxide layers: barrier oxide layers and porous oxide layers. The type and nature of the electrolyte used in this process determine the type of oxide layer growth on the metal surface. Research shows that utilization of an anodizing process increases bone-forming cell proliferation and adhesion [316, 317]. The titanium surface reacts with oxygen in the surrounding atmosphere and spontaneously forms a dense TiO_2 layer with a thickness of approximately 1.5–10 nm. This oxide layer is responsible for the outstanding biocompatibility of Ti implants. However, the natural oxide layer can be easily damaged and is not ideal for bone adhesion and bone formation in the early stages of the bone consolidation process. Bioactivity is also highly dependent on subsurface topography at micro and macro scales. Many efforts have been made to improve osseointegration by engineering the surface properties of titanium implants with methods such as anodization. Some studies have reported that artificial growth of oxide layer thickness leads to an increased bone response and improved biocompatibility. An increase in the anodizing voltage leads to the growth of layer thickness, increased roughness, and changes in the composition of the surface phase.

The production of titanium oxide on the surface is influenced by various factors such as temperature, electric current, and the chemical composition of the electrolytic solution. To achieve titanium anodizing, solutions such as sulfuric acid, phosphoric acid, and acetic acid are commonly used. Anodization in neutral environments creates a compact layer with nanometer pores, which is required for medical applications [318].

4.1.3.3. Plasma Electrolytic Oxidation Methods

Plasma electrolytic oxidation, or MAO, is a new surface engineering method to modify the surfaces of light metals such as aluminum, titanium, and magnesium, as well as metals such as bismuth, hafnium, tantalum, tungsten, zirconium, and niobium, by creating a ceramic oxide coating on their surface. This process occurs in an electrolytic bath and requires a voltage of several hundred volts, resulting in the formation of plasma. Plasma is an important and necessary part of the process that allows the sparking phenomenon to occur on the metal surface. The sparking phenomenon causes the metal to change into the base metal's oxide, allowing electrolyte compounds to enter the film. These compounds then grow and sinter, forming a condensed quasi-ceramic coating on the surface and strengthening the oxide layer. The main benefits of this process include excellent adhesion to the substrate, increased resistance to corrosion, erosion, and abrasion, and improved hardness, thermal stability, electrical properties, and biocompatibility in biomaterials. This method produces microporous oxide layers that are suitable substrates for anchoring bone cells [319]. When this technique was used to coat tantalum as a valuable metal in orthopedic and dental implants, the coated implants showed much higher wettability (the contact angle decreased from 86° to 9°), increasing MG63 cell adhesion and proliferation. MAO-produced HA typically has a low crystallinity. To improve this feature, subsequent hydrothermal treatment [308], ultrasonic assistance [320], or immersion in SBF [321] techniques are used.

4.1.4. *Physical and Electrophysical Methods*

Physical vapor deposition (PVD) refers to a set of vacuum deposition methods in which a solid material is vaporized in a vacuum environment and placed on the substrate as a thin layer. These techniques are environmentally friendly and have high biocompatibility and mechanical properties, making them suitable for the preparation of temperature-sensitive substrates [322]. Among the disadvantages of PVD are the coating of parts with a complex geometric shape, the need for a vacuum, and the high temperature required for the coating environment.

4.1.4.1. Thermal Evaporation Methods

Thermal evaporation (TE) is a simple method of creating a thin film using PVD. In this method, by heating the target material in a high vacuum chamber (less than 10^{-5} Torr), the vapor pressure of the material increases on its surface, and a thin layer of the material is formed on the substrate in the chamber. Thin layers of titanium oxide, titanium, and calcium phosphate produced by this method have been used to adapt the chemical properties and topography of biomedical materials. The surface of the coating is typically rough and porous due to the presence of plasma chemical reactions in the fine discharge channels. Titanium and its alloys are inert, and therefore, the chemical bond formed with bone tissue is limited. This can reduce the osseointegration of an implant and, on occasion, has been associated with the failure of the implant. To increase bioactivity, titanium and its alloys are coated with various surface modification methods such as TE. The bioactive behavior of the coatings obtained by this technique is reported to be much more favorable than methods such as MAO due to the uniform and dense distribution of HA formed on the surface [323].

4.1.4.2. Sputter Coating Methods

Sputtering is one of the vapor phase deposition methods used for producing metal films on the nano- to micro-scale. To perform the deposition process in a vacuum using sputtering, it is necessary to shoot the coating substance toward the target material in the plasma environment. The desired gas to be used in this process must have two characteristics: first, its weight must be enough to affect the target substance's atom, and second, it must not enter into a chemical reaction with the target substance. According to the aforementioned cases, the gases used in the sputtering process are inert (e.g., argon, xenon), where argon gas is the most commonly used in this process [324]. Research in this area reported that implants coated with sputter showed increased bone contact rates in goats. Histological examination revealed a stronger bone response to sputter HA-coated implants. Certainly, HA greatly promotes the initial bone reaction adjacent to dental implants [325].

4.1.4.3. Ion Implantation Methods

Ion implantation is a process in material engineering in which the ions of some materials can be implanted in another material and change the physical properties of that material. The TiN [326] and TiC [327] layers formed on the surface of a Ti_6Al_4V alloy improve its compatibility and bioactivity (through increased cell adhesion). Adding Zn to the surface of Mg alloys improves their corrosion resistance [328]. A study showed that Mg, a crucial metal correlated to bone strength, was added to the surface of micro/nanostructured titanium through ion implantation. Rat BM-MSCs were employed to assess cellular reactions, such as proliferation, bone growth, and differentiation, on the surface of the material. A higher enhancement in the dissemination and proliferative ability of rBMMSCs was noted on the surfaces of magnesium-implanted micro/nanostructures in comparison to the control plates. Furthermore, osteocalcin, osteopontin, and alkaline phosphatase gene expression increased on both surfaces and in their surrounding extracts. Greater levels of Mg ions were linked to improved cellular reactions, indicating that Mg ions played a role in stimulating the differentiation of rBMMSCs into osteoblasts [329].

4.1.4.4. Laser Cladding Methods

In this process, laser rays completely melt the metal or alloy powder and inject it onto the substrate surface, which also undergoes surface melting. Notably, the laser coating of S520 BG onto commercially pure titanium caused martensitic transformation on the surface of the piece, eliminating the potential toxicity of medical implants [330].

4.1.5. *3D Printing*

3D printing technology involves a series of processes in which materials are bonded together in a controlled manner to create a 3D object. Usually, this is done layer by layer. Types of 3D printing methods include fuse deposition modeling, vat photopolymerization, powder bed fusion, directive energy deposition, PolyJet, binder Jet, and sheet lamination. The most common of which is the FDM method for the development of bioactive coatings [302]. The use of 3D printing techniques to produce a coating, as a general solution, has not yet been refined. Some studies indicate the growing use of this method in various fields of tissue engineering and drug release systems [331]. For example, 3D printing was used to modify the surface of titanium alloy substrates with biofunctional multilayer polymer coatings. Selected polymers were loaded with the therapeutic agent, amorphous calcium phosphate (ACP), and vancomycin to promote bone integrity and antibacterial activity. The coatings showed a uniform ACP-containing deposition pattern and increased cell adhesion onto the titanium alloy substrate surface [332]. TiAlV and AISI 316 LVM stainless steel alloys coated with cellulose nanofibril suspension, alginate, carboxymethylcellulose, and clindamycin, using a 3D printer method, showed that they have good potential for use in orthopedic implants and in the long-term release of antibiotics at the prosthetic site [333].

4.2. *Bioactive Coating Materials*

To repair bone defects, it is necessary to use biomaterials that are both compatible with the body and strong enough to support the bone. However, traditional metallic implants show a limited ability to promote biological activity. Bioactive coatings can be applied to implants to address this issue. These coatings contain active ingredients that are released at the implant site in a controlled manner (**Figure 5**). Ceramics, glasses, polymers, biomolecules, and composites promote cell differentiation, proliferation, gene and tissue regeneration, and the release of bioactive molecules to target postoperative complications [334].

4.2.1. *Inorganic Coatings*

In the field of medicine, repairing bone defects is a complex task that requires the use of biomaterials that are not only compatible with the body but also strong enough to support the bone and promote biological activity.

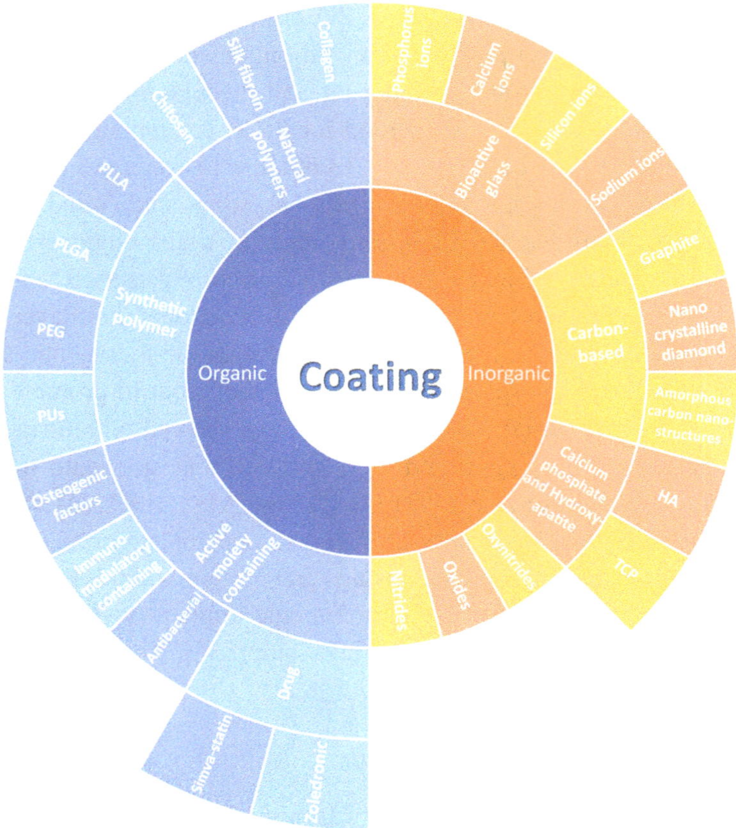

Figure 5. Bioactive coating materials applied for use in hard tissue applications.

One important aspect is that the bone implant material used must promote rapid cell adhesion and bone cell anchorage. This can be achieved through the development of inorganic coatings. In the following section, various inorganic bioactive coating materials are discussed, and their features are summarized in **Figure 6**.

4.2.1.1. Nitrides

Because of their exceptional features, nitride coatings have been highlighted as an important coating option for the surface modification of orthopedic implants. Metal nitride coatings, such as TaN, NbN, ZrN, and

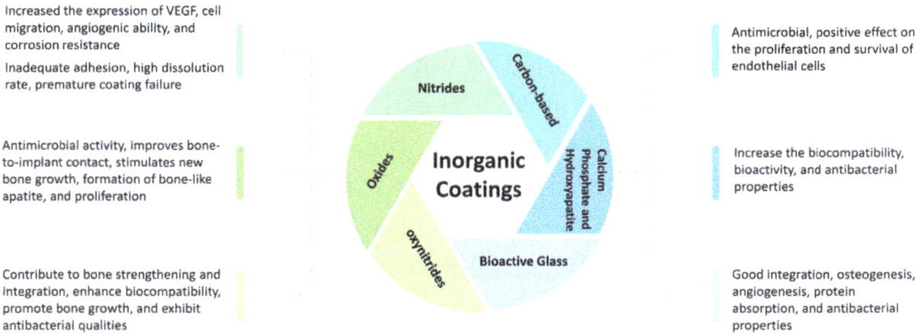

Figure 6. Characteristics of inorganic coatings used as bioactive coatings developed for medical applications.

TiN, have been studied as protective layers against the wear and corrosion of medical implant surfaces [335]. Nitride coatings are very biocompatible, and the human body appears to tolerate them without causing an inappropriate immune response [336]. Because of their bioinertness, TiN films are reported to be well accepted by living tissue [337]. In addition, these coatings are resistant to abrasion and prevent the diffusion of metal ions into body fluids [338, 339]. The corrosion resistance of TiN coatings is reported to be eight times the corrosion resistance of Ti [340]. Also, doping copper with this coating has been shown to lead to an increase in antibacterial properties. In this respect, TiCuN increased the expression of VEGF, cell migration, and angiogenic ability [341]. These coatings have several disadvantages, including inadequate adhesion and a high dissolution rate, which can lead to premature coating failure [342].

4.2.1.2. Oxides

It is well known that metal-containing nano oxides (Fe_3O_4, TiO_2, CuO, ZnO) have antibacterial characteristics. Titanium dioxide modified with reduced graphene oxide (rGO) exhibited antimicrobial activity against *Escherichia coli* when under artificial sunlight. TiO_2/rGO photocatalysts showed higher antibacterial activity than unmodified TiO_2 [343]. In addition to their antimicrobial characteristics, coating an implant surface with TiO_2 nanoparticles was shown to improve bone-to-implant contact and stimulate new bone growth adjacent to the implant [344]. Titanium oxide nanoparticles have been reported to improve the formation of bone-like apatite and the proliferation of MG-63 cells [345]. Adding CuO to a HA/hardystonite composite has been shown to improve the formation of the HA layer onto the sublayer and increase its electrical conductivity. This may play a significant role in improving fracture healing. The increase in electrical conductivity of this nanocomposite was reported to be caused by an increase in the number of charge carriers (due to the presence of copper ions) [346]. Furthermore, the antibacterial effects of CuO nanoparticles have been successfully assessed against two Gram-positive bacterial strains (*Staphylococcus aureus* and *Bacillus cereus*) as well as two Gram-negative bacterial strains (*E. coli* and *Pseudomonas aeruginosa*) [347]. Zinc oxide nanoparticles exert their antibacterial action *via* mechanisms including cell membrane disruption, protein and DNA binding, the generation of ROS, interference with bacterial DNA replication, and alteration of gene expression [348]. As such, nanoparticles composed of ZnO have potent antibacterial characteristics. Through generating ROS, including superoxide radicals, hydrogen peroxide, and hydroxyl radicals, bacterial DNA, proteins, and cell membranes are damaged, which ultimately leads to bacterial cell death [349, 350]. By altering the size, shape, and surface properties of ZnO nanoparticles, their antibacterial activity may be further enhanced. Specifically, smaller ZnO nanoparticles have displayed enhanced antibacterial activity as a result of their larger surface area and reactivity [348, 351]. Further, ZnO can increase apatite deposition on the surface of HA scaffolds, subsequently increasing the surface roughness and providing a suitable substrate for cell proliferation [352].

4.2.1.3. Oxynitrides

The presence of nitrogen in oxynitride coatings makes them very promising for medical implants because they contribute to bone strengthening and integration, enhance biocompatibility, promote bone growth, and exhibit antibacterial qualities to prevent infection [353–355]. Having a hydrophilic surface is very important for cell proliferation, and these coatings generally increase the hydrophilicity of the surface. Hardness, adhesion, corrosion resistance, minimal coating dissolution, and inertness in bodily fluids are some of the desirable features that have been made possible by coating metal substrates with oxynitrides. Researchers have discovered that increasing the oxygen content of a TiN coating decreased particle size, created an inert layer on the substrate, and ultimately boosted the corrosion resistance of the coating when in a salt solution [359]. Applying a TiN/TiO_2 gradient coating on Ti [355], stainless steel [357], or CoCr [358] alloy substrates improved their biocompatibility, wear resistance, and ability to promote bone cell development. The mechanism of action of a TiNOx coating is not well known, but it can be attributed to the presence of nitric oxide species on the surface.

4.2.1.4. Carbon-Based Coatings

Due to their high biocompatibility and mechanical qualities, amorphous carbon nanostructures, such as graphite-like carbon, pyrolytic carbon, diamond-like carbon (DLC), nanocrystalline diamond, and graphite, are all used in the medical field. Coatings based on DLC have been used on substrates made of silicon [359] and titanium [360], and because of their wear resistance, hardness, surface roughness, and adhesion strength, improvements to the properties of the original substrate have been achieved. As a result of their anti-fouling properties, carbon-based coatings, including graphene or CNTs, may lessen the chance of infection by preventing the accumulation of bacteria on the implant surface [361]. As mentioned, to make metal implants more resistant to corrosion, scientists utilize carbon-based coatings. These coatings are reported to not only extend the life of the implant but also aid in avoiding the release of hazardous metal ions [362]. An *in vivo* study investigated TiO_2 coated with a DLC film and showed adequate viability and no inflammatory reaction, thereby confirming this coating as biocompatible [363]. Several studies showed that Ag, Cu [364], F [365], and Si [366] doping into DLC coatings can deliver strong antimicrobial properties that are effective against a wide range of Gram-positive and Gram-negative bacteria. Unfortunately, this advantage has been accompanied by a decrease in the mechanical performance of the coating. Also, Si doping has a very positive effect on the proliferation and survival of endothelial cells because the polarity and wettability of the examined surfaces increased with the increased Si concentration, and therefore cell adhesion and proliferation were strengthened [364]. The biocompatibility and bioactivity of nanodiamonds have been reported [367]. These biomaterials have high wear resistance and a low friction coefficient, which makes them useful as protective coatings [368]. Since these coatings react with the cell wall of *P. aeruginosa*, they are able to prevent the adhesion of bacteria [369]. Further, several studies have been conducted to assess the ability of graphene oxide to promote bone hMSC differentiation. Graphene oxide preserved endogenous BMPs and subsequently released them to promote the osteogenic differentiation of hMSCs. The high specific surface area of graphene oxide nanoplates led to an increase in the loading capacity of BMPs and acted as a BMP storage [370, 371]. This material, together with HA and CS, has been used as a titanium coating and has increased the adhesion strength of the coating to the substrate surface [372].

4.2.1.5. Calcium Phosphate and Hydroxyapatite

As mentioned earlier, calcium phosphate is a family of materials and minerals containing calcium ions (Ca^{2+}) with inorganic phosphate anions. Calcium phosphate is found in many organisms, for example, in bone mineral and tooth enamel. Apatite is an impure and complex form of calcium phosphate. Calcium phosphate coatings (e.g., TCP, HA) are used to increase the biocompatibility and bioactivity of metal implants [373]. HA and TCP have different crystallization, stability, solubility, ion release, and mechanical properties [374]. Unlike highly crystalline HA, TCP-based coatings have high solubility in aqueous environments, which reduces the stability of the coating and may ultimately contribute to aseptic loosening [375]. HA is a bioactive substance, and it works by releasing calcium and phosphate ions and stimulating mineralization [376]. In addition to promoting implant and tissue integrity, an HA coating may also prevent ion diffusion into the living environment [377]. HA has poor mechanical properties, displays a lack of good adhesion to a metal surface, and has low corrosion resistance [378]. As a result of residual thermal stress, which is influenced by the difference between the coating's thermal coefficient and that of the metal sublayer, these coatings often develop cracks or become flaky [379]. A dispersed phase added to the coating structure is one potential approach that has been suggested to address these shortcomings. For example, HA coatings that include TiO_2 are more resistant to corrosion and have lower solubility [380]. The addition of Al_2O_3-SiO_2 has been shown to improve adhesion strength and wettability [381]. Also, the addition of zinc, magnesium, copper, strontium, silicon, manganese, and fluorine can be effective in promoting bone regeneration [382–385]. Zinc supplementation has been shown to increase alkaline phosphatase activity and stimulate bone formation by osteoblasts [386]. Magnesium has an antimicrobial effect due to the increase in pH caused by its degradation [387]. Strontium ions increase bone attachment to the implant surface and do this through promoting the proliferation of osteoblasts and accelerating the synthesis of bone matrix, thereby reducing bone loss [388]. Finally, the addition of silver to an HA coating was shown to increase implant biocompatibility and its antibacterial properties [389].

4.2.1.6. Bioactive Glass

BGs consist of bioceramic materials that promote rapid bone regeneration by releasing silicon, calcium, phosphorus, and sodium ions into the body [390]. Bioglass® 45S5 was first introduced in 1969 as the initial form of bioglass [391]. Among the most known biological glasses are Cerabone®, Biosilicate®, Ceravital®, and Bioverit® [392]. Various forms, such as bulk materials, powders, composites, and porous scaffolds, have been presented [393]. The key characteristic of a BG is the formation of a coating layer composed of phosphate, calcium, and silica at the surface which may increase their biological properties [393, 394]. Because of their bioactivity and biocompatibility, BG scaffolds are reported to integrate within bone. In several studies, BGs were compared with materials including HA, and their superiority in terms of promoting new bone growth is reported [395, 396]. In addition to osteogenesis, these materials also have angiogenic, protein absorption, and antibacterial properties [397]. They have been shown to promote angiogenesis by stimulating fibroblasts, osteoblasts, and endothelial cells to release GFs. Additionally, the presence of alkaline ions causes an antibacterial effect. Despite these benefits, they are not as mechanically strong as other ceramics. In this regard, additives including ZrO_2 and B_2O_3 have been shown to increase their resistance to corrosion, fatigue, and low tensile strength [398, 399]. These additives can improve the elastic modulus, hardness, and fracture toughness of BGs.

4.2.2. *Organic Coatings*

Recently, many researchers have become interested in polymer coatings because they are easy to manufacture, nontoxic, resistant to corrosion, and cost-effective. Polymers have mechanical properties that are not as strong as those of ceramics and metals. However, ceramic and metal materials have reported limitations, such as an inappropriate rate of deterioration and, in some cases, potential inflammatory reactions [400]. Organic coatings are designed to imitate the remarkable composition and structure of bone, making them highly compatible physiologically, as represented in **Figure 7**. By mimicking nature, these coatings can promote the adhesion, growth, and differentiation of bone-forming cells on the surface of implants, which ultimately leads to a stronger integration between the implant and the bone [401].

4.2.2.1. Synthetic Polymers

Polylactic glycolic acid, polyurethanes, polyethylene glycol, PCL, poly-L-lactic acid, and polymethyl methacrylate are the most common synthetic polymers used as biomaterials. These polymers are often not hydrophilic and do not have antibacterial activity [402]. Their lack of hydrophilicity also leads to a decrease in cell adhesion. To improve the performance of these materials in medical applications, they are often used as composites with other compounds or particles. For example, researchers found that coating titanium implants with a mixture of polyurethane, 20% graphene by weight, and 2% TCP increased cellular responsiveness and antibacterial activity [403]. PCL is hydrophobic, which limits its use in bioactivity enhancement applications. However, when combined with alginate, PCL demonstrated more biological activity than pure PCL in terms of osteogenic differentiation, cell survival, and calcium deposition. The addition of alginate to the PCL scaffold ensured higher hydrophilicity [404]. As previously stated, the function of HA is to enhance

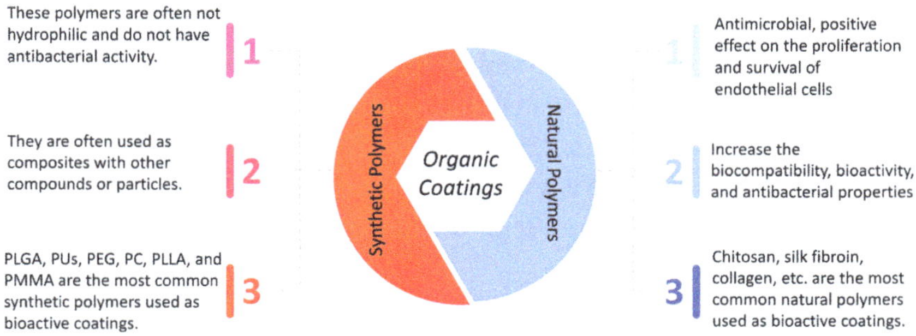

Figure 7. Characteristics of organic coatings used as bioactive coatings developed for medical applications.

mineralization and bone attachment to the implant surface. Results following the testing of a PCL/HA scaffold revealed that primary human BM-MSCs expressed mRNA for collagen type I and osteocalcin, and the quantity of extracellular calcium deposition rose when compared to PCL scaffolds. Moreover, experiments conducted in live organisms showed enhanced bone growth in a model of a calvarial defect in mice [405].

4.2.2.2. Natural Polymers

Natural polymers such as CS, SF, and collagen are used in bioactive coatings. CS is one of the most widely used natural polymers in various applications, including the coating of orthopedic implants, whose bone conduction properties have been proven [406]. CS/graphene oxide coatings on an Mg alloy surface have been used to improve its anticorrosion properties as well as increase the adhesion and proliferation of endothelial cells through enhancing the expression of VEGF [407].

SF is a fibrous protein with very favorable mechanical properties and made in the form of filaments by a large group of insects. The unique structure of silk, variety of processing, biocompatibility, availability in various forms, ability to be sterilized, appropriate surface chemistry, and controlled degradability have made silk a unique material in medical applications. The coating of SF reinforced with cellulose nanocrystals was investigated to increase corrosion protection and the biocompatibility of Mg-based alloys in orthopedic implant applications. Compared to the unmodified Mg alloy, the cellular compatibility of the coated alloy was significantly improved and showed excellent adhesion and spreading of human embryonic osteoblasts on the coating surface. This may have occurred because the degradation products of SF are its constituent amino acids and do not acidify the environment. Therefore, SF shows less immunogenicity (the immune response of the human body that is stimulated by a foreign substance) [408].

Collagen is one of the most abundant proteins in the body and is the main component of connective tissues, including skin, bone, and cartilage. Collagen strengthens and maintains the integrity of these tissues. This protein is suitable for coating metal surfaces, as they enhance communication with ECM proteins. ECM components play an active role in controlling cellular processes and interactions, making the modification of implant surfaces with ECM components highly desirable. Coating Mg alloys with a combination of calcium phosphate and collagen can significantly improve the biocompatibility and corrosion resistance of this alloy [409]. This coating also aids by controlling the Mg degradation rate and thus its potential toxicity. The collagen coating sealed the cracks and pores in a CaP coating and significantly increased its corrosion resistance. Since the CaP/collagen coating composition is similar to bone, it is reported to enhance the adhesion, proliferation, and differentiation of osteoblasts and shows excellent biocompatibility and osteoinduction [409]. A PDA/dicalcium phosphate dihydrate/collagen composite coating also provided similar results to a calcium phosphate/collagen coating when applied to an Mg alloy surface in terms of corrosion resistance and osteogenic differentiation ability [410]. It has also been reported that the binding of Mg ions to collagen can promote the proliferation and differentiation of osteoblasts through the expression of integrins and downstream signaling pathways. The potential mechanisms of this action are through activation *via* the integrin $\alpha2\beta1$-FAK-ERK1/2 protein-coupled receptor pathway [411].

4.2.3. *Active Moiety-Containing Coatings*

Materials such as GFs, chemokines, and drugs are known as cell-active materials and are used on the surface of orthopedic implants because these materials can effectively improve surface biocompatibility and osseointegration [302]. The active parts of these coatings can include drugs, osteogenic factors, immunomodulatory factors, and antibacterial films [412].

4.2.3.1. Drug-Containing Coatings

Zoledronic acid and simvastatin are bone-inducing drugs that cause faster bone formation and implant stabilization [413, 414]. The use of zoledronic acid within the coated surface reduced the activity of osteoclasts and apoptosis, but simvastatin increased the differentiation of MSCs into osteoblasts, decreased osteoblast apoptosis, and upregulated BMP-2. Biomimetic calcium phosphate coatings can be functionalized as a drug delivery system, by which osteoinductive agents such as BMPs are incorporated to enhance the osteoconductive properties of calcium phosphate coatings [415].

4.2.3.2. The Coating Containing Osteogenic Factors

A coating with osteogenic factors is a type of bioactive coating that includes elements capable of diffusing and stimulating osteogenic activity. The coatings enable bone cells to attach themselves, multiply, and differentiate on the surface of the orthopedic or dental implant [413]. The positive stimulating effect of osteogenic factors such as BMPs on the proliferation and differentiation of bone cells has been proven by several researchers [416, 417]. BMPs have been used in combination with HA, dopamine/gelatin, and collagen, among others. Most of the results indicated the facilitation of cell proliferation and increased osteogenesis adjacent to the implant [418].

4.2.3.3. Immunomodulatory Coatings

One of the reasons for the failure of implants in the body is the host's immune response. One of the effective methods to increase the success of an implant is *via* surface modification, which is explained in detail in the previous sections. Additionally, another effective strategy involves precisely adjusting biocompatibility through the delivery of safety factors, which allows the surface modification elements to perform their proper function. Interleukin 4 has been used to regulate the immune response of macrophages and can induce the polarization of M2 macrophages, thereby promoting the osteogenic differentiation of BM-MSCs *in vivo* and *in vitro* through increased BMP-2 expression [419].

4.2.3.4. Antibacterial Coatings

An ideal antibacterial coating destroys pathogens during initial contact and prevents infection in the short and long term. In addition to the various metal ion approaches described in the previous sections, other compounds, including iodine, chlorhexidine, dimethyl-amino dodecyl methacrylate, and dimethyl-amino ethyl methacrylate, also elicit antibacterial activity [420]. The mechanism of action of these compounds varies, for example, chlorhexidine is absorbed on the surface of the bacteria and destroys the permeability of the membrane [421]. While dimethylaminoethyl methacrylate inhibits the growth of bacteria and causes bone differentiation [422].

5. Conclusion

Bone grafting is a frequently used treatment that aims to encourage the body to produce new bone in areas where it is lacking or injured. Yet, there are drawbacks to standard grafting methods, such as insufficient graft supply, risk of immunological response, and the need for extra treatments. Due to their osteogenic capacity, osteoinduction, and osteoconduction features, autologous bone grafts generated from the patient's own body are popular in orthopedic and dental medicine. Mineralized, fresh-frozen, and dECM are the three main types of allografts, that is, human donor bone transplants. Although dentists employ xenogenous bone grafts, that is, transplants of non-resorbable bone tissue from one species to another, they encounter ethical, religious, and health concerns. Regenerative medicine and tissue engineering are changing the game when it comes to fixing and regenerating broken bones. In BTE, scaffolds are used to provide an ideal setting for cell proliferation and differentiation, thereby regenerating bone tissue. Artificial materials called alloplastic scaffolds may supplement or even completely replace the body's natural bone tissue. Alloplastic scaffolds often include HA, which provides a supportive environment for the proliferation of bone cells. It is also possible to restore bone deficiencies with other bioceramics that mimic the mineral component of bone. Also, BTE shows potential for natural and synthetic polymer-based scaffolds. Both natural and synthetic polymers are employed; however, natural polymers show improved cell adherence, while synthetic polymers elicit controlled degradation. Scaffolds made of composites provide targeted therapeutic delivery while simulating the properties of natural bone. Many researchers are interested in studying the biodegradability and multifunctionality of metal scaffolds because of their superior mechanical properties, but they also have downsides such as stress shielding and limited degradability. To enhance tissue ingrowth, porous titanium scaffolds have been manufactured for use in bone tissue restoration using advanced methods such as 3D printing. According to the basic concepts of personalized medicine, every person has distinctive traits that need tailored solutions to their health issues. To create one-of-a-kind scaffolds, CAD/CAM software uses CT scans of bone abnormalities to create blocks of xenogenic or alloplastic materials. Different methods exist for bone tissue regeneration to improve treatment efficiency, including implanting scaffolds containing vasculogenic factors, encapsulating GFs, and altering scaffold surfaces. In addition to cell-based, gene-based, and immunological therapies, multifunctional scaffolds provide support for a wide range of other treatments. Research has shown that MNPs, bioactive chemicals, nanofillers, and drug carriers may enhance bone regeneration and promote the formation of osteoblasts. Incorporating GFs into biodegradable scaffolds improves blood vessel formation and function, which in turn stimulates osteogenesis and angiogenesis, two processes that aid in bone tissue regeneration. A smart scaffold could be created by combining active, stimuli-responsive biomaterials, which allow for tailored therapy administration and early illness detection. Besides, oxygen-releasing scaffolds could help progenitor cells to overcome hypoxia conditions. Improving mechanical, tribological, and biocompatibility features may be achieved by surface modification and coating, which could be critical for implant design. While inorganic coatings exhibit antimicrobial and protective properties, polymeric coatings are being considered due to their low production costs and simplicity.

In this chapter, we present contemporary methods used to augment bone regeneration, as well as highlight advancements and modification techniques that can improve various aspects of the biomaterials currently utilized in BTE. This includes their mechanical, chemical, and, mostly their biological properties. However, and into the future, further research is needed to develop smart and autonomous scaffolding approaches, as well as other strategies that carefully mimic and stimulate the body's healing process to ensure rapid and complete healing, no matter the clinical scenario.

References

1. Šromová V, Sobola D, Kaspar P. A brief review of bone cell function and importance. *Cells*. 2023;12(21):2576.
2. Perić Kačarević Ž, Rider P, Alkildani S, Retnasingh S, Pejakić M, Schnettler R, et al. An introduction to bone tissue engineering. *Int. J. Artif. Organs*. 2020;43(2):69–86.
3. Dimitriou R, Jones E, McGonagle D, Giannoudis PV. Bone regeneration: Current concepts and future directions. *BMC Med.* 2011;9:1–10.
4. Oryan A, Alidadi S, Moshiri A, Maffulli N. Bone regenerative medicine: Classic options, novel strategies, and future directions. *J. Orthop. Surg. Res.* 2014;9(1):18.
5. Fesseha H, Fesseha Y. Bone grafting, its principle and application: A review. *Osteol. Rheumatol. Open J.* 2020;1(1):43–50.
6. Pendharkar SS. Alloplastic bone grafts in maxillofacial surgery-an overview. *J. Dent. Spec.* 2024;12(1):3–6.
7. Balaji VR, Manikandan D, Ramsundar A. Bone grafts in periodontics. *Matrix Sci. Med.* 2020;4(3):57–63.
8. Lee SS, Du X, Kim I, Ferguson SJ. Scaffolds for bone-tissue engineering. *Matter*. 2022;5(9):2722–59.
9. Abdelaziz AG, Nageh H, Abdo SM, Abdalla MS, Amer AA, Abdal-Hay A, et al. A review of 3D polymeric scaffolds for bone tissue engineering: Principles, fabrication techniques, immunomodulatory roles, and challenges. *Bioengineering*. 2023;10(2):204.
10. Wang F, Cai X, Shen Y, Meng L. Cell-scaffold interactions in tissue engineering for oral and craniofacial reconstruction. *Bioact. Mater.* 2023;23:16–44.

11. Murphy CM, O'Brien FJ, Little DG, Schindeler A. Cell-scaffold interactions in the bone tissue engineering triad. *Eur. Cell Mater.* 2013;26:120–32.
12. Percival KM, Paul V, Husseini GA. Recent advancements in bone tissue engineering: Integrating smart scaffold technologies and bio-responsive systems for enhanced regeneration. *Int. J. Mol. Sci.* 2024;25(11):6012.
13. Ferraz MP. Bone grafts in dental medicine: An overview of autografts, allografts and synthetic materials. *Materials*. 2023;16(11):4117.
14. Zhang J, Li S, He H, Han L, Zhang S, Yang L, et al. Clinical guidelines for indications, techniques, and complications of autogenous bone grafting. *Chin. Med. J. (Engl.)*. 2024;137(1):5–7.
15. Schmidt AH. Autologous bone graft: Is it still the gold standard? *Injury*. 2021;52(Suppl 2):S18–S22.
16. Jakoi AM, Iorio JA, Cahill PJ. Autologous bone graft harvesting: A review of grafts and surgical techniques. *Musculoskelet. Surg*. 2015;99(3):171–78.
17. Roberts TT, Rosenbaum AJ. Bone grafts, bone substitutes and orthobiologics: The bridge between basic science and clinical advancements in fracture healing. *Organogenesis*. 2012;8(4):114–24.
18. Donos N, Akcali A, Padhye N, Sculean A, Calciolari E. Bone regeneration in implant dentistry: Which are the factors affecting the clinical outcome? *Periodontol. 2000*. 2023;93(1):26–55.
19. Battafarano G, Rossi M, De Martino V, Marampon F, Borro L, Secinaro A, et al. Strategies for bone regeneration: From graft to tissue engineering. *Int. J. Mol. Sci.* 2021;22(3):1128.
20. Finkemeier CG. Bone-grafting and bone-graft substitutes. *J. Bone Joint Surg. Am.* 2002;84(3):454–64.
21. Lombardo JA, Russell N, He J, Larson MJ, Walsh WR, Mundis GMM Jr, et al. Autograft cellular contribution to spinal fusion and effects of intraoperative storage conditions. *Spine. (Phila Pa 1976)*. 2023;48(16):1181–89.
22. Sönmez TT, Prescher A, Salama A, Kanatas A, Zor F, Mitchell D, et al. Comparative clinicoanatomical study of ilium and fibula as two commonly used bony donor sites for maxillofacial reconstruction. *Br. J. Oral Maxillofac. Surg.* 2013;51(8):736–41.
23. Kumar P, Vinitha B, Fathima G. Bone grafts in dentistry. *J. Pharm. Bioallied Sci.* 2013;5(Suppl 1):S125–S127.
24. Baldwin P, Li DJ, Auston DA, Mir HS, Yoon RS, Koval K. Autograft, allograft, and bone graft substitutes: Clinical evidence and indications for use in the setting of orthopaedic trauma surgery. *J. Orthop. Trauma*. 2019;33(4):203–13.

25. Harasen G. Stimulating bone growth in the small animal patient: Grafts and beyond!. *Can. Vet. J.* 2011;52(2):199–200.
26. Perez JR, Jose J, Mohile NV, Boden AL, Greif DN, Barrera CM, et al. Limb salvage reconstruction: Radiologic features of common reconstructive techniques and their complications. *J. Orthop.* 2020;21:183–91.
27. Bumbasirevic M, Stevanovic M, Bumbasirevic V, Lesic A, Atkinson HDE. Free vascularised fibular grafts in orthopaedics. *Int. Orthop.* 2014;38(6): 1277–82.
28. Zhang Z, Hao Z, Xian C, Fang Y, Cheng B, Wu J, et al. Neuro-bone tissue engineering: Multiple potential translational strategies between nerve and bone. *Acta Biomater.* 2022;153:1–12.
29. Xiao L, Liu J, Yan F, Xiao Y. Peripheral sensory nerve regeneration: Novel target in bone tissue engineering. *Brain-X.* 2024;2(3):e71.
30. Chen S, Zhou X, Li T, He C. Vascularization and innervation for bone tissue engineering. *Acc. Mater. Res.* 2024;5(9):1121–33.
31. Liu S, Liu S, Li S, Liang B, Han X, Liang Y, et al. Nerves within bone and their application in tissue engineering of bone regeneration. *Front. Neurol.* 2022;13:1085560.
32. Sun W, Ye B, Chen S, Zeng L, Lu H, Wan Y, et al. Neuro-bone tissue engineering: Emerging mechanisms, potential strategies, and current challenges. *Bone Res.* 2023;11(1):65.
33. Pfister BJ, Gordon T, Loverde JR, Kochar AS, Mackinnon SE, Cullen DK. Biomedical engineering strategies for peripheral nerve repair: Surgical applications, state of the art, and future challenges. *Crit. Rev. Biomed. Eng.* 2011;39(2):81–124.
34. Safa B, Buncke G. Autograft substitutes: Conduits and processed nerve allografts. *Hand Clin.* 2016;32(2):127–40.
35. Pape H-C, Tarkin IS. Reamer irrigator aspirator: A new technique for bone graft harvesting from the intramedullary canal. *Oper. Tech. Orthop.* 2008;18(2):108–13.
36. Yee MA, Hundal RS, Perdue AM, Hake ME. Autologous bone graft harvest using the reamer-irrigator-aspirator. *J. Orthop. Trauma.* 2018;32(Suppl 1): S20–s21.
37. Tajabadi M, Barghamadi H, Orimi HG, Gholami M, Pasandideh Z. Musculoskeletal regenerative nanomedicine: Current therapies, translational hurdles, and future directions. In: *Nanoengineering in Musculoskeletal Regeneration.* Amsterdam, Netherlands: Elsevier, 2020:237–72.

38. Araújo CRG, Astarita C, D'Aquino R, Pelegrine AA. Evaluation of bone regeneration in rat calvaria using bone autologous micrografts and xenografts: Histological and histomorphometric analysis. *Materials. (Basel).* 2020;13(19):4284.
39. Zhang Z, Gan Y, Guo Y, Lu X, Li X. Animal models of vertical bone augmentation. *Exp. Ther. Med.* 2021;22(3):919.
40. Blanc-Sylvestre N, Bouchard P, Chaussain C, Bardet C. Pre-clinical models in implant dentistry: Past, present, future. *Biomedicines*. 2021;9(11):1538.
41. Beer AJ, Tauro TM, Redondo ML, Christian DR, Cole BJ, Frank RM. Use of allografts in orthopaedic surgery: Safety, procurement, storage, and outcomes. *Orthop. J. Sports Med.* 2019;7(12):2325967119891435.
42. Miron RJ. Optimized bone grafting. *Periodontol. 2000*. 2024;94(1):143–60.
43. Steijvers E, Ghei A, Xia Z. Manufacturing artificial bone allografts: A perspective. *Biomater. Transl.* 2022;3(1):65–80.
44. Sohn H-S, Oh J-K. Review of bone graft and bone substitutes with an emphasis on fracture surgeries. *Biomater. Res*. 2019;23:9.
45. Moore MA, Samsell B, McLean J. Allograft tissue safety and technology. In: *Biologics in Orthopaedic Surgery*. 2019:49–62.
46. Ciszyński M, Dominiak S, Dominiak M, Gedrange T, Hadzik J. Allogenic bone graft in dentistry: A review of current trends and developments. *Int. J. Mol. Sci.* 2023;24(23):16598.
47. Grover V, Kapoor A, Malhotra R, Sachdeva S. Bone allografts: A review of safety and efficacy. *Indian J. Dent. Res*. 2011;22(3):496.
48. Zhang X, Chen X, Hong H, Hu R, Liu J, Liu C. Decellularized extracellular matrix scaffolds: Recent trends and emerging strategies in tissue engineering. *Bioact. Mater*. 2022;10:15–31.
49. Amirazad H, Dadashpour M, Zarghami N. Application of decellularized bone matrix as a bioscaffold in bone tissue engineering. *J. Biol. Eng*. 2022; 16(1):1.
50. Eastlund T. Viral infections transmitted through tissue transplantation. In: Kennedy JF, Phillips GO, Williams PA (eds). *Sterilisation of Tissues Using Ionising Radiations*. Amsterdam: Elsevier, 2005:255–78.
51. Fischer M, Bortel E, Schoon J, Behnke E, Hesse B, Weitkamp T, et al. Cold physical plasma treatment optimization for improved bone allograft processing. *Front. Bioeng. Biotechnol.* 2023;11:1264409.
52. Wheeler DL, Enneking WF. Allograft bone decreases in strength in vivo over time. *Clin. Orthop. Relat. Res.* 2005;435:36–42.

53. Kauke-Navarro M, Noel OF, Knoedler L, Knoedler S, Panayi AC, Stoegner VA, et al. Novel strategies in transplantation: Genetic engineering and vascularized composite allotransplantation. *J. Surg. Res.* 2023;291:176–86.
54. Luo X, Zhang J, Zou S, Wang X, Chen G, Li Z, et al. Bone fragment co-transplantation alongside bone marrow aspirate infusion protects kidney transplant recipients. *Front. Immunol.* 2021;12:630710.
55. Boyan BD, Weesner TC, Lohmann CH, Andreacchio D, Carnes DL, Dean DD, et al. Porcine fetal enamel matrix derivative enhances bone formation induced by demineralized freeze dried bone allograft in vivo. *J. Periodontol.* 2000;71(8):1278–86.
56. Rocha LR, Dias RB, Fernandes MBC, Prinz R, Eirado TP, Costa IS, et al. A new option for bone regeneration: A rapid methodology for cellularization of allograft with human bone marrow stromal cells with in vivo bone-forming potential. *Injury*. 2023;54(Suppl 6):110777.
57. Coquelin L, Fialaire-Legendre A, Roux S, Poignard A, Bierling P, Hernigou P, et al. In vivo and in vitro comparison of three different allografts vitalized with human mesenchymal stromal cells. *Tissue Eng. Part A*. 2012;18(17–18):1921–31.
58. Schwartz Z, Mellonig JT, Carnes Jr DL, de la Fontaine J, Cochran DL, Dean DD, et al. Ability of commercial demineralized freeze-dried bone allograft to induce new bone formation. *J. Periodontol.* 1996;67(9):918–26.
59. Schwartz Z, Somers A, Mellonig JT, Carnes Jr DL, Dean DD, Cochran DL, et al. Ability of commercial demineralized freeze-dried bone allograft to induce new bone formation is dependent on donor age but not gender. *J. Periodontol.* 1998;69(4):470–78.
60. Nazeer J, Singh R, Suri P, Mouneshkumar CD, Bhardwaj S, Iqubal MA, et al. Evaluation of marginal bone loss around dental implants in cigarette smokers and nonsmokers. A comparative study. *J. Fam. Med. Prim. Care.* 2020;9(2):729–34.
61. Levin L, Schwartz-Arad D. The effect of cigarette smoking on dental implants and related surgery. *Implant Dent.* 2005;14(4):357–61.
62. Pius AK, Toya M, Gao Q, Lee ML, Ergul YS, Chow SK-H, et al. Effects of aging on osteosynthesis at bone-implant interfaces. *Biomolecules.* 2023;14(1):52.
63. Bertl K, Ebner M, Knibbe M, Pandis N, Kuchler U, Ulm C, et al. How old is old for implant therapy in terms of early implant losses? *J. Clin. Periodontol.* 2019;46(12):1282–93.

64. Griffin KS, Davis KM, McKinley TO, Anglen JO, Chu TM, Boerckel JD, et al. Evolution of bone grafting: Bone grafts and tissue engineering strategies for vascularized bone regeneration. *Clin. Rev. Bone Miner. Metab.* 2015;13:232–44.
65. Zecha PJ, Schortinghuis J, van der Wal JE, Nagursky H, van den Broek KC, Sauerbier S, et al. Applicability of equine hydroxyapatite collagen (eHAC) bone blocks for lateral augmentation of the alveolar crest. A histological and histomorphometric analysis in rats. *Int. J. Oral Maxillofac. Surg.* 2011;40(5):533–42.
66. Bracey DN, Seyler TM, Jinnah AH, Lively MO, Willey JS, Smith TL, et al. A decellularized porcine xenograft-derived bone scaffold for clinical use as a bone graft substitute: A critical evaluation of processing and structure. *J. Funct. Biomater.* 2018;9(3):45.
67. Bauermeister A, Maatz R. A method of bone maceration; results in animal experiments. *J. Bone Joint Surg. Am.* 1957;39-A(1):153–66.
68. Bracey DN, Cignetti NE, Jinnah AH, Stone AV, Gyr BM, Whitlock PW, et al. Bone xenotransplantation: A review of the history, orthopedic clinical literature, and a single-center case series. *Xenotransplantation.* 2020;27(5): e12600.
69. Correia F, Pozza DH, Gouveia S, Felino AC, Faria-Almeida R. Advantages of porcine xenograft over autograft in sinus lift: A randomised clinical trial. *Materials (Basel).* 2021;14(12):3439.
70. Correia F, Gouveia S, Felino AC, Faria-Almeida R, Pozza D. Maxillary sinus augmentation with xenogenic collagen-retained heterologous cortico-cancellous bone: A 3-year follow-up randomized controlled trial. *Dent. J.* 2024;12(2):33.
71. Calasans-Maia M, Resende R, Fernandes G, Calasans-Maia J, Alves AT, Granjeiro JM. A randomized controlled clinical trial to evaluate a new xenograft for alveolar socket preservation. *Clin. Oral Implants Res.* 2014; 25(10):1125–30.
72. Amid R, Kheiri A, Kheiri L, Kadkhodazadeh M, Ekhlasmandkermani M. Structural and chemical features of xenograft bone substitutes: A systematic review of in vitro studies. *Biotechnol. Appl. Biochem.* 2021;68(6): 1432–52.
73. Campana V, Milano G, Pagano E, Barba M, Cicione C, Salonna G, et al. Bone substitutes in orthopaedic surgery: From basic science to clinical practice. *J. Mater. Sci. Mater. Med.* 2014;25(10):2445–61.

74. Hawthorne WJ. Ethical and legislative advances in xenotransplantation for clinical translation: Focusing on cardiac, kidney and islet cell xenotransplantation. *Front. Immunol.* 2024;15:1355609.
75. Bayliss G. Practical ethical concerns in allocation of pig kidneys to humans. *Clin. Kidney J.* 2022;15(12):2161–68.
76. de Azambuja Carvalho PH, de Oliveira Ciaramicolo N, Júnior OF, Pereira-Filho VA. Clinical and laboratorial outcomes of xenogeneic biomaterials: Literature review. *Front. Oral Maxillofac. Med.* 2021;5:8.
77. Barbeck M, Udeabor SE, Lorenz J, Kubesch A, Choukroun J, Sader RA, et al. Induction of multinucleated giant cells in response to small sized bovine bone substitute (Bio-Oss™) results in an enhanced early implantation bed vascularization. *Ann. Maxillofac. Surg.* 2014;4(2):150–7.
78. Valencia-Llano CH, López-Tenorio D, Grande-Tovar CD. Biocompatibility assessment of two commercial bone xenografts by in vitro and in vivo methods. *Polymers. (Basel)*. 2022;14(13):2672.
79. Kloss FR, Kämmerer PW, Kloss-Brandstätter A. First clinical case report of a xenograft-allograft combination for alveolar ridge augmentation using a bovine bone substitute material with hyaluronate (Cerabone(®) Plus) combined with allogeneic bone granules (Maxgraft(®)). *J. Clin. Med.* 2023;12(19):6214.
80. Wang T, Krieger J, Huang C, Das A, Francis MP, Ogle R, et al. Enhanced osseous integration of human trabecular allografts following surface modification with bioactive lipids. *Drug Deliv. Transl. Res.* 2016;6(2): 96–104.
81. Qiu Z-Y, Chen C, Wang X-M, Lee I-S. Advances in the surface modification techniques of bone-related implants for last 10 years. *Regen. Biomater.* 2014;1(1):67–79.
82. Chokwattananuwat N, Suttapreyasri S. Surface-modified deproteinized human demineralized tooth matrix for bone regeneration: Physicochemical characterization and osteoblast cell biocompatibility. *Regen. Biomater.* 2024;11:rbae030.
83. Dhavalikar P, Jenkins D, Rosen N, Kannapiran A, Salhadar K, Shachaf O, et al. Hydroxyapatite nanoparticle-modified porous bone grafts with improved cell attachment. *J. Mater. Chem. B.* 2023;11(44):10651–64.
84. Sarinnaphakorn L, Di Silvio L. Surface-modified titanium to enhance osseointegration in dental implants. In: Di Silvio L (ed) *Cellular Response to Biomaterials*. Amsterdam: Elsevier, 2009:572–88.
85. Wei Z, Reisdorf RL, Thoreson AR, Jay GD, Moran SL, An K-N, et al. Comparison of autograft and allograft with surface modification for flexor

tendon reconstruction: A canine in vivo model. *J. Bone Joint Surg. Am.* 2018;100(7):e42.
86. Wang J, Cui Y, Zhang B, Sun S, Xu H, Yao M, et al. Polydopamine-modified functional materials promote bone regeneration. *Mater. Des.* 2024;238:112655.
87. Huang S, Liang N, Hu Y, Zhou X, Abidi N. Polydopamine-assisted surface modification for bone biosubstitutes. *BioMed Res. Int.* 2016;2016(1):2389895.
88. Zhu Q, Jiao H, Zhao X, Tang Y, Zhao K, Gou X. Hydroxyapatite formation in biomimetic synthesis with the interface of a pDA@SIS membrane. *RSC Adv.* 2022;12(21):13209–19.
89. Tao C, Jin M, Yao H, Wang D-A. Dopamine based adhesive nano-coatings on extracellular matrix (ECM) based grafts for enhanced host-graft interfacing affinity. *Nanoscale.* 2021;13(43):18148–59.
90. Mercado-Pagán ÁE, Stahl AM, Shanjani Y, Yang Y. Vascularization in bone tissue engineering constructs. *Ann. Biomed. Eng.* 2015;43(3):718–29.
91. Tsigkou O, Pomerantseva I, Spencer JA, Redondo PA, Hart AR, O'Doherty E, et al. Engineered vascularized bone grafts. *Proc. Natl. Acad. Sci. U S A.* 2010;107(8):3311–16.
92. Saghiri M-A, Asatourian A, Garcia-Godoy F, Sheibani N. The role of angiogenesis in implant dentistry part II: The effect of bone-grafting and barrier membrane materials on angiogenesis. *Med. Oral Patol. Oral Cir. Bucal.* 2016;21(4):e526–e537.
93. Wu V, Schulten EAJM, Helder MN, Ten Bruggenkate CM, Bravenboer N, Klein-Nulend J. Bone vitality and vascularization of mandibular and maxillary bone grafts in maxillary sinus floor elevation: A retrospective cohort study. *Clin. Implant Dent. Relat. Res.* 2023;25(1):141–51.
94. Cohn Yakubovich D, Tawackoli W, Sheyn D, Kallai I, Da X, Pelled G, et al. Computed tomography and optical imaging of osteogenesis-angiogenesis coupling to assess integration of cranial bone autografts and allografts. *JoVE (J. Vis. Exp.).* 2015;106:e53459.
95. Rombouts C, Jeanneau C, Camilleri J, Laurent P, About I. Characterization and angiogenic potential of xenogeneic bone grafting materials: Role of periodontal ligament cells. *Dent. Mater. J.* 2016;35(6):900–07.
96. Hu K, Olsen BR. The roles of vascular endothelial growth factor in bone repair and regeneration. *Bone.* 2016;91:30–8.
97. Detsch R, Stoor P, Grünewald A, Roether JA, Lindfors NC, Boccaccini AR. Increase in VEGF secretion from human fibroblast cells by bioactive glass S53P4 to stimulate angiogenesis in bone. *J. Biomed. Mater. Res. A.* 2014;102(11):4055–61.

98. Huang J, Lu J, Liu Z, Jin J, Xie C, Zheng Y, et al. Covalent immobilization of VEGF on allogeneic bone through polydopamine coating to improve bone regeneration. *Front. Bioeng. Biotechnol.* 2022;10:1003677.
99. Zhao J, Zhou C, Xiao Y, Zhang K, Zhang Q, Xia L, et al. Oxygen generating biomaterials at the forefront of regenerative medicine: Advances in bone regeneration. *Front. Bioeng. Biotechnol.* 2024;12:1292171.
100. Suvarnapathaki S, Wu X, Zhang T, Nguyen MA, Goulopoulos AA, Wu B, et al. Oxygen generating scaffolds regenerate critical size bone defects. *Bioact. Mater.* 2022;13:64–81.
101. Díaz-Vegas A, Campos CA, Contreras-Ferrat A, Casas M, Buvinic S, Jaimovich E, et al. ROS production via P2Y1-PKC-NOX2 is triggered by extracellular ATP after electrical stimulation of skeletal muscle cells. *PloS One*. 2015;10(6):e0129882.
102. Schmelter M, Ateghang B, Helmig S, Wartenberg M, Sauer H. Embryonic stem cells utilize reactive oxygen species as transducers of mechanical strain-induced cardiovascular differentiation. *FASEB J.* 2006;20(8):1182–4.
103. Sart S, Song L, Li Y. Controlling redox status for stem cell survival, expansion, and differentiation. *Oxid. Med. Cell. Longev.* 2015;2015(1):105135.
104. Hsu EL, Stock SR. Growth factors, carrier materials, and bone repair. *Handb. Exp. Pharmacol.* 2020;262:121–56.
105. Chen R, Wang J, Liu C. Biomaterials act as enhancers of growth factors in bone regeneration. *Adv. Funct. Mater.* 2016;26(48):8810–23.
106. Lieberman JR, Daluiski A, Einhorn TA. The role of growth factors in the repair of bone: Biology and clinical applications. *J. Bone Joint. Surg. Am.* 2002;84(6):1032–44.
107. Gross SM, Rotwein P. Quantification of growth factor signaling and pathway cross talk by live-cell imaging. *Am. J. Physiol. Cell Physiol.* 2017;312(3): C328–C340.
108. Jing Z, Liang Z, Yang L, Du W, Yu T, Tang H, et al. Bone formation and bone repair: The roles and crosstalk of osteoinductive signaling pathways. *Process Biochem.* 2022;118:252–62.
109. Wei Q, Holle A, Li J, Posa F, Biagioni F, Croci O, et al. BMP–2 signaling and mechanotransduction synergize to drive osteogenic differentiation via YAP/TAZ. *Adv. Sci. (Weinh).* 2020;7(15):1902931.
110. Shimono K, Oshima M, Arakawa H, Kimura A, Nawachi K, Kuboki T. The effect of growth factors for bone augmentation to enable dental implant placement: A systematic review. *Jpn. Dent. Sci. Rev.* 2010;46(1):43–53.

111. Keranmu D, Nuermuhanmode N, Ainiwaer A, Guli, Taxifulati D, Shan W, et al. Clinical application of concentrate growth factors combined with bone substitute in Alveolar ridge preservation of anterior teeth. *BMC Oral Health*. 2022;22(1):54.
112. Cicciù M. Growth factor applied to oral and regenerative surgery. *Int. J. Mol. Sci*. 2020;21(20):7752.
113. Burger MG, Grosso A, Briquez PS, Born GME, Lunger A, Schrenk F, et al. Robust coupling of angiogenesis and osteogenesis by VEGF-decorated matrices for bone regeneration. *Acta. Biomater.* 2022;149:111–25.
114. Gillman CE, Jayasuriya AC. FDA-approved bone grafts and bone graft substitute devices in bone regeneration. *Mater. Sci. Eng. C Mater. Biol. Appl*. 2021;130:112466.
115. Bessho K, Kusumoto K, Fujimura K, Konishi Y, Ogawa Y, Tani Y, et al. Comparison of recombinant and purified human bone morphogenetic protein. *Br. J. Oral Maxillofac. Surg*. 1999;37(1):2–5.
116. Jung RE, Glauser R, Schärer P, Hämmerle CH, Sailer HF, Weber FE. Effect of rhBMP-2 on guided bone regeneration in humans. *Clin. Oral Implants Res*. 2003;14(5):556–68.
117. Kaigler D, Avila G, Wisner-Lynch L, Nevins ML, Nevins M, Rasperini G, et al. Platelet-derived growth factor applications in periodontal and peri-implant bone regeneration. *Expert Opin. Biol. Ther*. 2011;11(3):375–85.
118. Tavelli L, Ravidà A, Barootchi S, Chambrone L, Giannobile WV. Recombinant human platelet-derived growth factor: A systematic review of clinical findings in oral regenerative procedures. *JDR Clin. Trans. Res*. 2021 Apr;6(2):161–73.
119. Pokhrel S. Hydroxyapatite: preparation, properties and its biomedical applications. *Adv. Chem. Eng. Sci*. 2018;8(04):225–40.
120. Cheah CW, Al-Namnam NM, Lau MN, Lim GS, Raman R, Fairbairn P, et al. Synthetic material for bone, periodontal, and dental tissue regeneration: where are we now, and where are we heading next?. *Materials (Basel)*. 2021;14(20):6123.
121. Fukuba S, Okada M, Nohara K, Iwata T. Alloplastic bone substitutes for periodontal and bone regeneration in dentistry: Current status and prospects. *Materials (Basel)*. 2021;14(5):1096.
122. Özcolak B, Erenay B, Odabaş S, Jandt KD, Garipcan B. Effects of bone surface topography and chemistry on macrophage polarization. *Sci. Rep*. 2024;14(1):12721.

123. Roseti L, Parisi V, Petretta M, Cavallo C, Desando G, Bartolotti I, et al. Scaffolds for bone tissue engineering: State of the art and new perspectives. *Mater. Sci. Eng. C Mater. Biol. Appl.* 2017;78:1246–62.
124. Gao C, Lai Y, Cheng L, Cheng Y, Miao A, Chen J, et al. PIP2 alteration caused by elastic modulus and tropism of electrospun scaffolds facilitates altered BMSCs proliferation and differentiation. *Adv. Mater.* 2023;35(18): e2212272.
125. Pandey A, Kannaiyan J, Chhabra H, Palaniyandi M, Rajangam B, Suriya Narayanan S. Biological and synthetic scaffold: An extra cellular matrix for constructive tissue engineering. *Int. J. Med. Res. Rev.* 2016;4(10):1882–96.
126. Tajvar S, Hadjizadeh A, Samandari SS. Scaffold degradation in bone tissue engineering: An overview. *Inter. Biodeterior. Biodegrad.* 2023;180:105599.
127. Yuan H, Fernandes H, Habibovic P, de Boer J, Barradas AMC, de Ruiter A, et al. Osteoinductive ceramics as a synthetic alternative to autologous bone grafting. *Proc. Natl. Acad. Sci. U S A.* 2010;107(31):13614–9.
128. Nevins M, Nevins ML, Schupbach P, Kim SW, Lin Z, Kim DM. A prospective, randomized controlled preclinical trial to evaluate different formulations of biphasic calcium phosphate in combination with a hydroxyapatite collagen membrane to reconstruct deficient alveolar ridges. *J. Oral Implantol.* 2013;39(2):133–9.
129. Goetz LH, Schork NJ. Personalized medicine: motivation, challenges, and progress. *Fertil Steril.* 2018;109(6):952–63.
130. Cruz N, Gil Mur J, Paulo Tondela J. Custom-made alloplastic and xenogenic scaffolds for bone augmentation — 1st year clinical outcomes. *Clin. Oral Implants Res.* 2018;29(S17):11–13.
131. He J, Li K, Wu T, Chen J, Li S, Zhang X. Research progress in degradable metal–based multifunctional scaffolds for bone tissue engineering. *MedComm–Biomater. App.* 2023;2(4):e60.
132. Li S, Cui Y, Liu H, Tian Y, Wang, Fan Y, et al. Application of bioactive metal ions in the treatment of bone defects. *J. Mater. Chem. B.* 2022;10(45): 9369–88.
133. Wei X, Zhou W, Tang Z, Wu H, Liu Y, Dong H, et al. Magnesium surface-activated 3D printed porous PEEK scaffolds for in vivo osseointegration by promoting angiogenesis and osteogenesis. *Bioact. Mater.* 2023;20:16–28.
134. Li P, Dai J, Li Y, Alexander D, Čapek J, Geis-Gerstorfer J, et al. Zinc based biodegradable metals for bone repair and regeneration: Bioactivity and molecular mechanisms. *Mater. Today Bio.* 2024;25:100932.

135. Xia D, Qin Y, Guo H, Wen P, Lin H, Voshage M, et al. Additively manufactured pure zinc porous scaffolds for critical-sized bone defects of rabbit femur. *Bioact. Mater.* 2023;19:12–23.
136. Li K, Hu D, Zhang X, Li J, Huang S, Ji H, et al. Mg-incorporated micro/nano-topographical calcium silicate coatings with enhanced osteogenic properties and reduced inflammatory reactions. *Discov. Mater.* 2023;3(1):16.
137. Liu H, Chen H, Han Q, Sun B, Liu Y, Zhang A, et al. Recent advancement in vascularized tissue-engineered bone based on materials design and modification. *Mater. Today Bio.* 2023;23:100858.
138. Xiang H, Dai X, Xu W, Li S, Yang X, Huang Z, et al. Cryogenic 3D printing of bifunctional silicate nanoclay incorporated scaffolds for promoted angiogenesis and bone regeneration. *Mater. Des.* 2022;223:111220.
139. Peng B, Xu H, Song F, Wen P, Tian Y, Zheng Y. Additive manufacturing of porous magnesium alloys for biodegradable orthopedic implants: Process, design, and modification. *J. Mater. Sci. Technol.* 2023;182:79–110.
140. Sreenivasamurthy SA, Akhter FF, Akhter A, Su Y, Zhu D. Cellular mechanisms of biodegradable zinc and magnesium materials on promoting angiogenesis. *Biomater. Adv.* 2022;139:213023.
141. Al Sakkaf A, Jannuddi FS, Md Yusop AH, Nur H. Challenges in the use of fe-based materials for bone scaffolds applications: Perspective from in vivo biocorrosion. *Mater. Today Commun.* 2022;33:104564.
142. Wegener B, Behnke M, Milz S, Jansson V, Redlich C, Hermanns W, et al, Local and systemic inflammation after implantation of a novel iron based porous degradable bone replacement material in sheep model. *Sci. Rep.* 2021;11(1):12035.
143. Ulum MF, Nasution AK, Yusop AH, Arafat A, Kadir MRA, Juniantito V, et al. Evidences of in vivo bioactivity of fe-bioceramic composites for temporary bone implants. *J. Biomed. Mater. Res.B. Appl. Biomater.* 2015;103(7):1354–65.
144. Rabeeh VPM, Rahim SA, Kinattingara Parambath SK, Rajanikant GK, Hanas T. Iron–gold composites for biodegradable implants: In vitro investigation on biodegradation and biomineralization. *ACS Biomater. Sci. Eng.* 2023;9(7):4255–68.
145. Carluccio D, Demir AG, Caprio L, Previtali B, Bermingham MJ, Dargusch MS. The influence of laser processing parameters on the densification and surface morphology of pure fe and Fe-35Mn scaffolds produced by selective laser melting. *J. Manuf. Process.* 2019;40:113–21.

146. Chen H, Zhou S, Dong B, Jin J, Liu T, Guan P. A general rule for transition metals doping on magnetic properties of Fe-based metallic glasses. *J. Alloys Compd.* 2020;819:153062.
147. Shuai C, Cheng Y, Yang W, Feng P, Yang Y, He C, et al. Magnetically actuated bone scaffold: Microstructure, cell response and osteogenesis. *Compos. Part B Eng.* 2020;192:107986.
148. Laubach M, Hildebrand F, Suresh S, Wagels M, Kobbe P, Gilbert F, et al. The concept of scaffold-guided bone regeneration for the treatment of long bone defects: Current clinical application and future perspective. *J. Funct. Biomater.* 2023;14(7):341.
149. Zuo W, Yu L, Lin J, Yang Y, Fei Q. Properties improvement of titanium alloys scaffolds in bone tissue engineering: a literature review. *Ann. Transl. Med.* 2021;9(15):1259.
150. Li Y, Liu H, Wang C, Yan R, Xiang L, Mu X, et al. 3D printing titanium grid scaffold facilitates osteogenesis in mandibular segmental defects. *NPJ Regen. Med.* 2023;8(1):38.
151. Alonzo M, Primo FA, Kumar SA, Mudloff JA, Dominguez E, Fregoso G, et al. Bone tissue engineering techniques, advances and scaffolds for treatment of bone defects. *Curr. Opin. Biomed. Eng.* 2021;17:100248.
152. Panda S, Biswas CK, Paul S. A comprehensive review on the preparation and application of calcium hydroxyapatite: A special focus on atomic doping methods for bone tissue engineering. *Ceram. int*, 2021;47(20):28122–44.
153. Özcan M, Hotza D, Fredel MC, Cruz A, Volpato CÂM. Materials and manufacturing techniques for polymeric and ceramic scaffolds used in implant dentistry. *J. Compos. Sci.* 2021;5(3):78.
154. Eppley BL, Pietrzak WS, Blanton MW. Allograft and alloplastic bone substitutes: A review of science and technology for the craniomaxillofacial surgeon. *J. Craniofac. Surg.* 2005;16(6):981–9.
155. Zhu W, Li W, Chen K, Feng B, Zhou L, Weng X, et al. Injectable and assembled 3D solid structure for free-to-fixed shape in bone reconstruction. *App. Mater. Today.* 2020;21:100823.
156. Matassi F, Nistri L, Chicon Paez D, Innocenti M. New biomaterials for bone regeneration. *Clin. Cases Miner Bone Metab.* 2011;8(1):21–4.
157. Huang J, Best SM. Ceramic biomaterials for tissue engineering. In: *Tissue Engineering using Ceramics and Polymers.* Amsterdam: Elsevier, 2022:3–40.
158. Meffert RM, Thomas JR, Hamilton KM, Brownstein CN. Hydroxylapatite as an alloplastic graft in the treatment of human periodontal osseous defects. *J. Periodontol.* 1985;56(2):63–73.

159. Yu X, Tang X, Gohil SV, Laurencin CT. Biomaterials for bone regenerative engineering. *Adv. Healthc. Mater.* 2015;4(9):1268–85.
160. Ros-Tárraga P, Mazón P, Rodríguez MA, Meseguer-Olmo L, De Aza PN. Novel resorbable and osteoconductive calcium silicophosphate scaffold induced bone formation. *Materials (Basel).* 2016;9(9):785.
161. Pearson JJ, Gerken N, Bae C, Lee KB, Satsangi A, McBride S, et al. In vivo hydroxyapatite scaffold performance in infected bone defects. *J. Biomed. Mater. Res. B. Appl. Biomater.* 2020;108(3):1157–66.
162. Zhao Y, Chen H, Ran K, Zhang Y, Pan H, Shangguan J, et al. Porous hydroxyapatite scaffold orchestrated with bioactive coatings for rapid bone repair. *Biomater. Adv.* 2023;144:213202.
163. Ong MM, Eber RM, Korsnes MI, MacNeil RL, Glickman GN, Shyr Y, et al.. Evaluation of a bioactive glass alloplast in treating periodontal intrabony defects. *J. Periodontol.* 1998;69(12):1346–54.
164. Crush J, Hussain A, Seah KTM, Khan WS. Bioactive glass: Methods for assessing angiogenesis and osteogenesis. *Front Cell Dev. Biol.* 2021;9: 643781.
165. Jahani B, Wang XN, Brooks A. Additive manufacturing techniques for fabrication of bone scaffolds for tissue engineering applications. *Recent Prog. Mater.* 2020;2(3):1–41.
166. Fu Q, Saiz E, Rahaman MN, Tomsia AP. Bioactive glass scaffolds for bone tissue engineering: State of the art and future perspectives. *Mater Sci. Eng. C Mater Biol. Appl.* 2011;31(7):1245–56.
167. Manoochehri H, Ghorbani M, Moosazadeh Moghaddam M, Nourani MR, Makvandi P, Sharifi E. Strontium doped bioglass incorporated hydrogel-based scaffold for amplified bone tissue regeneration. *Sci. Rep.* 2022; 12(1):10160.
168. Miri AK, Muja N, Kamranpour NO, Lepry WC, Boccaccini AR, Clarke SA, et al. Ectopic bone formation in rapidly fabricated acellular injectable dense collagen-bioglass hybrid scaffolds via gel aspiration-ejection. *Biomaterials.* 2016;85:128–41.
169. Sun T, Zhou K, Liu M, Guo X, Qu Y, Cui W, et al. Loading of BMP-2-related peptide onto three-dimensional nano-hydroxyapatite scaffolds accelerates mineralization in critical-sized cranial bone defects. *J.Tissue Eng. and Regen. Med.* 2018;12(4):864–77.
170. Li D, Huifang L, Zhao J, Yang Z, Xie X, Wei Z, et al. Porous lithium-doped hydroxyapatite scaffold seeded with hypoxia-preconditioned bone-marrow mesenchymal stem cells for bone-tissue regeneration. *Biomed. Mater.* 2018;13(5):055002.

171. Ribas RG, Schatkoski VM, do Amaral Montanheiro TL, de Menezes BRC, Stegemann C, Leite DMG, et al. Current advances in bone tissue engineering concerning ceramic and bioglass scaffolds: A review. *Ceram. Int.* 2019;45(17, Part A):21051–61.
172. Zhu Y, Yang Q, Yang M, Zhan X, Lan F, He J, et al. Protein corona of magnetic hydroxyapatite scaffold improves cell proliferation via activation of mitogen-activated protein kinase signaling pathway. *ACS Nano.* 2017;11(4):3690–3704.
173. Pasandideh Z, Tajabadi M, Javadpour J, Mirkazemi SM. The effects of Fe^{3+} and Co^{2+} substitution in $Ca_{10\text{-}x\text{-}y}Fe_xCo_y(PO_4)_6(OH)_2$ hydroxyapatite nanoparticles: Magnetic, antibacterial, and improved drug release behavior. *Ceram. Internat.* 2020;46(10, Part B):16104–18.
174. Arnold PM, Sasso RC, Janssen ME, Fehlings MG, Heary RF, Vaccaro AR, et al. I-actor™ bone graft vs autograft in anterior cervical discectomy and fusion: 2-year follow-up of the randomized single-blinded food and drug administration investigational device exemption study. *Neurosurgery.* 2018; 83(3):377–84.
175. Liu X, Ma PX. Polymeric scaffolds for bone tissue engineering. *Ann Biomed. Eng.* 2004;32(3):477–86.
176. Collins MN, Ren G, Young K, Pina S, Reis RL, Oliveira JM. Scaffold fabrication technologies and structure/function properties in bone tissue engineering. *Adv. Funct. Mater.* 2021;31(21):2010609.
177. Liu S, Zhang L, Li Z, Gao F, Zhang Q, Bianco A, et al. Materials-mediated in situ physical cues for bone regeneration. *Adv. Funct. Mater.* 2024;34(1): 2306534.
178. Liu Y, Lim J, Teoh S-H. Development of clinically relevant scaffolds for vascularised bone tissue engineering. *Biotechnol. Adv.* 2013;31(5):688–705.
179. Abbasi N, Hamlet S, Love RM, Nguyen N-T. Porous scaffolds for bone regeneration. *J. Sci. Adv. Mater. Dev.* 2020;5(1):1–9.
180. Yuan B, Zhou S-Y, Chen X-S. Rapid prototyping technology and its application in bone tissue engineering. *J. Zhejiang Univ. Sci. B.* 2017;18(4): 303–15.
181. De France KJ, Xu F, Hoare T. Structured macroporous hydrogels: Progress, challenges, and opportunities. *Adv. Healthc. Mater.* 2018;7(1).
182. Ma Y, Wang X, Su T, Lu F, Chang Q, Gao J. Recent advances in macroporous hydrogels for cell behavior and tissue engineering. *Gels.* 2022;8(10):606.
183. Fu J, Wiraja C, Muhammad HB, Xu C, Wang D-A. Improvement of endothelial progenitor outgrowth cell (EPOC)-mediated vascularization in

Gelatin-based hydrogels through pore size manipulation. *Acta Biomater.* 2017;58:225–37.
184. Han Y, Lian M, Wu Q, Qiao Z, Sun B, Dai K. Effect of pore size on cell behavior using melt electrowritten scaffolds. *Front. Bioeng. Biotechnol.* 2021;9:629270.
185. Turnbull G, Clarke J, Picard F, Riches P, Jia L, Han F, et al. 3D bioactive composite scaffolds for bone tissue engineering. *Bioact. Mater.* 2018;3(3): 278–314.
186. Leng Y, Yang F, Wang Q, Li Z, Yuan B, Peng C, et al. Material-based therapy for bone nonunion. *Mater. Des.* 2019;183:108161.
187. Álvarez-Chimal R, Arenas-Alatorre JÁ, Álvarez-Pérez MA. Nanoparticle-polymer composite scaffolds for bone tissue engineering: A review. *Eur. Polym. J.* 2024;213:113093.
188. Elyaderani AK, De Lama-Odría MD, Del Valle LJ, Puiggalí J. Multifunctional scaffolds based on emulsion and coaxial electrospinning incorporation of hydroxyapatite for bone tissue regeneration. *Int. J. Mol. Sci.* 2022; 23(23):15016.
189. Litowczenko J, Woźniak-Budych MJ, Staszak K, Wieszczycka K, Jurga S, Tylkowski B, et al. Milestones and current achievements in development of multifunctional bioscaffolds for medical application. *Bioact. Mater.* 2021;6(8):2412–38.
190. Zheng W, Bai Z, Huang S, Jiang K, Liu L, Wang X. The effect of angiogenesis-based scaffold of mesoporous bioactive glass nanofiber on osteogenesis. *Int. J. Mol. Sci.* 2022;23(20):12670.
191. Chen W, Xie G, Lu Y, Wang J, Feng B, Wang Q, et al. An improved osseointegration of metal implants by pitavastatin loaded multilayer films with osteogenic and angiogenic properties. *Biomaterials.* 2022;280:121260.
192. Huo S, Wang F, Lyu Z, Hong Q, Nie B, Wei J, et al. Dual-functional polyetheretherketone surface modification for regulating immunity and bone metabolism. *Chem. Eng. J.* 2021;426:130806.
193. Bai J, Wang H, Chen H, Ge G, Wang M, Gao A, et al. Biomimetic osteogenic peptide with mussel adhesion and osteoimmunomodulatory functions to ameliorate interfacial osseointegration under chronic inflammation. *Biomaterials.* 2020;255:120197.
194. Wu M, Chen F, Liu H, Wu P, Yang Z, Zhang Z, et al. Bioinspired sandwich-like hybrid surface functionalized scaffold capable of regulating osteogenesis, angiogenesis, and osteoclastogenesis for robust bone regeneration. *Mater. Today Bio.* 2022;17:100458.

195. Bello SA, Cruz-Lebrón J, Rodríguez-Rivera OA, Nicolau E. Bioactive scaffolds as a promising alternative for enhancing critical-size bone defect regeneration in the craniomaxillofacial region. *ACS Appl. Bio Mater.* 2023;6(11):4465–4503.
196. Wu G. Bioactive agents for functionalization of biomaterials for precise tissue engineering. *Front. Bioeng. Biotechnol.* 2023;11:1141827.
197. Cui Y, Wang J, Tian Y, Fan Y, Li S, Wang G, et al. Functionalized decellularized bone matrix promotes bone regeneration by releasing osteogenic peptides. *ACS Biomater. Sci. Eng.* 2023;9(8):4953–68.
198. Kaliva M, Chatzinikolaidou M, Vamvakaki M. Applications of smart multifunctional tissue engineering scaffolds. In: Wang Q (eds) *Smart Materials for Tissue Engineering: Applications.* London: The Royal Society of Chemistry, 2017.
199. Zhang K, Wang S, Zhou C, Cheng L, Gao X, Xie X, et al. Advanced smart biomaterials and constructs for hard tissue engineering and regeneration. *Bone Res.* 2018;6(1):31.
200. Montoya C, Du Y, Gianforcaro AL, Orrego S, Yang M, Lelkes PI. On the road to smart biomaterials for bone research: Definitions, concepts, advances, and outlook. *Bone Res.* 2021;9(1):12.
201. Badeau BA, Comerford MP, Arakawa CK, Shadish JA, DeForest CA. Engineered modular biomaterial logic gates for environmentally triggered therapeutic delivery. *Nat. Chem.* 2018;10(3):251–58.
202. Muzzio N, Moya S, Romero G. Multifunctional scaffolds and synergistic strategies in tissue engineering and regenerative medicine. *Pharmaceutics.* 2021;13(6):792.
203. Zhu T, Zhou H, Chen X, Zhu Y. Recent advances of responsive scaffolds in bone tissue engineering. *Front. Bioeng. Biotechnol.* 2023;11:1296881.
204. Wei H, Cui J, Lin K, Xie J, Wang X. Recent advances in smart stimuli-responsive biomaterials for bone therapeutics and regeneration. *Bone Res.* 2022;10(1):17.
205. da Silva Sergio LP, da Fonseca AS, Mencalha AL, de Paoli F. Photobiomodulation on extracellular matrix. *Laser Phys.* 2023;33(3):033001.
206. Raja IS, Kim C, Oh N, Park J-H, Hong SW, Kang MS, et al. Tailoring photobiomodulation to enhance tissue regeneration. *Biomaterials.* 2024;309:122623.
207. Furtado GS, Martin V, Araújo R, Gomes PS, Lago ADN. Osteoinductive activity of photobiomodulation in an organotypic bone model. *Photodiagnosis Photodyn. Ther.* 2024;45:103936.

208. Yaralı Çevik ZB, Karaman O, Topaloğlu N. Photobiomodulation therapy at red and near-infrared wavelengths for osteogenic differentiation in the scaffold-free microtissues. *J. Photochem. Photobiol. B.* 2023;238:112615.
209. Pomini KT, Buchaim DV, Bighetti ACC, Hamzé AL, Reis CHB, Duarte MAH, et al. Tissue bioengineering with fibrin scaffolds and deproteinized bone matrix associated or not with the transoperative laser photobiomodulation protocol. *Molecules.* 2023;28(1):407.
210. Kim J, Choi H-S, Kim Y-M, Song S-C. Thermo–responsive nanocomposite bioink with growth–factor holding and its application to bone regeneration. *Small.* 2023;19(9):e2203464.
211. Lavanya K, Chandran SV, Balagangadharan K, Selvamurugan N. Temperature- and pH-responsive chitosan-based injectable hydrogels for bone tissue engineering. Mater. Sci. Eng. *C. Mater. Biol. Appl.* 2020;111: 110862.
212. Saravanan S, Vimalraj S, Anuradha D. Chitosan based thermoresponsive hydrogel containing graphene oxide for bone tissue repair. *Biomed. Pharmacother.* 2018;107:908–17.
213. Rogina A, Ressler A, Matić I, Ferrer GG, Marijanović I, Ivanković M, et al. Cellular hydrogels based on pH-responsive chitosan-hydroxyapatite system. *Carbohydr. Polym.* 2017;166:173–82.
214. Wang L, Pang Y, Tang Y, Wang X, Zhang D, Zhang X, et al. A biomimetic piezoelectric scaffold with sustained Mg2+ release promotes neurogenic and angiogenic differentiation for enhanced bone regeneration. *Bioact. Mater.* 2023;25:399–414.
215. Jin L, Shan J, Hao Y, Wang Y, Liu L. Enhanced bone regeneration by low-intensity pulsed ultrasound and lipid microbubbles on PLGA/TCP 3D-printed scaffolds. *BMC Biotechnol.* 2023;23(1):13.
216. McCarthy C, Camci-Unal G. Low intensity pulsed ultrasound for bone tissue engineering. *Micromachines. (Basel).* 2021;12(12):1488.
217. Volarić D, Žauhar G, Chen J, Jerbić Radetić AT, Omrčen H, Raič A, et al. The effect of low-intensity pulsed ultrasound on bone regeneration and the expression of osterix and cyclooxygenase-2 during critical-size bone defect repair. *Int. J. Mol. Sci.* 2024;25(7):3882.
218. Puts R, Khaffaf A, Shaka M, Zhang H, Raum K. Focused low-intensity pulsed ultrasound (FLIPUS) mitigates apoptosis of MLO-Y4 osteocyte-like cells. *Bioengineering. (Basel).* 2023;10(3):387.
219. Basak S, Gopinath P. Ferrogels: A wonder material from mechanobiological perspective. *Curr. Opin. Biomed. Eng.* 2023;26:100449.

220. Choi Y, Kim C, Kim HS, Moon C, Lee KY. 3D printing of dynamic tissue scaffold by combining self-healing hydrogel and self-healing ferrogel. *Colloids Surf. B Biointerfaces.* 2021;208:112108.
221. Gebhart P, Attaran A, Wallmersperger T. Multiphysics modeling of porous ferrogels at finite strains. *Phys. Sci. Rev.* 2022;7(11):1209–35.
222. Blyakhman FA, Makarova EB, Shabadrov PA, Fadeyev FA, Shklyar TF, Safronov AP, et al. Magnetic nanoparticles as a strong contributor to the biocompatibility of ferrogels. *Phys. Met. Metallogr.* 2020;121(4):299–304.
223. Blyakhman FA, Safronov AP, Zubarev AY, Shklyar TF, Makeyev OG, Makarova EB, et al. Polyacrylamide ferrogels with embedded maghemite nanoparticles for biomedical engineering. *Results Phys.* 2017;7:3624–33.
224. Ravanbakhsh H, Bao G, Mongeau L. Carbon nanotubes promote cell migration in hydrogels. *Sci. Rep.* 2020;10(1):2543.
225. Awasthi S, Gaur JK, Bobji MS. Advanced ferrogels with high magnetic response and wear resistance using carbon nanotubes. *J. Alloys Compd.* 2020;848:156259.
226. Zhang Y, Dai J, Hang R, Yao X. Impact of surface biofunctionalization strategies on key effector cells response in polyacrylamide hydrogels for bone regeneration. *Biomater. Adv.* 2024;158(11):213768.
227. Duan G, Chang D, Zhang C, Li S, Liu X, Wang Z, et al. Biofunctionalisation strategies of material surface and the inspired biological effects for bone repair. *Biosurf. Biotribol.* 2024;10(2):17–41.
228. Iijima K, Otsuka H. Cell scaffolds for bone tissue engineering. *Bioengineering.(Basel).* 2020;7(4):119.
229. Perez JR, Kouroupis D, Li DJ, Best TM, Kaplan L, Correa D. Tissue engineering and cell-based therapies for fractures and bone defects. *Front. Bioeng. Biotechnol.* 2018;6:105.
230. Stamnitz S, Klimczak A. Mesenchymal stem cells, bioactive factors, and scaffolds in bone repair: From research perspectives to clinical practice. *Cells.* 2021;10(8):1925.
231. Venkataiah VS, Yahata Y, Kitagawa A, Inagaki M, Kakiuchi Y, Nakano M, et al. Clinical applications of cell-scaffold constructs for bone regeneration therapy. *Cells.* 2021;10(10):2687.
232. Riester O, Borgolte M, Csuk R, Deigner H-P. Challenges in bone tissue regeneration: Stem cell therapy, biofunctionality and antimicrobial properties of novel materials and its evolution. *Int. J. Mol. Sci.* 2020;22(1):192.
233. Kessler F, Arnke K, Eggerschwiler B, Neldner Y, Märsmann S, Gröninger O, et al. Murine iPSC-loaded scaffold grafts improve bone regeneration in critical-size bone defects. *Int. J. Mol. Sci.* 2024;25(10):5555.

234. Dave K, Gomes VG. Interactions at scaffold interfaces: Effect of surface chemistry, structural attributes and bioaffinity. *Mater. Sci. Eng. C.* 2019; 105:110078.
235. Zhang Q, Zhou J, Zhi P, Liu L, Liu C, Fang A, et al. 3D printing method for bone tissue engineering scaffold. *Med. Nov. Technol. Dev.* 2023;17:100205.
236. Yazdanpanah Z, Johnston JD, Cooper DML, Chen X. 3D bioprinted scaffolds for bone tissue engineering: State-of-the-art and emerging technologies. *Front. Bioeng. Biotechnol.* 2022;10:824156.
237. Han J, Park S, Kim JE, Park B, Hong Y, Lim JW, et al. Development of a scaffold-on-a-chip platform to evaluate cell infiltration and osteogenesis on the 3D-printed scaffold for bone regeneration. *ACS Biomater. Sci. Eng.* 2023;9(2):968–77.
238. Luo D, Chen B, Chen Y. Stem cells-loaded 3D-printed scaffolds for the reconstruction of alveolar cleft. *Front. Bioeng. Biotechnol.* 2022;10:939199.
239. de Leeuw AM, Graf R, Lim PJ, Zhang J, Schädli GN, Peterhans S, et al. Physiological cell bioprinting density in human bone-derived cell-laden scaffolds enhances matrix mineralization rate and stiffness under dynamic loading. *Front. Bioeng. Biotechnol.* 2024;12:1310289.
240. Chai N, Zhang J, Zhang Q, Du H, He X, Yang J, et al. Construction of 3D printed constructs based on microfluidic microgel for bone regeneration. *Compos. Part B Eng.* 2021;223:109100.
241. Khan MUA, Aslam MA, Abdullah MFB, Stojanović GM. Current perspectives of protein in bone tissue engineering: Bone structure, ideal scaffolds, fabrication techniques, applications, scopes, and future advances. *ACS Appl. Bio Mater.* 2024;7(8):5082–5106.
242. Boddepalli Y, Chava N, Gadiraju S, Pachchava KS, Kotikalapudi K, Siddiqui N. A review on growth factor loaded scaffolds for rapid healing of bone tissue: Life sciences — biotechnology. *Int. J. Life Sci. Pharma Res.* 2023;13(5):L176–L198.
243. Tollabi M, Poursalehi Z, Mehrafshar P, Bakhtiari R, Sarmadi VH, Tayebi L, et al. Insight into the role of integrins and integrins-targeting biomaterials in bone regeneration. *Connect. Tissue Res.* 2024;65(5): 343–63.
244. Zhou X, Zhang Q, Chen L, Nie W, Wang W, Wang H, et al. Versatile nanocarrier based on functionalized mesoporous silica nanoparticles to codeliver osteogenic gene and drug for enhanced osteodifferentiation. *ACS Biomater. Sci. Eng.* 2019;5(2):710–23.
245. Visser R, Rico-Llanos GA, Pulkkinen H, Becerra J. Peptides for bone tissue engineering. *J. Control. Release.* 2016;244:122–35.

246. Ye Z, Zhu X, Mutreja I, Boda SK, Fischer NG, Zhang A, et al. Biomimetic mineralized hybrid scaffolds with antimicrobial peptides. *Bioact. Mater.* 2021;6(8):2250–60.
247. Gharaei R, Tronci G, Goswami P, Wynn Davies RP, Kirkham J, Russell SJ. Biomimetic peptide enriched nonwoven scaffolds promote calcium phosphate mineralisation. *RSC Adv.* 2020;10(47):28332–342.
248. Richardson SW, Kolbe HJ, Duncan R. Potential of low molecular mass chitosan as a DNA delivery system: Biocompatibility, body distribution and ability to complex and protect DNA. *Int. J. Pharm.* 1999;178(2):231–43.
249. Laird NZ, Acri TM, Tingle K, Salem AK. Gene- and RNAi-activated scaffolds for bone tissue engineering: Current progress and future directions. *Adv. Drug Deliv. Rev.* 2021;174:613–27.
250. Raftery RM, Tierney EG, Curtin CM, Cryan S-A, O'Brien FJ. Development of a gene-activated scaffold platform for tissue engineering applications using chitosan-pDNA nanoparticles on collagen-based scaffolds. *J. Control. Release.* 2015;210:84–94.
251. Grath A, Dai G. Direct cell reprogramming for tissue engineering and regenerative medicine. *J. Biol. Eng.* 2019;13(1):14.
252. Yoon J-Y, Mandakhbayar N, Hyun J, Yoon DS, Patel KD, Kang K, et al. Chemically-induced osteogenic cells for bone tissue engineering and disease modeling. *Biomaterials.* 2022;289:121792.
253. Yamamoto K, Sato Y, Honjo K, Ichioka H, Oseko F, Sowa Y, et al. Generation of directly converted human osteoblasts that are free of exogenous gene and xenogenic protein. *J. Cell. Biochem.* 2016;117(11):2538–45.
254. Sato Y, Yamamoto K, Horiguchi S, Tahara Y, Nakai K, Kotani S-I, et al. Nanogel tectonic porous 3D scaffold for direct reprogramming fibroblasts into osteoblasts and bone regeneration. *Sci. Rep.* 2018;8(1):15824.
255. Malek-Khatabi A, Javar HA, Dashtimoghadam E, Ansari S, Hasani-Sadrabadi MM, Moshaverinia A. In situ bone tissue engineering using gene delivery nanocomplexes. *Acta. Biomater.* 2020;108:326–36.
256. Khorsand B, Nicholson N, Do A-V, Femino JE, Martin JA, Petersen E, et al. Regeneration of bone using nanoplex delivery of FGF-2 and BMP-2 genes in diaphyseal long bone radial defects in a diabetic rabbit model. *J. Control. Release.* 2017;248:53–59.
257. Lackington WA, Gomez-Sierra MA, González-Vázquez A, O'Brien FJ, Stoddart MJ, Thompson K. Non-viral gene delivery of interleukin-1 receptor antagonist using collagen-hydroxyapatite scaffold protects rat BM-MSCs from IL-1β-mediated inhibition of osteogenesis. *Front. Bioeng. Biotechnol.* 2020;8:582012.

258. Xue X, Hu Y, Deng Y, Su J. Recent advances in design of functional biocompatible hydrogels for bone tissue engineering. *Adv. Funct. Mater.* 2021;31(19):2009432.
259. Guo L, Liang Z, Yang L, Du W, Yu T, Tang H, et al. The role of natural polymers in bone tissue engineering. *J. Control. Release.* 2021;338:571–82.
260. Nguyen LH, Annabi N, Nikkhah M, Bae H, Binan L, Park S, et al. Vascularized bone tissue engineering: Approaches for potential improvement. *Tissue Eng. Part B Rev.* 2012;18(5):363–82.
261. Liu X, Rahaman MN, Hilmas GE, Bal BS. Mechanical properties of bioactive glass (13–93) scaffolds fabricated by robotic deposition for structural bone repair. *Acta Biomater.* 2013;9(6):7025–34.
262. Saberi A, Kouhjani M, Mohammadi M, Hosta-Rigau L. Novel scaffold platforms for simultaneous induction osteogenesis and angiogenesis in bone tissue engineering: A cutting-edge approach. *J. Nanobiotechnol.* 2023; 21(1):351.
263. Kaigler D, Wang Z, Horger K, Mooney DJ, Krebsbach PH. VEGF scaffolds enhance angiogenesis and bone regeneration in irradiated osseous defects. *J. Bone Miner. Res.* 2006;21(5):735–44.
264. Dashnyam K, Buitrago JO, Bold T, Mandakhbayar N, Perez RA, Knowles JC, et al. Angiogenesis-promoted bone repair with silicate-shelled hydrogel fiber scaffolds. *Biomater. Sci.* 2019;7(12):5221–31.
265. Elefteriou F. Impact of the autonomic nervous system on the skeleton. *Physiol. Rev.* 2018;98(3):1083–1112.
266. Tao R, Mi B, Hu Y, Lin S, Xiong Y, Lu X, et al. Hallmarks of peripheral nerve function in bone regeneration. *Bone Res.* 2023;11(1):6.
267. Wang Q, Qin H, Deng J, Xu H, Liu S, Weng J, et al. Research progress in calcitonin gene-related peptide and bone repair. *Biomolecules.* 2023; 13(5):838.
268. Li J, Shang G, Wang Y, Wang X, Ji Y, Li Y. Therapeutic effects of calcitonin gene-related peptide-modified bone marrow mesenchymal stem cells combined with autogenous bone grafting for treatment of osteonecrosis of the femoral head in rabbits. *Biochem. Eng. J.* 2020;153:107399.
269. Hao Z, Ren L, Zhang Z, Yang Z, Wu S, Liu G, et al. A multifunctional neuromodulation platform utilizing Schwann cell-derived exosomes orchestrates bone microenvironment via immunomodulation, angiogenesis and osteogenesis. *Bioact. Mater.* 2023;23:206–22.
270. Wang T, Li W, Zhang Y, Xu X, Qiang L, Miao W, et al. Bioprinted constructs that simulate nerve–bone crosstalk to improve microenvironment for bone repair. *Bioact. Mater.* 2023;27:377–93.

271. Kuhn MR, Haffner-Luntzer M, Kempter E, Reber SO, Ichinose H, Vacher J, et al. Myeloid cell-derived catecholamines influence bone turnover and regeneration in mice. *Front. Endocrinol.(Lausanne).* 2022;13:997745.
272. Tschaffon-Müller MEA, Kempter E, Steppe L, Kupfer S, Kuhn MR, Gebhard F, et al. Neutrophil-derived catecholamines mediate negative stress effects on bone. *Nat. Commun.* 2023;14(1):3262.
273. Li S, Li Z, Yang J, Ha Y, Zhou X, He C. Inhibition of sympathetic activation by delivering calcium channel blockers from a 3D printed scaffold to promote bone defect repair. *Adv. Healthc. Mater.* 2022;11(16):e2200785.
274. Touri M, Moztarzadeh F, Abu Osman NA, Dehghan MM, Milan PB, Farzad-Mohajeri S, et al. Oxygen-releasing scaffolds for accelerated bone regeneration. *ACS Biomater. Sci. Eng.* 2020;6(5):2985–94.
275. Haixia X, Peng Z, Jiezhao L, Huiling G, Xie C, Yihan W, et al. 3D-printed magnesium peroxide-incorporated scaffolds with sustained oxygen release and enhanced photothermal performance for osteosarcoma multimodal treatments. *ACS Appl. Mater. Interfaces.* 2024;16(8):9626–39.
276. Pei Z, Montagne K, Namiki A, Shinohara M, Ushida T, Furukawa KS. Printable oxygen–generating biodegradable scaffold for thicker tissue–engineered medical products. *Artif. Organs.* 2024;48(4):402–07.
277. Wang Z, Chen T, Li X, Guo B, Liu P, Zhu Z, et al. Oxygen-releasing biomaterials for regenerative medicine. *J. Mater. Chem. B.* 2023;11(31):7300–20.
278. Augustine R, Gezek M, Bostanci NS, Nguyen A, Camci-Unal G. Oxygen-generating scaffolds: One step closer to the clinical translation of tissue engineered products. *Chem. Eng. J.* 2023;455(Pt 2):140783.
279. Teh SW, Koh AE-H, Tong JB, Wu X, Samrot AV, Rampal S, et al. Hypoxia in bone and oxygen releasing biomaterials in fracture treatments using mesenchymal stem cell therapy: A review. *Front. Cell Dev. Biol.* 2021;9:634131.
280. Domingo-Lopez DA, Levey RE, Brennan B, Carroll O, Gale SE, Millman JR, et al. A predictive oxygen durability model to analyze oxygen consumption of insulin producing cells encapsulated within a highly oxygenated hydrogel. *Adv. Mater. Technol.* 2023;8(1):2200643.
281. Abdi SIH, Ng SM, Lim JO. An enzyme-modulated oxygen-producing micro-system for regenerative therapeutics. *Int. J. Pharm.* 2011;409(1–2):203–5.
282. Kang JI, Park KM, Park KD. Oxygen-generating alginate hydrogels as a bioactive acellular matrix for facilitating wound healing. *J. Ind. Eng. Chem.* 2019;69:397–404.

283. Huh J-S. Functionalized biomaterials-oxygen releasing scaffolds. *J. Biotechnol. Biomater.* 2015;5(2):1.
284. Farris AL, Rindone AN, Grayson WL. Oxygen delivering biomaterials for tissue engineering. *J. Mater. Chem. B.* 2016;4(20):3422–32.
285. Augustine R, Camci-Unal G. Scaffolds with high oxygen content support osteogenic cell survival under hypoxia. *Biomater. Sci.* 2023;11(16): 5560–75.
286. Khorshidi S, Karimi-Soflou R, Karkhaneh A. A hydrogel/particle composite with a gradient of oxygen releasing microparticle for concurrent osteogenic and chondrogenic differentiation in a single scaffold. *Colloids Surf. B. Biointerfaces.* 2021;207:112007.
287. Forget A, Staehly C, Ninan N, Harding FJ, Vasilev K, Voelcker NH, et al. Oxygen-releasing coatings for improved tissue preservation. *ACS Biomater. Sci. Eng.* 2017;3(10):2384–90.
288. Rahmati M, Silva EA, Reseland JE, Heyward CA, Haugen HJ. Biological responses to physicochemical properties of biomaterial surface. *Chem. Soc. Rev.* 2020;49(15):5178–5224.
289. Thouless MD. Cracking and delamination of coatings. *J. Vac. Sci. Technol. A.* 1991;9(4):2510–15.
290. Mozetič M. Surface modification to improve properties of materials. *Materials. (Basel).* 2019;12(3):441.
291. Anselme K, Ploux L, Ponche A. Cell/material interfaces: Influence of surface chemistry and surface topography on cell adhesion. *J. Adhes. Sci. Technol.* 2010;24(5):831–52.
292. Hu X, Wang T, Li F, Mao X. Surface modifications of biomaterials in different applied fields. *RSC Adv.* 2023;13(30):20495–511.
293. Mitra SP. Protein adsorption on biomaterial surfaces: Subsequent conformational and biological consequences — A review. *J. Surf. Sci. Technol.* 2020;36(1–2):7–38.
294. Fromhold Jr A. Space-charge modification of the ionic currents for oxide growth. *Solid State Ion.* 1995;75:229–39.
295. Pereira HF, Cengiz IF, Silva FS, Reis RL, Oliveira JM. Scaffolds and coatings for bone regeneration. *J. Mater. Sci. Mater. Med.* 2020;31:1–16.
296. Safaei M, Mohammadi H, Beddu S, Mozaffari HR, Rezaei R, Sharifi R, et al. Surface topography steer soft tissue response and antibacterial function at the transmucosal region of titanium implant. *Int. J. Nanomed.* 2024; 19:4835–56.

297. Perez RA, Mestres G. Role of pore size and morphology in musculo-skeletal tissue regeneration. *Mater. Sci. Eng. C. Mater. Biol. Appl.* 2016;61:922–39.
298. Fröhlich E. The role of surface charge in cellular uptake and cytotoxicity of medical nanoparticles. *Int. J. Nanomed.* 2012;7:5577–91.
299. Nishino M, Matsuzaki I, Musangile FY, Takahashi Y, Iwahashi Y, Warigaya K, et al. Measurement and visualization of cell membrane surface charge in fixed cultured cells related with cell morphology. *PLoS One.* 2020;15(7):e0236373.
300. Silva-Bermudez P, Rodil SE. An overview of protein adsorption on metal oxide coatings for biomedical implants. *Surf. Coat. Technol.* 2013;233: 147–58.
301. Bodhak S, Bose S, Bandyopadhyay A. Role of surface charge and wettability on early stage mineralization and bone cell–materials interactions of polarized hydroxyapatite. *Acta Biomater.* 2009;5(6):2178–88.
302. Nikolova MP, Apostolova MD. Advances in multifunctional bioactive coatings for metallic bone implants. *Materials. (Basel).* 2022;16(1):183.
303. Bokov D, Jalil AT, Chupradit S, Suksatan W, Ansari MJ, Shewael IH, et al. Nanomaterial by sol–gel method: Synthesis and application. *Adv. Mater. Sci. Eng.* 2021;2021(1):5102014.
304. Jokanović V, Vilotijević M, Jokanović B, Jenko M, Anžel I, Stamenković D, et al. Investigations of corrosion on the surface of titanium substrate caused by combined alkaline and heat treatment. *Corros. Sci.* 2014;82:180–90.
305. Singh A, Singh G, Chawla V. Characterization and mechanical behaviour of reinforced hydroxyapatite coatings deposited by vacuum plasma spray on SS-316L alloy. *J. Mech. Behav. Biomed. Mater.* 2018;79:273–82.
306. Demnati I, Parco M, Grossin D, Fagoaga I, Drouet C, Barykin G, et al. Hydroxyapatite coating on titanium by a low energy plasma spraying mini-gun. *Surf. Coat. Technol.* 2012;206(8–9):2346–53.
307. Hikku GS, Arthi C, Robert RBJ, Jeyasubramanian K, Murugesan R. Calcium phosphate conversion technique: A versatile route to develop corrosion resistant hydroxyapatite coating over Mg/Mg alloys based implants. *J. Magnes. Alloys.* 2022;10(7):1821–45.
308. Zhang Y, Luo S, Wang Q, Ramachandran CS. Effect of hydrothermal treatment on the surface characteristics and bioactivity of HAP based MAO coating on Ti-6Al-4V alloy. *Surf. Coat. Technol.* 2023;464:129566.
309. Benčina M, Iglič A, Mozetič M, Junkar I. Crystallized TiO_2 nanosurfaces in biomedical applications. *Nanomaterials. (Basel).* 2020;10(6):1121.

310. Giavaresi G, Ambrosio L, Battiston GA, Casellato U, Gerbasi R, Finia M, et al. Histomorphometric, ultrastructural and microhardness evaluation of the osseointegration of a nanostructured titanium oxide coating by metal-organic chemical vapour deposition: An in vivo study. *Biomaterials.* 2004; 25(25):5583–91.
311. Fini M, Giardino R, Borsari V, Torricelli P, Rimondini L, Giavaresi G, et al. In vitro behaviour of osteoblasts cultured on orthopaedic biomaterials with different surface roughness, uncoated and fluorohydroxyapatite-coated, relative to the in vivo osteointegration rate. *Int. J. Artif. Organs.* 2003;26(6): 520–28.
312. Rehman MAU, Bastan FE, Nawaz A, Nawaz Q, Wadood A. Electrophoretic deposition of PEEK/bioactive glass composite coatings on stainless steel for orthopedic applications: An optimization for in vitro bioactivity and adhesion strength. *Int. J. Adv. Manuf. Technol.* 2020;108:1849–62.
313. Djošić M, Janković A, Mišković-Stanković V. Electrophoretic deposition of biocompatible and bioactive hydroxyapatite-based coatings on titanium. *Materials. (Basel).* 2021;14(18):5391.
314. Rojaee R, Fathi M, Raeissi K. Comparing nanostructured hydroxyapatite coating on AZ91 alloy samples via sol-gel and electrophoretic deposition for biomedical applications. *IEEE Trans. Nanobioscience.* 2014;13(4): 409–14.
315. Uicich FC, Merlo JL, Redersdorff IE, Herrera Seitz MK, Pastore JI, Ballarre J. Optimized electrophoretic deposition of chitosan/mesoporous glass nanoparticles with gentamicin on titanium implants: Enhancing hemocompatibility and antibacterial activity. *ACS Appl. Bio Mater.* 2024; 7(7):4642–53.
316. Manjaiah M, Laubscher RF. Effect of anodizing on surface integrity of grade 4 titanium for biomedical applications. *Surf. Coat. Technol.* 2017;310: 263–72.
317. Knapic D, Minenkov A, Luczak W, Zrinski I, Kleber C, Hild S, et al. Hindrance of osteoblast cell adhesion on titanium by surface nanostructuring. *Surf. Interfaces.* 2024;46:103990.
318. Jáquez-Muñoz JMJ, Gaona-Tiburcio C, Mendez CT, Carrera-Ramirez MG, Baltazar-Zamora MA, Hurtado GS, et al. Corrosion of anodized titanium alloys. *Coatings.* 2024;14(7):809.
319. Ahangari A, Mokhtarzade A, Mahmoodi M. In vitro tribological behavior and corrosion resistance of SiO2/TiO2/ZrO2 coatings formed on the tantalum

substrate using plasma electrolytic oxidation for orthopedic implant applications. *Mater. Chem. Phys.* 2023;308:128210.

320. Wen X, Liu X, Xi F, Zhang X, Kang Y. Micro-arc oxidation (MAO) and its potential for improving the performance of titanium implants in biomedical applications. *Front. Bioeng. Biotechnol.* 2023;11:1282590.
321. Ghamsarizade R, Mohammadloo HE, Roshan S. Modification of hydroxyapatite coatings for implant applications. In: *Biomaterials-Properties, Production and Devices.* New York: Nova Science Publishers, 2023:1.
322. Zarka M, Dikici B, Niinomi M, Ezirmik KV, Nakai M, Yilmazer H. A systematic study of β-type Ti-based PVD coatings on magnesium for biomedical application. *Vacuum.* 2021;183:109850.
323. Durdu S, Aktug SL, Korkmaz K, Yalcin E, Aktas S. Fabrication, characterization and in vitro properties of silver-incorporated TiO2 coatings on titanium by thermal evaporation and micro-arc oxidation. *Surf. Coat. Technol.* 2018;352:600–08.
324. Colligon J, Vishnyakov V. Thin films: Sputtering, PVD methods, and applications. In: *Surface and Interface Science* (1st ed., Vol 9). Hoboken: Wiley, 2020:1–55.
325. Vercaigne S, Wolke JGC, Naert I, Jansen JA. Bone healing capacity of titanium plasma–sprayed and hydroxylapatite–coated oral implants. *Clin. Oral Implants Res.* 1998;9(4):261–71.
326. Mu J, Wang H, Qin B, Zhang Y, Chen L, Zeng C. Improved wear and corrosion resistance of biological compatible TiZrNb films on biomedical Ti6Al4V substrates by optimizing sputtering power. *Surf. Coat. Technol.* 2021;428:127866.
327. Wei G, Tan M, Attarilar S, Li J, Uglov VV, Wang B, et al. An overview of surface modification, a way toward fabrication of nascent biomedical Ti–6Al–4V alloys. *J. Mater. Res. Technol.* 2023;24:5896–5921.
328. Zhao Y, Jamesh MI, Li WK, Wu G, Wang C, Zheng Y, et al. Enhanced antimicrobial properties, cytocompatibility, and corrosion resistance of plasma-modified biodegradable magnesium alloys. *Acta Biomater.* 2014;10(1): 544–556.
329. Wang G, Li J, Zhang W, Xu L, Pan H, Wen J, et al. Magnesium ion implantation on a micro/nanostructured titanium surface promotes its bioactivity and osteogenic differentiation function. *Int. J. Nanomed.* 2014;9: 2387–98.
330. Bajda S, Liu Y, Tosi R, Cholewa-Kowalska K, Krzyzanowski M, Dziadek M, et al. Laser cladding of bioactive glass coating on pure titanium substrate

with highly refined grain structure. *J. Mech. Behav. Biomed. Mater.* 2021; 119:104519.

331. Algahtani MS, Mohammed AA, Ahmad J, Saleh E. Development of a 3D printed coating shell to control the drug release of encapsulated immediate-release tablets. *Polymers.* 2020;12(6):1395.
332. Adarkwa E, Roy A, Ohodnicki J, Lee B, Kumta PN, Desai S. 3D printing of drug-eluting bioactive multifunctional coatings for orthopedic applications. *Int. J. Bioprint.* 2023;9(2):661.
333. Maver T, Mastnak T, Mihelič M, Maver U, Finšgar M. Clindamycin-based 3D-printed and electrospun coatings for treatment of implant-related infections. *Materials.* 2021;14(6):1464.
334. Kravanja KA, Finšgar M. A review of techniques for the application of bioactive coatings on metal-based implants to achieve controlled release of active ingredients. *Mater. Des.* 2022;217:110653.
335. Hübler R, Cozza A, Marcondes TL, Souza RB, Fiori FF. Wear and corrosion protection of 316-L femoral implants by deposition of thin films. *Surf. Coat. Technol.* 2001;142–144:1078–83.
336. van Hove RP, Sierevelt IN, van Royen BJ, Nolte PA. Titanium–nitride coating of orthopaedic implants: A review of the literature. *Biomed. Res. Int.* 2015;2015(1):485975.
337. Kao C-T, Ding S-J, Chen Y-C, Huang TH. The anticorrosion ability of titanium nitride (TiN) plating on an orthodontic metal bracket and its biocompatibility. *J. Biomed. Mater. Res.* 2002;63(6):786–92.
338. Gobbi SJ, Gobbi VJ, Reinke G, Rocha Y. Orthopedic implants: Coating with TiN. *Biomed. J. Sci. Tech. Res.* 2019;16(1):11740–742.
339. Malikian R, Maruthainar K, Stammers J, Wilding CP, Blunn GW. Four station knee simulator wear testing comparing titanium niobium nitride with cobalt chrome. *J. Bioeng. Biomed. Sci.* 2013;3(3).
340. Uddin GM, Jawad M, Ghufran M, Saleem MW, Raza MA, Rehman ZU, et al. Experimental investigation of tribo-mechanical and chemical properties of TiN PVD coating on titanium substrate for biomedical implants manufacturing. *Int. J. Adv. Manuf. Technol.* 2019;102:1391–1404.
341. Liu H, Zhang X, Jin S, Zhao Y, Ren L, Yang K. Effect of copper-doped titanium nitride coating on angiogenesis. *Mater. Lett.* 2020;269: 127634.
342. Correa Filho L, Schmidt S, López A, Cogrel M, Leifer K, Engqvist H, et al. The effect of coating density on functional properties of SiN_x coated implants. *Materials. (Basel).* 2019;12(20):3370.

343. Wanag A, Rokicka P, Kusiak-Nejman E, Kapica-Kozar J, Wrobel RJ, Markowska-Szczupak A, et al. Antibacterial properties of TiO_2 modified with reduced graphene oxide. *Ecotoxicol. Environ. Saf.* 2018;147:788–93.
344. Ballo AM, Bjöörn D, Astrand M, Palmquist A, Lausmaa J, Thomsen P. Bone response to physical–vapour–deposited titanium dioxide coatings on titanium implants. *Clin. Oral Implants Res.* 2013;24(9):1009–17.
345. Fan X, Wang W, Jiang N, Qi B, Li G, Peng Z, et al. Non-cytotoxic and bioactive nanocomposite film of natural Arabic gum incorporating TiO_2 nanoparticles for bone tissue regeneration. *J. Saudi Chem. Soc.* 2023; 27(5):101713.
346. Youness RA, Ibrahim MA, Taha MA. Evaluation of the electrical and dielectric behavior of the apatite layer formed on the surface of hydroxyapatite/hardystonite/copper oxide hybrid nanocomposites for bone repair applications. *Ceram. Int.* 2022;48(14):19837–850.
347. Khalaji AD, Pazhand Z, Kiani K, Machek P, Jarosova M, Mazandarani R. CuO nanoparticles: Preparation, characterization, optical properties, and antibacterial activities. *J. Mater. Sci. Mater. Electron.* 2020;31:11949–954.
348. Gudkov SV, Burmistrov DE, Serov DA, Rebezov MB, Semenova AA, Lisitsyn. A mini review of antibacterial properties of ZnO nanoparticles. *Front. Phys.* 2021;9:641481.
349. Mendes CR, Dilarri G, Forsan CF, Sapata VMR, Lopes PRM, de Moraes PB, et al. Antibacterial action and target mechanisms of zinc oxide nanoparticles against bacterial pathogens. *Sci. Rep.* 2022;12(1):2658.
350. Sirelkhatim A, Mahmud S, Seeni A, Kaus NHM, Ann LC, Bakhori SKM, et al. Review on zinc oxide nanoparticles: Antibacterial activity and toxicity mechanism. *Nano-Micro Lett.* 2015;7:219–42.
351. Babayevska N, Przysiecka Ł, Iatsunskyi I, Nowaczyk G, Jarek M, Janiszewska E, et al. ZnO size and shape effect on antibacterial activity and cytotoxicity profile. *Sci. Rep.* 2022;12(1):8148.
352. Heidari F, Bazargan-Lari R, Razavi M, Fahimipour F, Vashaee D, Tayebi L. Nano–hydroxyapatite and nano–hydroxyapatite/zinc oxide scaffold for bone tissue engineering application. *Int. J. Appl. Ceram. Technol.* 2020;17(6): 2752–61.
353. Fenker M. Properties of oxynitride thin films for bio-medical applications. In: Vaz F (ed) *Metallic Oxynitride thin Films by Reactive Sputtering and Related Deposition Methods: Processes, Properties and Applications.* United Arab Emirates: Bentham Science Publishers, 2013:254–64.

354. Senocak TC, Ezirmik KV, Aysin F, Ozek NS, Cengiz S. Niobium-oxynitride coatings for biomedical applications: Its antibacterial effects and in-vitro cytotoxicity. *Mater. Sci. Eng. C. Mater. Biol. Appl.* 2021;120:111662.
355. Banakh O, Moussa M, Matthey J, Pontearso A, Cattani-Lorente M, Sanjines R, et al. Sputtered titanium oxynitride coatings for endosseous applications: Physical and chemical evaluation and first bioactivity assays. *Appl. Surf. Sci.* 2014;317:986–93.
356. Pana I, Braic V, Dinu M, Braic V, Massima Mouele ES, Parau AC, et al. In vitro corrosion of titanium nitride and oxynitride-based biocompatible coatings deposited on stainless steel. *Coatings.* 2020;10(8):710.
357. Rieder P, Scherrer S, Filieri A, Wiskott HWA, Durual S. TiNOx coatings increase human primary osteoblasts proliferation independently of the substrate: A short report. *Bio. Mater. Eng.* 2012;22(5):277–81.
358. Durual S, Rieder P, Garavaglia G, Filieri A, Cattani-Lorente M, Scherrer SS, et al. TiNOx coatings on roughened titanium and CoCr alloy accelerate early osseointegration of dental implants in minipigs. *Bone.* 2013;52(1): 230–37.
359. Zhang M, Xie T, Qian X, Zhu Y, Liu X. Mechanical properties and biocompatibility of ti-doped diamond-like carbon films. *ACS Omega.* 2020;5(36): 22772–7.
360. Granek A, Monika M, Ozimina D. Diamond-like carbon films for use in medical implants. In: *AIP Conference Proceedings.* Melville: AIP Publishing, 2018.
361. Sousa-Cardoso F, Teixeira-Santos R, Mergulhão FJM. Antifouling performance of carbon-based coatings for marine applications: A systematic review. *Antibiotics. (Basel).* 2022;11(8):1102.
362. Pukha VE, Glukhov AA, Belmesov AA, Kabachkov EN, Khodos II, Khadem M, et al. Corrosion-resistant nanostructured carbon-based coatings for applications in fuel cells based on bipolar plates. *Vacuum.* 2023;218: 112643.
363. Wachesk CC, Seabra SH, Dos Santos TAT, Trava-Airoldi VJ, Lobo AO, Marciano FR. In vivo biocompatibility of diamond-like carbon films containing TiO_2 nanoparticles for biomedical applications. *J. Mater. Sci. Mater. Med.* 2021;32(9):117.
364. Birkett M, Zia AW, Devarajan DK, Soni, Panayiotidis MI, Joyce TJ, et al. Multi-functional bioactive silver-and copper-doped diamond-like carbon coatings for medical implants. *Acta Biomater.* 2023;167:54–68.

365. Yonezawa K, Kawaguchi M, Kaneuji A, Ichiseki T, Iinuma Y, Kawamura K, et al. Evaluation of antibacterial and cytotoxic properties of a fluorinated diamond-like carbon coating for the development of antibacterial medical implants. *Antibiotics. (Basel).* 2020;9(8):495.
366. Bociaga D, Sobczyk-Guzenda A, Komorowski P, Balcerzak J, Jastrzebski K, Przybyszewska K, et al. Surface characteristics and biological evaluation of Si-DLC coatings fabricated using magnetron sputtering method on Ti6Al7Nb substrate. *Nanomaterials. (Basel).* 2019;9(6):812.
367. Pan F, Khan M, Ragab AH, Javed E, Alsalmah HA, Khan I, et al. Recent advances in the structure and biomedical applications of nanodiamonds and their future perspectives. *Mater. Des.* 2023;233:112179.
368. Terranova ML. Key challenges in diamond coating of titanium implants: Current status and future prospects. *Biomedicines.* 2022;10(12):3149.
369. Medina O, Nocua J, Mendoza F, Gómez-Moreno R, Ávalos J, Rodríguez C, et al. Bactericide and bacterial anti-adhesive properties of the nanocrystalline diamond surface. *Diamond Relat. Mater.* 2012;22:77–81.
370. Li Z, Xiang S, Lin Z, Li EN, Yagi H, Cao G, et al. Graphene oxide-functionalized nanocomposites promote osteogenesis of human mesenchymal stem cells via enhancement of BMP-SMAD1/5 signaling pathway. *Biomaterials.* 2021;277:121082.
371. Wang Q, Li M, Cui T, Wu R, Guo F, Fu M, et al. A novel zwitterionic hydrogel incorporated with graphene oxide for bone tissue engineering: Synthesis, characterization, and promotion of osteogenic differentiation of bone mesenchymal stem cells. *Int. J. Mol. Sci.* 2023;24(3):2691.
372. Malavika C, Thomas P, Jose AJ. Graphene: Promising nanoplatform for biomedical applications. In: Holban A-M, Grumezescu AM (eds) *Materials for Biomedical Engineering.* Netherland: Elsevier, 2019.307–22.
373. Gao J, Su Y, Qin Y-X. Calcium phosphate coatings enhance biocompatibility and degradation resistance of magnesium alloy: Correlating in vitro and in vivo studies. *Bioact. Mater.* 2021;6(5):1223–29.
374. Zerankeshi MM, Mofakhami S, Salahinejad E. 3D porous HA/TCP composite scaffolds for bone tissue engineering. *Ceram. Int.* 2022;48(16): 22647–663.
375. Rey C, Combes C, Drouet C, Glimcher MJ. Tricalcium phosphate-based ceramics. In: Kokubo T (ed) *Bioceramics and their Clinical Applications.* Netherland: Elsevier, 2008:326–66.
376. de Melo CCDSB, Cassiano FB, Bronze-Uhle ÉS, Stuani VT, Bordini EAF, Gallinari MO, et al. Mineral–induced bubbling effect and biomineralization

as strategies to create highly porous and bioactive scaffolds for dentin tissue engineering. *J. Biomed. Mater. Res. B Appl. Biomater.* 2022;110(8):1757–70.
377. Doymus B, Kerem G, Karatas AY, Kok FN, Önder S. A functional coating to enhance antibacterial and bioactivity properties of titanium implants and its performance in vitro. *J. Biomater. Appl.* 2021;35(6):655–69.
378. Guo Y, Li G, Xu Y, Xu Z, Gang M, Sun G, et al. The microstructure, mechanical properties, corrosion performance and biocompatibility of hydroxyapatite reinforced ZK61 magnesium-matrix biological composite. *J. Mech. Behav. Biomed. Mater.* 2021;123:104759.
379. Sankar M, Suwas S, Balasubramanian S, Manivasagam G. Comparison of electrochemical behavior of hydroxyapatite coated onto WE43 Mg alloy by electrophoretic and pulsed laser deposition. *Surf. Coat. Technol.* 2017;309: 840–48.
380. Mirak M, Alizadeh M, Ghaffari M, Ashtiani MN. Characterization, mechanical properties and corrosion resistance of biocompatible Zn-HA/TiO2 nanocomposite coatings. *J. Mech. Behav. Biomed. Mater.* 2016;62: 282–90.
381. Ebrahimi N, Sedaghat Ahangari Hossein Zadeh A, Vaezi MR, Mozafari M. A new double-layer hydroxyapatite/alumina-silica coated titanium implants using plasma spray technique. *Surf. Coat. Technol.* 2018;352:474–82.
382. Xia W, Chang J, Engqvist H. Biological effect of ions in calcium phosphates on bone regeneration. In: *The World Scientific Encyclopedia of Nanomedicine and Bioengineering II: Bioimplants, Regenerative Medicine, and Nano-Cancer Diagnosis and Phototherapy Volume 3: Design of Bioactive Materials for Bone Repair And Regeneration.* World Scientific Publishing, 2021:125–46.
383. Zhao Q, Ni Y, Wei H, Duan Y, Chen J, Xiao Q, et al. Ion incorporation into bone grafting materials. *Periodontol. 2000.* 2024;94(1):213–30.
384. Habibovic P, Barralet J. Bioinorganics and biomaterials: Bone repair. *Acta Biomater.* 2011;7(8):3013–26.
385. Ratnayake JTB, Mucalo M, Dias GJ. Substituted hydroxyapatites for bone regeneration: A review of current trends. *J. Biomed. Mater. Res. B Appl. Biomater.* 2017;105(5):1285–99.
386. Sadighi A, Roshan MM, Moradi A, Ostadrahimi A. The effects of zinc supplementation on serum zinc, alkaline phosphatase activity and fracture healing of bones. *Saudi Med. J.* 2008;29(9):1276–79.
387. Emelyanenko AM, Kaminsky VV, Pytskii IS, Emelyanenko KA, Domantovsky AG, Chulkova EV, et al. Antimicrobial activity and

degradation of superhydrophobic magnesium substrates in bacterial media. *Metals.* 2021;11(7):1100.

388. Liu X, Huang H, Zhang J, Sun T, Zhang W, Li Z. Recent advance of strontium functionalized in biomaterials for bone regeneration. *Bioengineering. (Basel).* 2023;10(4):414.
389. Xie C-M, Lu X, Wang K-F, Meng F-Z, Jiang O, Zhang H-P, et al. Silver nanoparticles and growth factors incorporated hydroxyapatite coatings on metallic implant surfaces for enhancement of osteoinductivity and antibacterial properties. *ACS Appl. Mater. Interfaces.* 2014;6(11):8580–89.
390. Sun A, Thakur A, Thakur P. Bio-ceramics and bio-glasses for orthopedics and tissue engineering. In: Suhag D, Thakur A, Thakur P (eds), *Integrated Nanomaterials and their Applications.* London: Springer, 2023:177–200.
391. Hench LL. The future of bioactive ceramics. *J. Mater. Sci. Mater. Med.* 2015;26(2):86.
392. Montazerian M, Dutra Zanotto E. History and trends of bioactive glass–ceramics. *J. Biomed. Mater. Res. A.* 2016;104(5):1231–49.
393. Cannio M, Bellucci D, Roether JA, Boccaccini DN, Cannillo V. Bioactive glass applications: A literature review of human clinical trials. *Materials. (Basel).* 2021;14(18):5440.
394. Farooq I, Imran Z, Farooq U, Leghari A, Ali H, Dada OA. Bioactive glasses — structure and applications. In: Khurshid Z, Najeeb S, Zafar M, Sefat F (eds) *Advanced Dental Biomaterials.* Netherland: Elsevier, 2019:453–76.
395. Lin JC, Kuo KL, Ding SJ. Plasma–sprayed hydroxyapatite–bioactive glass composites on Ti6A14V. In: *Proceedings of The 17th Annual Conference on Composites and Advanced Ceramic Materials: Ceramic Engineering and Science Proceedings.* Hoboken: Wiley Online Library, 1993.
396. Zhang M, Pu X, Chen X, Yin G. In-vivo performance of plasma-sprayed CaO–MgO–SiO_2-based bioactive glass-ceramic coating on Ti–6Al–4V alloy for bone regeneration. *Heliyon.* 2019;5(11):e02824.
397. Zahid S, Shah AT, Jamal A, Chaudhry AA, Khan AS, Khan AF, et al. Biological behavior of bioactive glasses and their composites. *RSC Adv.* 2016;6(74):70197–214.
398. Kang T-Y, Seo J-Y, Ryu J-H, Kim K-M, Kwon J-S. Improvement of the mechanical and biological properties of bioactive glasses by the addition of zirconium oxide (ZrO_2) as a synthetic bone graft substitute. *J. Biomed. Mater. Res. A.* 2021;109(7):1196–1208.
399. Deilmann L, Winter O, Cerrutti B, Bradtmüller H, Herzig C, Limbeck A, et al. Effect of boron incorporation on the bioactivity, structure, and

mechanical properties of ordered mesoporous bioactive glasses. *J. Mater. Chem. B.* 2020;8(7):1456–65.
400. Echeverria Molina MI, Malollari KG, Komvopoulos K. Design challenges in polymeric scaffolds for tissue engineering. *Front. Bioeng. Biotechnol.* 2021;9:617141.
401. Fraioli R, Rechenmacher F, Neubauer S, Manero JM, Gil J, Kessler H, et al. Mimicking bone extracellular matrix: Integrin-binding peptidomimetics enhance osteoblast-like cells adhesion, proliferation, and differentiation on titanium. *Colloids Surf. B Biointerfaces.* 2015;128:191–200.
402. Daniel S. Biodegradable polymeric materials for medicinal applications. In: Thomas S, Balakrishnan P. (eds) *Green Composites.* Singapore: Springer, 2021:351–72.
403. Szaraniec B, Pielichowska K, Pac E, Menaszek E. Multifunctional polymer coatings for titanium implants. *Mater. Sci. Eng. C. Mater. Biol Appl.* 2018; 93:950–57.
404. Donnaloja F, Jacchetti E, Soncini M, Raimondi MT. Natural and synthetic polymers for bone scaffolds optimization. *Polymers.* 2020;12(4):905.
405. Chuenjitkuntaworn B, Inrung W, Damrongsri D, Mekaapiruk K, Supaphol P, Pavasant P. Polycaprolactone/hydroxyapatite composite scaffolds: Preparation, characterization, and in vitro and in vivo biological responses of human primary bone cells. *J. Biomed. Mater. Res. A.* 2010;94(1):241–51.
406. Stępniewski M, Martynkiewicz J, Gosk J. Chitosan and its composites: Properties for use in bone substitution. *Polim. Med.* 2017;47(1):49–53.
407. Pan C, Xu R, Chen J, Zhang Q, Deng L, Hong Q. A CO-releasing coating based on carboxymethyl chitosan-functionalized graphene oxide for improving the anticorrosion and biocompatibility of magnesium alloy stent materials. *Int. J. Biol. Macromol.* 2024;271(pt 2):132487.
408. Asadi H, Ghalei S, Handa H, Ramasamy RP. Cellulose nanocrystal reinforced silk fibroin coating for enhanced corrosion protection and biocompatibility of Mg-based alloys for orthopedic implant applications. *Prog. Org. Coat.* 2021;161:106525.
409. Guo Y, Su Y, Gu R, Zhang Z, Li G, Lian J, et al. Enhanced corrosion resistance and biocompatibility of biodegradable magnesium alloy modified by calcium phosphate/collagen coating. *Surf. Coat. Technol.* 2020;401:126318.
410. Guo Y, Jia S, Qiao L, Su Y, Gu R, Li G, et al. Enhanced corrosion resistance and biocompatibility of polydopamine/dicalcium phosphate dihydrate/collagen composite coating on magnesium alloy for orthopedic applications. *J. Alloys Compd.* 2020;817:152782.

411. Nie X, Sun X, Wang C, Yang J. Effect of magnesium ions/Type I collagen promote the biological behavior of osteoblasts and its mechanism. *Regen. Biomater.* 2020;7(1):53–61.
412. Zhang BGX, Myers DE, Wallace GG, Brandt M, Choong PFM. Bioactive coatings for orthopaedic implants — recent trends in development of implant coatings. *Int. J. Mol. Sci.* 2014;15(7):11878–921.
413. Mo X, Zhang D, Liu K, Zhao X, Li X, Wang W. Nano-hydroxyapatite composite scaffolds loaded with bioactive factors and drugs for bone tissue engineering. *Int. J. Mol. Sci.* 2023;24(2):1291.
414. Zhang B, Zhou Z, Zhang Y, Miu Y, Jin C, Ding W, et al. A sugary solution: Harnessing polysaccharide-based materials for osteoporosis treatment. *Carbohydr. Polym.* 2024;345:122549.
415. Lin X, Chen J, Lio Y, Pathak JL, Li H, Liu Y. Biomimetic calcium phosphate coating as a drug delivery vehicle for bone tissue engineering: A mini-review. *Coatings.* 2020;10(11):1118.
416. Bal Z, Kushioka J, Kodama J, Kaito T, Yoshikawa H, Korkusuz P, et al. BMP and TGFβ use and release in bone regeneration. *Turk. J. Med. Sci.* 2020;50(S1–2):1707–22.
417. Toosi S, Behravan J. Osteogenesis and bone remodeling: A focus on growth factors and bioactive peptides. *Biofactors.* 2020;46(3):326–40.
418. Sarian MN, Iqbal N, Sotoudehbagha P, Razavi M, Ahmed QU, Sukotjo C, et al. Potential bioactive coating system for high-performance absorbable magnesium bone implants. *Bioact. Mater.* 2022;12:42–63.
419. Zhao D-W, Zuo K-Q, Wang K, Sun Z-Y, Lu Y-P, Cheng L, et al. Interleukin-4 assisted calcium-strontium-zinc-phosphate coating induces controllable macrophage polarization and promotes osseointegration on titanium implant. *Mater. Sci. Eng. C. Mater. Biol. Appl.* 2021;118:111512.
420. Meenakshi S, Dureja S, Raghunath N, Gowda DV, Osmani RA. Advances in polymeric materials for dental and biomedical applications. In: *Handbook of Biodegradable Polymers.* Singapore: Jenny Stanford Publishing, 2024: 575–649.
421. Nourbakhsh F, Lotfalizadeh M, Badpeyma M, Shakeri A, Soheili V. From plants to antimicrobials: Natural products against bacterial membranes. *Phytother. Res.* 2022;36(1):33–52.
422. Khademi R, Kharaziha M. Antibacterial and osteogenic doxycycline imprinted bioglass microspheres to combat bone infection. *ACS Appl. Mater. Interfaces.* 2024;16(25):31966–82.

https://doi.org/10.1142/9789819819645_0005

Chapter 5

Tissue-Specific Biomaterials for Use in Musculoskeletal Tissue Engineering

Golara Kafili*[,1], Abdolreza Simchi[1,2,3]

[1]*Center for Nanoscience and Nanotechnology, Institute for Convergence Science and Technology, Sharif University of Technology, P.O. Box 14588-89694, Tehran, Iran*
[2]*Department of Materials Science and Engineering, Sharif University of Technology, P.O. Box 11365-11155, Tehran, Iran*
[3]*Center for BioScience and Technology, Institute for Convergence Science and Technology, Sharif University of Technology, P.O. Box 14588-89694, Tehran, Iran*

Chapter Outline

***Corresponding author:** Golara Kafili, Center for Nanoscience and Nanotechnology, Institute for Convergence Science and Technology, Sharif University of Technology, P.O. Box 14588-89694, Tehran, Iran. E-mail: g_kafili@yahoo.com

Abstract

Musculoskeletal disorders significantly affect an individual's socio-physiological well-being, often limiting their daily activities. Due to the shortage of autologous and allogenic grafts, there is an urgent need for tissue-engineered constructs (TECs) to aid in regenerating damaged musculoskeletal tissues. While a variety of natural and synthetic polymers have been employed in fabricating TECs, each material has its own set of advantages and limitations. However, none of these materials fully replicate the biochemical cues of native tissues. In this context, decellularized extracellular matrix (dECM) materials have shown great promise by closely mimicking the biochemical and biophysical characteristics of their tissue of origin. Specifically, dECMs derived from musculoskeletal tissues offer a valuable approach to regenerating musculoskeletal injuries due to their inherent tissue-specific bioactive components. This chapter reviews various types of scaffolds and TECs constructed from musculoskeletal dECMs, detailing their fabrication methods, functions, advantages, and limitations. It also highlights recent advancements and explores practical strategies to overcome existing challenges. The information provided aims to offer a comprehensive understanding of tissue-specific biomaterials for a broad audience with a background in biomedical engineering and biomedicine.

1. The Musculoskeletal System: Anatomy and Extracellular Matrix Composition

Modern society increasingly experiences musculoskeletal-related conditions as a result of sedentary lifestyles, population aging, and unsafe livelihoods [1]. Musculoskeletal disorders, including degenerative diseases (e.g., degenerative osteoarthritis [OA]), tumor resections, immune-mediated degradation, and infectious conditions causing defects in musculoskeletal-related tissues, can severely affect a patient's quality of life and restrict physical activity [2]. Hence, people suffering from musculoskeletal diseases face serious challenges, including lack of independence, fatigue, pain, limited movement, and a restricted quality of life accompanied by physiological and psychological burdens [3].

The musculoskeletal system, the body's locomotor structure, comprises various tissues, including bone, cartilage, tendon, ligament, and skeletal muscle [4]. Each of these components plays a crucial role in providing structural strength, stability, and mobility. For example, cartilage is a hard tissue within the musculoskeletal system, notable for being avascular and lacking neural innervation [5]. The extracellular matrix (ECM) of cartilage is mostly composed of collagen type II and glycosaminoglycans (GAGs). Aging is the main cause of many cartilage degenerative diseases, such as OA, which are mostly observed in the hip, shoulder, and knee joints. In severe cases, the treatment of OA relies on surgery for the employment of a joint prosthesis that can eventually induce extreme pain, inflammation, and even infection in patients and may even require a second surgery due to the limited lifespan of prosthetics [6]. The meniscus, a fibrocartilaginous tissue with a rubbery nature located in the knee joint, acts as a lubricating unit to diminish the friction between the tibia and femur [7]. The lack of adequate blood flow due to aging inhibits the functionality of the meniscus in elderly people [8]. The younger generation may also face serious meniscus injuries, such as tears during sports or due to other incidents [9]. Considering the limited blood supply, the self-healing capacity of the meniscus upon damage is inadequate [10]. Therefore, the main treatment modalities include surgical interventions, such as autologous or allograft transplantation or the use of an artificial implant. Nonetheless, graft transplantations may encounter shape or size mismatches, thus requiring new methods for patient-specific and custom-designed three-dimensional (3D)-printed scaffolds [11].

Tendons are robust tissues primarily composed of collagen that function to connect skeletal muscles to bones [12]. They are known for their exquisite tensile strength, enabling the movement of skeletal tissues. Therefore, tendon injuries, including rupture, strain, and tears, induce intensive inflammation that often takes a long time to resolve on its own [13]. Ligaments are soft tissues that connect two bones. Their ECM is primarily composed of collagen type I (i.e., about 75% of dry weight) and some noncollagenous proteins (e.g., elastin) accompanied by GAGs and proteoglycans [14]. The hierarchical organization of collagenous components within the tendon and ligament ECM contributes to their mechanical stiffness [15]. Entheses are interfacial tissues that connect ligaments and tendons to bone and enable force transmission between the hard (i.e., bone) and the soft tissues with their undeniable mechanical mismatch [16].

As such, the musculoskeletal system is a multi-tissue system in which each tissue plays an important and distinguishable part in the maintenance of body strength and movement. Presenting details about every aspect of the whole system is out of the scope of this chapter. Therefore, among all tissues within the musculoskeletal system, this chapter will mainly focus on bone as a hard tissue and skeletal muscle as a representative of a soft tissue. As shown in **Figure 1**, bone is a hard tissue with a hierarchical structure that supports body movement and is composed of essential minerals [3]. Bone is composed of osteon units, which are generated by the organization of concentric parallel lamellar sheets around blood vessels [17]. Within the lamellae, collagen fibers are arranged parallel to each other. Finally, these mineralized collagen fibers are also organized by the alignment of hydroxyapatite crystals within self-assembled collagen subunits. The ECM of bone tissue is a complex mixture of organic (40%) and inorganic (60%) components. The organic portion consists of 90% fibrous collagen type I and 10% noncollagenous components, including glycoproteins (e.g., osteopontin, osteocalcin, thrombospondin, R-spondins, and osteonectin) [18]. The needle-like hydroxyapatite crystals ($Ca_5(PO_4)_3OH$) arranged between collagen fibers form the inorganic component of bone ECM [3]. There are different growth factors (GFs) in the bone matrix, such as vascular endothelial growth factor (VEGF) and bone morphogenetic protein-2 (BMP-2), and several types of cells, including osteoprogenitor cells, osteoblasts, osteoclasts, and osteocytes [4]. Upon the formation of a microcrack within the bone structure, osteoclasts and osteoblasts communicate, and new ECM is secreted to remodel the damaged tissue [19].

There are three main groups of muscles in the body: skeletal, cardiac, and smooth muscles [20]. Skeletal muscle is composed of muscle fibers, muscle cells, blood vessels, and nerves, forming ~40% of an adult's body weight and aiding with the movement of the skeletal system [21]. The skeletal muscles are bound to the bone with the help of tendons. Skeletal muscles, controlled by the somatic nervous system, can contract and relax voluntarily [20]. The vascular networks within the skeletal muscle transport oxygen and nutrients and exchange metabolites and waste products [22]. Skeletal muscle possesses a very complex hierarchical arrangement (**Figure 1**). The muscle bundles are composed of fascicle units that in turn are composed of muscle fibers. Muscle fibers contain multinucleated cells, and their well-organized bundles support the mechanical strength of skeletal muscle [23]. The muscle fibers may vary in diameter between 10 and 100 μm and in length between a few millimeters and centimeters [24]. Skeletal muscle fibers comprise a striated structure due to repeating contractile subunits called sarcomeres, which are composed of myosin and actin protein filaments. The muscle fibers are wrapped by a connective tissue named the endomysium [25]. The fascicles are axially well-organized structures covered by another connective tissue called the

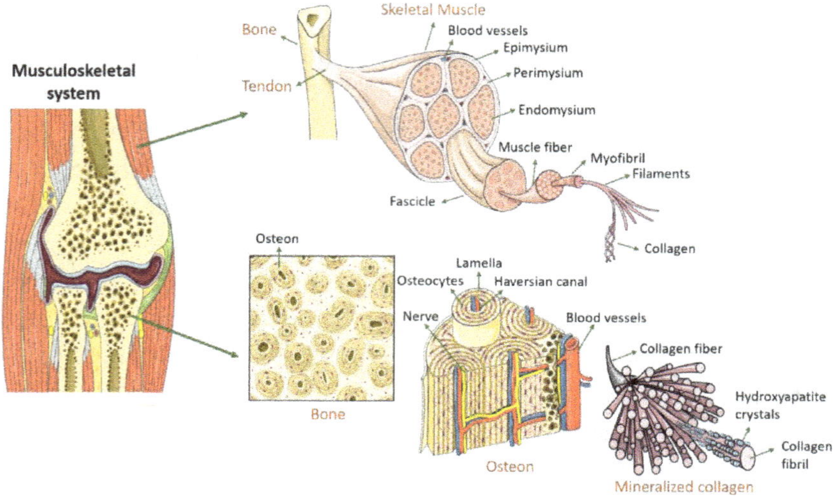

Figure 1. A scheme of the hierarchical structure of the bone and skeletal muscle. The information used in the construction of the images is adapted from ref. [29, 30]. The images were drawn by Servier Medical Art (Les Laboratories Servier), licensed under Creative Commons Attribution 4.0.

perimysium. Finally, the whole muscle mass is enclosed by a sheath of connective tissue named the epimysium [4]. It is also important to point out that skeletal muscle tissue possesses distinctive cell populations, including endothelial cells, neurons, fibroblasts, macrophages, and inherent stem cells (i.e., satellite cells) [25, 26]. Satellite cells, known as mononucleated quiescent cells, are located beneath the basal membrane in the sarcolemma membrane [27]. These muscle tissue-specific stem cells are quiescent in normal tissues, but they activate upon a muscular injury and contribute to muscle regeneration by differentiating into myoblasts [28].

The ECM of skeletal muscles is located at the position of the basement membrane covering the muscle fibers, which are composed of two sublayers, namely, the inner basal lamina and the outer reticular lamina [26]. It also contains a heterogeneous mix of structural and adhesive proteins such as elastin, collagen (i.e., collagen I, III, IV, V, VI, VII, XII, XIV, and XVIII), keratin, fibronectin, laminin, GAGs, and proteoglycans (e.g., heparan sulfate, lumican, decorin, biglycan, perlecan, and agrin), as well as various GFs and cytokines [25, 31, 32]. Immunohistochemical (IHC) staining of native skeletal muscle tissues has shown that collagen type IV, laminin, and fibronectin are mostly localized in the endomysium and epimysium surrounding the muscle fibers [33]. BMP, basic fibroblast GF, epidermal GF, hepatocyte growth factor (HGF), insulin-like growth factor-1 (IGF-1), insulin-like growth factor binding protein-4 (IGFBP-4), transforming growth factor-beta-1 (TGF-β1), TGF-β3, platelet-derived growth factor (PDGF), and VEGF are among the prominent GFs and cytokines within the skeletal muscle-derived decellularized extracellular matrix (SMdECM) [34].

This book provides an overview of clinically relevant diagnostic techniques and imaging technologies for musculoskeletal diseases and conditions. It also highlights current preclinical and clinical medications and treatments aimed at repairing and restoring musculoskeletal disorders. As a contemporary and highly significant topic in the field, this chapter will focus on tissue-specific sources of biomaterials for musculoskeletal tissue engineering (TE) and regeneration. Different kinds of biomaterials and nanomaterials, various types of scaffolds and grafts, and artificial constructs for the engineering or regeneration of musculoskeletal diseases are covered in other chapters. In this chapter, the anatomy and ECM composition of tissues in the musculoskeletal system are first introduced. Then, general examples of musculoskeletal disorders are highlighted, and their current treatment approaches, with their potential advantages and drawbacks, are also presented. Following this, the tissue-specific decellularized extracellular matrix (dECM), as a prominent source of biomaterial for use in musculoskeletal tissue engineering and regenerative medicine (TERM) applications, is introduced. The subsequent sections introduce general treatment modalities for musculoskeletal diseases and provide more insights into how the implementation of processed tissue-derived biomaterials can actively contribute to improved regeneration outcomes. Accordingly, the substantial processing and fabrication methods, including the *in situ* formation of hydrogels, electrospinning of dECM-based solutions, 3D printing of scaffolds containing dECM components, and bioprinting of cell-embedded dECM bioinks, are discussed. The engineering and therapeutic advantages of each method along with their possible shortcomings are explored. Finally, some biomedical interventions to address current challenges regarding the intrinsic characteristics of dECM-based scaffolds and methods to enhance their innate properties are briefly explained. This chapter provides up-to-date information for a wide range of readers, including medical experts, engineers, biologists, chemists, and professionals from multidisciplinary fields.

2. Regeneration of Musculoskeletal Deficiencies

In the case of manageable musculoskeletal injuries, the inherent regenerative capacity of most musculoskeletal tissues is often adequate to restore the tear or defect site [1]. However, in extended and severe injuries, external interventions are critical to regulating the proper reconstruction of functional tissue. For instance, bone is capable of repairing itself in the case of small fractures [3]. Nonetheless, as the severity of the defect condition or size expands, the bone can no longer fully regenerate itself. Although autologous bone grafts are the gold standard treatment for large-scale bone defects, the limited availability of a donor site as well as its infection and morbidity impose serious burdens. As another important example within the musculoskeletal system, skeletal muscle tissue is also known to self-regenerate in the cases of mild-to-moderate muscle injuries [22]. This ability is related to satellite stem cell activation and their self-renewal capacity. However, the traumatic loss of muscle tissue impairs its function. Moreover, in the case of volumetric muscle loss (VML), tumor ablation, and degenerative diseases, the injured site cannot be self-regenerated due to the extreme loss of host stem cells and ECM components [28]. If the muscle loss exceeds 20% of its content, the innate regenerative capacity of muscle tissue will not be enough to recover the injury [33]. These conditions may be followed by a prolonged immune response and enhanced secretion by fibroblasts, leading to the deposition of fibrotic tissue in the defect site [35]. Consequently, the inability of the fibrotic muscle site to contract impairs the force production by muscle tissue and leads to a lack in muscular functionality. Current treatment approaches to repair VML include the transplantation of autologous muscle flaps or grafts [24]. However, the limited availability of donor tissue and the possible side effects at the donor site (e.g., the loss of functionality and risk of infection or necrosis) are the leading challenges [36]. The use of xenografts and allografts is also limited by the high risk of severe immune responses that can lead to graft failure and/or the risk of the transmission of infectious diseases [24]. Therefore, the fabrication of functional scaffolds or tissue-engineered substitutes is required to restore musculoskeletal deficiency.

TE has enabled the reconstruction of damaged tissues by providing scaffolds that can mechanically support the injured area during the healing process and even deliver bioactive components to encourage the quality of the regeneration process by activating endogenic or exogenic cells [37]. For instance, bone scaffolds exhibit important features to promote osteoconduction and osteoinduction, provide sufficient mechanical properties to withstand external loads, and possess a well-matched biodegradability rate with the regeneration rate of new bone tissue [38]. A proper scaffold for skeletal muscle TE should provide topographical cues to guide the formation of elongated multinucleated myotubes, as well as biochemical cues to encourage the myogenic differentiation and maturation of tissue-engineered constructs (TECs) [34]. Furthermore, providing access to vascular and neural networks is essential for the successful regeneration and maturation of tissues [24]. Both natural and synthetic materials have been exploited for the fabrication of scaffolds to recover musculoskeletal defects and injuries. Collagen, alginate, silk, gelatin, hyaluronic acid, and chitosan are among the widely used examples of natural biopolymers, which have shown promising results on the regeneration of target tissues owing to their bioactivity and availability of cell-binding motifs in some cases [26]. Nevertheless, despite the biocompatibility of natural polymers, the lack of sufficient mechanical and rheological properties alleviates their potential for the construction of scaffolds, especially in load-bearing tissues, such as bone [39]. As a result, synthetic polymers (e.g., polycaprolactone [PCL], poly(lactide-co-glycolide) [PLGA], polylactic acid [PLA], polyethylene glycol, and polyurethane) have been introduced for the manufacturing of mechanically robust scaffolds with prolonged degradation rates. Yet, poor cell adhesion and inherent hydrophobicity of most synthetic polymers attenuate their biofunctionality and contribution to tissue repair [40]. Despite the advantages provided by each of these groups of materials, their lack of integration with the host tissue may impair the expected therapeutic results [41]. Therefore, the materials derived from the target native tissue can enhance the regeneration of injured tissue by providing similar biochemical components and a higher level of mimicry with the host microenvironment [40]. To this end, tissue-derived ECM biomaterials have drawn great attention in the last decade due to their inherent biocompatibility, low immunogenicity, and tissue-specific functionality, which serves the restoration of injured tissues [42]. For instance, using decellularized bone tissue as a bone substitute can enhance the regeneration of the defect site by providing a similar ECM composition to native tissue. The preserved organic and inorganic components within a bone-derived decellularized extracellular matrix (BdECM) are known for their regulatory function toward several cell activities that affect the bone remodeling process [4].

2.1. *Decellularized Tissue-Derived Biomaterials for Musculoskeletal Tissue Engineering*

Many studies have shown that decellularized tissue-specific ECM-derived materials hold great promise in TE and the regeneration of musculoskeletal injuries [3, 24, 43]. The biochemical cues preserved in tissue-derived biomaterials are known for their regulatory functions on cell activities, such as cell growth, proliferation, migration, and differentiation [21]. Examples include laminin, which promotes myoblast adhesion and myogenesis; collagen type IV, which supports myoblast adhesion and migration; and chondroitin sulfate, which impedes myoblast differentiation [23]. This section discusses the advantages of BdECM- and SMdECM-derived scaffolds for treating bone and skeletal muscle defects, respectively.

The GFs within the ECM contribute to tissue-specific differentiation, such as myogenic differentiation and osteogenic differentiation [44]. This, in turn, affects the regeneration of injured tissue. However, the remaining antigenic cellular components in the native tissues, such as cellular proteins, lipids, and nucleic acids, can cause severe immune responses and lead to implant rejection; hence, they must be removed by applying a decellularization process [45, 46]. So far, various decellularization methods, including physical, chemical, biological, and a combination, have been used to decellularize native tissues [47]. The physical techniques mainly include shaking, cycles of freeze-thawing, and mincing. The chemical methods involve ionic, nonionic, or zwitterionic detergents; hypertonic or hypotonic solutions; acid or basic solutions; organic solvents; and chelating agents [1]. Enzymatic reagents (e.g., trypsin, nucleases, and lipase) have been examined as biological decellularization techniques [40]. More details regarding decellularization techniques, including their mechanism of action and possible side effects on the remaining ECM components, are summarized in **Table 1**. In most cases, a successful removal of cellular components and surface antigens cannot be achieved by a solo reagent. Hence, using a combination of techniques and reagents is highly recommended for effective decellularization of the target tissue [3].

For the processing of dECM biomaterials, tissues can be obtained from different sources, including animals (e.g., porcine, bovine, mouse, and monkey) or humans. Among animal sources, porcine-derived tissues are often considered the most frequently used source due to their close anatomical and physiological similarity to human tissues [24]. However, the risk of transmission of porcine retrovirus infection to humans is undeniable. The tissues derived from humans cause the least of challenges, while the shortage of cadaveric donors restricts their availability [48]. For musculoskeletal TE and regeneration, several forms of dECM biomaterials have been exploited. For example, the simplest form of SMdECM is skeletal muscle tissue pieces cut from native tissues and then decellularized to be used as SMdECM tissue pieces or tissue sheets [23]. Despite the promising therapeutic outcomes, the dECM tissue pieces/sheets can suffer from shape and size mismatch when needed to repair irregular-shaped defects [32]. Another technique involves solubilizing dECM to fabricate fibrous scaffolds by electrospinning [21]. The dECM solution for electrospinning can be a pristine dECM solution or a blended solution with synthetic polymers to enhance spinability [32]. The processing of dECM tissues into a hydrogel form through enzymatic digestion in a mildly acidic environment followed by pH neutralization and salt-balancing has been used as a promising technique to obtain temperature-sensitive hydrogels [49, 50]. Neutralized dECM pre-gel solutions can be used as an injectable hydrogel to form a solid gel by incubation at the physiologic temperature of the body [37]. The SMdECM hydrogels can be utilized as injectable hydrogels to fill irregularly shaped tissue defects or be used for intramuscular injection as a minimally invasive therapy [10]. Alternatively, dECM-derived hydrogels can serve as a carrier for bioactive and therapeutic molecules and components (e.g., drugs, GFs,

Table 1. Different types of decellularization techniques, reagents, and their specific functions.

Method	**Agent/Procedure**	**Function**	**Disadvantages**	**Advantages**	**Ref.**
Physical techniques	Freezing and thawing cycles	Lysis of cell membrane through formed ice crystals	Disruption of protein components within ECM; attenuate mechanical properties	Aiding cell removal and separation of various layers of tissues	[1, 54]
	Mincing/chopping	Increasing surface area for better function of decellularization agents	-	Facilitating the infiltration of decellularization agents	[55]
	Mechanical agitation	Facilitating the decellularization process and dissociation of cells from the basement membrane	Alteration of ECM composition	Enhancing cell removal efficiency	[2]
	Sonication	Disruption of the cell membrane through the formation of cavitation bubbles and induction of shear stress	Damage to tissues; denaturation of protein components	Facilitating the infiltration of adjunct decellularization agents	[2]
	Scrapping	Manual detachment of cells	Damaging basement membrane	Assisting separation of undesired tissue sublayers	[56]
	NTIRE	Induction of surface pores on cell membranes through electrical pulses	Toxicity of used solvents	Assisting leakage of intracellular components; maintaining ECM structure	[1]

	High hydrostatic pressure	Disruption of the cell membrane by high pressures applied to tissue	Damage to ECM proteins	Aiding cell removal	[54]
	Supercritical fluid	Cell removal by enhancing chemical exposure	-	Aiding removal of cellular residues; better preservation of bioactive components within ECM	[1, 40]
Chemical techniques	Triton X-100	Breaking lipid–lipid and protein–lipid interactions with minor effect on protein–protein interactions	Disruption of structural features within native tissues; troublesome removal of chemical remnants from dECM	Removal of membrane components and intracellular residues; causing less damage to ECM structure compared to other detergents	[40, 54]
	Sodium dodecyl sulfate	Solubilization of cell membrane; breaking protein–protein interactions	Loss of protein components, GAGs, and GFs within ECM; troublesome removal of chemical remnants from dECM	Enhanced removal of membrane components and intracellular remnants	[1]
	Sodium deoxycholate	Solubilization of cell membrane; breaking protein–protein interactions	Denaturation of protein components within ECM; troublesome removal of chemical remnants from dECM	Removal of membrane components and intracellular remnants	[40]

(Continued)

Table 1. *(Continued)*

Method	Agent/Procedure	Function	Disadvantages	Advantages	Ref.
	CHAPS	Disruption of lipid–lipid, lipid–protein, and DNA–protein interactions	Insufficient removal of intracellular constituents	Less detrimental effects on ECM proteins as compared to ionic and nonionic detergents	[2]
	NaCl	Osmotic shock-induced cell lysis	Difficulty in removal of DNA fragments	Assisting the detachment of cells from ECM proteins; maintaining the protein content of ECM	[54]
	Tris-HCl	Lysis of cellular components by osmotic stress	Difficulty in removal of DNA fragments	Preservation of GAGs	[1]
	Glycerol	Dehydration and lysis of cellular components; removal of lipids	Possible impairment of ECM structure	Preventing calcification upon implantation of dECM materials by removal of phospholipids during decellularization	[57]
	Ethanol	Lysis of cellular components; removal of lipids	Alteration of structural features of ECM; not efficient enough for thick and dense tissues	Aiding cell removal by dehydration and solubilization of cells; antimicrobial activity	[40]

	Isopropyl alcohol	Removal of lipids	Precipitation of proteins	Dissociation of lipids from tissues containing high lipid content, such as adipose and bone	[55]
	Sodium hydroxide	Disruption of collagenous components	Attenuating mechanical properties; disturbing ECM integrity	High cell removal efficiency	[1]
	Peracetic acid	Solubilizing nucleic acids and cytoplasmic components	Disruption of ECM; loss of GAGs	Assisting removal of cellular and nuclear components; sterilization	[40]
	EDTA	Assisting the dissociation of cells through the separation of metal ions	Not efficient enough as a solo decellularization agent; environmental concerns of separated metal ions	Improving the quality of decellularization in combination with other agents	[40]
	EGTA	Assisting the dissociation of cells from proteins	Not efficient enough as a solo decellularization agent; denature of ECM proteins	Improving the quality of decellularization in combination with other agents	[2]
Biological techniques	Trypsin	Breaking protein–cell interactions; dissociation of cells from ECM	Detrimental for proteins, especially collagen and elastin; protease activity; diminishing mechanical strength; not sufficient as a solo decellularization agent	Facilitating infiltration of adjunct decellularization agents	[54]

(Continued)

Table 1. *(Continued)*

Method	Agent/Procedure	Function	Disadvantages	Advantages	Ref.
	Nucleases (DNase, RNase)	Breaking nucleic acids into smaller fragments	Difficult removal from remaining dECM material	Assisting removal of cellular fragments; causing less immunogenicity	[40]
	Dispase	Cleavage of peptides	Disruption of ECM	Specific function on collagen type IV and fibronectin	[54]
	Lipase	Targeting of phospholipids of cell membrane	Difficult removal of lipid residues	Preserving ECM components, including proteins and GAGs	[1]
	Collagenase	Assisting cell removal by disruption of collagen fibrils	Removal of structural proteins	-	[56]

and nanoparticles) to target the treatment site and promote the regeneration capacity [3]. Besides, the dECM-derived scaffolds may be embedded with tissue-specific cell types to augment tissue regeneration. Although these approaches provide promising results for the regeneration of musculoskeletal impairments, the finite source of biopsies from donor tissues (as the cell source) and the requirement for excessive cell expansion limit the quick therapeutic outcome [3]. Some studies have pursued an *in situ* muscle regeneration process using cell-free SMdECM scaffolds for the recruitment of endogenous stem cells or progenitor cells by stimulating their activation and differentiation [1, 32, 51]. It is believed that chemotactic factors secreted from SMdECM trigger endogenous stem cells to migrate into the site of injury and contribute to the reconstruction of defects [24]. Successfully stimulating endogenous stem/progenitor cells and controlling their fate are key players in achieving the targeted therapeutic outcomes. Despite the promising results expected from the migration of recruited cells into SMdECM scaffolds, the disorganized muscle fibers within these scaffolds mitigate the functionality of regenerated tissue [22]. To solve this issue, prefabricated bioprinted TECs with aligned encapsulated cells may serve well [52]. Herein, dECM hydrogels can be employed as a cell-embedded bioink to fabricate TECs with more complex, custom-designed geometries. Nowadays, 3D bioprinting of cell-encapsulated dECM bioinks has been considered a trending and promising approach for fabricating functional TECs as tissue substitutes to treat musculoskeletal injuries [53]. All these fabrication procedures involving SMdECM/BdECM materials will be described in detail in the following section.

3. Processing and Fabrication of Decellularized Extracellular Matrix–Based Biomaterials for Bone and Muscle Tissue Engineering

dECM-based biomaterials have proven to be valuable for engineering tissue-like constructs due to their intrinsic tissue-specific biochemical cues. It is also known that topographical cues are critical in regulating cell alignment to modulate their specific characteristics, such as directing the myogenesis of muscle cells [58]. Therefore, attempts have been made to use these materials as whole decellularized tissues, organs, or tissue pieces (e.g., dECM sheets and particles) [23, 59]. Alternatively, processing into dECM solutions for electrospinning, injectable dECM hydrogels for minimally invasive therapy, or precursors for 3D printing/bioprinting has been studied [32, 46, 58]. For example, electrospinning [21] and 3D bioprinting [53] have been employed to provide biophysical cues to augment the myogenic functionality of cells and guide the biomimetic anisotropic arrangement of muscle fibers. The fabrication of uniaxially nanofibrous dECM-based scaffolds *via* electrospinning and micropatterned scaffolds *via* 3D printing/bioprinting techniques will be thoroughly explored in the following sections, highlighting the synergistic effects of biochemical and biophysical cues in biofabricated dECM-based constructs.

3.1. *Scaffolds Derived from Whole Tissue/Organ Decellularization*

The perfusion decellularization technique *via* the innate vasculature of the tissue of origin has shown promising outcomes in removing cellular components from large intact tissues or organs to produce large-scale scaffolds containing tissue-specific biochemical cues [60]. Using this decellularization technique enables the preservation of the original size and volume of the target tissue/organ and allows the treatment of clinically relevant-scale defects or injuries. Zhang *et al.* [33] prepared a muscle scaffold with inherent vascular networks through perfusion decellularization of a porcine rectus abdominis. This method aided in preserving the original innate architecture and structural features of the native muscle tissue. The treatment of partial-thickness abdominal wall defects in rats with perfusion-decellularized skeletal muscle graft was followed by infiltration of mononucleated cells and a few populations of multinucleated cells around the implant. Eight weeks postsurgery, more neo-muscle fibers, neo-vessels, and peripheral innervation were observed in decellularized muscle graft-treated groups as compared to the control group. The innervation of treated defects might be a result of infiltrated Schwann cells into the preserved neural channels within the decellularized skeletal muscle graft.

Several studies have shown that BdECM scaffolds retain the porous microstructure, rigidity, stiffness, and roughness of native bone tissue, which play a significant role in guiding the differentiation of cells to the osteogenic lineage [2]. The preserved innate structural features in BdECM scaffolds therefore present the native bone tissue features and can provoke cellular activities by affecting both cell–cell and cell–ECM interactions. Sladkova *et al.* [61] seeded human-induced pluripotent stem cell-derived mesodermal progenitor cells on BdECM scaffolds obtained from bovine and human sources and dynamically cultured the engineered constructs for 5 weeks in a perfusion bioreactor. Despite minor changes in the structure and composition of these two sources of BdECM scaffolds derived from either animal or human tissue, growth and mineralization were alike. This study affirmed that bovine BdECM scaffolds have significant potential for use as human bone grafts.

3.2. *Tissue Pieces: Decellularized Extracellular Matrix Sheets and Particles*

Nakada *et al.* [23] used longitudinal SMdECM-sliced sheets for the culture of C2C12 myoblasts. The results showed that myoblasts were well adhered to the SMdECM sheets and exhibited a spindle-like morphology. The phalloidin staining of cell-seeded SMdECM sheets showed the development of filopodia and lamellipodia in the adhered cells. Changing the culture medium to a differentiation medium also induced myotube formation that aligned with the orientation of the SMdECM sheet. Overall, the inherent longitudinal orientation of SMdECM sheets guided the formation of aligned myotubes. Due to the active interaction between myocytes and the SMdECM sheets, these tissue pieces can serve as simple yet bioactive platforms for studying cell functions, such as cell migration or differentiation.

Powdered BdECM has extensively been exploited as an additive material for enhancing the mechanical and biological properties of bone scaffolds [18, 62]. It was shown that increasing BdECM content by up to 30% increased the mechanical properties of 3D-printed PCL-based composite scaffolds [59]. BdECM also improved cell adhesion onto scaffolds compared to PCL-only scaffolds and enhanced the expression of osteogenic genes even in the absence of soluble osteogenic factors. Moreover, the human adipose stem cell (hASC)-seeded 3D-printed PCL scaffolds reinforced with BdECM particles exhibited more bone regeneration in murine calvarial defects at 1 and 3 months postimplantation. In another study, the effect of different additive particles, including tricalcium phosphate (TCP), hydroxyapatite, BdECM, and Bio-Oss® (BO, a commercially available bovine xenograft bone substitute in which the organic constituents of bone have been removed), was studied on the mechanical and biological properties of 3D-printed PCL scaffolds using a fused deposition modeling technique [63]. In this comparative study, collagen type I and osteocalcin expression levels were significantly higher in the PCL/BdECM/BO group than in those containing hydroxyapatite or TCP.

3.3. *Decellularized Extracellular Matrix-Based Electrospun Scaffolds*

Electrospinning is a well-developed technique for fabricating nano- and micro-fibrous scaffolds to mimic the structural features of the ECM in native tissues. Electrospinning enables the fabrication of both randomly oriented (RO) and aligned fibrous scaffolds, where each of these fiber orientations may serve well for specific biomedical and TE approaches [21]. The aligned fibers are known to guide myogenic differentiation and myotube formation [64]. The porous structure of electrospun scaffolds also contributes to the transfer of nutrients and the exchange of metabolic waste products [32]. Patel *et al.* [28] investigated the effect of aligned electrospun scaffolds made from an SMdECM–PCL blend and PCL-only scaffolds on muscle regeneration in marine models with partial-thickness VML injuries. A higher expression of myogenin (a myogenic differentiation marker) in the blend group compared to the PCL-only scaffold was shown. This finding supports the effect of SMdECM on the differentiation of host stem cells. However, the force production in the treated VML injuries with the SMdECM–PCL blend was not sufficient, possibly due to the lack of innervation between regenerated myofibers within the 28 days of treatment. Smoak *et al.* [21] prepared electrospun SMdECM scaffolds of random orientation collected on a stationary plate, with intermediate-to-extremely aligned fibers using a rotating collector drum with differing rotating speeds

(**Figures 2a-i** and **2a-ii**). Comparing aligned scaffolds with RO fibrous scaffolds has revealed that the alignment of fibers enhances the adhesion and growth of C2C12 cells on the scaffold surface. Quantitative analysis of myotube formation on cell-laden glutaraldehyde (GA)-crosslinked SMdECM scaffolds cultured in an induction medium (**Figure 2a-iii**) has indicated that more aligned myotubes are formed on highly aligned fibrous scaffolds (**Figure 2a-iv**). To evaluate the effect of micro- and nano-topographical features on the engineering of muscle-like structures, scaffolds were made using a combination of 3D printing and electrospinning techniques [58]. A multiscale composite scaffold composed of electrospun nanofibrous methacrylated skeletal muscle-derived decellularized extracellular matrix (SMdEMA) on a 3D-printed PLGA-micropatterned scaffold was fabricated to mimic the basal lamina of the skeletal muscle. The electrospinning setup and photocrosslinking parameters for the subsequent crosslinking of electrospun mats (ultraviolet [UV] light, 400 mW.cm^{-2}) are shown in **Figure 2b-i.** Examination of the effect of SMdEMA concentration showed that the 10 wt% solution produced stable nanofibrous scaffolds (**Figure 2b-ii**). The multiscale scaffolds were fabricated by depositing uniaxially aligned nanofibrous SMdEMA onto printed micropatterned PLGA struts (**Figure 2b-iii**). The micropatterned PLGA struts were separately fabricated by 3D printing a PLGA/polyvinyl alcohol (PVA) mixture with a ratio of 7:3 at 150°C, followed by PVA leaching. Two control groups were also fabricated, which included (i) micropatterned PLGA covered with gelatin methacryloyl (GelMA) nanofibers to compare with the effect of tissue-specific components within SMdEMA and (ii) nonpatterned PLGA coated with SMdEMA to compare the effect of micropatterned PLGA on cell behavior (**Figure 2b-iv**). Pattern-guided muscle progenitor cells, uniaxially stretched parallel to the direction of fibers in the scaffolds, were observed. The cells exhibited multipolar morphology on the nonpatterned scaffold. Immunofluorescence (IF) staining of myosin heavy chains (MHCs) was carried out to determine the myogenic differentiation of muscle progenitor cells. As shown in **Figure 2b-v**, the MHCs were uniaxially aligned in multiscale patterned scaffolds, while a multipolar random arrangement was observed in the nonpatterned control group. These results implied the guidance effect of nano/micro patterns of scaffolds on the myogenic function of muscle cells. Moreover, a higher level of MHCs was

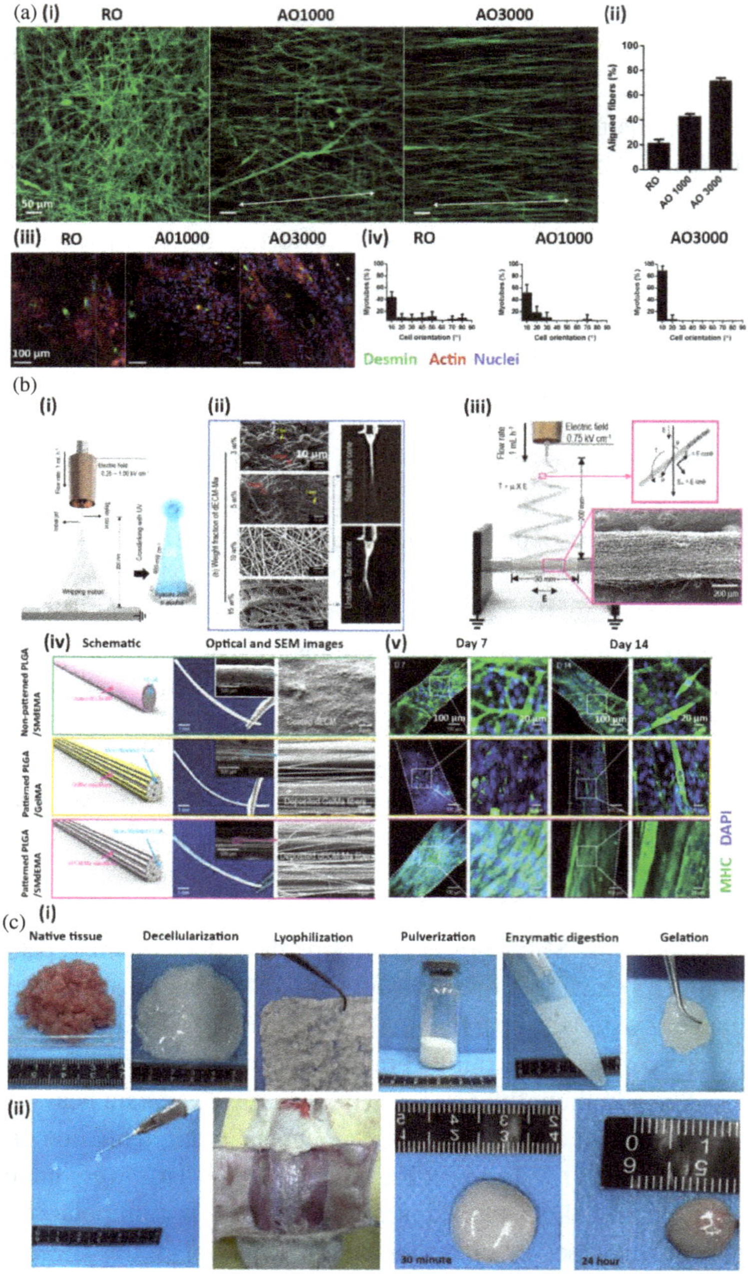

Figure 2. (*Continued*)

detected in SMdEMA-coated micropatterned PLGA scaffolds. This finding also affirmed that tissue-specific biochemical cues within SMdEMA supported the myogenic differentiation of muscle progenitor cells better than frequently used polymers, such as GelMA, without tissue-specific components. Overall, the multiscale composite scaffold composed of micropatterned PLGA covered with uniaxially aligned SMdEMA nanofibers showed myogenic activity due to the synergistic effects of guidance over micro/nano features and tissue-specific biochemical cues provided by an SMdEMA component [58].

Although the electrospinning technique provides control over fiber alignment in fibrous scaffolds, which contributes to cell fate, the two-dimensionality of electrospun scaffolds and partial cell penetration limit

Figure 2. (***Continued on facing pages***) (a) Electrospun SMdECM scaffolds with different degrees of fiber orientation to control cellular activities [Reprinted from ref. [21], Copyright 2021, with permission from The American Association for the Advancement of Science (AAAS)]. **(a-i)** Confocal images of electrospun SMdECM scaffolds with RO fibers collected on a stationary plate, intermediate aligned fibers obtained with a rotating collector at a speed of 1,000 rpm (AO1000), and extremely aligned fibers obtained with a rotating collector at a speed of 3,000 rpm (AO3000); double-headed arrows indicate the fiber direction. **(a-ii)** Graph representing fiber alignment. **(a-iii)** IF staining of myotube formation (green color: desmin; red color: actin; and blue color: nuclei); double-headed arrows indicate the direction of myotube alignment. **(a-iv)** Graph representing myotube alignment of cell-laden GA-crosslinked SMdECM fibrous scaffolds cultured for 7 days in an induction medium. **(b)** Fabrication of multiscale composite scaffold for alignment and maturation of muscle progenitor cells [Reprinted with permission from ref. [58], Copyright 2019, American Chemical Society]. **(b-i)** Electrospinning and photocrosslinking setup of SMdEMA nanofibrous scaffolds. **(b-ii)** SEM images of electrospun scaffolds with different SMdEMA concentrations. **(b-iii)** Schematic representation of electrospinning setup over fibrillated PLGA struts using an electrostatic torque accompanied by the representative SEM image. **(b-iv)** Schematic representation and optical/SEM images of three groups, including PLGA coated with SMdEMA hydrogel, micropatterned PLGA deposited with nanofibrous GelMA, and micropatterned PLGA deposited with nanofibrous SMdEMA. **(b-v)** DAPI/MHC IF images of three scaffold groups after 7 and 14 days of culture. **(c)** Formation of SMdECM-derived hydrogel [Reprinted from ref. [46], Copyright (2016), with permission from John Wiley and Sons]. **(c-i)** Processing steps of injectable and temperature-sensitive SMdECM hydrogel. **(c-ii)** Injectability and *in situ* gelation of SMdECM pre-gel solution at physiologic temperature assessed by subcutaneous injection to the abdomen of rats.

their capability to mimic the 3D microenvironment experienced by cells in native tissues [21]. Conversely, dECM-derived hydrogels provide a 3D microenvironment for encapsulated cells [46]. Therefore, *in situ* forming dECM hydrogels have been exploited as a minimally invasive method for the recovery of damaged or injured tissues. Cell-encapsulated dECM hydrogels have also been trending in the last decade for the biofabrication of TECs to mimic the biochemically and anatomically relevant characteristics of native target tissues. These approaches will be discussed in more detail in the following subsections.

3.4. *In Situ Forming Decellularized Extracellular Matrix–Based Hydrogels*

Neutralized dECM pre-gel solutions are a versatile class of minimally invasive therapeutic approaches that can be applied as injectable hydrogels *in vivo* [65]. These hydrogels are temperature-sensitive and turn into a solid gel form following incubation at 37°C [66]. As shown in **Figure 2c-i**, the skeletal muscle should be decellularized, lyophilized, and ground to form a dry powder. The SMdECM powder is then digested in the presence of the enzyme pepsin and then neutralized and incubated at physiologic temperature to form a stable gel network. Fu *et al.* [46] investigated the injectability of an SMdECM pre-gel solution and demonstrated its ability to undergo *in situ* gelation at body temperature (**Figure 2c-ii**). The SMdECM pre-gel solution was injected subcutaneously into the abdomen of rats. The analysis of the sacrificed animals indicated that a minimum incubation time of 30 min at body temperature was required to solidify the SMdECM solution. Improved hydrogel shape retention was observed 24 hours after injection. The structural integrity and biocompatibility of the injectable SMdECM hydrogels provide a strong foundation for their potential use in regenerating injured skeletal muscle tissue through minimally invasive therapy.

Sarcopenia is a degenerative muscle disease associated with muscle loss due to immobility or aging. An *et al.* [25] developed an injectable cell-free hybrid hydrogel composed of aldehyde-modified hyaluronic acid conjugated with pyrogallol groups (AH-PG) and SMdECM for treating sarcopenia. The study showed that the self-crosslinkable hydrogel activates endogenous satellite stem cells (Pax7+/MyoD+ cells) and myocytes (Pax7–/MyoD+ cells), thereby treating mouse models with disuse-induced muscle atrophy. This study supports the effect of a cell-free AH-PG/SMdECM hydrogel in recruiting endogenous satellite stem cells to contribute to muscle regeneration *via* proliferation, migration, and differentiation. Furthermore, the impact of a hybrid hydrogel was assessed on muscle recovery in an age-related muscle atrophy model. Histological examination revealed that larger muscle fibers were formed in the hybrid hydrogel-treated group compared to the phosphate-buffered saline-treated and SMdECM-treated groups. Overall, the hybrid AH-PG/SMdECM hydrogel showed promising muscle mass recovery, vascularization, and innervation in both age-related and disuse muscle atrophy models. Wang *et al.* [67] developed an *in situ*–forming photocurable composite hydrogel composed of silk fibroin methacryloyl (SilMA) and SMdECM. The composite hydrogel possessed an interconnected porous structure that facilitated the transportation of oxygen and nutrients and the exchange of metabolites necessary for cell survival. The benefits from the tissue-specific biochemical cues delivered by an SMdECM hydrogel actively contributed to regulating muscle cell growth. However, the decellularization and enzymatic digestion processes mitigate the final mechanical properties of SMdECM hydrogels, and as such, they fall way behind the mechanical performance of native skeletal muscle tissue. The addition of SilMA to SMdECM could enhance the mechanical properties to around 10 kPa, which is in the same order as native skeletal muscle tissue. The composite hydrogel's degradation rate was also reduced compared to an SMdECM-only hydrogel.

Another study showed that BdECM hydrogels promote the osteogenic differentiation of mesenchymal stem cells (MSCs) and adipose stem cells (ASCs) and support new bone formation after transplantation [68]. BdECM hydrogels also encouraged the osteogenic differentiation of C2C12 and mouse primary calvarial cells, both in the presence and absence of osteogenic medium [43]. The expression of osteogenic markers, including osteocalcin and osteopontin, was also enhanced due to the regulatory function of biochemical cues preserved in BdECM hydrogels, thereby confirming the promotion of cell differentiation toward the osteogenic lineage. The osteogenic induction of BdECM hydrogels on dental pulp stem cells was further exhibited by the enhanced expression of Runt-related transcription factor 2 and bone sialoprotein in comparison to collagen type I hydrogels [69]. However, the demineralization process using acidic treatment coupled with the decellularization process leads to the loss of inherent mineral content (e.g., calcium-based and phospho-based components), which significantly diminishes the mechanical properties of BdECM hydrogels compared to native bone tissue [41].

3.5. *Three-Dimensional-Printed Scaffolds Incorporated with Decellularized Extracellular Matrix Materials*

3D printing is an additive manufacturing technique that has been extensively applied for the fabrication of custom-designed and patient-specific scaffolds based on the defect parameters measured using magnetic resonance imaging or computed tomography scans [63]. This approach allows control over the general anatomical and interconnected porous structure within the 3D-printed construct to regulate cellular behavior and nutritional transport [70]. It is noteworthy that 3D printing is distinct from the bioprinting technique in the very important aspect that it does not include direct incorporation of viable cells into the inks, while the cell-laden bioinks are utilized for bioprinting [40]. Nevertheless, cell seeding on scaffolds postprinting can always be carried out. Both natural and synthetic polymers have been successfully employed for the 3D printing of dECM-incorporated scaffolds for TE applications [18, 41]. Recently, gelatin hydrogel scaffolds reinforced with BdECM particles with a mean diameter of 100 μm were fabricated using 3D printing technology (**Figures 3a-i and 3a-ii**) [18]. Varying concentrations of BdECM (1, 3, and 5% w/v) were incorporated into gelatin hydrogel. It was shown that increasing the BdECM content improved the mechanical modulus, while printability and shape fidelity were diminished beyond 5% w/v BdECM (**Figure 3a-iii**). The 3D-printed scaffolds also supported the viability, adhesion, and proliferation of MC3T3 cells, due to the bioactivity of collagen and hydroxyapatite components preserved within the BdECM particles.

dECM-derived hydrogels are another example of natural biomaterials that can be used as ink materials for the 3D printing of scaffolds for targeted TERM applications [71]. It has been shown that the intrinsic components within a BdECM hydrogel, including various proteins, GFs, GAGs, and cytokines, can effectively enhance the regeneration of damaged bone tissue [68]. However, the mechanical strength of a BdECM hydrogel cannot replicate the mechanical properties of native bone [72]. In other words, despite the biocompatibility and cell-friendly microenvironment provided by 3D-printed scaffolds composed of natural polymers, their mechanical durability does not satisfy the criteria for hard tissues, such as load-bearing bone [73]. Hence, scaffolds fabricated by the 3D printing of synthetic thermoplastic polymers (e.g., PCL, PLGA, and PLA) have been considered a reasonable alternative **(Figure 3b-i)**. Recently, 3D-printed PCL scaffolds with a diameter of 6 mm were implanted into 8 mm rat calvarial defects **(Figure 3b-ii)** [41]. Herein, the gap between the bone defect and scaffold was filled with either a BdECM hydrogel, β-TCP powder, or the slurry-like material composed of β-TCP dispersed in a BdECM hydrogel. TCP is an osteoconductive bioceramic that possesses a chemical composition similar to the minerals of native bone tissue [74]. Although BdECM provides a complex mixture of various tissue-specific biochemical cues, the decellularization and demineralization processes reduce the calcium and phosphate content of native bone tissue. Therefore, the combination of BdECM and TCP can be considered an appropriate option to replicate the similar composition of native bone. Notably, the most accelerated bone regeneration was yielded by the TCP–BdECM scaffold **(Figures 3b-ii and 3b-iii)** [41]. In another study [70], the synergistic effect of β-TCP and a BdECM hydrogel was evaluated in 3D-printed porous PCL or PCL/β-TCP-based scaffolds filled with BdECM hydrogel. The BdECM hydrogel aims to compensate for the lack of cell adhesion on the hydrophobic PCL scaffold surface. The alkaline phosphatase expression of MC3T3-E1 cells seeded on the 3D-printed scaffolds determined that incorporating both β-TCP and BdECM significantly promoted early osteogenic differentiation compared to scaffolds containing only one of these additive components. Alizarin red S staining also confirmed improved results during late osteogenic differentiation in the PCL/β-TCP/BdECM scaffold. Overall, the combination of β-TCP as an inorganic material with a BdECM hydrogel as an organic biomaterial is a promising approach to support osteogenic differentiation *in vitro* and to augment bone regeneration *in vivo* [41, 70].

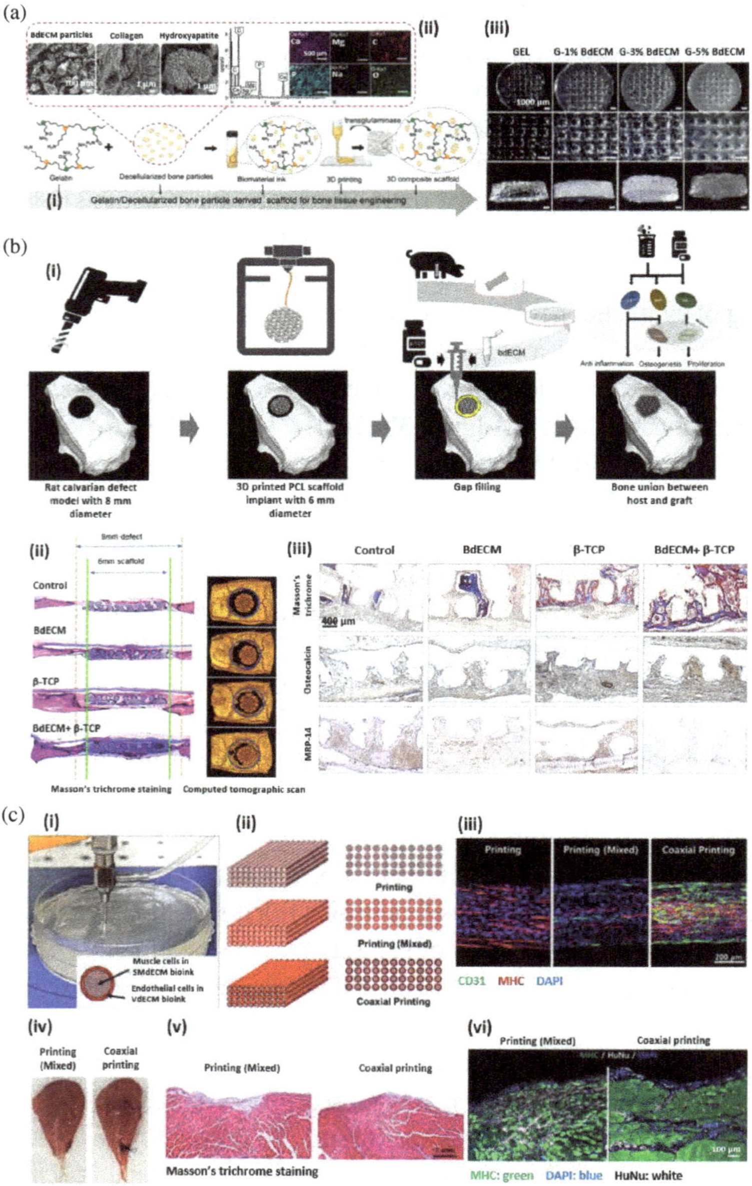

Figure 3. (*Continued*)

3.6. *Decellularized Extracellular Matrix–Based Bioprinted Tissue-Engineered Constructs*

Although the 3D printing process provides a practical route for fabricating custom-designed scaffolds, the lack of cells embedded in the ink biomaterial restricts its potential for an active regenerating process or biomimicking the target tissues [40]. Cell-laden bioprinting offers a spectacular opportunity to recapitulate tissue-specific biophysical cues of native tissues and organs [75]. It also enables the positioning of different cell-laden bioinks in anatomically relevant, predetermined locations to mimic

Figure 3. (***Continued on facing pages***) (**a**) Incorporation of BdECM particles into natural scaffolds for bone TE applications [Reprinted from ref. [18], Copyright (2022), with permission from Elsevier]. (**a-i**) Schematic representation of a BdECM-incorporated gelatin ink for 3D printing of a bone scaffold. (**a-ii**) SEM images of BdECM particles composed of collagen and hydroxyapatite crystals. (**a-iii**) Top and side view photographs of 3D-printed gelatin-based scaffolds containing various concentrations of BdECM particles. (**b**) Synergistic osteogenic activity of a BdECM hydrogel and β-TCP particles for treating bone fractures [Reproduced with permission from Yun *et al.* [41], *International Journal of Molecular Sciences*, published by MDPI, 2021]. (**b-i**) Schematic representation of bone defects treated with 3D-printed PCL scaffolds in combination with a BdECM hydrogel, β-TCP powder, or β-TCP-incorporated BdECM hydrogel. (**b-ii**) Masson's trichrome staining and computed tomographical scanning of bone defects treated with different groups. In Masson's trichrome staining, red stains represent soft tissue, and blue stains represent the newly formed bone tissue, which was intensified in the BdECM/β-TCP treatment group. (**b-iii**) Histological analysis using Masson's trichrome staining and IHC examination using osteocalcin and MRP-14 staining of bone defects implanted with different groups of 3D-printed scaffolds. (**c**) Bioprinting of pre-vascularized muscle constructs for the treatment of VML injury [Reprinted from ref. [22], Copyright (2019), with permission from Elsevier]. (**c-i**) Bioprinting of pre-vascularized constructs through a coaxial nozzle consisting of muscle cells embedded within an SMdECM bioink in the core and an endothelial cell-encapsulated VdECM bioink in the shell. (**c-ii**) Three types of bioprinted constructs made from (1) hSMC-embedded SMdECM bioink, (2) a mixed hSMC-encapsulated SMdECM and a HUVEC-encapsulated VdECM, and (3) a coaxial construct composed of hSMC-encapsulated SMdECM as the core and a HUVEC-encapsulated VdECM as the shell. (**c-iii**) IF imaging of 3D-bioprinted constructs. (**c-iv**) The gross observation of VML-injured models treated with pre-vascularized mixed and coaxial bioprinted constructs. (**c-v**) Histological Masson's trichrome staining of treated injured muscles. (**c-vi**) IF staining of treated injured muscles.

the architectural features of target tissue [24]. Lee *et al.* [76] used a methacrylated bone-derived decellularized extracellular matrix (BdEMA)–sodium alginate composite hydrogel to improve the biological activity and rapid photocrosslinking ability of BdEMA in combination with the appropriate processability of alginate. The results revealed that the 3D-bioprinted construct containing BdEMA not only supported the viability and proliferation of encapsulated cells but also promoted higher mineralization rates. Even though two crosslinking approaches using $CaCl_2$ aerosol spraying and UV photocrosslinking were applied, the mechanical modulus of the 3D-bioprinted construct (90.4 ± 14.9 MPa) was still much lower than that of the native bone tissue (10.9–34.3 GPa for cortical bone and 0.01–1.61 GPa for cancellous bone [4]).

SMdECM-derived hydrogels are suitable for encapsulating muscle cells without compromising their viability and biological functionality [36]. Therefore, they have paved the way for use as a tissue-specific bioink for 3D bioprinting applications. Choi *et al.* [53] developed functional skeletal muscle constructs with various shapes and pore designs by bioprinting a C2C12 cell–encapsulated SMdECM bioink inside a PCL framework, which served as supporting constraints. The constructs were incubated at 37°C for 60 min to allow gelation of the SMdECM bioink. Confocal IF images affirmed the uniform distribution of aligned cells inside the printed patterns. Fluorescence imaging of MHCs also showed that the bioprinted constructs supported myotube formation even more than a collagen bioink. The striated band patterns observed in the constructs further confirmed myotube maturation, contributing to the contractile function of muscular constructs. Quantitative analysis of morphometric characteristics indicated that tissue-specific SMdECM significantly enhanced myotube length, width, area, and fusion index compared to a collagen bioink. Therefore, the SMdECM bioink could facilitate the formation of multinucleated aligned muscle fibers with functional contractile behavior upon electrical stimulation [53]. However, the low mechanical and rheological properties of the bioink limited the resolution of large-scale tissue constructs with featured architectural elements. To overcome this shortcoming, another study [22] showed bioprinting complex structures into a gelatin granules–PVA bath to fabricate myoblast-cell-embedded constructs for VML treatment (**Figure 3c-i**). This technique enabled bioprinting volumetric intricate constructs without needing a supporting framework printed from synthetic polymers. Treatment of a VML defect model with three groups of either an SMdECM hydrogel, an SMdECM sponge, or a bioprinted SMdECM construct showed that the bioprinted construct provided the best therapeutic outcome in terms of muscle contractility. However, this approach resulted in only about a 70% improvement in functionality compared to the uninjured control group. These findings highlighted the necessity of additional considerations on bioprinted constructs to further improve the medically expected functions. Therefore, three further bioprinted groups — (i) human skeletal muscle cells (hSMCs)-encapsulated SMdECM bioink, (ii) a mixture of hSMC-encapsulated SMdECM and HUVEC-encapsulated vascular-derived decellularized extracellular matrix (VdECM) bioink, and (iii) a bioprinted core–shell fibrillar construct composed of a hSMC-encapsulated SMdECM bioink (as the core material) and a HUVEC-encapsulated VdECM bioink (as the shell material) — were fabricated to investigate the effect of pre-vascularization on the functionality of treated VML injuries (**Figure 3c-ii**). IF staining of MHCs within the constructs revealed the formation of aligned myotubes in all three bioprinted groups, while endothelial network formation was significantly enhanced in the coaxially bioprinted group (**Figure 3c-iii**). The expression of MHC and CD31 in the mixed bioprinted group appeared distinct from each other, suggesting the contrariwise effect of myotube and endothelial cells on each other's growth during co-culture. Nevertheless, the compartmentalized design of the coaxially bioprinted constructs inhibited this effect by promoting myotube formation in the core part and endothelial network formation in the shell. Both mixed and coaxial pre-vascularized constructs were implanted in VML injuries, and a large portion of muscle volume was recovered in both treatment groups (**Figure 3c-iv**). Meanwhile, Masson's trichrome histological staining showed that more fibrotic tissue (i.e., scar) was deposited in the treated group with a mixed bioprinted construct (**Figure 3c-v**). Although newly formed muscle fibers were observed in both treated groups with pre-vascularized bioprinted constructs, they were better distributed in the coaxial bioprinted group (**Figure 3C-vi).** In another work, dual photocrosslinking and thermal crosslinking processes were used to enhance the mechanical and rheological properties of SMdECM bioinks [77]. This process enabled 3D bioprinting of various intricate structures, such as lattices, planes, cylindrical patterns, and more anatomically relevant geometries, including the nose and ear. It was shown that the dual crosslinking approach enhanced the structural integrity of printed plane constructs, which showed proper flexibility and could be folded without getting torn.

Recent studies denote that taking advantage of both biochemical and biophysical (i.e., topographical) cues may exhibit a synergistic effect on developing functional myotubes [34, 52]. Accordingly, uniaxially patterned scaffolds were fabricated by bioprinting the SMdEMA–PVA mixture, followed by leaching out the aligned PVA as the sacrificial component during the first 24 hours of the culture period [34]. The SMdEMA composition in the 3D-bioprinted constructs with or without topographical features supported the elongation of encapsulated myoblast cells relative to GelMA (as the control group). Long-term culture of the bioprinted constructs showed that the structures fabricated using SMdEMA with uniaxially topographical cues supported the formation and maturation of multinucleated myotubes in the direction of the printing path. Moreover, the IF staining of bioprinted constructs with sarcomeric α-actinin determined distinctive striated sarcomeres in SMdEMA-containing structures regardless of topographical features as opposed to the GelMA group containing topographical cues.

Studies have shown that electrical stimulation has an enormous effect on cellular activities, such as myogenic differentiation of myoblasts, morphological changes, and uniaxial alignment of cells by regulating membrane potential or ion transportation [78]. Cells are capable of sensing extrinsic electrical fields *via* voltage-gated ion channels that can affect their cytoskeletal organization, migration, proliferation, and differentiation through the activation of a number of signaling pathways [79]. However, applying a strong electrical field (i.e., >1 $kV.mm^{-1}$) or an electrical field for a long time (e.g., >2 s) can potentially damage the cell membrane and cause cell death [52]. In an innovative study, the bioprinting of skeletal muscle constructs was coupled with *in situ* electrical stimulation, designated as the E-printing process [52]. An electrical field of 0.7 $kV.mm^{-1}$ was applied between the nozzle tip and the ground during the bioprinting process of a photocrosslinkable hASC-laden SMdEMA bioink. Examination of the bioprinted constructs with or without *in situ* electrical stimulation showed that more aligned F-actin fibers were developed in electrically stimulated bioprinted constructs. Striated muscle fibers were only developed in E-printed muscle constructs, regardless of the culture in the growth medium or myogenic medium, which was not observed in nonstimulated alternatives.

4. Modulating the Inherent Properties of Decellularized Extracellular Matrix–Based Biomaterials for Bone and Muscle Tissue Engineering

4.1. *Exogenous Bioactive Components for Enhancement of the Regenerating Capacity*

As discussed in previous sections, dECM biomaterials provide a unique cell-friendly microenvironment that cannot be replicated by simply mixing an extensive range of tissue-specific biomolecules and components. However, the decellularization and digestion process of dECM materials has been shown to diminish their intrinsic biochemical cues [80]. For instance, the decellularization of bone tissue as a bone substitute biomaterial has exhibited less osteoinductivity compared to intact bone [81]. Yet, the decellularization of native tissues as a source of biomaterial is inevitable due to the intense immunological responses associated with the innate cellular components, which lead to host rejection of the transplanted scaffold [1]. As a result, the inclusion of bioactive therapeutic agents, such as GFs, into dECM-based scaffolds is considered a promising route to compensate for this loss in the bioactive components, thereby boosting the development and regeneration of target tissues [82]. The FDA approved PDGF for the treatment of ankle fusion. It exerts an indirect effect on bone regeneration within large defects by recruiting stem cells into the defect site and promoting their migration and proliferation [83]. Rindone *et al.* [62] developed a biomimetic delivery system to attach PDGF to heparin-conjugated BdECM (HC-BdECM) particles that enabled the sustained release of PDGF over a 21-day period. The implantation of a PCL-fibrin graft containing HC-BdECM/PDGF into a murine critical-size bone defect over a 12-week study period encouraged mineral deposition and bone formation due to the activation of osteogenic signaling that was induced by the sustained release of PDGF. Developing vascularized bone grafts coupled with osteogenic properties is crucial for inhibiting osteonecrosis upon implantation [84]. The hydrogels utilized as bone substitutes mostly lack vascularization due to their dense structure, which hampers the proper transportation of nutrients and metabolites [85]. Wu *et al.* [86] fabricated a porous bone-mimetic hydrogel based on GelMA–polyethylene oxide (PEO) containing demineralized bone matrix (DBM) particles, as an osteogenic ingredient, and PLGA-encapsulated VEGF microspheres, as an angiogenic ingredient. The interconnected micropores within hydrogels were prepared by the photocrosslinking of GelMA and the subsequent leaching of the PEO component to satisfy mass transport. The osteogenic-angiogenic porous hydrogel supported the viability, migration, and osteogenic differentiation of MSCs *in vitro* and encouraged vascularized bone regeneration *in vivo*. The vascularization of an implanted porous hydrogel, as opposed to a nonporous equivalent, was supported by (i) easier infiltration of host blood vessels into the porous hydrogel network and (ii) enhanced angiogenesis due to the sustained release of VEGF. Platelet-rich plasma (PRP), as a plasma-related product, is considered a rich source of various GFs and cytokines, such as TGF-β, IGF, and PDGF [87]. It has been shown that the incorporation of PRP under negative pressure into a BdECM bone substitute stimulates higher levels of new bone formation within a critical-size radial defect compared to empty or PRP-free-treated defects [81]. The lack of calcium and phosphate constituents within DBM is known to limit its application as an efficient bone graft [88]. Inorganic osteoconductive materials, such as TCP, bioglass, and hydroxyapatite crystals, have shown promising results in compensating for the loss of minerals within DBM and BdECM scaffolds [72, 89]. Incorporating TCP in the form of a powder or granule into a BdECM hydrogel containing DBM particles showed similar *in vitro* results in terms of the promotion of osteogenesis [88]. However, the implantation of hydrogels into a femoral defect in a rabbit model determined that the incorporation of granular TCP into the hydrogel scaffold supported bone regeneration, while the TCP powder itself stimulated the formation of fibrous dysplasia. This observation was attributed to the sustained release of calcium and phosphate from the granules of TCP over the bone-regenerating period. Besides, the granules of TCP could better activate osteoblasts and encourage angiogenesis for improved bone repair *in vivo* [90].

Recent studies have shown that incorporating a myogenic-inducing factor (i.e., IGF-1) into a scaffold affected the migration, proliferation, and differentiation of muscle satellite cells, myoblasts, and muscle progenitor cells, thereby promoting the regeneration of injured muscle tissue [91]. It was also shown that the controlled and sustained release of IGF-1 from a scaffold into the injury site over the regeneration period influenced its functionality. *In vitro* assays on nonwoven fibrous poly(L-lactic acid) (PLLA) embedded within an SMdECM hydrogel with or without IGF-1 **(Figures 4a-i and 4a-ii)** showed that incorporating IGF-1 enhanced the myogenic differentiation of C2C12 cells when cultured in differentiation medium [36]. Treatment of a rabbit tibialis anterior muscle defect with an SMdECM-embedded PLLA scaffold for 2 months showed that IGF-1 decreased the infiltration of inflammatory cells and reduced collagen deposition **(Figure 4a-iii)**. IHC staining of MHC in implanted scaffolds also affirmed that IGF-1 enhanced the formation of myofibers. Furthermore, in another study [31], loading IGFBP-3-conjugated IGF-1 into the SMdECM tissue enhanced its half-life. Although the burst release of IGF-1 up to day 1 was observed in both IGF-1-loaded and IGF-1/IGFBP-3-loaded scaffolds, the formation of the IGF-1/IGFBP-3 complex prolonged the release of IGF-1 from SMdECM scaffolds for up to 28 days. It was proposed that the initial burst release activated myoblasts, while the extended release of the remaining IGF-1 over time promoted cell proliferation and migration [31].

The ECM composition is tissue-specific and may vary significantly between different tissue origins; thereby, the ECM composition of a specific tissue type obtained from different animals and species may show distinctive characteristics [92]. This fact implies the importance of the selected animal/human source on the therapeutic properties of derived dECM TECs [93]. Thrombospondin-2 (TSP2) is known for its antiangiogenic properties [94]. Studies have shown that dECM hydrogels derived from genetically engineered mice lacking TSP2 can enhance angiogenesis during wound healing without the need for exogenic proangiogenic factors [95]. Recently, SMdECM hydrogels derived from skeletal muscle

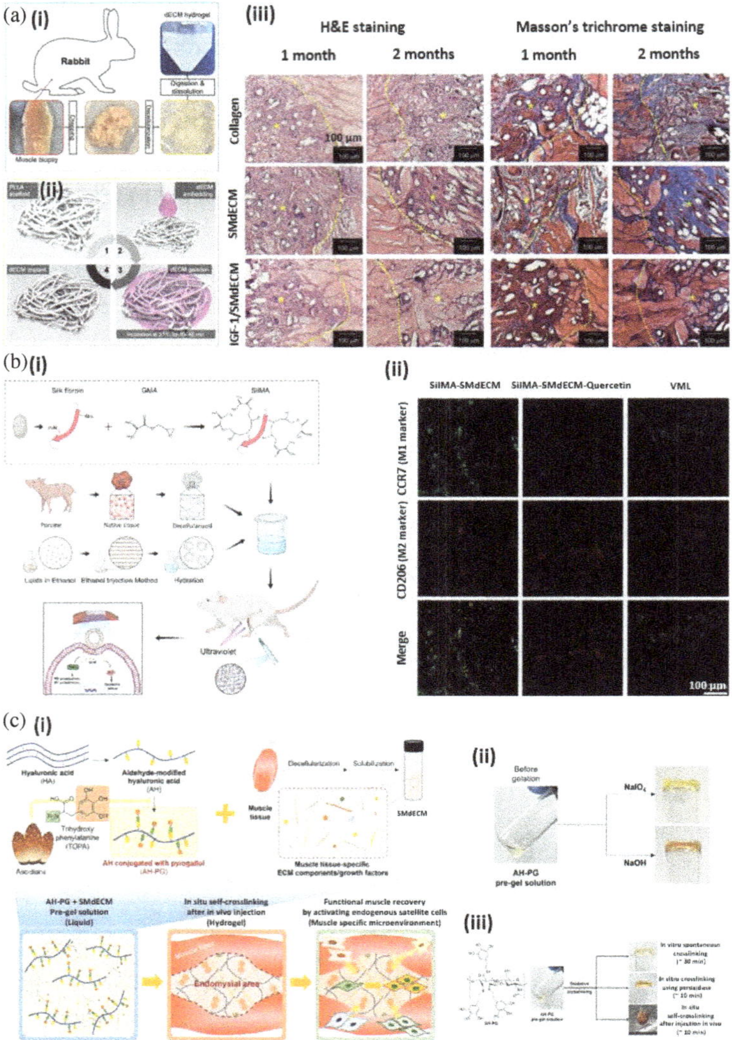

Figure 4. (a) The effect of an IGF-1-loaded SMdECM-based scaffold on muscle regeneration [Reprinted from ref. [36], Copyright (2019), with permission from Elsevier]. **(a-i)** Preparation of a hydrogel from decellularized skeletal muscle tissue. **(a-ii)** Schematic representation of various fabrication steps for scaffolds, including (1) a PLLA scaffold, (2) embedding of an SMdECM pre-gel solution, (3) inducing thermal gelation by incubating the SMdECM-loaded PLLA scaffold at 37 °C for 30–45 min, and (4) implantation of a scaffold. **(a-iii)** Histological staining of implanted PLLA scaffolds filled with collagen hydrogel, SMdECM hydrogel, or IGF-1-loaded SMdECM after 1 and 2 months (*illustrates

tissue from two different murine strains (i.e., C57BL/6J WT and TSP2KO mice) were prepared [92]. Proteomic analyses showed that some ECM components, such as collagenous proteins, were differently expressed in the skeletal muscles derived from the two genotypes. A tube formation assay using HUVECs determined that more tubes were formed within an SMdECM hydrogel derived from TSP2KO mice than WT mice. The *in situ* SMdECM hydrogel gelation technique was employed by subcutaneous injection of SMdECM pre-gel solutions. The IF staining of CD31 and α-smooth muscle actin indicated that vessels were only formed in animals treated with SMdECM hydrogels derived from TSP2KO mice. The results of this study affirm that removing TSP2 in genetically engineered mice promotes the formation of neovessels in defects treated with TSP2KO-derived dECM hydrogels.

4.2. *Regulating the Immune Responses of Decellularized Extracellular Matrix Materials*

Macrophages form a major component of the immune cell population and are classified as (i) M1 macrophages with pro-inflammatory activity and (ii) M2 macrophages with anti-inflammatory and pro-healing activity [67]. M1 macrophages are known to influence the activation and migration of satellite cells, while M2 macrophages facilitate the differentiation

←

Figure 4. (***Continued on facing pages***) the implanted region, and empty circle spaces within images are attributed to remaining PLLA scaffolds). **(b)** Immunoregulation of muscle tissue regeneration through the incorporation of quercetin as an antioxidant agent [Reprinted from ref. [67], Copyright (2022), with permission from Elsevier]. **(b-i)** Schematic representation of the preparation of photocrosslinkable SilMA–SMdECM hydrogel incorporated with quercetin-loaded liposomes for treating VML injuries in the rat model. **(b-ii)** IF imaging of CCR7 as the M1 marker and CD206 as the M2 marker for detecting macrophage polarization 14 days postoperation. **(c)** Development of a hybrid self-crosslinking hydrogel for muscle regeneration [Reprinted from ref. [25], Copyright (2024), with permission from Elsevier]. **(c-i)** Schematic representation of an *in situ* self-crosslinking AH-PG hydrogel containing SMdECM as a tissue-specific bioactive component for recovery of muscle injuries. **(c-ii)** Crosslinking of AH-PG hydrogel using oxidizing agents. **(c-iii)** Oxidative crosslinking of an AH-PG pre-gel solution under various *in vitro* or *in vivo* conditions.

of satellite cells and promote myotube formation [28]. Therefore, the polarization of macrophages toward the M2 phase is an important factor that affects the regeneration of muscle injuries. In this regard, treating VML injuries with electrospun SMdECM–PCL scaffolds showed a prolonged presence of M1 macrophages at the injury site, as evaluated by the expression of inducible nitric oxide synthase, followed by the onset of anti-inflammatory M2 macrophages at the later stage of treatment (i.e., 28 days), which expressed arginase [28]. These results propose the possible inherent immunomodulating effect of the SMdECM scaffold. Inflammation within large muscle defects, such as those occurring with VML, forms oxidant components (e.g., reactive oxygen species [ROS]) at the injured site, which hampers muscle tissue regeneration due to oxidative stress [96]. Quercetin is a natural polyphenol flavonoid compound with antioxidant and inflammation-suppressive properties [97]. Wang *et al.* [67] introduced quercetin-loaded liposomes into a composite SilMA–SMdECM hydrogel to mitigate oxidative stress through ROS clearance and regulate the polarization of macrophages during muscle regeneration (**Figure 4b-i**). Treatment of VML injuries with the quercetin-loaded SilMA–SMdECM hydrogel showed less collagen deposition and more muscle fiber regeneration than the hydrogel without quercetin. The IF images of treated VML injuries 14 days postoperation revealed that the incorporation of quercetin-loaded liposomes into the SilMA–SMdECM hydrogel increased the expression of CD206 (i.e., a surface marker on M2 macrophages) and decreased the expression of CCR7 (i.e., a surface marker on M1 macrophages), representing a shift from the M1 to M2 phenotype (**Figure 4b-ii**). The ROS scavenging properties of quercetin were also confirmed by comparing the IF staining of ROS following VML injury.

4.3. *Mechanical Reinforcement of Bone and Muscle Decellularized Extracellular Matrix Materials*

dECM hydrogels have successfully been adopted for TE applications due to their unique properties, including biocompatibility, tissue-specific biochemical and biophysical cues, and low immunogenicity [37]. However, their limited mechanical strength and stability upon exposure to decellularization solutions and subsequent enzymatic digestion pose challenges for fabricating constructs with complex geometries [34]. Besides, the thermally induced crosslinking of dECM hydrogels is a time-consuming phenomenon that may deteriorate the shape fidelity of printed constructs [77]. So far, different approaches, including the incorporation of supplementary natural polymers [75], reinforcement using nanomaterials [42], utilization of supportive frameworks made from synthetic thermoplastic materials [53], and crosslinking of the dECM network [98], have been utilized to improve the strength of dECM-derived biomaterials for better fit to expected therapeutic outcomes. In the following sections, two methods of chemical crosslinking and photocrosslinking will be presented and discussed.

4.3.1. *Conventional Crosslinking Using Chemical Reagents*

The thermally crosslinked dECM-derived hydrogels lack suitable mechanical properties and may degrade quickly in the grafted site, interfering with the expected time for full regeneration [28]. Smoak *et al.* [21] chemically crosslinked electrospun SMdECM scaffolds through exposure to GA vapor. The degree of crosslinking was assessed by determining the level of free amine groups using the ninhydrin assay. The study showed that exposure to GA vapor for 30 min resulted in 70.4% ± 4.7% crosslinking, while increasing the exposure time to 24 hours led to almost 100% crosslinking. The higher crosslinking density of electrospun scaffolds was reflected in their higher tensile modulus. However, GA crosslinking imposed adverse effects on cellular activities since the cells on the 24-hour crosslinked scaffolds were less confluent compared to uncrosslinked and 30-min crosslinked counterparts. This might be due to the fewer free amine groups available on 24-hour crosslinked scaffolds since the free amine groups are known for their positive effect on cell adhesion. Furthermore, no myotube formation was observed for C2C12 cells seeded on 24-hour crosslinked scaffolds cultured in a differentiation induction medium. Nevertheless, the 30-minute crosslinked scaffold with highly aligned architecture led to better myotube alignment, emphasizing the synergistic effect of both fiber alignment of the scaffold and proper mechanical properties. In a study conducted by An *et al.* [25], a self-crosslinkable hybrid hydrogel was designed by combining AH-PG with

SMdECM (**Figure 4c-i**). The AH-PG constituent of the hybrid hydrogel enhanced the stability, delayed biodegradation, and provided tissue adhesiveness, while the SMdECM provided the muscle tissue-specific bioactive cues necessary for muscle regeneration. As shown in **Figure 4c-ii**, self-crosslinking of AH-PG could be initiated by adding $NaIO_4$ or by increasing the pH to 7.5 (e.g., using NaOH) [25]. *In situ* and *in vivo* oxidative crosslinking of the hydrogel was also feasible, possibly due to the presence of peroxidase enzymes or ROS within the body (**Figure 4c-iii**). The results of these studies affirmed that a similar oxidative crosslinking ability could be attained using 0.6–6 $U.mL^{-1}$ horseradish peroxidase without imposing toxicity in C2C12 cells *in vitro*.

4.3.2. *Rapid Crosslinking via Photosensitive Moieties*

Kim *et al.* [34] used a methacrylated SMdECM hydrogel (SMdEMA) to enable rapid photocrosslinking of dECM-derived hydrogels in the presence of a photoinitiator (e.g., Irgacure 2959). Their results showed that altering the photocrosslinking parameters, such as the degree of methacrylation or light intensity, can enhance the viscoelastic properties. For instance, increasing the methacrylation degree from 30% to 80% at a constant concentration (i.e., 3 wt%) significantly enhanced the mechanical modulus after light exposure. Increasing UV power from 181 to 410 $mW.cm^{-2}$ not only influenced the same parameter but also improved the printability of the lattice constructs. However, the possible side effects of the photocrosslinking process on cell viability should be considered, as results indicated cell death after the exposure of the cell-laden SMdEMA hydrogels to light intensities higher than 300 $mW.cm^{-2}$. Kim *et al.* [52] used an *in situ* photocrosslinking method for hASC-laden SMdEMA bioinks by coupling a transparent Teflon tube to the nozzle tip. It was shown that applying UV intensities higher than 500 $mW.cm^{-2}$ increased the risk of cell death due to the experience of higher wall–shear stresses as a result of enhanced viscosity and mechanical moduli.

Modifying dECM materials with methacrylic groups is the most frequent approach to enable photocrosslinkability. However, this modification is highly prone to diminish the bioactivity of dECM materials while inducing cytotoxicity [99]. Recently, Yeleswarapu *et al.* [77] introduced a photocrosslinking process for SMdECM hydrogels that does not involve chemical modification. They showed that the incorporation of Eosin Y as a photosensitizer, triethanolamine (TEA) as a co-initiator, and N-vinylpyrrolidone (NVP) as an accelerator comonomer into an unmodified SMdECM hydrogel improved mechanical properties upon exposure to light at a wavelength of 515 nm. This technique provided initial structural stability for bioprinting the SMdECM bioink to crosslink the outer surfaces of constructs. However, subsequent thermal processing is required to crosslink the inner parts through the self-assembly of collagenous components. The lack of sufficient crosslinking of the whole construct upon exposure to light might be due to the nonmodified dECM hydrogel since this photocrosslinking setup has shown better results for methacrylic functionalized corneal dECM hydrogels [98, 100]. The concentrations of the photocrosslinking agents (i.e., Eosin Y, TEA, and NVP) also require careful adjustment because the cell viability and morphology are highly affected by these agents. For instance, it was shown that lower cell viability and a round morphology were observed at concentrations higher than 0.03 mM [77]. Although dual crosslinking of SMdECM hydrogels significantly enhanced the mechanical properties, they still did not match the mechanical strength of native tissue. The selection of the photoinitiator is also important because each material is activated upon exposure to a specific range of light wavelengths. For instance, Irgacure 2959 is UV-sensitive, while Eosin Y is visible light responsive, which is a safer approach to avoid cell harm [101]. However, Eosin Y is a type II photoinitiator that lacks adequate crosslinking kinetics, thereby requiring a co-initiator and comonomer to accelerate the photocrosslinking process [77]. On the contrary, Irgacure is a type I photoinitiator that does not require the need for co-agents. In conclusion, each photoinitiator has its pros and cons. Therefore, the selection of a photoinitiator requires attention to every aspect of the photocrosslinking process, including the light source, cell viability, and crosslinking kinetics.

5. Applications and Prospects

The dECM-derived biomaterials have made progressive strides toward TERM by presenting innate biochemical and biophysical cues (i.e., nano- and micro-structural features) similar to native tissues [37]. The inherent biochemical cues preserved within dECM play a key role in regulating cellular activities, such as survival, viability, proliferation, migration, and differentiation into the intended lineage [70]. However, some critical requirements should be considered during the preparation of dECM biomaterials to ensure a balance between the envisioned properties. It is of utmost importance to make sure that cellular components and cell-associated antigens have been removed successfully from the target tissue to inhibit immune responses upon implantation [2]. It should also be noted that exposure to different decellularization reagents can mitigate the structural strength of the dECM material compared to the native tissue [3]. Besides, processing into a hydrogel form through enzymatic digestion may further decrease the mechanical properties. Mimicking the mechanical properties of the target tissue is critical in regulating cellular activities *in vitro* and restoring tissue functionality *in vivo* [1]. Therefore, chemical crosslinking, for example, using GA as the crosslinker agent [21], has shown promising effects in improving the mechanical properties of SMdECM scaffolds. However, the residual unreacted crosslinking agents are highly susceptible to inducing cytotoxicity and hampering biological properties [3]. Thus, it is essential to implement new modification approaches, such as photocrosslinking, to enhance both the structural integrity and mechanical durability of dECM biomaterials. The decellularization process may further influence the content of bioactive components within the dECM and lead to the loss of a portion of its components depending on the type and concentration of decellularization agents [40]. Hence, replenishing some types of bioactive components or GFs into dECM scaffolds may enhance their biomedical outcomes and repairing capacity [36].

The topographical features of scaffolds are known to guide the formation and organization of tissue-specific cells and have been adopted as a promising approach in the engineering of musculoskeletal constructs [34]. For example, the contractile function of the muscle cells in engineered skeletal muscle tissue-like constructs highly depends on the guidance of cells within engineered patterns [58]. Some fabrication techniques, such as electrospinning and 3D bioprinting, have shown reliable results in generating desired topographical cues [52]. 3D-bioprinted TECs made from dECM bioinks can also be used as *in vitro* modeling platforms for studying pathological conditions [40]. The bioprinted models, recapitulating physiological characteristics of the target tissue, can also be used for drug screening applications to explore the best combination of drugs to cure the intended condition [4]. Neuronal integration during muscle regeneration, through the interaction between myofibers formed in TECs and the neural network of host tissue, is a key factor in determining the functionality of recovered muscle tissue [52]. Applying electrical stimulation to tissue-engineered muscle-like constructs has shown promising results in the development of neuromuscular junctions [52]. Utilizing additional therapies, such as ultrasound, is reportedly useful in gaining some advantages to the medical outcomes of SMdECM-derived TECs for the regeneration of functional skeletal muscle tissues. Hence, it is worth further attention and focus in future studies [3].

The therapeutic function of different forms of dECM-derived scaffolds and TECs for treating musculoskeletal diseases has been examined *in vivo* in small animals, such as rats [3]. Yet, clinical studies on the employment of dECM for the recovery of musculoskeletal defects are in the early stage, and more clinical trials are required to translate these achievements from the laboratory into the clinic for the repair of human musculoskeletal injuries [102]. So far, the FDA-approved ECM-based grafts, including DBM, have shown promising clinical outcomes and bring hope for the approval of more tissue-specific dECM biomaterials in the near future [54]. However, the successful removal of immunogenic cellular components from dECM products should still be assessed meticulously because of failures that have occurred. For example, the remaining cells within commercial heart valves (i.e., the SynerGraft valve) led to the deaths of three patients [2]. Therefore, improved standardization testing is required to confirm the reproducibility and safety of dECM-based products when obtaining regulatory approval [1].

6. Conclusions

The musculoskeletal diseases caused by aging or traumatic accidents significantly affect both the physical activity and mental well-being of individuals. Musculoskeletal tissues possess excellent self-healing ability upon manageable injuries. However, in the case of critical-size defects, the inherent self-repair capacity is not adequate to recover whole tissue damage. In most cases, the injury is refilled with fibrotic tissue that lacks the intrinsic functionality of the target tissue. Autografts and allografts are gold standard medical treatments, but they are faced with a serious lack of supply. Therefore, the TECs containing pro-healing factors have been successfully adopted for the recruitment of resident stem cells to contribute to the regeneration of large-scale tissue loss. Among various biomaterials, the tissue-specific ECM materials (i.e., bone-derived ECM and skeletal muscle-derived ECM), introduced in this chapter, bring immense hope for functional TERM applications of bone and skeletal muscle, respectively. The potential of different types of dECM-based scaffolds, including decellularized tissue pieces, *in situ* forming injectable hydrogels, electrospun scaffolds, 3D-printed grafts, and bioprinted TECs, was presented and discussed. This chapter sheds light on the exquisite and unique function of tissue-specific dECM-based scaffolds in the regeneration of musculoskeletal injuries that could not be achieved by any other alternative candidate. Meanwhile, the decellularization and enzymatic digestion processes could pose significant challenges regarding inadequate mechanical and rheological properties for the fabrication of scaffolds with intricate biomimetic designs, as well as the loss of some inherent bioactive components, diminishing expected therapeutic outcomes. Therefore, the implementation of exogenous mediators (e.g., GFs), external stimulations (e.g., electrical fields and topographical cues), and additional crosslinking approaches (e.g., photocrosslinking) for fostering a more reassuring microenvironment using dECM materials should be explored. In summary, this chapter provided in-depth information about the applicability of dECM biomaterials for treating musculoskeletal diseases and provided potential solutions and road maps addressing their current shortcomings.

References

1. Liu H, Xing F, Yu P, Lu R, Ma S, Shakya S, et al. Biomimetic fabrication bioprinting strategies based on decellularized extracellular matrix for musculoskeletal tissue regeneration: Current status and future perspectives. *Mater. Des.* 2024;243:113072.

2. Zhang X, Chen X, Hong H, Hu R, Liu J, Liu C. Decellularized extracellular matrix scaffolds: Recent trends and emerging strategies in tissue engineering. *Bioact. Mater.* 2022;10:15–31.
3. Luo R, Hu R, Xu J, Yu P, Wu X, Zhe M, et al. Decellularized extracellular matrix as a promising biomaterial for musculoskeletal tissue regeneration. *Nanotechnol. Rev.* 2023;12(1):20230151.
4. Park W, Gao G, Cho DW. Tissue-specific decellularized extracellular matrix bioinks for musculoskeletal tissue regeneration and modeling using 3D bioprinting technology. *Int. J. Mol. Sci.* 2021;22(15):7837.
5. Wang Y, Pereira R, Peach C, Huang B, Vyas C, Bartolo P. Robotic in situ bioprinting for cartilage tissue engineering. *Int. J. Extreme Manuf.* 2023;5(3):032004.
6. Kwon H, Brown W, Lee C, Wang D, Paschos N, Hu J, et al. Surgical and tissue engineering strategies for articular cartilage and meniscus repair. *Nat. Rev. Rheumatol.* 2019;15(9):550–70.
7. Yun H, Song B, Shin D, Yin X, Truong M, Noh S, et al. Fabrication of decellularized meniscus extracellular matrix according to inner cartilaginous, middle transitional, and outer fibrous zones result in zone-specific protein expression useful for precise replication of meniscus zones. *Mater. Sci. Eng. C.* 2021;128:112312.
8. Wang B, Barceló X, Von Euw S, Kelly D. 3D printing of mechanically functional meniscal tissue equivalents using high concentration extracellular matrix inks. *Mater. Today Bio.* 2023;20:100624.
9. Li Z, Yan W, Zhao F, Wang H, Cheng J, Duan X, et al. Regional specific tunable meniscus decellularized extracellular matrix (MdECM) reinforced bioink promotes anisotropic meniscus regeneration. *Chem. Eng. J.* 2023;473:145209.
10. Chae S, Lee SS, Choi YJ, Hong DH, Gao G, Wang JH, et al. 3D cell-printing of biocompatible and functional meniscus constructs using meniscus-derived bioink. *Biomaterials.* 2021;267:120466.
11. Xia B, Kim D-H, Bansal S, Bae Y, Mauck RL, Heo S-J. Development of a decellularized meniscus matrix-based nanofibrous scaffold for meniscus tissue engineering. *Acta Biomater.* 2021;128:175–85.
12. Jin H, Kang Y, Gao H, Lin Z, Huang D, Zheng Z, et al. Decellularization-based modification strategy for bioactive xenografts promoting tendon repair. *Adv. Healthcare Mater.* 2024;13(4):2302660.
13. Anjum S, Li T, Saeed M, Ao Q. Exploring polysaccharide and protein-enriched decellularized matrix scaffolds for tendon and ligament repair: A review. *Int. J. Biol. Macromol.* 2023;254(Pt 2):127891.

14. McKee TJ, Perlman G, Morris M, Komarova SV. Extracellular matrix composition of connective tissues: A systematic review and meta-analysis. *Sci. Rep.* 2019;9(1):10542.
15. Eisner LE, Rosario R, Andarawis-Puri N, Arruda EM. The role of the non-collagenous extracellular matrix in tendon and ligament mechanical behavior: A review. *J. Biomech. Eng.* 2022;144(5):050801.
16. Blaudez F, Ivanovski S, Hamlet S, Vaquette C. An overview of decellularisation techniques of native tissues and tissue engineered products for bone, ligament and tendon regeneration. *Methods.* 2020;171:28–40.
17. Olszta MJ, Cheng X, Jee SS, Kumar R, Kim YY, Kaufman MJ, et al. Bone structure and formation: A new perspective. *Mater. Sci. Eng. R.* 2007; 58(3–5):77–116.
18. Kara A, Distler T, Polley C, Schneidereit D, Seitz H, Friedrich O, et al. 3D printed gelatin/decellularized bone composite scaffolds for bone tissue engineering: Fabrication, characterization and cytocompatibility study. *Mater. Today Bio.* 2022;15:100309.
19. Xu J, Yu L, Liu F, Wan L, Deng Z. The effect of cytokines on osteoblasts and osteoclasts in bone remodeling in osteoporosis: A review. *Front. Immunol.* 2023;14:1222129.
20. Cho D-W, Kim BS, Jang J, Gao G, Han W, Singh NK. *3D Bioprinting.* Berlin: Springer; 2019.
21. Smoak MM, Hogan KJ, Grande-Allen KJ, Mikos AG. Bioinspired electrospun dECM scaffolds guide cell growth and control the formation of myotubes. *Sci. Adv.* 2021;7(20):eabg4123.
22. Choi YJ, Jun YJ, Kim DY, Yi HG, Chae SH, Kang J, et al. A 3D cell printed muscle construct with tissue-derived bioink for the treatment of volumetric muscle loss. *Biomaterials.* 2019;206:160–9.
23. Nakada S, Yamashita Y, Akiba S, Shima T, Arikawa-Hirasawa E. Myocyte culture with decellularized skeletal muscle sheet with observable interaction with the extracellular matrix. *Bioengineering.* 2022;9(7):309.
24. Baiguera S, Del Gaudio C, Di Nardo P, Manzari V, Carotenuto F, Teodori L. 3D printing decellularized extracellular matrix to design biomimetic scaffolds for skeletal muscle tissue engineering. *Biomed Res. Int.* 2020;2020(1): 2689701.
25. An S, Jeon EJ, Kim M, Han SY, Song YS, Jeon J. Endomysium-permeable muscle extracellular matrix composite hydrogel for promoting functional muscle recovery in muscle atrophy. *Chem. Eng. J.* 2024;485:149906.

26. Boso D, Maghin E, Carraro E, Giagante M, Pavan P, Piccoli M. Extracellular matrix-derived hydrogels as biomaterial for different skeletal muscle tissue replacements. *Materials.* 2020;13(11):2483.
27. Seale P, Sabourin LA, Girgis-Gabardo A, Mansouri A, Gruss P, Rudnicki MA. Pax7 is required for the specification of myogenic satellite cells. *Cell.* 2000;102(6):777–86.
28. Patel KH, Talovic M, Dunn AJ, Patel A, Vendrell S, Schwartz M, et al. Aligned nanofibers of decellularized muscle extracellular matrix for volumetric muscle loss. *J. Biomed. Mater. Res. B.* 2020;108(6):2528–37.
29. Zhu G, Zhang T, Chen M, Yao K, Huang X, Zhang B, et al. Bone physiological microenvironment and healing mechanism: Basis for future bone-tissue engineering scaffolds. *Bioact. Mater.* 2021;6(11):4110–40.
30. Zhang W, Liu Y, Zhang H. Extracellular matrix: An important regulator of cell functions and skeletal muscle development. *Cell Biosci.* 2021; 11(1):65.
31. Shapiro L, Elsangeedy E, Lee H, Atala A, Yoo JJ, Lee SJ. In vitro evaluation of functionalized decellularized muscle scaffold for in situ skeletal muscle regeneration. *Biomed. Mater.* 2019;14(4):045015.
32. Smoak MM, Han A, Watson E, Kishan A, Grande-Allen KJ, Cosgriff-Hernandez E. Fabrication and characterization of electrospun decellularized muscle-derived scaffolds. *Tissue Eng. C.* 2019;25(5):276–87.
33. Zhang J, Hu ZQ, Turner NJ, Teng SF, Cheng WY, Zhou HY, et al. Perfusion-decellularized skeletal muscle as a three-dimensional scaffold with a vascular network template. *Biomaterials.* 2016;89:114–26.
34. Kim W, Lee H, Lee J, Atala A, Yoo JJ, Lee SJ, et al. Efficient myotube formation in 3D bioprinted tissue construct by biochemical and topographical cues. *Biomaterials.* 2020;230:119632.
35. Hurtgen BJ, Ward CL, Garg K, Pollot BE, Goldman SM, McKinley TO, et al. Severe muscle trauma triggers heightened and prolonged local musculoskeletal inflammation and impairs adjacent tibia fracture healing. *J. Musculoskelet. Neuronal Interact.* 2016;16(2):122–34.
36. Lee H, Ju YM, Kim I, Elsangeedy E, Lee JH, Yoo JJ, et al. A novel decellularized skeletal muscle-derived ECM scaffolding system for in situ muscle regeneration. *Methods.* 2020;171:77–85.
37. Kafili G, Niknejad H, Tamjid E, Simchi A. Amnion-derived hydrogels as a versatile platform for regenerative therapy: From lab to market. *Front. Bioeng. Biotechnol.* 2024;12:1358977.

38. Wang P, Gong Y, Zhou G, Ren W, Wang X. Biodegradable implants for internal fixation of fractures and accelerated bone regeneration. *ACS Omega.* 2023;8(31):27920–31.
39. Visscher DO, Farré-Guasch E, Helder MN, Gibbs S, Forouzanfar T, van Zuijlen PP, et al. Advances in bioprinting technologies for craniofacial reconstruction. *Trends Biotechnol.* 2016;34(9):700–10.
40. Kafili G, Kabir H, Kandeloos AJ, Golafshan E, Ghasemi S, Mashayekhan S, et al. Recent advances in soluble decellularized extracellular matrix for heart tissue engineering and organ modeling. *J. Biomater. Appl.* 2023; 38(5):577–604.
41. Yun S, Choi D, Choi DJ, Jin S, Yun WS, Huh JB, et al. Bone fracture-treatment method: Fixing 3D-printed polycaprolactone scaffolds with hydrogel type bone-derived extracellular matrix and β-tricalcium phosphate as an osteogenic promoter. *Int. J. Mol. Sci.* 2021;22(16):9084.
42. Kafili G, Tamjid E, Niknejad H, Simchi A. Development of printable nano-engineered composite hydrogels based on human amniotic membrane for wound healing application. *J. Mater. Sci.* 2023;58(30):12351–72.
43. Alom N, Peto H, Kirkham GR, Shakesheff KM, White LJ. Bone extracellular matrix hydrogel enhances osteogenic differentiation of C2C12 myoblasts and mouse primary calvarial cells. *J. Biomed. Mater. Res. B.* 2018; 106(2):900–8.
44. Sicari BM, Rubin JP, Dearth CL, Wolf MT, Ambrosio F, Boninger M, et al. An acellular biologic scaffold promotes skeletal muscle formation in mice and humans with volumetric muscle loss. *Sci. Transl. Med.* 2014;6(234): 234ra58–234ra58.
45. Badylak SF, Gilbert TW. Immune response to biologic scaffold materials. *Semin. Immunol.* 2008;20(2):109–16.
46. Fu Y, Fan X, Tian C, Luo J, Zhang Y, Deng L, et al. Decellularization of porcine skeletal muscle extracellular matrix for the formulation of a matrix hydrogel: A preliminary study. *J. Cell. Mol. Med.* 2016;20(4):740–9.
47. Gilbert TW, Sellaro TL, Badylak SF. Decellularization of tissues and organs. *Biomaterials.* 2006;27(19):3675–83.
48. Porzionato A, Sfriso MM, Pontini A, Macchi V, Petrelli L, Pavan PG, et al. Decellularized human skeletal muscle as biologic scaffold for reconstructive surgery. *Int. J. Mol. Sci.* 2015;16(7):14808–31.
49. Kafili G, Tamjid E, Niknejad H, Simchi A. Effect of pepsin digestion time on the properties of temperature sensitive human amniotic membrane derived hydrogel. *Modares J. Biotechnol.* 2023;13(3):113–31.

50. Kafili G, Tamjid E, Niknejad H, Simchi A. Concentration modulated microstructure and rheological properties of nanofibrous hydrogels derived from decellularized human amniotic membrane for 3D cell culture. *J. Mater. Sci.: Mater. Eng.* 2024;19(1):12.
51. Barajaa MA, Otsuka T, Ghosh D, Kan HM, Laurencin CT. Development of porcine skeletal muscle extracellular matrix–derived hydrogels with improved properties and low immunogenicity. *Proc. Natl. Acad. Sci. U.S.A.* 2024;121(19):e2322822121.
52. Kim W, Lee H, Lee CK, Kyung JW, An SB, Han I, et al. A bioprinting process supplemented with in situ electrical stimulation directly induces significant myotube formation and myogenesis. *Adv. Funct. Mater.* 2021; 31(51):2105170.
53. Choi Y-J, Kim TG, Jeong J, Yi H-G, Park JW, Hwang W, et al. 3D cell printing of functional skeletal muscle constructs using skeletal muscle-derived bioink. *Adv. Healthcare Mater.* 2016;5(20):2636–45.
54. Golebiowska AA, Intravaia JT, Sathe VM, Kumbar SG, Nukavarapu SP. Decellularized extracellular matrix biomaterials for regenerative therapies: Advances, challenges and clinical prospects. *Bioact. Mater.* 2024;32:98–123.
55. McInnes AD, Moser MA, Chen X. Preparation and use of decellularized extracellular matrix for tissue engineering. *J. Funct. Biomater.* 2022;13(4):240.
56. Allu I, Sahi AK, Koppadi M, Gundu S, Sionkowska A. Decellularization techniques for tissue engineering: Towards replicating native extracellular matrix architecture in liver regeneration. *J. Funct. Biomater.* 2023;14(10):518.
57. Gadre M, Kasturi M, Agarwal P, Vasanthan K. Decellularization and their significance for tissue regeneration in the era of 3D bioprinting. *ACS Omega.* 2024;9(7):7375–92.
58. Lee H, Kim WJ, Lee J, Yoo JJ, Kim GH, Lee SJ. Effect of hierarchical scaffold consisting of aligned dECM nanofibers and poly (lactide-co-glycolide) struts on the orientation and maturation of human muscle progenitor cells. *ACS Appl. Mater. Interfaces.* 2019;11(43):39449–58.
59. Hung BP, Naved BA, Nyberg EL, Dias M, Holmes CA, Elisseeff JH, et al. Three-dimensional printing of bone extracellular matrix for craniofacial regeneration. *ACS Biomater. Sci. Eng.* 2016;2(10):1806–16.
60. Crapo PM, Gilbert TW, Badylak SF. An overview of tissue and whole organ decellularization processes. *Biomaterials.* 2011;32(12):3233–43.
61. Sladkova M, Cheng J, Palmer M, Chen S, Lin C, Xia W, et al. Comparison of decellularized cow and human bone for engineering bone grafts with human induced pluripotent stem cells. *Tissue Eng. Part A.* 2019;25(3–4):288–301.

62. Rindone AN, Kachniarz B, Achebe CC, Riddle RC, O'Sullivan AN, Dorafshar AH, et al. Heparin-conjugated decellularized bone particles promote enhanced osteogenic signaling of PDGF-BB to adipose-derived stem cells in tissue engineered bone grafts. *Adv. Healthcare Mater.* 2019;8(10):1801565.
63. Nyberg E, Rindone A, Dorafshar A, Grayson WL. Comparison of 3D-printed poly-ε-caprolactone scaffolds functionalized with tricalcium phosphate, hydroxyapatite, bio-oss, or decellularized bone matrix. *Tissue Eng. Part A.* 2017;23(11–12):503–14.
64. Patel KH, Dunn AJ, Talovic M, Haas GJ, Marcinczyk M, Elmashhady H, et al. Aligned nanofibers of decellularized muscle ECM support myogenic activity in primary satellite cells in vitro. *Biomed. Mater.* 2019;14(3):035010.
65. Vurat MT, Parmaksiz M, Elçin AE, Elçin YM. Bioactive composite hydrogels as 3D mesenchymal stem cell encapsulation environment for bone tissue engineering: In vitro and in vivo studies. *J. Biomed. Mater. Res. A.* 2023;111(2):261–77.
66. Kafili G, Tamjid E, Niknejad H, Simchi A. Development of injectable hydrogels based on human amniotic membrane and polyethyleneglycol-modified nanosilicates for tissue engineering applications. *Eur. Polym. J.* 2022;179:111566.
67. Wang Y, Wei X, Wang L, Qian Z, Liu H, Fan Y. Quercetin-based composite hydrogel promotes muscle tissue regeneration through macrophage polarization and oxidative stress attenuation. *Compos. Part B.* 2022;247:110311.
68. Cheng CW, Solorio LD, Alsberg E. Decellularized tissue and cell-derived extracellular matrices as scaffolds for orthopaedic tissue engineering. *Biotechnol. Adv.* 2014;32(2):462–84.
69. Paduano F, Marrelli M, White LJ, Shakesheff KM, Tatullo M. Odontogenic differentiation of human dental pulp stem cells on decellularized extracellular matrix scaffolds. *J. Biomater. Sci. Polym. Ed.* 2017;28(8):730–48.
70. Kim J-Y, Ahn G, Kim C, Lee J-S, Lee I-G, An S-H, et al. Synergistic effects of beta tri-calcium phosphate and porcine-derived decellularized bone extracellular matrix in 3D-printed polycaprolactone scaffold on bone regeneration. *Macromol. Biosci.* 2018;18(6):1800025.
71. van der Heide D, Cidonio G, Stoddart MJ, D'Este M. 3D printing of inorganic-biopolymer composites for bone regeneration. *Biofabrication.* 2022;14(4):042003.
72. Aytekin E, Vurat MT, Elçin AE, Elçin YM. Decellularized bone matrix/45S5 bioactive glass biocomposite hydrogel-based constructs with angiogenic

and osteogenic properties: Ex ovo and ex vivo evaluations. *Macromol. Biosci.* 2024;24(4):2300295.
73. Saroia J, Yanen W, Wei Q, Zhang K, Lu T, Zhang B. A review on biocompatibility nature of hydrogels with 3D printing techniques, tissue engineering application and its future prospective. *Bio-Des. Manuf.* 2018;1:265–79.
74. Wang Y, Liu C, Song T, Cao Z, Wang T. 3D printed polycaprolactone/β-tricalcium phosphate/carbon nanotube composite–Physical properties and biocompatibility. *Heliyon.* 2024;10(5):e26071.
75. Kafili G, Tamjid E, Niknejad H, Simchi A. Development of bioinspired nanocomposite bioinks based on decellularized amniotic membrane and hydroxyethyl cellulose for skin tissue engineering. *Cellulose.* 2024;31(5):1–25.
76. Lee J, Hong J, Kim W, Kim GH. Bone-derived dECM/alginate bioink for fabricating a 3D cell-laden mesh structure for bone tissue engineering. *Carbohydr. Polym.* 2020;250:116914.
77. Yeleswarapu S, Dash A, Chameettachal S, Pati F. 3D bioprinting of tissue constructs employing dual crosslinking of decellularized extracellular matrix hydrogel. *Biomater. Adv.* 2023;152:213494.
78. Thrivikraman G, Boda SK, Basu B. Unraveling the mechanistic effects of electric field stimulation towards directing stem cell fate and function: A tissue engineering perspective. *Biomaterials.* 2018;150:60–86.
79. Naskar S, Kumaran V, Basu B. Reprogramming the stem cell behavior by shear stress and electric field stimulation: Lab-on-a-chip based biomicrofluidics in regenerative medicine. *Regen. Eng. Transl. Med.* 2019;5:99–127.
80. Kort-Mascort J, Flores-Torres S, Peza-Chavez O, Jang JH, Pardo LA, Tran SD, et al. Decellularized ECM hydrogels: Prior use considerations, applications, and opportunities in tissue engineering and biofabrication. *Biomater. Sci.* 2023;11(2):400–31.
81. Leng Y, Abdullah A, Wendt MK, Calve S. Hyaluronic acid, phosphatidylserine, and water content in cartilage as targets for cartilage preservation strategies. *Ann. Transl. Med.* 2020;8(5).
82. Park S, Rahaman KA, Kim YC, Jeon H, Han HS. Fostering tissue engineering and regenerative medicine to treat musculoskeletal disorders in bone and muscle. *Bioact. Mater.* 2024;40:345–65.
83. Buza III JA, Einhorn T. Bone healing in 2016. *Clin. Cases Miner. Bone Metab.* 2016;13(2):101.
84. Millikan PD, Karas V, Wellman SS. Treatment of osteonecrosis of the femoral head with vascularized bone grafting. *Curr. Rev. Musculoskelet. Med.* 2015;8:252–59.

85. Huebsch N, Lippens E, Lee K, Mehta M, Koshy ST, Darnell MC, et al. Matrix elasticity of void-forming hydrogels controls transplanted-stem-cell-mediated bone formation. *Nat. Mater.* 2015;14(12):1269–77.
86. Wu X, Huo Y, Ci Z, Wang Y, Xu W, Bai B, et al. Biomimetic porous hydrogel scaffolds enabled vascular ingrowth and osteogenic differentiation for vascularized tissue-engineered bone regeneration. *Appl. Mater. Today.* 2022;27:101478.
87. El-Sharkawy H, Kantarci A, Deady J, Hasturk H, Liu H, Alshahat M, et al. Platelet-rich plasma: Growth factors and pro-and anti-inflammatory properties. *J. Periodontol.* 2007;78(4):661–9.
88. Kang HJ, Park SS, Tripathi G, Lee BT. Injectable demineralized bone matrix particles and their hydrogel bone grafts loaded with β-tricalcium phosphate powder and granules: A comparative study. *Mater. Today Bio.* 2022;16:100422.
89. Roldan L, Isaza C, Ospina J, Montoya C, Domínguez J, Orrego S, et al. A comparative study of HA/DBM compounds derived from bovine and porcine for bone regeneration. *J. Funct. Biomater.* 2023;14(9):439.
90. Kang HJ, Makkar P, Padalhin AR, Lee GH, Im SB, Lee BT. Comparative study on biodegradation and biocompatibility of multichannel calcium phosphate based bone substitutes. *Mater. Sci. Eng. C.* 2020;110:110694.
91. Ten Broek RW, Grefte S, Von den Hoff JW. Regulatory factors and cell populations involved in skeletal muscle regeneration. *J. Cell. Physiol.* 2010;224(1):7–16.
92. Chen Z, Huang Y, Xing H, Tseng T, Edelman H, Perry R, et al. Novel muscle-derived extracellular matrix hydrogel promotes angiogenesis and neurogenesis in volumetric muscle loss. *Matrix Biol.* 2024:127:38–47.
93. Hernandez MJ, Yakutis GE, Zelus EI, Hill RC, Dzieciatkowska M, Hansen KC, et al. Manufacturing considerations for producing and assessing decellularized extracellular matrix hydrogels. *Methods.* 2020;171:20–7.
94. Zhang X, Lawler J. Thrombospondin-based antiangiogenic therapy. *Microvasc. Res.* 2007;74(2–3):90–9.
95. Morris AH, Lee H, Xing H, Stamer DK, Tan M, Kyriakides TR. Tunable hydrogels derived from genetically engineered extracellular matrix accelerate diabetic wound healing. *ACS Appl. Mater. Interfaces.* 2018;10(49): 41892–901.
96. San Emeterio CL, Hymel LA, Turner TC, Ogle ME, Pendleton EG, York WY. Nanofiber-based delivery of bioactive lipids promotes pro-regenerative

inflammation and enhances muscle fiber growth after volumetric muscle loss. *Front. Bioeng. Biotechnol.* 2021;9:650289.

97. Lesjak M, Beara I, Simin N, Pintać D, Majkić T, Bekvalac K, et al. Antioxidant and anti-inflammatory activities of quercetin and its derivatives. *J. Funct. Foods.* 2018;40:68–75.
98. Yazdanpanah G, Jalilian E, Shen X, Anwar KN, Jiang Y, Jabbehdari S, et al. The effect of decellularization protocols on characterizations of thermoresponsive and light-curable corneal extracellular matrix hydrogels. *Sci. Rep.* 2023;13(1):8145.
99. Rothrauff BB, Coluccino L, Gottardi R, Ceseracciu L, Scaglione S, Goldoni L, et al. Efficacy of thermoresponsive, photocrosslinkable hydrogels derived from decellularized tendon and cartilage extracellular matrix for cartilage tissue engineering. *J. Tissue Eng. Regen. Med.* 2018;12(1):e159–e170.
100. Yazdanpanah G, Shen X, Nguyen T, Anwar KN, Jeon O, Jiang Y, et al. A light-curable and tunable extracellular matrix hydrogel for in situ suture-free corneal repair. *Adv. Funct. Mater.* 2022;32(24):2113383.
101. Yang J, Tan Q, Li K, Liao J, Hao Y, Chen Y. Advances and trends of photoresponsive hydrogels for bone tissue engineering. *ACS Biomater. Sci. Eng.* 2024;10(4):1921–45.
102. Dziki J, Badylak S, Yabroudi M, Sicari B, Ambrosio F, Stearns K, et al. An acellular biologic scaffold treatment for volumetric muscle loss: Results of a 13-patient cohort study. *NPJ Regen. Med.* 2016;1(1):16008.

https://doi.org/10.1142/9789819819645_0006

Chapter 6

Smart and Degradable Biomaterials

Bahar Gok[1], Ozan Barıs Kurtur[1], Nisanur Cakmakci[1], Tuba Okur[2], Kubra Aranci[3], Pinar Inan[4], Serda Kecel Gunduz[5], Yasemin Budama-Kilinc[6,*]

[1]*Department of Bioengineering, Graduate School of Natural and Applied Science, Yildiz Technical University, İstanbul 34220, Turkey*
[2]*Department of Bioengineering, Faculty of Engineering, Gebze Technical University, Kocaeli 41400, Turkey*
[3]*Department of Bioengineering, Graduate School of Natural and Applied Science, Marmara University, Kadıköy 34722, Turkey*
[4]*Department of Biology, Graduate School of Natural and Applied Science, Canakkale Onsekiz Mart University, Çanakkale 17100, Turkey*
[5]*Physics Department, Faculty of Science, Istanbul University, Istanbul 34134, Turkey*
[6]*Department of Bioengineering, Faculty of Chemical and Metallurgical Engineering, Yildiz Technical University, Istanbul 34220, Turkey*

Chapter Outline

---

* **Corresponding author:** Yasemin Budama-Kilinc, Department of Bioengineering, Faculty of Chemical and Metallurgical Engineering, Yildiz Technical University, Istanbul 34220, Turkey. E-mail: yaseminbudama@gmail.com

Abstract

Smart biomaterials are capable of responding to changes in physiological parameters or external stimuli, such as ionic effects, pH, light, temperature, electric fields, and magnetic fields. Due to these properties, smart biomaterials have a wide range of applications, which attracts the attention of researchers. For example, they can be used as intelligent drug delivery systems that can release therapeutic agents using stimuli such as temperature, pH, and light in a controlled manner. Materials that respond to a magnetic field can be used as imaging agents in the form of nanoparticles, or they can support the development of bone cells as magnetically responsive tissue-engineered scaffolds. Bioabsorbable materials can be used as scaffolds that degrade along with cell proliferation, differentiation, and tissue formation and may obviate the need for surgical removal of permanent materials in orthopedic applications. On the other hand, materials that respond to electrochemical stimuli can be developed as smart devices that release drugs in a controlled manner or promote bone cell differentiation or mineral deposition onto tissue scaffolds. In this chapter, we provide a summary of the use of polymers, metals, and ceramics and discuss their unique properties and applications as smart biomaterials.

1. Introduction

Biomaterials have been extensively researched over the last few decades [1]. Some of these biomaterials are classified as substances that react to chemical stimuli, including changes in pH and chemical concentrations; physical stimuli, including heat, magnetic fields, light, and electric fields [2–4]; and biological stimuli such as glucose, enzymes, and inflammation [5, 6]. These biomaterials are also referred to as "smart biomaterials" [7] or "environmentally responsive biomaterials" [8, 9]. Smart biomaterials aim to deliver drugs in a controlled manner at the right place and the right time and offer prospects for a broad range of drug delivery applications. Therefore, they play an important role in developing selective treatments [10]. In this sense, pH-sensitive polymers have gained excellent academic and commercial interest over the past two decades [3]. Smart biomaterials have played an important role in the development of novel medical devices for cancer treatment and diagnosis. For example, magnetic nanoparticles (MNPs) are being utilized to improve hyperthermia treatments and enhance immunoassay, magnetic separation, magnetic resonance imaging (MRI) diagnostics, and cellular labeling [11]. Among the various tumor-targeted nanomaterials investigated, pH-sensitive polymeric materials have become a widely used approach in cancer diagnosis and treatment strategies. This results from pathophysiological properties of tumor tissues, which exhibit a lower pH compared to normal healthy tissues [12, 13]. Smart polymers can also generate heat or promote bone cell attachment to scaffold surfaces. Furthermore, cell proliferation and differentiation are reported to be promoted using ultrasound, light, electrical stimulation, and magnetic fields, thereby augmenting bone regeneration [6]. Shape memory biomaterials have been investigated for use in the development of minimally invasive surgical medical devices [14, 15]. These materials allow a medical device to be inserted in a compressed form, after which they expand upon reaching the desired physiological location. Such biomaterials can be used in the development of stents for vascular or urological applications. These stents are highly important not only for their mechanical properties but also for their ability to release drugs at the targeted and located site [16]. Biosensors based on smart biomaterials have also attracted great interest. They have been used in forensic analysis and clinical diagnosis, as their properties change in response to variations in the concentration of certain analytes [17]. In addition, biosensors and actuators have been combined and used for insulin delivery and in glucose sensing [18].

As a result, smart biomaterials offer interesting solutions for drug delivery, cancer therapy and diagnosis, tissue engineering, actuator stimulation, and protein folding. Patients may adapt better to smart polymers because they are generally flexible, rigid, and strong. These materials can also maintain drug stability and drug levels within the therapeutic window [16, 19–21]. In this chapter, the latest developments in smart biomaterials are reviewed, with a focus on their applications in the musculoskeletal field.

2. Shape Memory Polymers

Shape memory polymers (SMPs) are smart polymers that can alter their macroscopic characteristics, such as shape and color, in response to external stimuli and then revert to their initial condition when the effect of the external stimulus has passed [22]. It has both a temporary form and a stored (permanent) form. Thus, SMPs sensitive to stimuli can regain their original (or permanent) shape when exposed to external stimuli [23]. Factors such as heat, light, magnetic fields, electrical fields, and pH are considered external stimuli [24]. The shape memory effect has two essential prerequisites that must be met. One factor is that the polymer possesses a stable network structure, while another is that it can change shape upon stimulation and contains critical sites that allow it to return to its original configuration once the stimulus is removed [25]. The type of physical–chemical cross-link, its ratio and density, and the stability of the polymer network (i.e., the interaction of macromolecules with one another) influence the polymer's initial shape. The occurrence of the reversible shapeshift, or the creation of the transient shape, is caused by critical nodes in the polymeric network [26]. The main advantage of SMPs is that they are light and inexpensive. In addition, their optimal biodegradability, simple manufacturing process, low density, and easily adjustable glass transition temperature are all beneficial [27, 28]. The elongation behavior is also an important property for shape memory biomaterials. These materials can be extended significantly by external effects such as applied stress or temperature changes. This extension occurs through changes in the molecular structure of the polymer. When heated, the polymer chains become more flexible, and elongation occurs.

Elongation, combined with the shape memory mechanism, allows the polymer to return to its original shape at a certain temperature or with a triggering effect (e.g., an increase in temperature). This process allows the polymer to maintain its memory even after long-term deformation. Their elongation properties make SMPs usable in a wide range of applications, from medical to automotive. For example, medical stents can be compact when deployed and expand to take the desired shape when exposed to body temperature. The elongation capacity of SMPs, combined with high flexibility, increases the material's resistance to deformation. This supports the mechanical strength and longevity of the materials [29–31]. On the contrary, SMPs have poor stress and load memory. SMP composites are created and can be given unique properties, such as high toughness and high impact resistance, to overcome these drawbacks [25, 32].

There are two effects imparted by SMPs. They are the shape memory effect and the ability to change shape. Both of these effects are built *via* the polymer network [33]. However, the mechanisms that underlie active movement vary. For both of these effects, functional groups sensitive to environmental factors are located within the structure of the polymer or polymer domains. Movement is then triggered by an appropriate stimulus. There are differences in the movement of these effects in terms of geometry, the degree of recovery of the material, and the degree of freedom that determines the measure of the external effect [34]. SMPs possess a molecular network structure with at least two different phases. The phase with the highest thermal transition (Tperm) is the temperature that must be reached to form the physical cross-links responsible for the permanent shape [35, 36]. On the other hand, switching segments are the segments that can soften after a specific transition temperature (Ttrans) and are in charge of the transitory form. In some circumstances, this is both the melting temperature (Tm) and the glass transition temperature (Tg) [37]. Reaching Ttrans (while staying below Tperm) smoothes out those switching parts. Thus, it activates the switching by allowing the material to return to its permanent shape (**Figure 1**).

Below the Ttrans temperature, the flexibility of the segments is limited. When Tm is selected to program SMPs, voltage-induced crystallization of the switching segment must first be achieved [38, 39]. This voltage then rises above Tm and is cooled below Tm, so the program can start.

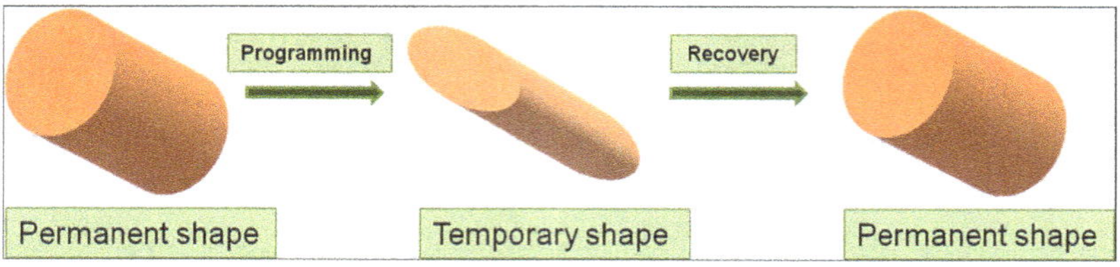

Figure 1. Schematic representation of the one-way shape memory effect under the thermal factor. With the programming process, the permanent shape is transferred to the temporary shape. Exposing the polymer to a temperature above Ttrans during the deformation allows the permanent shape to be regained.

These crystallites form covalent network points that prevent the natural helical structure of the polymer from regenerating [38]. The hard–soft segment ratio is mostly between 5:95 and 95:5. However, the optimum ratio is between 20:80 and 80:20. SMPs are typically highly viscoelastic, and there are many models and analysis methods for these polymers [40].

SMPs have a wide range of applications. There has been a high interest, especially in areas such as biomedical, textiles, electronics, and packaging. Tissue-compatible fibers produced with SMPs can be used as smart suture threads during surgery [41, 42]. These materials are preferred due to their self-compacting feature. This feature has increased the use of SMPs in the field of biomedicine. Implants required for surgery can be administered into the body through a small incision. These implants undergo a shape change when they reach body temperature [41]. Such materials are hydrolytically degradable. Therefore, they can contribute to the production of multifunctional substances. In certain applications, the aim is to use degradable implants, thereby removing the need for a second surgical procedure to remove the traditionally used nondegradable material from the body [43]. In addition, with the use of actively movable polymers in this process, remote control or controlled drug release can be achieved after implantation [44]. SMPs can also be used to make customized prosthetics. These polymers can react to body heat and transform into the desired shape, creating more comfortable and functional prosthetics. They can be used in wound closure procedures as a replacement for sutures or staples and can be activated at body temperature to close the wound. They can also be used as stabilizers or support structures that help bones stay in the correct position during fracture treatment. These polymers change shape during the healing process, allowing the bone to stay in the correct position. Finally, the flexibility and memory properties of SMPs are being investigated for improving functionality in materials such as medical devices, stents, or other implants [45–47].

3. Piezoelectric Materials

Piezoelectricity was discovered by utilizing the symmetrical property of crystal materials and the generation of electrical signals with changing temperatures [48, 49]. Natural and synthetic piezoelectric materials are used in many fields today. After the discovery of barium titanate (BT) and lead–zirconate–titanate (PZT) synthetic ceramic materials, both easy to manufacture and showing better piezoelectric properties, the importance and application areas of piezoelectric materials have further developed [48]. Over time, piezoelectric devices have been used in communications and sonar technologies, as well as in lighters, watches, optical devices, aerospace, large-scale robots, electronics, and ultrasonic imaging in health care [48, 50–52]. Piezoelectric materials are considered smart materials because of their ability to convert the direct piezoelectric effect to the inverse piezoelectric effect [53]. In recent years, research on the development and use of smart materials has gained importance [53, 54]. Piezoelectric scaffolds are a type of smart material that can generate electrical signals in response to applied stress, increasing tissue regeneration by stimulating signaling pathways [54]. This is especially important for improving cell activity in nerve tissue regeneration. A key advantage of piezoelectric scaffolds is that an electric potential can be generated under the action of mechanical forces without the need for electrodes [55]. In recent years, piezoelectric materials have been investigated for tissue engineering applications, where electroactive scaffolds have been shown to improve the repair and regeneration of tissues [53, 56]. Studies particularly focus on the relationship between the piezoelectric effect and bone and musculoskeletal repair and state-of-the-art piezoelectric materials (polymers, ceramics, and their composites), as well as manufacturing pathways for producing piezoelectric scaffolds and their therapies in tissue repair [57–59].

Electrical stimulation from piezoelectric scaffolds can promote tissue repair and regeneration in specific ways [60]. Therefore, well-optimized piezoelectric scaffolds can generate suitable bioelectric signals similar to those of the natural extracellular matrix found in bone and cartilage tissue [61]. Bone, cartilage, dentin, tendon, and keratin tissues all have piezoelectric capabilities [62]. Therefore, electroactive scaffolds that mimic the piezoelectric coefficients of natural tissues may be a suitable alternative for the repair and regeneration of skeletal tissues such as bone and cartilage. There are many piezoelectric ceramics with high piezoelectric coefficients [63]. Lead-free barium titanate is often used as an alternative material in tissue engineering applications [53]. As a result, when piezoelectric materials are integrated into cells or tissue as scaffolds, they act as tissue stimulators to promote the differentiation of desired cells. Recent research shows that it is important to investigate the use of piezoelectric materials for implantable devices due to their biocompatibility [52, 59].

4. Magnetic Materials

Magnetic materials are composed of elements that exhibit ferromagnetic or ferrimagnetic properties. A ferromagnetic property is associated with a permanent magnetic moment, which means ferromagnetic materials will retain their magnetization even after the external magnetic field is removed [64, 65]. Currently, nine elements exhibit ferromagnetic properties; three of them are transition group metals: iron (Fe), nickel (Ni), and cobalt (Co), while the other six are rare-earth metals: gadolinium, terbium, dysprosium, holmium, erbium, and thulium [66]. However, only Fe, Ni, and Co have ferromagnetic properties at or above room temperature [64, 65]. Therefore, magnetic materials are often produced from these three elements (Fe, Ni, and Co) [66]. Magnetic materials can directly or indirectly create magnetic fields, which are closely related to the survival and evolution of organisms on Earth [67, 68]. Each cell, tissue, organ, and organism has magnetic fields of its own, and they can interact with different magnetic fields created by magnetic materials [69, 70]. Therefore, various scientific studies have focused on the possible health benefits of magnetic materials on organisms [71]. In recent years, the use of magnetism-induced materials (MIMs) is gaining great interest for their potential applications, such as tissue repair, regeneration, and the treatment of diseases. According to new studies, magnetic fields are effective in increasing the interaction between cells as well as shortening the cell proliferation cycle. It may activate associated signaling pathways and excite a range of sensitive receptors on the cell surface to increase cell activity, leading to the formation of new tissue [72]. In addition, it has been demonstrated that a magnetic field accelerates the healing of defects by influencing cell metabolic behavior, such as proliferation and adhesion, thereby increasing the integration of implants and the calcium content of newly formed bone. The application of a magnetic field in combination with growth factors/signaling factors/drugs in bone restoration applications has shown a proven synergistic effect [73]. For this purpose, the magnetic materials have been designed as nanoparticles, films, scaffolds, and implants to meet different needs [72].

4.1. *Magnetic Nanoparticles*

MNPs are a type of nanomaterial composed of iron oxides, pure metals, and their alloys. They may be manipulated by an external magnetic field and have beneficial effects on repairing living organisms, either through their application alone or when combined with the appropriate magnetic field [74]. Due to the biocompatible and nontoxic properties of MNPs, their use in biomedical applications, such as nuclear magnetic imaging, targeted drug delivery, hyperthermia, gene therapy, and cell and tissue targeting, has been extensively reviewed [68, 75]. MNPs are increasingly playing an important role in bone tissue engineering (BTE) applications. In particular, iron-based nanoparticles such as iron oxide nanoparticles (IONPs) have been extensively researched for biomedical applications because of their superior biocompatibility, safety, and unique magnetic properties [76–78]. The main mechanism of IONPs involves their deposition on the surface of the cell membrane under a magnetic field, followed by endocytosis by the cells. After the IONPs enter the cell through endocytosis, the physiological function of the cell can be modified. If an external magnetic field is applied to MNPs, they will be rapidly magnetized. The synergistic combination of magnetic particles and the magnetic field promotes their bone rebuilding capacity by activating intracellular pathways that facilitate osteogenesis [79]. MNPs are not only involved in activating the biochemical pathways of cells but also play a role as delivery vehicles for therapeutics and in gene transfection techniques [80, 81]. Moreover, MNPs can serve as MRI contrast agents for tracking implanted cells, monitoring scaffold degradation, and supporting bone regeneration [82]. Although MNPs are versatile, their biggest drawback is their easy agglomeration due to high surface energy. MNPs may lose their well-recognized biological impact because of this agglomeration. Indeed, dispersion problems and a reduction in cellular uptake have been reported following MNP aggregation. However, these problems can be reduced using new anti-agglomeration methods such as surface coating, washing with an organic solvent, freeze-drying, ultrasonics, and use of anti-agglomeration surfactants. It has been reported that a surfactant, also known as a surface modifier, is more powerful in preventing agglomeration [83–86]. MNPs have a distinct advantage over other materials in that they are more stable in terms of their physical and chemical characteristics, as well as their cost of manufacturing [87]. Therefore, they are important for bone tissue repair and regeneration applications.

4.2. *Magnetic Scaffolds*

Magnetic scaffolds are developed as a result of the combination of MNPs and different types of biomaterials [88, 89]. A magnetic environment is produced within scaffolds loaded with MNPs [76]. In particular, the magnetic stimulation of IONPs within a bone scaffold has been investigated and shown to encourage the formation of bone *via* increased stem cell activity [90]. The incorporated IONPs interact with surface receptors and stimulate osteogenic-related signaling pathways when exposed to an alternating magnetic field [88]. Furthermore, engineered scaffolds can display osteoconductive and osteoinductive properties [91]. Recent studies have confirmed that a magnetic scaffold promotes the migration of growth factors and stem cells, promoting bone restoration and regeneration [92].

In addition to the biological performance of MNPs, the mechanical strength of scaffolds has been improved through the inclusion of MNPs within the scaffold. Several studies have reported that the concentration of MNPs within the scaffold contributes toward improving the mechanical properties of the scaffolds [76, 93, 94]. Another important task of magnetic scaffolds is to act as carriers for bioagents. Under an external magnetic field, magnetic scaffolds have been reported to release bioagents that can be absorbed by tissues during tissue regeneration. Studies have termed magnetic scaffolds as fixed "stations." Adjusting the scaffolds to the specific needs of the healing tissue provides a unique opportunity for BTE applications, and the controlled release of bioagents from magnetic scaffolds facilitates tissue regeneration and angiogenesis. Therefore, magnetic scaffolds are a superior option to conventional ones for bone tissue regeneration and repair and may provide significant benefits to patients [95].

To promote appropriate repair performance, MNPs and magnetic scaffolds need to be artificially controlled after their implantation. Therefore, these materials must be designed to exhibit magnetic responsiveness under an externally applied magnetic field. Generally, MNPs are responsive to magnetic fields, and when they are incorporated into a scaffold, they impart this ability to the scaffold. Materials that respond to magnetic fields are also called "smart biomaterials" [96]. The biggest advantage of using smart MNPs and scaffolds in BTE is that they have instructive/inductive or stimulating effects on cells and tissues due to the magnetic field effect [97]. In addition, smart magnetic-field-stimuli-responsive materials (MNPs and MNP-incorporated scaffolds) have high controllability, which is in high demand for bone tumor ablation and local bone regeneration [6]. Even though many studies have investigated the use of MIMs for applications in bone tissue regeneration, and numerous successes have been reported, there is still a lot of work to be done. First, new synthesis methods are needed to reduce cytotoxicity and improve the biocompatibility of the available MIMs. Second, improved techniques are required to produce MIM-based materials that are highly functional toward their biological purposes. Third, more relevant *in vitro* and *in vivo* experimental techniques are required to detect and investigate the biocompatibility and cytotoxicity of MIMs. Finally, MNP-based composites have great potential as contrast agents for MRI, and further investigations into their diagnostic and therapeutic applications are necessary [98]. Despite all of this, using magnetic technology to promote bone tissue repair and regeneration has great significance and could help solve related clinical bone repair issues.

5. pH-Sensitive Polymers

pH-sensitive polymers, an important class of smart biomaterials, respond to pH by undergoing structural changes such as *via* solubility, surface activity, configuration, and chain conformation [3]. The stimulus-sensitive properties of these polymers are of great interest for many applications, such as tissue engineering, drug delivery, gene delivery, industrial coatings, personal care, oil exploration, and water remediation [99–104]. For this reason, they have become very popular in recent years, and new studies using this technology continue to be published [105–110]. pH-sensitive polymers can possess linear, nonlinear branched, or network structures [111]. Depending on their structure, they can exhibit self-assembly behaviors [3], swelling [112], or shrinkage [112, 113]. Recently, pH-sensitive polymers have received significant attention in bone and musculoskeletal systems for their use in drug delivery systems and tissue engineering [104, 114, 115]. Osteoporosis, a metabolic bone disease, leads to the breakdown of the bone structure due to excessive osteoclast activity *via* a localized decrease in the pH level within the bone microenvironment. Similarly, bone fractures and infections also lead to pH changes in the microenvironment. Following a bone fracture, the pH reduces to 6.8 within the first few days of healing, with a tendency to increase toward alkaline conditions in the following weeks. Infections, such as osteomyelitis, can also affect the microenvironmental pH. An infection can cause a decrease in pH during the early stages of infection and then an increase during the later chronic stage. These pH changes have a significant effect on bone regeneration and osteoblast activity [116]. In this context, pH-sensitive polymeric biomaterials can be used to deliver osteogenic and antibacterial drugs [117]. Deng *et al.* developed a bilayer polydopamine coating for application to the bone implant surfaces. Silver nanoparticles were applied to the first layer and apatite to the second layer [118]. In response to bacterial infection, the coating released Ag^+, Ca^{2+}, and PO_4^{3-} ions. Polyetheretherketone scaffolds modified with the bilayer coating showed superior antibacterial and osteogenic activity *in vitro* and bone ingrowth into infected bone defects *in vivo*. George *et al.* developed a pH-responsive injectable oligo[poly(ethylene glycol)fumarate]–dopamine hydrogel [119]. The results suggest that this hydrogel is a promising injectable bone scaffold material that reduces the displacement of bone implants by adhering to the bone structure.

The contents of endosomes (pH: 4.9–6.0) and lysosomes (pH: 4.0–4.5) are acidic and are often involved in the endocytosis of nanoparticles by osteoclasts. These features within osteoclasts highlight a potential treatment-targeted strategy using pH-sensitive drug delivery systems for conditions characterized by excessive bone resorption [120]. Gong *et al.* developed chitosan (CS)-coated mesoporous silica nanoparticles (MSNs) loaded with pH-sensitive naringin (CS@MSNs-Na) to suppress osteoclast activity. In this regard, bone marrow–derived macrophages were used to induce osteoclasts, and their ability to inhibit osteoclasts *in vitro* was observed following co-culture with CS@MSNs-Na. Moreover, it was reported that the nanoparticles inhibited osteoclast activity and thereby promoted bone regeneration in an *in vivo* rat bone defect model [121]. In another study, a pH-sensitive bisphosphonate (BP)-based nanocomposite hyaluronic acid hydrogel (HA-BP) was developed to regulate osteoclast activity and enhance bone regeneration. The developed hydrogel provided controlled BP release in an acidic pH environment and enabled *in vivo* bone tissue regeneration [122]. Gan *et al.* developed CS/MSNs containing pH-sensitive bone morphogenetic protein-2 (BMP-2) and dexamethasone (Dex). The results showed that after the nanoparticles were delivered to the cells, the lower pH triggered Dex release following the initial release of BMP-2. In addition, the nanoparticles significantly increased osteoblast differentiation *in vivo* over a 4-week period [123].

In addition to the "normal" tissue and intracellular pH range, different physiological and pathological conditions exhibit varying pH levels. For example, bacterial infections produce acidic pus with a pH between 6.0 and 6.6. When a tissue becomes inflamed, the pH can range between 6.0 and 7.0 [124]. Therefore, pH-sensitive polymers are potentially very important for the treatment of bacterial infection and tissue inflammation. In a study to enhance the osteointegration of an implant *in vitro* and *in vivo*, the authors developed titanium dioxide nanotubes coated with osteogenic growth peptide-loaded zeolitic imidazolate framework-67 (TNT-ZIF-67@OGP) and showed that these pH-sensitive implants exhibited potent antimicrobial and anti-inflammatory properties in the early phase of implantation [125]. Bonadies *et al.* synthesized resveratrol (RSV)-loaded electrospun polylactic acid (PLA) membranes (PLA-RSV2) and evaluated their antibacterial and antibiofilm potential [126]. The findings revealed that PLA-RSV membranes release RSV only at pH levels below 5.5 (i.e., during an oral bacterial infection) and act as a drug reservoir under neutral pH. These results showed that it is a promising candidate for preventing implant-associated infections. Lei *et al.* developed a pH-sensitive multilayer film for the controlled release of ibuprofen targeting implant infections [127]. The results reported that the release of ibuprofen in the film was sensitive to a narrow pH (pH: 6.8–7.4) and exhibited antibacterial properties. Wu *et al.* designed a pH-sensitive photodynamic nanosystem by decorating Rose Bengal (RB) polydopamine nanoparticles with polymyxin B (PMB) and gluconic acid (GA) (RB@PMB@GA NPs) for the treatment of biofilm-associated infections [128]. RB@PMB@GA NPs exhibited good biofilm penetration under acidic conditions, as well as robust stability and biocompatibility at physiological pH. Chen *et al.* developed a microfluidic CS-based device for pH-sensitive drug delivery to bone tissue following a bacterial infection. This study reported that minocycline release in the acidic microenvironment of infected sites using a pH-sensitive PDMAEMA hydrogel both combated infection and promoted osteoblast proliferation. The study showed that the device inhibited the growth of *Staphylococcus aureus (S. aureus)* and *Streptococcus mutans* and had no toxic effects on MC3T3-E1 osteoblasts. As such, this study represents a promising therapeutic approach for treating infectious bone defects [129]. Zhang *et al.* developed a pH-sensitive topical drug carrier consisting of a core–shell microsphere with a borate glass (BG) core and a mesoporous hydroxyapatite (HA) shell (BG-HA), coated with CS. Its ability to inhibit bone infection and promote bone tissue regeneration was investigated. While vancomycin release was negligible in a neutral environment, the pores in the HA shell opened due to the swelling of CS in an acidic environment, thus enabling drug release. Furthermore, vancomycin-loaded BG-HA@CS exhibited highly effective antibacterial activity against *S. aureus* and

Escherichia coli (E.coli). The results indicated that BG-HA@CS is a multifunctional system that could provide self-regulated drug release, control the acidic environment at the bone infection site, and promote bone tissue regeneration [130].

6. Bioresorbable Metals

Biodegradable or bioresorbable materials are of increasing interest for use as biomedical implants and devices designed to perform temporary functions in the body. When bioresorbable materials chemically react with biofluids, they can produce biocompatible and soluble end products. In this way, the material both eliminates the need for surgical removal and aids in the restoration of the damaged tissue [131]. Metals possess higher ductility, toughness, impact resistance, and wear resistance properties than other biomaterials. In this context, metals stand out as more favorable candidates for load-bearing orthopedic applications, such as joint replacements, bone plates, and screws, as well as for suture wires, pacemakers, coronary stents, and dental implants [132]. Metals are preferred as bioresorbable materials because they show improved biocompatibility and mechanical strength compared to polymers [133]. Bioresorbable metals, such as magnesium (Mg), zinc (Zn), tungsten (W), and molybdenum (Mo), have well-known roles in temporary orthopedic materials, vascular implants, and bioresorbable electronics [131].

6.1. *Bioresorbable Metals in Orthopedics*

In orthopedics, metal materials have been used for many years to produce temporary or permanent devices such as joint replacement implants, bone plates, pins, and screws [134]. For these applications, commonly used materials include cobalt-chromium alloy, titanium-based alloys, and 316L stainless steel. However, they have significant disadvantages, including their lack of bioactivity, high modulus, and altered wear and corrosion resistance compared to bone [135]. In addition, implants typically have a finite lifespan when implanted into the body. This situation has led researchers to investigate materials that will provide mechanical support for new tissue formation and biodegrade over time [136]. Bioresorbable implant materials are an attractive alternative. This is largely due to the risks observed following the insertion of permanent implants, especially in childhood. These risks include metallic ion release and related toxicological problems, osteolysis, and difficulties in surgical removal when the implant has fully integrated into bone [137]. Windhagen *et al.* evaluated the efficacy of Mg-based screws (MgYREZr) and standard titanium screws following a chevron osteotomy for treating patients with hallux valgus ($n = 26$) [138]. They determined no significant differences in the outcome between the two screws in terms of the Hallux score, pain rating scale, or range of motion of the first metatarsophalangeal joint. Furthermore, the study showed that the Mg-based screws did not cause reactions such as foreign body reaction, osteolysis, or systemic inflammation. The authors also stated no significant differences between the groups in which the two screws were applied separately in terms of laboratory findings or radiographic results, and therefore, biodegradable Mg-based screws were equivalent to their titanium counterparts. Grün *et al.* investigated the degradation behavior of ZX00, a bioresorbable Mg–Zn–Ca alloy, in both small and large animal models [137]. They observed no adverse effects on bone formation and ingrowth at 6, 12, and 24 weeks postimplantation, with no fibrotic or sclerotic encapsulation adjacent to the implant. They also showed that the implant exhibited a similar homogeneous and slow degradation rate in both animal models. Furthermore, a clinical research study that investigated fracture reduction and fixation using ZX00 screws reported excellent clinical and functional results [139]. As such, implants produced using bioabsorbable metals continue to take their place in the market. For example, the RemeOs™ trauma screw, produced by Bioretec and containing Mg, Zn, and Ca, was approved by the US Food and Drug Administration in 2023 and has taken its place in the US market [140, 141].

6.2. *Bioresorbable Metal Tissue Scaffolds*

The development of three-dimensional (3D) tissue scaffolds for defect repair plays an important role in tissue regeneration and has attracted a lot of attention in the field over recent decades. Ideally, a biodegradable scaffold should have sufficient porosity, interconnectivity, bioactivity, and biocompatibility, thereby not producing any toxic products during its degradation. Finally, the rate of degradation should be compatible with tissue regeneration [142, 143]. Furthermore, the scaffolds must have sufficient mechanical properties to withstand the mechanical forces that may occur during the implantation procedure and not collapse during the patient's daily activities. However, achieving adequate stiffness and mechanical strength, and maintaining these properties during the patient's recovery period and as the scaffold degradation process occurs, is the biggest challenge for biodegradable scaffolds [142]. In this context, polymers are seen as very favorable materials to provide these properties in scaffolds due to their ease of processing, biocompatibility, and biodegradability [142]. However, the poor mechanical properties of these polymers remain the main limitation for their use as scaffolds. Polymers may lose their mechanical integrity and mass during the decomposition process, and since porous polymeric structures are quite weak, they may not achieve properties such as sufficient strength and Young's modulus, which are especially needed in hard tissue applications [144]. Cheng *et al.* fabricated Mg scaffolds of the same porosity but with different pore sizes using a traditional fabrication method — the titanium wire space holder method [145]. The authors observed that by altering the pore orientation within the scaffold, the mechanical characteristics could be modified to more accurately mimic the range found in native human cancellous bone. The *in vitro* and *in vivo* studies conducted showed that osteoblastic differentiation, cytocompatibility, and the inflammatory response of the scaffold were beneficial for tissue regeneration. The study also showed that the scaffold had almost completely degraded and had been replaced by newly formed bone. He *et al.* fabricated scaffolds consisting of a Zn outer shell and Fe core layer (Fe@Zn) *via* a template-assisted electrodeposition technique [146]. This study showed that the fabricated scaffolds exhibited mechanical properties and structures similar to human cancellous bone. Notably, the degradation rate of the scaffold could be adjusted by varying the thickness of the Zn and Fe layers. The scaffold delivered 95% and 100% efficacy against *S. aureus* and *E. coli*, respectively. Although the scaffold exhibited a mild inflammatory response, substantial amounts of new bone formation and growth were measured within the scaffold structure. Yao *et al.* used NaCl particles and a vacuum heating-press sintering method to create Zn scaffolds [147]. The findings revealed that the porosity of the Zn scaffolds ranged from 11.3% to 63.3%. In addition, the compressive yield strength (14.2–73.7 MPa) and compressive elastic modulus (1.9–6.7 GPa) of the scaffold were comparable to those of cancellous bone (2–12 MPa and 0.1–5 GPa). In addition, the authors reported that the porous structure stimulated osteoblast proliferation and significantly accelerated the rate of scaffold degradation. Xia *et al.* used specialized laser powder bed fusion technology to create pure Zn porous scaffolds with diamond structures [148]. The findings demonstrated that the compressive strength and hardness of pure Zn porous scaffolds were comparable to those of cancellous bone and that their degradation rates were comparatively advantageous for bone regeneration. In addition, they showed *via in vivo* studies that pure Zn scaffolds hold promise for applications that involve restoring tissue within large bone defects. Wang *et al.* created a composite material consisting of Mg, nano-HA, and polylactic acid and utilized it to create customized scaffolds for bone repair using 3D printing (fused deposition modeling) [149]. The outcomes demonstrated that the scaffold could stimulate osteogenesis and angiogenesis and had the appropriate mechanical, processable, and degradable qualities. In addition, it was reported that this composite scaffold has potential for clinical development and application, satisfying the complex requirements for treating critical-sized trabecular bone defects in load-bearing animals.

7. Electrochemical Biomaterials

Electroactive biomaterials, which belong to a new generation of smart biomaterials, allow for the direct transmission of electrical, electrochemical, and electromechanical stimuli to cells [150, 151]. Biomaterials that respond to electrochemical stimuli can be used for many purposes, including drug delivery, monitoring, and efficacy evaluation. The development of electrochemically stimulated miniature electrical systems and circuits has become very attractive, especially for health challenges that require intermittent drug dosing on demand over a long period of time [152]. It has been reported that materials with such properties can be developed as absorbable or implantable devices for controlled drug release *via* electrochemical stimulation and can provide advantages in the treatment of various diseases [153, 154].

Electrochemical techniques and technologies are being investigated to enhance implant biocompatibility [155], characterization [156, 157], and performance evaluation [158]. Furthermore, the development of electrochemical biosensors for the determination of analytes such as superoxide and C-terminal telopeptide of type 1 collagen, which are known to be markers in disorders related to the musculoskeletal system, has been the subject of previous research [159, 160]. Indeed, the development of electrochemical smart biomaterials for use in musculoskeletal tissue engineering applications is at the forefront of research. Huang *et al.* integrated carboxylated carbon nanotubes and BMP-2 within a chemically cross-linked carboxymethyl CS hydrogel to monitor bone regeneration [161]. The study reported that the scaffold exhibited electrochemical response signals sensitive to the amount of osteogenic differentiation and tissue mineralization at both cellular and animal levels. The study also found that the inclusion of BMP-2 into the scaffold synergistically induced new bone formation with the carbon nanotubes. Furthermore, the development of biomaterials in which drug delivery can be electrochemically triggered has been possible using intrinsically conducting polymers such as polypyrrole [162]. Cao *et al.* designed electroactive surfaces that could mimic the initial process of trabecular bone formation by immobilizing chondrocyte-derived plasma membrane nanofragments (PMNFs) [163]. The polypyrrole-based electroactive surface dynamically controlled the presentation of PMNFs on the surface *via* electrochemical redox switching and promoted bone mineral formation with differing morphologies within 2 days.

8. Ultraviolet-Triggered Agent Release

Light is an agent that delivers therapeutic activity and has been used since ancient times. Early civilizations believed that sunlight enhanced the healing properties of medicinal plants. On the other hand, the microbe-killing effect of the sun was also discovered, and notably, one type of tuberculosis was shown to be eradicated *via* light [111]. In modern medicine, light is used to treat diseases ranging from skin conditions to depression. These applications include controlled release systems and photodynamic therapy, which utilize different wavelengths of light [20]. Light is a beneficial option for stimuli-responsive biomaterials compared to temperature or pH because of its tolerability. Therefore, several studies have sought to develop controlled release systems that can be triggered by light. For example, the release profile of a light-based system has been shown to be tunable according to exposure time, beam diameter, light intensity, and wavelength. Light is composed of different wavelengths, such as ultraviolet (UV) light, visible light, and near-infrared (NIR), and each application may require a specific wavelength. Notably, UV and visible light cannot successfully penetrate tissue deeper than 1 cm due to scattering and absorption by hemoglobin and water. This means that organs will receive only a limited amount of UV light, but NIR can penetrate deeper into tissues up to a depth of 2 cm [111]. UV light is found between the X-ray and visible regions on the spectrum scale. There are different classes of UV light; vacuum UV light ranges from 40 to 190 nm, far UV light from 190 to 220 nm, UVC is from 220-290 nm, UVB is from 290-320 nm and UVA is from 320-400 nm. In addition, UV light sources are divided into natural and artificial. For example, halogen lights, fluorescent lights, germicidal lamps, and laser types are artificial sources, while the sun is a natural UV source and induces vitamin D production in the body [164].

Light-triggered controlled release systems mostly use UV light to release substances because the short wavelength is appropriate to disrupt the biomaterial, thereby releasing the agent. UV light can photocleave covalent bonds. Photolabile bonds can be used to bind the carrier and release agent, or the carrier itself can be composed of photolabile bonds. These bonds can be used in many systems from nanoparticles (**Figure 2**) to hydrogels [165–167]. For instance, UV-triggered liposomal structures require photolabile lipids, or selective degradation can be achieved in hydrogels by applying different wavelengths of light. Furthermore, these systems are used for various applications in the body, including in BTE.

Bone tissue may require a comparably higher amount and longer frequency of drug delivery because it possesses a dense and occluded structure compared to other tissue types. Controlled release drug delivery is a

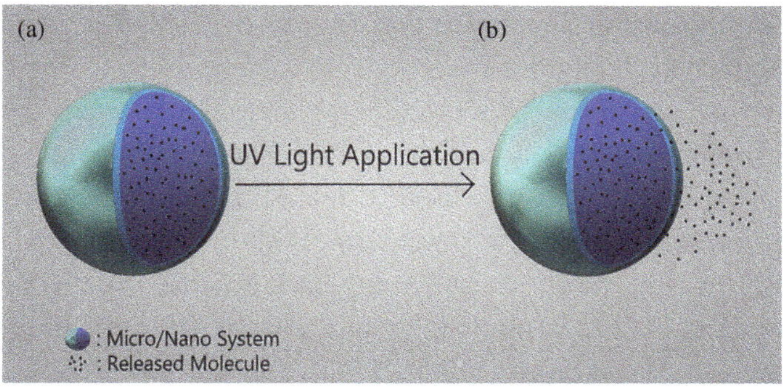

Figure 2. Schematic representation of UV-triggered controlled release system. (a) Nano/micro system before UV light application. (b) Nano/micro system after UV light application.

method designed to decrease drug excretion levels and increase bioavailability [168]. Many UV-triggered controlled release systems have been reported in the literature. A study by Gan *et al.* investigated human mesenchymal stem cells (hMSCs) and their osteogenic differentiation. In this study, noncoding microRNA (Chol-miR-26a) modified with UV-degradable cholesterol ester bonds was investigated. With the aid of these bonds, an injectable poly(ethylene glycol) (PEG) hydrogel, modified with a copper-free click reaction, was filled with Chol-miR-26a. Upon UV irradiation, Chol-c-miR-26a was selectively released from the hydrogel. Compared to the control group, it was concluded that the designed system improved osteogenic differentiation and had the potential to augment bone repair within bone defects [169]. Another study related to photodegradable hydrogels aimed to stimulate the osteogenic differentiation of hMSCs *via* the release of an siRNA molecule. In this study, an increase in gene expression was measured to confirm hMSC differentiation. Due to the anionic structure of the RNA molecule, a polyethyleneimine molecule was used to create a charge balance for cell internalization. On-demand stimulation was created by exposing the PEG hydrogel to UV light. Study controls were also included, and the UV light was used to better understand the release profile, while another control system investigated the effects without UV stimulation. The results showed that the osteogenic differentiation of hMSCs increased due to the acceleration of siRNA release from the UV-applied system [170]. A further study used pNIPAm-*co*-nitrobenzyl methacrylate (pNIPAm-*co*-NBMA) microgels, which produced copolymerization using a free radical precipitation polymerization method. A Dex molecule, which induces hMSC differentiation to osteoblasts, was used as the release agent. In this study, a UV light-triggered mechanism was used to release the Dex molecule, and a non-UV-triggered mechanism was also used to compare the control release profile. The results of the study showed that UV light induced hMSC osteogenesis in a controlled manner. Also notably, the microgel did not appear to be toxic to the hMSCs [171].

UV light is easily tunable for targeted use due to the variety of changeable parameters it accommodates. However, these parameters create both advantages and disadvantages. The penetration length and wavelength can be both an advantage and a disadvantage. However, it is clear that UV-triggered release applications are very effective for BTE and regeneration studies.

9. Future Aspects

Smart biomaterials are receiving increasing attention in medicine and the medical field due to their ability to respond to different external stimuli. These materials may offer interesting solutions in many areas, including diagnostics, disease treatment, drug delivery systems, and tissue engineering. They are considered very suitable for therapeutic use due to their ability to maintain the stability and dosage levels of drugs. In this context, it is predicted that smart materials have the potential to overcome various unmet medical challenges and may provide significant developments in the diagnosis and treatment of diseases in the near future. It is hoped that the relevant materials will deliver important properties such as promoting the repair and regeneration process in patients, thereby increasing quality of life.

References

1. Kowalskı PS, Bhattacharya C, Afewerkı S, Langer R. Smart biomaterials: Recent advances and future directions. *ACS Biomater. Sci. Eng.* 2022;4:3809–17.

2. Ebara M. Smart polymers for biomedical applications. In: Wakayama Y, Ariga K (eds) *System-Materials Nanoarchitectonics*. New York: Springer, 2022.
3. Kocak G, Tuncer C, Bütün V. pH-responsive polymers. *Polym. Chem.* 2017;8:144–176.
4. Tarıq A, BHawanı SA, Alotaıbı KM, Moheman A. Smart biopolymers and their applications. In: *Smart Polymer Nanocomposites*. Amsterdam: Elsevier, 2021.
5. Gayathrı V, Jaısankar SN, Samanta D. Temperature and pH responsive polymers: Sensing applications. *J. Macromol. Sci., Part A:Pure Appl. Chem.* 2021;59(2):1–29.
6. Weı H, Cuı J, Lın K, Xıe J, Wang X. Recent advances in smart stimuli-responsive biomaterials for bone therapeutics and regeneration. *Bone Res.* 2022;10:1–19.
7. Kaıth BS. Kumar R. Psyllium polysaccharide-based hydrogels as smart biomaterials. *Mater. Today: Proc.* 2022;53:244–46.
8. Gawade PM, Shadısh JA, Badeau BA, Deforest CA. Logic-based delivery of site-specifically modified proteins from environmentally responsive hydrogel biomaterials. *Adv. Mater.* 2019;31:1902462.
9. Fu Z, Ouyang L, Xu R, Yang Y, Sun W. Responsive biomaterials for 3D bioprinting: A review. *Mater. Today* 2022;52:112–32.
10. Sha S. An overview on smart polymers as the backbone to hard tissue formation. *SPAST Abst.* 2021;1.
11. karımı Z, Karımı L, Shokrollahı H. Nano-magnetic particles used in biomedicine: Core and coating materials. *Mater. Sci. Eng. C* 2013;33: 2465–75.
12. Gharehdaghı Z, Rahımı R, Naghıb SM, Molaabası F. Fabrication and application of copper metal–organic frameworks as nanocarriers for pH-responsive anticancer drug delivery. *J. Iran. Chem. Soc.* 2022:1–11.
13. Tang H, Zhao W, Yu J, Lı Y, Zhao C. Recent development of pH-responsive polymers for cancer nanomedicine. *Molecules* 2018;24:4.
14. Karger-Kocsıs J. Recent advances in shape memory polymers and composites: A review. *J. Mater. Sci.* 2008;43:254–69.
15. Delaey J, Dubruel P, Van Vlıerberghe S. Shape-memory polymers for biomedical applications. *Adv. Funct. Mater.* 2020;30:1909047.
16. Dawood NMZ, Saeed BB. Smart pharmaceutical polymers classification and applications: A review. *ACE.* 2021:1:7–17.
17. Thammakhet C, Thavarungkul P. Kanatharana P. Development of an on-column affinity smart polymer gel glucose sensor. *Anal. Chim. Acta.* 2011;695:105–12.

18. Brahım S, Narınesıngh D, Guıseppı-elıe A. Bio-smart hydrogels: Co-joined molecular recognition and signal transduction in biosensor fabrication and drug delivery. *Biosens. Bioelectron.* 2022;17:973–81.
19. Hoffman AS, Stayton PS, Press O, Murthy N, Lackey CA, Cheung C, et al. Design of “smart” polymers that can direct intracellular drug delivery. *Polym. Adv. Technol.* 2022;13:992–9.
20. James HP, John R, Alex A, Anoop K. Smart polymers for the controlled delivery of drugs–a concise overview. *Acta Pharm. Sin. B.* 2014;4:120–7.
21. Bellınger AM, Jafarı M, Grant TM, Zhang S, Slater HC, Wenger EA, et al. Oral, ultra–long-lasting drug delivery: Application toward malaria elimination goals. *Sci. Transl. Med.* 2016;8:365ra157.
22. Lendleın A, Schmıdt AM, Langer, R. AB-polymer networks based on oligo (ε-caprolactone) segments showing shape-memory properties. *Proc. Natl. Acad. Sci.* (2001);98:842–7.
23. Yang B, Huang W, Lı C, Lı LJP. Effects of moisture on the thermo-mechanical properties of a polyurethane shape memory. *Polymer.* 2006;47:1348–56.
24. Lendleın A, Kelch S. Shape-memory polymers. *Angew. Chem. Int. Ed.* 2002;41: 2034–57.
25. Meng H, Lı GJP. A review of stimuli-responsive shape memory polymer composites. *Polymer.* 2013;54:2199–2221.
26. Canbay CA, Ünlü N. Production and characterization of shape memory polymeric nanocomposite materials. *J. Mol. Struct.* 2021;1227:129708.
27. Behl M, Razzaq MY, Lendleın A. Multifunctional shape-memory polymers. *Adv. Mater.* 2010;22:3388–3410.
28. Meng Q, Hu J. A review of shape memory polymer composites and blends. *Compos. Part A. Appl. Sci. Manuf.* 2009;40:1661–72.
29. Xıa Y, He Y, Zhang F, Lıu Y, Leng J. A review of shape memory polymers and composites: Mechanisms, materials, and applications. *Adv. Mater.* 2021;33:2000713.
30. Hager MD, Bode S, Weber C, Schubert US. Shape memory polymers: Past, present and future developments. *Prog. Polym. Sci.* 2015;49:3–33.
31. Wagermaıer W, Kratz K, Heuchel M, Lendleın A. Characterization methods for shape-memory polymers. In: *Shape-Memory Polymers.* 2010: 97–145.
32. Zhu Y, Hu J, Choı KF, Yeung KW, Meng Q, Chen, S. Crystallization and melting behavior of the crystalline soft segment in a shape-memory polyurethane ionomer. *J. Appl. Polym. Sci.* 2008;107:599–609.

33. Nguyen TD, Qı HJ, Castro F, Long KN. A thermoviscoelastic model for amorphous shape memory polymers: Incorporating structural and stress relaxation. *J. Mech. Phys. Solids* 2008;56:2792–814.
34. Leı M, Chen Z, Lu H, Yu KJNR. Recent progress in shape memory polymer composites: Methods, properties, applications and prospects. *Nanotechnol. Rev.* 2019;8:327–51.
35. Fan J, Lı G. High enthalpy storage thermoset network with giant stress and energy output in rubbery state . *Nat. Cmmun.* 2018;9:1–8.
36. Ortega AM, Kasprzak SE, Yakackı CM, Dıanı J, Greenberg AR, Gall K. Structure–property relationships in photopolymerizable polymer networks: Effect of composition on the crosslinked structure and resulting thermomechanical properties of a (meth) acrylate-based system. *J. Appl. Polym. Sci.* 2008;110:1559–72.
37. Safranskı DL, Gall KJP. Effect of chemical structure and crosslinking density on the thermo-mechanical properties and toughness of (meth) acrylate shape memory polymer networks. *Polymer.* 2008;49:4446–55.
38. Lı Y, Lıu ZJP. A novel constitutive model of shape memory polymers combining phase transition and viscoelasticity. *Polymer* 2018;143:298–308.
39. Pan Z, Zhou Y, Z N, Lıu Z. A modified phase-based constitutive model for shape memory polymers. *Polym. Int.* 2018;67:1677–83.
40. Chan BQY, Lıow SS, Loh XJ. Organic–inorganic shape memory thermoplastic polyurethane based on polycaprolactone and polydimethylsiloxane. *RSC Adv.* 2016;6:34946–54.
41. Hussaın F, Hojjatı M, Okamoto M, Gorga RE. Polymer-matrix nanocomposites, processing, manufacturing, and application: An overview. *J. Comp. Mater.* 2006;40:1511–75.
42. Thostenson ET, Lı C, Chou TW. Nanocomposites in context. *Compos. Sci. Technol.* 2005;65:491–516.
43. Gunes IS, Jana SC. Shape memory polymers and their nanocomposites: A review of science and technology of new multifunctional materials. *J. Nanosci. Nanotechnol.* 2008;8:1616–37.
44. Madbouly SA, Lendleın, A. Shape-memory polymer composites. In: *Shape-Memory Polymers.* 2009:41–95.
45. Chen Y, Chen C, Rehman HU, Zheng X, Lı H, Lıu H, et al. Shape-memory polymeric artificial muscles: Mechanisms, applications and challenges. *Molecules.* 2020;25:4246.
46. Dayyoub T, Maksımkın AV, Fılıppova OV, Tcherdyntsev VV, Telyshev DV. Shape memory polymers as smart materials: A review. *Polymers.* 2022;14:3511.

47. Li T, Chen L, Yuan Y, Shı R. The current status, prospects, and challenges of shape memory polymers application in bone tissue engineering. *Polymers.* 2023;15:556.
48. Akgün M. *Piezoelektrik özellikli, polimer nano kompozit malzeme geliştirilmesi ve titreşim sensörü olarak kullanilabilirliğinin incelenmesi.* Yüksek lisans Uludağ Üniversitesi; 2018.
49. Tıchý J, Erhart J, Kıttınger E, Prívratská J. *Fundamentals of Piezoelectric sensorics: Mechanical, dielectric, and thermodynamical properties of piezoelectric materials.* Berlin: Springer Science & Business Media, 2010.
50. Dagdevıren C, Yang BD, Su Y, Tran PL, Joe P, Anderson E, et al. Conformal piezoelectric energy harvesting and storage from motions of the heart, lung, and diaphragm. *Proc. Natl Acad. Sci.* 2014;111:1927–32.
51. Gan J, Zhang X. A review of nonlinear hysteresis modeling and control of piezoelectric actuators. *AIP Adv.* 2019;9:040702.
52. Shın DM, Hong SW, Hwang YH. Recent advances in organic piezoelectric biomaterials for energy and biomedical applications. *Nanomaterials.* 2020;10:123.
53. Jacob J, More N., Kalıa K, Kapusettı G. Piezoelectric smart biomaterials for bone and cartilage tissue engineering. *Inflamm. Regen.* 2018;38:1–11.
54. Zaszczynska A, Sajkıewıcz P, Gradys A. Piezoelectric scaffolds as smart materials for neural tissue engineering. *Polymers.* 2020;12:161.
55. Steel EM, Sundararaghavan HG. Electrically conductive materials for nerve regeneration. *Neural Engineering.* New York: Springer.
56. Wu S, Chen MS, Maurel P, Lee YS, Bunge MB, Arınzeh TL. Aligned fibrous PVDF-TrFE scaffolds with Schwann cells support neurite extension and myelination in vitro. *J. Neural Eng.* 2018;15:056010.
57. Tandon B, Blaker JJ, Cartmell SH. Piezoelectric materials as stimulatory biomedical materials and scaffolds for bone repair. *Acta Biomater.* 2018;73:1–20.
58. Lıu PJ, Wang K, Lı L, Zhang R, Xu ZG. Lead-free piezoelectric materials for musculoskeletal tissue engineering. *Mater. Today Sustain.* 2023; 22:100393.
59. Weı Y, Lıang, Y, Qı K, Gu Z, Yan B, Xıe H. Exploring the application of piezoelectric ceramics in bone regeneration. *J. Biomater. Appl.* 2024; 39:409–20.
60. Mınary-Jolandan M, Yu MF. Nanoscale characterization of isolated individual type I collagen fibrils: Polarization and piezoelectricity. *Nanotechnology.* 2009;20:085706.

61. Barbosa F, Ferreıra FC, Sılva JC. Piezoelectric electrospun fibrous scaffolds for bone, articular cartilage and osteochondral tissue engineering. *Int. J. Mol. Sci.* 2022;23:2907.
62. Bassett CAL. Biologic significance of piezoelectricity. *Calcif. Tissue Res.* 1967;1:252–72.
63. Cıofanı G, Rıcottı L, Canale C, D'alessandro D, Berrettını S, Mazzolaı, B, et al. Effects of barium titanate nanoparticles on proliferation and differentiation of rat mesenchymal stem cells. *Colloids Surf. B: Biointerfaces.* 2013;102:312–20.
64. Kong LB, Lıu L, Yang Z, Lı S, Zhang T, Wang C. Theory of ferrimagnetism and ferrimagnetic metal oxides. In: Stojanovic B (eds) *Magnetic, Ferroelectric, and Multiferroic Metal Oxides.* Amsterdam: Elsevier, 2018.
65. Shahrı MM. Magnetic materials and magnetic nanocomposites for biomedical application. In: Henry D (ed) *Harnessing Nanoscale Surface Interactions: Contemporary Synthesis, Applications and Theory.* Amsterdam: Elsevier, 2019.
66. Szymczak H. Magnetic materials and applications. In: Bassanı F, Lıedl GL, Wyder P. (eds.) *Encyclopedia of Condensed Matter Physics.* Oxford: Elsevier.
67. Pan D, Caruthers SD, Senpan A, Schmıeder AH, Wıcklıne SA, Lanza GM. Revisiting an old friend: Manganese-based MRI contrast agents. *Wiley Interdiscip. Rev.:Nanomed. Nanobiotechnol.* 2011;3:162–73.
68. Clavıjo-Jordan V, Kodıbagkar VD, Beeman SC Hann BD, Bennett KM. Principles and emerging applications of nanomagnetic materials in medicine. *Wiley Interdiscip. Rev.:Nanomed. Nanobiotechnol.* 2012;4:345–65.
69. Lohmann KD, Placıdı M, Schmıckler H. Q-monitoring in LEP. 1988.
70. Peng J, Zhao J, Long Y, Xıe Y, Nıe J, Chen L. Magnetic materials in promoting bone regeneration. *Front. Mater.* 2019;6:268.
71. Dashnyam K, Perez RA, Sıngh RK, Lee EJ, Kım HW. Hybrid magnetic scaffolds of gelatin–siloxane incorporated with magnetite nanoparticles effective for bone tissue engineering. *RSC Adv.* 2014;4:40841–51.
72. Sengupta S, Mıchalek M, Galusek D, Boccaccını AR. Magnetic bioactive materials for bone regeneration and tissue engineering. *FunGlass School 2019/part*, 2019.
73. Ansarı M. Bone tissue regeneration: Biology, strategies and interface studies. *Prog. Biomater.* 2019;8:223–37.
74. Subramanıan M, Mıaskowskı A, Jenkıns SI, Lım J, Dobson J. Remote manipulation of magnetic nanoparticles using magnetic field gradient to promote cancer cell death. *Appl. Phys. A* 2019;125:226.

75. Sıngh RK, Patel KD, Lee JH, Lee EJ, Kım JH, Kım TH, et al. Potential of magnetic nanofiber scaffolds with mechanical and biological properties applicable for bone regeneration. *PLoS One.* 2014;9:e91584.
76. Dasarı A, Xue J, Deb S. Magnetic nanoparticles in bone tissue engineering. *Nanomaterials.* 2022;12:757.
77. O'Grady K. Progress in applications of magnetic nanoparticles in biomedicine. *J. Phys. D:Appl. Phys.* 2009;42:220301.
78. Lı Y, Ye D, Lı M, Ma M, Gu N. Adaptive materials based on iron oxide nanoparticles for bone regeneration. *Chem. Phys. Chem.* 2018;19:1965–79.
79. Theruvath AJ, Nejadnık H, Muehe AM, Gassert F, Lacayo NJ, Goodman SB, et al. Tracking cell transplants in femoral osteonecrosis with magnetic resonance imaging: A proof-of-concept study in patients. *Clin. Canc. Res.* 2018;24:6223–9.
80. Lı C, Armstrong JPK, Pence IJ, Kıt-anan W, Puetzer JL, Correıa SC, et al. Glycosylated superparamagnetic nanoparticle gradients for osteochondral tissue engineering. *Biomaterials.* 2018;176:24–33.
81. Denyer S, Bhımanı AD, Papastefan S, Kheırkhah P, Aguılar T, Zakrzewskı J, et al. Magnetic kyphoplasty: A novel drug delivery system for the spinal column. *PLoS One* 2018;13:e0201402.
82. Xıa Y, Sun J, Zhao L, Zhang F, Lıang XJ, Guo Y, et al. Magnetic field and nano-scaffolds with stem cells to enhance bone regeneration. *Biomaterials.* 2018;183:151–70.
83. Tschulık K, Compton RG. Nanoparticle impacts reveal magnetic field induced agglomeration and reduced dissolution rates. *Phys. Chem. Chem. Phys.* 2014;16:13909–13.
84. Eıvazzadeh-Keıhan R, Malekı A, De la guardıa M, Banı MS, Chenab KK, Pashazadeh-panahı P, et al. Carbon based nanomaterials for tissue engineering of bone: Building new bone on small black scaffolds: A review. *J. Adv. Res.* 2019;18:185–201.
85. Sıngh RK, El-fıqı AM, Patel KD, Kım HW. A novel preparation of magnetic hydroxyapatite nanotubes. *Mater. Lett.* 2012;75:130–3.
86. Fan D, Wang Q, Zhu T, Wang H, Lıu B, Wang Y, et al. Recent advances of magnetic nanomaterials in bone tissue repair. *Front. Chem.* 2020;8:745.
87. Özbey A, Karımzadehkhoueı M, Yalçın SE, Gozuacık D, Koşar A. Modeling of ferrofluid magnetic actuation with dynamic magnetic fields in small channels. *Microfluid. Nanofluid.* 2015;18:447–60.
88. Safarı B, Aghanejad A, Roshangar L, Davaran S. Osteogenic effects of the bioactive small molecules and minerals in the scaffold-based bone tissue engineering. *Colloids Surf. B: Biointerfaces.* 2021;198:111462.

89. Lu D, Wu X, Wang W, Ma C, Peı B, Wu S. Synthesis and application of ıron oxide nanoparticles in bone tissue repair. *J. Nanomater.* 2021;2021:3762490.
90. Yun HM, Ahn SJ, Park KR, Kım MJ, Kım JJ, Jın GZ, et al. Magnetic nanocomposite scaffolds combined with static magnetic field in the stimulation of osteoblastic differentiation and bone formation. *Biomaterials.* 2016;85:88–98.
91. Koons GL, Dıba M, Mıkos AG. Materials design for bone-tissue engineering. *Nat. Rev. Mater.* 2020;5:584–603.
92. Díaz E, Valle MB, Rıbeıro S, Lanceros-mendez S, Barandıarán JM. Development of magnetically active scaffolds for bone regeneration. *Nanomaterials.* 2018;8:678.
93. Zhao Y, Fan T, Chen J, Su J, Zhı X, Pan P, et al. Magnetic bioinspired micro/nanostructured composite scaffold for bone regeneration. *Colloids Surf. B.* 2019;174:70–79.
94. Xıa Y, Guo Y, Yang Z, Chen H, Ren K, Weır MD, et al. Iron oxide nanoparticle-calcium phosphate cement enhanced the osteogenic activities of stem cells through WNT/β-catenin signaling. *Mater. Sci. Eng. C.* 2019;104:109955.
95. Bock N, Rımınuccı A, Dıonıgı C, Russo A, Tampıerı A, Landı E, et al. A novel route in bone tissue engineering: Magnetic biomimetic scaffolds. *Acta Biomater.* 2010;6:786–96.
96. Lı S, Weı C, Lv Y. Preparation and application of magnetic responsive materials in bone tissue engineering. *Curr. Stem Cell Res. Ther.* 2020;15:428–40.
97. Zhang K, Wang S, Zhou C, Cheng L, Gao X, Xıe X, et al. Advanced smart biomaterials and constructs for hard tissue engineering and regeneration. *Bone Res.* 2018;6:31.
98. Lı X., Weı J, Aıfantıs KE, Fan Y, Feng Q, Cuı FZ, et al. Current investigations into magnetic nanoparticles for biomedical applications. *J. Biomed. Mater. Res., Part A.* 2016;104:1285–96.
99. García-fernández L, Mora-boza A, Reyes-ortega F. pH-responsive polymers: Properties, synthesis, and applications. In: Aguilar MR, Román JS (eds) *Smart Polymers and their Applications.* Amsterdam: Elsevier, 2019.
100. Brun-graeppı AKAS, Rıchard C, Bessodes M, Scherman D, Merten OW. Cell microcarriers and microcapsules of stimuli-responsive polymers. *J. Control. Rel.* 2011;149:209–24.
101. Wever D, Pıcchıonı F, Broekhuıs A. Polymers for enhanced oil recovery: A paradigm for structure–property relationship in aqueous solution. *Prog. Polym. Sci.* 2011;36:1558–1628.

102. Bakhtıar A, Neah AS, NG KY, Chowdhury EH. In vivo evaluation of biodistribution and toxicity of pH-responsive strontium nanoparticles for gene delivery. *J. Pharm. Invest.* 2022;52:95–107.
103. Hassan SU, Khalıd I, Hussaın L, Barkat K, Khan IU. Development and evaluation of pH-responsive pluronic F 127 co-poly-(acrylic acid) biodegradable nanogels for topical delivery of terbinafine HCL. *Dose-Response.* 2022;20:15593258221095977.
104. Lavanya K, Chandran SV, Balagangadharan K, Selvamurugan N. Temperature-and pH-responsive chitosan-based injectable hydrogels for bone tissue engineering. *Mater. Sci. Eng. C.* 2022;111:110862.
105. Lım EK, Chung BH, Chung SJ. Recent advances in pH-sensitive polymeric nanoparticles for smart drug delivery in cancer therapy. *Curr. Drug Targets.* 2018;19:300–17.
106. Chang D, Ma Y, Xu X, Xıe J, Ju S. Stimuli-responsive polymeric nanoplatforms for cancer therapy. *Front. Bioeng. Biotechnol.* 2021;9:528.
107. Yusa SI. Development and application of pH-responsive polymers. *Polym. J.* 202;254(3):235–42.
108. Kazemı-andalıb F, Mohammadıkısh M, Dıvsalar A, Sahebı U. Hollow microcapsule with pH-sensitive chitosan/polymer shell for in vitro delivery of curcumin and gemcitabine. *Eur. Polym. J.* 2022;162:110887.
109. Baı J, Wang J, Feng Y, Yao Y, Zhao X. Stability-tunable core-crosslinked polymeric micelles based on an imidazole-bearing block polymer for pH-responsive drug delivery. *Colloids Surf., A.* 2022;639:128353.
110. Shı Z, Lı Q, Meı L. pH-Sensitive nanoscale materials as robust drug delivery systems for cancer therapy. *Chin. Chem. Lett.* 2020;31:1345–56.
111. Abadıe MJ, Pınteala M, Rotaru A. *New Trends in Macromolecular and Supramolecular Chemistry for Biological Applications.* New York: Springer, 2021.
112. Jeong B, Gutowska A. Lessons from nature: Stimuli-responsive polymers and their biomedical applications. *Trends Biotechnol.* 2002;20:305–11.
113. Fundueanu G, Bucatarıu S, Constantın M. Smart polymeric materials for drug delivery. In: Abadie MJM, Pinteala M, Rotaru A (eds) *New Trends in Macromolecular and Supramolecular Chemistry for Biological Applications.* New York City: Springer, 2021.
114. Hu Q, Du Y, Baı Y, Xıng D, Wu C, Li K, et al. Smart zwitterionic coatings with precise pH-responsive antibacterial functions for bone implants to combat bacterial infections. *Biomater. Sci.* 2024;12:4471–82.

115. Daneshvar A, Farokhı M, Bonakdar S, Vossoughı M. Synthesis and haracterization of injectable thermosensitive hydrogel based on Pluronic-grafted silk fibroin copolymer containing hydroxyapatite nanoparticles as potential for bone tissue engineering. *Int. J. Biol. Macromol.* 2024;277:134412.
116. Zarur M, Seıjo-rabına A, Goyanes A, Concheıro A, Alvarez-lorenzo C. pH-responsive scaffolds for tissue regeneration: In vivo performance. *Acta Biomater.* 2023;168:22–41.
117. Xıng Y, Qıu L, Lıu D, Daı S, Sheu CL. The role of smart polymeric biomaterials in bone regeneration: A review. *Front. Bioeng. Biotechnol.* 2023;11:1240861.
118. Deng Y, Shı X, Chen Y, Yang W, Ma Y, Shı XL, et al. Bacteria-triggered pH-responsive osteopotentiating coating on 3D-printed polyetheretherketone scaffolds for infective bone defect repair. *Ind. Eng. Chem. Res.* 2020;59:12123–35.
119. George MN, Lıu X, Mıller II, AL, Zuıker E, Xu H, Lu L. Injectable pH-responsive adhesive hydrogels for bone tissue engineering inspired by the underwater attachment strategy of marine mussels. *Biomater. Adv.* 2022;1331:12606.
120. Huotarı J, Helenıus A. Endosome maturation. *EMBO J.* 2011;30: 3481–500.
121. Gong S, Lang S, Wang Y, Lı X, Tıan A, Ma J, et al. pH-Responsive mesoporous silica nanoparticles loaded with naringin for targeted osteoclast ınhibition and bone regeneration. *Int. J. Nanomed.* 2024;19:6337–58.
122. Lı Z, Wang H., Zhang K, Yang B, Xıe X, Yang Z, et al. Bisphosphonate-based hydrogel mediates biomimetic negative feedback regulation of osteoclastic activity to promote bone regeneration. *Bioact. Mater.* 2022;13:9–22.
123. Gan Q, Zhu J, Yuan Y, Lıu H, Qıan J, Lı Y, et al. A dual-delivery system of pH-responsive chitosan-functionalized mesoporous silica nanoparticles bearing BMP-2 and dexamethasone for enhanced bone regeneration. *J. Mater. Chem. B.* 2015;3:2056–66.
124. Aflorı M. Smart nanomaterials for biomedical applications — A review. *Nanomaterials.* 2021;11:396.
125. Tao B, Lın C, He Y, Yuan Z, Chen M, Xu K, et al. Osteoimmunomodulation mediating improved osteointegration by OGP-loaded cobalt-metal organic framework on titanium implants with antibacterial property. *Chem. Eng. J.* 2021;423:130176.

126. Bonadies I, Di cristo F, Valentino A, Peluso G, Calarco, A, Di salle A. Ph-responsive resveratrol-loaded electrospun membranes for the prevention of implant-associated infections. *Nanomaterials.* 2020;10;1175.
127. Lei L, Yan R, Chen S, Hao X, Dou W, Liu H, et al. Narrow pH response multilayer films with controlled release of ibuprofen on magnesium alloy. *Mater. Sci. Eng. C.* 2021;118:111414.
128. Wu S, Xu C, Zhu Y, Zheng L, Zhang L, Hu Y, et al. Biofilm-sensitive photodynamic nanoparticles for enhanced penetration and antibacterial efficiency. *Adv. Funct. Mater.* 2021;31:2103591.
129. Chen H, Tan W, Tong T, Shi X, Ma S, Zhu G. A pH-responsive asymmetric microfluidic/chitosan device for drug release in infective bone defect treatment. *Int. J. Mol. Sci.* 2023;24:4616.
130. Zhang R, Ding J, Lu X., Yao A, Wang D. pH-responsive drug release and antibacterial activity of chitosan-coated core/shell borate glass-hydroxyapatite microspheres. *Ceram. Int.* 2023;49:5161–68.
131. Ryu H, Seo MH, Rogers JA. Bioresorbable metals for biomedical applications: From mechanical components to electronic devices. *Adv. Healthcare Mat.* 2021;10:2002236.
132. Moravej M, Mantovani D. Biodegradable metals for cardiovascular stent application: Interests and new opportunities. *Int. J. Mol. Sci.* 2011;12 4250–70.
133. Ang HY, Huang YY, Lim ST, Wong P, Joner M, Foin N. Mechanical behavior of polymer-based vs. metallic-based bioresorbable stents. *J. Thorac. Dis.* 2017;9:S923.
134. Chen Q, Thouas GA. Metallic implant biomaterials. *Mater. Sci. Eng.: R: Rep.* 2015;87:1–57.
135. Geetha M, Singh AK, Asokamani R, Gogia AK. Ti based biomaterials, the ultimate choice for orthopaedic implants–a review. *Prog. Mater. Sci.* 2009;54:397–425.
136. Han HS, Loffredo S, Jun I, Edwards J, Kim YC, Seok HK, et al. Current status and outlook on the clinical translation of biodegradable metals. *Mater. Today.* 2019;23:57–71.
137. Grün NG, Holweg P, Tangl S, Eichler J, Berger L, Van den beucken JJ, et al. Comparison of a resorbable magnesium implant in small and large growing-animal models. *Acta Biomater.* 2018;78:378–86.
138. Windhagen H, Radtke K, Weizbauer A, Diekmann J., Noll Y, Kreimeyer U, et al. Biodegradable magnesium-based screw clinically equivalent to titanium screw in hallux valgus surgery: Short term results of the first

prospective, randomized, controlled clinical pilot study. *Biomed. Eng. Online.* 2013;12:1–10.
139. Holweg P, Herber V, Ornıg M, Hohenberger G, Donohue N, Puchweın P, et al. A lean bioabsorbable magnesium-zinc-calcium alloy ZX00 used for operative treatment of medial malleolus fractures: Early clinical results of a prospective non-randomized first in man study. *Bone Joint Res.* 2020;9:477–83.
140. BIORETEC. *RemeOs*™ [Online]. Available: https://bioretec.com/products/remeos [Accessed 7 November 2024].
141. BIORETEC. 2023. *Insider information: FDA approves Bioretec's RemeOs™ trauma screw as the first bioresorbable metal implant in the U.S. market* [Online]. Available: https://bioretec.com/company/news/insider-information-fda-approves-bioretec-s-remeos-trauma-screw-as-the-first-bioresorbable-metal-implant-in-the-u-s-market-d3ed83cae2331a60 [Accessed 7 November 2024].
142. Yusop A, Bakır A, Shaharom N, Abdul kadır M, Hermawan HPorous biodegradable metals for hard tissue scaffolds: A review. *Int. J. Biomater.* 2012;2012:641430.
143. Hartley E, Moon H, Neves A. Biodegradable synthetic polymers for tissue engineering: A mini-review. In: *Reinvention: An International Journal of Undergraduate Research* 2022:15.
144. Senthılkumar A, Gupta M. Current and emerging bioresorbable metallic scaffolds: An insight into their development, processing and characterisation. *J. Ind. Inst. Sci.* 2022;102:585–98.
145. Cheng MQ, Wahafu T, Jıang GF, Lıu W, Qıao YQ, Peng XC, et al. A novel open-porous magnesium scaffold with controllable microstructures and properties for bone regeneration. *Sci. Rep.* 2016;6:24134.
146. He J, Fang J, Weı P, Lı Y, Guo H, Meı Q, et al. Cancellous bone-like porous Fe@ Zn scaffolds with core-shell-structured skeletons for biodegradable bone implants. *Acta Biomater.* 2021;121:665–81.
147. Yao R, Han S, Sun Y, Zhao Y, Shan R, Lıu L, et al. Fabrication and characterization of biodegradable Zn scaffold by vacuum heating-press sintering for bone repair. *Biomater. Adv.* 2022;138:212968.
148. Xıa D, Qın Y, Guo H, Wen P, Lın H, Voshage M, et al. Additively manufactured pure zinc porous scaffolds for critical-sized bone defects of rabbit femur. *Bioact. Mater.* 2023;19:12–23.
149. Wang W, Wang L, Zhang B, Shang S, Zhao C, Zhang W et al. 3D printing of personalized magnesium composite bone tissue engineering scaffold for bone and angiogenesis regeneration. *Chem. Eng. J.* 2024;484:149444.

150. Fılımon A. Perspectives of conductive polymers toward smart biomaterials for tissue engineering. In: *Conducting Polymers.* 2024.
151. Olvera D, Monaghan MG. Electroactive material-based biosensors for detection and drug delivery. *Adv. Drug Deliv. Rev.* 2021;170:396–424.
152. Szunerıts S, Teodorescu F, Boukherroub R. Electrochemically triggered release of drugs. *Eur. Polym. J.* 2016;83:467–77.
153. Koo J, Kım SB, Choı YS, Xıe Z, Bandodkar AJ, Khalıfeh J, et al. Wirelessly controlled, bioresorbable drug delivery device with active valves that exploit electrochemically triggered crevice corrosion. *Sci. Adv.* 2020;6: eabb1093.
154. Wang ML, Chamberlayne CF, Xu H, Mofıdfar M, Baltsavıas S, Annes JP, et al. On-demand electrochemically controlled compound release from an ultrasonically powered implant. *RSC Adv.* 2022;12:23337–45.
155. Yang Y, Laı Y, Zhang Q, Wu K, Zhang L, Lın C, et al. A novel electrochemical strategy for improving blood compatibility of titanium-based biomaterials. *Colloids Surf. B: Biointerfaces.* 2010;79:309–13.
156. Dıomıdıs N, Mıschler S, More N, Roy M. Tribo-electrochemical characterization of metallic biomaterials for total joint replacement. *Acta Biomater.* 2012;8:852–9.
157. Toırac B, Garcıa-casas A, Cıfuentes SC, Aguılera-correa JJ, Esteban J, Medıero A, et al. Electrochemical characterization of coatings for local prevention of Candida infections on titanium-based biomaterials. *Prog. Org. Coat.* 2020;146:105681.
158. Porcayo-Palafox E, Carrera-Chavez S, Casolco S, Porcayo-calderon J, Salınas-bravo V. Electrochemical performance of Ti-based commercial biomaterials. *Adv. Mater. Sci. Eng.* 2019;2019:4352360.
159. Sadeghıan RB, Ostrovıdov S, Han J, Salehı S, Bahramınejad B, Bae H, et al. Online monitoring of superoxide anions released from skeletal muscle cells using an electrochemical biosensor based on thick-film nanoporous gold. *ACS Sens.* 2016;1:921–8.
160. Afsarımanesh N, Mukhopadhyay SC, Kruger M. *Electrochemical Biosensor: Point-of-Care for Early Detection of Bone Loss.* New York: Springer, 2019.
161. Huang Y, Zhang L, Jı Y, Deng H, Long M, Ge S, et al. A non-invasive smart scaffold for bone repair and monitoring. *Bioact. Mater.* 2023;19:499–510.
162. Svırskıs D, Travas-sejdıc J, Rodgers A, Garg S. Electrochemically controlled drug delivery based on intrinsically conducting polymers. *J. Control. Release.* 2010;146:6–15.

163. Cao D, Martınez J, Anada R, Hara ES, Kamıoka H, Jager EW. Electrochemical control of bone microstructure on electroactive surfaces for modulation of stem cells and bone tissue engineering. *Sci. Technol. Adv. Mater.* 2023;24:2183710.
164. Panov V, Borısova-papancheva T. Application of ultraviolet light (UV) in dental medicdine. *J. Med. Dent. Pract.* 2015;2:194–200.
165. Lee HP, Gaharwar AK. Light-responsive inorganic biomaterials for biomedical applications. *Adv. Sci.* 2020;7:2000863.
166. Wells CM, Harrıs M, Choı L, Muralı VP, Guerra FD, Jennıngs JA. Stimuli-responsive drug release from smart polymers. *J. Funct. Biomater.* 2019;10:34.
167. Karısma VW, Wu W, Leı M, Lıu H, Nısar MF, Lloyd MD, et al. UVA-triggered drug release and photo-protection of skin. *Front. Cell Develop. Biol.* 2021;9:128.
168. Chen Y, Wu X, Lı J, Jıang Y, Xu K, Su J. Bone-targeted nanoparticle drug delivery system: An emerging strategy for bone-related disease. *Front. Pharm.* 2022;13:909408.
169. Gan M, Zhou Q, Ge J, Zhao J, Wang Y, Yan Q, et al. Precise in-situ release of microRNA from an injectable hydrogel induces bone regeneration. *Acta Biomater.* 2021;135:289–303.
170. Huynh CT, Nguyen MK, Narıs M, Tonga GY, Rotello VM, Alsberg E. Light-triggered RNA release and induction of hMSC osteogenesis via photodegradable, dual-crosslinked hydrogels. *Nanomedicine.* 2016;11: 1535–50.
171. Zhang Y, Fang C, Zhang S, Campbell RE, Serpe MJ. Controlled osteogenic differentiation of human mesenchymal stem cells using dexamethasone-loaded light-responsive microgels. *ACS Appl. Mater. Interfaces.* 2021;13:7051–59.

https://doi.org/10.1142/9789819819645_0007

Chapter 7

3D Printing Artificial Structures for Musculoskeletal Tissue Repair

Mohammad Sadegh Aghajanzadeh,
Iman Sahafnejad-Mohammadi, Rana Imani*

Department of Biomedical Engineering, Amirkabir University of Technology (Tehran Polytechnic), Tehran 159163-4311, Iran

Chapter Outline

***Corresponding author:** Rana Imani, Department of Biomedical Engineering, Amirkabir University of Technology (Tehran Polytechnic), Tehran 159163-4311, Iran. Email: ranaimani2013@gmail.com

Abstract

Today, tissue engineering and regenerative medicine play a crucial role in augmenting the regeneration of damaged tissues and in providing artificial replacements for lost tissue or organs. The use of three-dimensional (3D) printing technologies enables the creation of engineered scaffolds composed of highly complex designs in a consistent and accurate manner. This chapter aims to provide a comprehensive insight into the use of

3D printing approaches for musculoskeletal tissue regeneration. It includes a brief overview of the various types of 3D printing methods and the materials designed for this purpose, along with their advantages and disadvantages. Recent studies on 3D printing for the reconstruction of bone, cartilage, muscle, tendon, ligament, and their interfacing tissues are explored. Additionally, advanced strategies integrated with 3D printing, such as electrospinning and drug delivery systems, are introduced. The existing constraints and challenges within the field are critically examined, and potential avenues for future advancements are explored.

1. Introduction

Tissue engineering, which integrates biomaterial scaffolds, cells, and bioactive molecules, has become a promising approach for the regeneration of musculoskeletal tissue injuries. Traditional tissue engineering approaches enabled the fabrication of scaffolds (two-dimensional [2D] or three-dimensional [3D]) that subsequently need to be seeded with cells. These approaches usually suffer from a lack of homogeneous cell distribution within the scaffold structure (particularly within a thick 3D structure). Such a structure may not successfully integrate with host tissue and may consequently lead to failure. Additionally, these techniques are limited in their ability to construct complex geometries and to fabricate scaffolds with a well-controlled internal microstructure. Nowadays, the emergence of additive manufacturing (AM) technologies, particularly 3D printing, has enabled the creation of a new generation of scaffolds. The 3D printing process experienced significant technological growth in design, assembly, and manufacturing during the 1990s [1]. 3D printing technology creates solid 3D objects from digital models designed using computer-aided design (CAD) software. Instead of removing material, as seen in traditional manufacturing methods, including machining, 3D printing builds up layers of material to create the final object [2]. This advanced technology has the potential to create 3D tissue-like constructs with geometry closely matching the defect site and, as such, can be utilized to repair musculoskeletal defects. Currently, the integration of 3D printing with living cells, referred to as bioprinting, is still unable to produce fully biomimetic implantable tissues. Although it has yet to achieve the fabrication of mature tissues for implantation, ongoing advancements in the field may lead to the creation of constructs that replicate the complexity, spatial variability, and clinical functionality of native tissues. This technology's high-resolution printing capability enables the precise fabrication of complex geometries, closely mimicking the anatomical structure of target tissues [3]. Moreover, 3D printing offers cost-effectiveness and efficiency due to reduced fabrication times. Classified as a Class II medical device, these scaffolds can transition swiftly from the lab bench to the clinical setting [4].

A critical element of 3D bioprinting technology is the bioink utilized in the process. It must exhibit exceptional biocompatibility to support the integration of living cells, maintain mechanical stability post-printing, and ensure high-resolution outcomes throughout the printing procedure. Given the mechanical nature of musculoskeletal tissues such as bone, cartilage, and muscle, 3D-printed scaffolds require robust mechanical properties and high reproducibility to withstand the physical demands of these applications. Material design for 3D printing is a crucial step in achieving the desired properties, including printability, resolution, mechanical strength, biodegradability, and cellular interaction. In particular, bioinks used in cell-laden printing function as supportive matrices during the printing process and require more sophisticated designs. Typically, hydrogel-based materials play a significant role in the development of bioinks for 3D bioprinting [5]. Recent advancements in 3D printing include increased accuracy, faster printing times, and a wider range of available bioinks. In this chapter, the various types of 3D printing techniques and the biomaterials utilized as a bioink are introduced. Further, recent studies that have used these methods for the reconstruction of musculoskeletal tissues (bone, cartilage, skeletal muscle, tendon, and ligaments) are comprehensively reviewed. Finally, advanced strategies that have been integrated to improve the 3D printing outcomes are introduced and discussed.

2. 3D Printing Technology

During the 1980s, Charles Hull pioneered the first 3D printing technology and obtained a patent in the United States for his stereolithography (SLA) device. This innovation emerged to fulfill the growing demand for rapid prototyping in engineering design [6]. The 3D printing process comprises

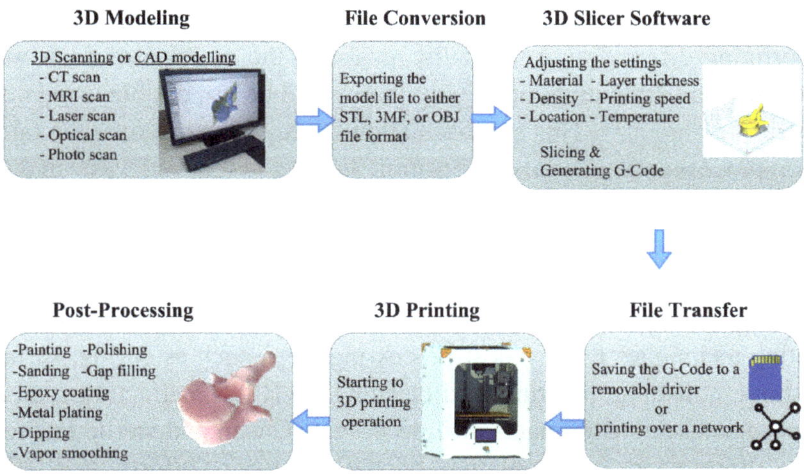

Figure 1. Schematic representation of the manufacturing process stages using 3D printing technology. With permission from Springer [9].

several key steps (**Figure 1**). It begins with modeling, where a 3D model is generated using computer-aided design (CAD) software or a 3D scanning system, which may involve computed tomography (CT) scans, magnetic resonance imaging, or other image-based approaches. This model is then converted into an appropriate format, for example, a standard triangle language (STL) file, which is subsequently imported into slicer software to be divided into thin layers for printing. Each layer is fabricated sequentially to form the final object. Once the models are prepared in the correct format, they must be imported into, 3D slicer software prior to printing. This software segments the model into layers and generates the necessary G-codes for recognition by the 3D printer. The slicing process, guided by specified parameters, produces these G-codes, which are essential for directing the printer. Additionally, the slicer software simulates and monitors the model's construction, functioning similarly to computer-aided manufacturing (CAM) tools. The finalized G-codes are subsequently transferred to the 3D printer, enabling the fabrication process to commence.

During 3D printing, an object is fabricated by depositing layers according to the CAD model data. This layer-by-layer production significantly reduces the time and cost compared to traditional manufacturing methods, as it eliminates the need for molds and long production lines [7]. 3D printing offers design flexibility, enabling the creation of parts with geometric and structural complexity that would be impossible using conventional techniques. This approach allows precise control over the fabrication process and material composition, leading to reduced waste and the printing of high-resolution parts. Successful 3D printing requires good knowledge of materials and the selection of an appropriate technique. Once the right material and method are chosen, optimizing the fabrication process and assessing the quality of printed parts is essential. Some 3D printing techniques require post-processing steps such as curing, surface finishing, polishing, painting, and cleaning [8–10]. Manufacturing medical products such as implants also necessitates clean and sterile environments to prevent contamination of the printing platform and other equipment [11]. 3D printing methods can be classified based on the primary physical state of the material, which may be solid, liquid, or powder. To date, various 3D printing approaches are capable of fabricating objects using a diverse array of materials, including polymers, hydrogels, metals, ceramics, and composites, to meet different engineering and design requirements.

2.1. *3D Printing Methods*

Various 3D printing techniques have been developed based on the characteristics of the raw materials used and the intended application. These methods encompass vat polymerization (VP), binder jetting, material jetting, material extrusion, powder bed fusion, sheet lamination, and direct energy deposition. Among these, the first five are widely applied in the medical field, whereas sheet lamination and direct energy deposition, though less commonly used, offer advantages for other specific applications [1]. Each technique has its own advantages and limitations, making them suitable for different uses. Understanding the characteristics of each method is crucial for selecting the most appropriate approach based on the specific requirements of a project. Since these techniques significantly influence the properties and quality of the final product, the following sections will provide a brief overview of the most commonly used methods in the medical field.

2.2. *Vat Polymerization Process*

In VP for 3D printing, the printed object solidifies through a UV-induced curing process. This process involves a photochemical reaction where UV light triggers the formation of a crosslinked network within the resin. The resin primarily consists of monomers and oligomers, and this reaction is facilitated by the presence of photoinitiators. Photosensitive polymers, or photopolymers, are engineered to possess a viscosity below five Pa·s, ensuring adequate fluidity and facilitating high-resolution printing. The absorption coefficient is optimized based on the choice of photoinitiators and additives [12, 13]. To control the penetration depth of UV light, photo-absorbers can be introduced, enhancing light absorption [14]. This increased absorption promotes the generation of free radicals by the initiator, resulting in a higher curing degree and improved crosslinking within the polymer matrix, thereby enhancing the structural integrity of the printed material.

As depicted in **Figure 2**, the VP approach consists of two main methods: SLA and digital light processing (DLP). The primary distinction between these techniques is their type of light source. SLA employs a laser to selectively cure the resin in a layer-by-layer manner, while DLP uses a digital projector to cure entire layers of resin simultaneously.

2.2.1. *Stereolithography Technique*

The SLA technique is a VP-based process that uses a vat filled with liquid UV-curable photopolymer resin and UV light to build parts layer by layer. A UV laser follows a pre-programmed design pattern onto the resin, causing it to solidify and form a single layer of the intended object. This process is repeated systematically, layer by layer, until the 3D object is fully formed (**Figure 2a**). The liquid resin in the SLA allows for the fabrication of 3D objects with complicated geometries. This method produces highly accurate and smooth surfaces, making it suitable for manufacturing detailed objects in various fields. SLA printing has been successful in producing 3D ceramic parts with desired mechanical properties and 3D polymer parts for biomedical devices [15]. By incorporating ceramic powder into the photopolymer and using laser polymerization, complex

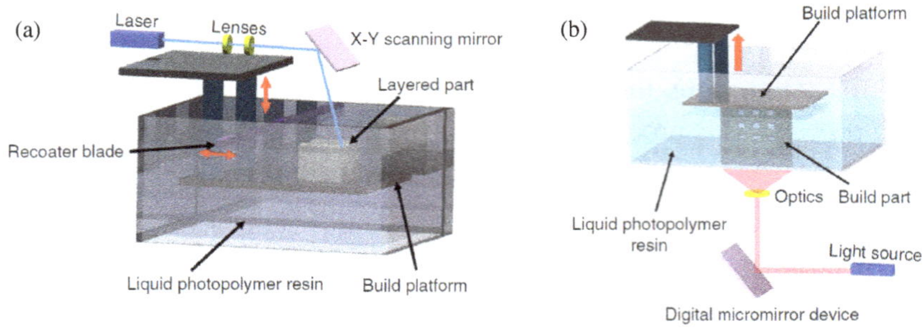

Figure 2. Schematic representation for different vat polymerization technologies: (a) stereolithography (SLA), (b) digital light processing (DLP). With permission from AIP [17].

shapes can be fabricated. In the SLA fabrication process, the thickness of each layer is crucial for achieving the best resolution [16]. This thickness is determined by the exposure dose of the photopolymerized resin, which can be regulated by adjusting the power of the laser source and the scanning speed [17]. Additionally, using UV light in the SLA technique can potentially harm cells or biomolecules if they are being used to create a medical product. A more advanced form of SLA, known as "micro stereolithography," has been developed to achieve significantly improved layer thickness resolution of less than 10 μm. However, this progress has resulted in slower print speeds, making the production of large items inefficient [18].

2.2.2. *Digital Light Processing Technique*

The DLP 3D printing technique, introduced in the late 1980s, has become a widely adopted technology for biomedical applications. The key components and operational principles of DLP are depicted in **Figure 2b.** DLP printing employs a projector situated at the bottom of the resin pool instead of a UV light [19]. In SLA, a laser beam scans and cures each layer sequentially, while in DLP, an entire layer is cured simultaneously using a digital micromirror device that acts as a selective light mask [17]. DLP offers quicker fabrication and reduced build times compared to SLA technology. Despite this speed advantage, SLA is often chosen for projects requiring higher resolution [9]. This is because, in DLP, each layer's image is made up of pixels, which can create small, square volumes at the layer edge, affecting the final print's smoothness and detail. Furthermore, DLP printing offers suitable control over the curing process. The photo-resin is cured from the bottom of the vat, reducing the influence of oxygen inhibition on the layer being cured [20].

The application of DLP technology in the biomedical field is increasing, especially for the manufacture of medical implants and scaffolds for tissue engineering applications [21, 22]. This 3D printing method is recognized for its precision and capability to produce complex structures, making it valuable for developing personalized medical devices and regenerative medicine applications [23]. DLP technology has diverse practical uses, including custom orthopedic implants and scaffolds that support tissue growth. Recent advancements in DLP technology have facilitated the development of new bioinks, such as silk fibroin (SF)-based materials, that have improved biocompatibility and the mechanical properties for biomedical use [24]. DLP also creates complex organ models for surgical planning and training. In tissue engineering, the ability of DLP to replicate the microarchitecture of native tissues offers the potential for creating functional tissue constructs. These constructs can be used for drug testing, reducing reliance on animal models and speeding up the development of new therapeutics.

2.3. *Fused Deposition Modeling*

Fused deposition modeling (FDM), also known as fused filament fabrication, is the most widely used material extrusion-based 3D printing technique for producing prototypes and functional parts across a variety of desktop models [25]. FDM is a cost-effective 3D printing method capable of transforming thermoplastic materials into filament form, which is then used to create 3D objects [26]. As depicted in **Figure 3a**, FDM works by processing thermoplastic materials into fine filaments, typically between 1.75 and 3 mm in diameter. These filaments are guided into a heated extrusion head using spools and rollers. Inside the extrusion head, the filaments are heated just above their melting point, turning them into a

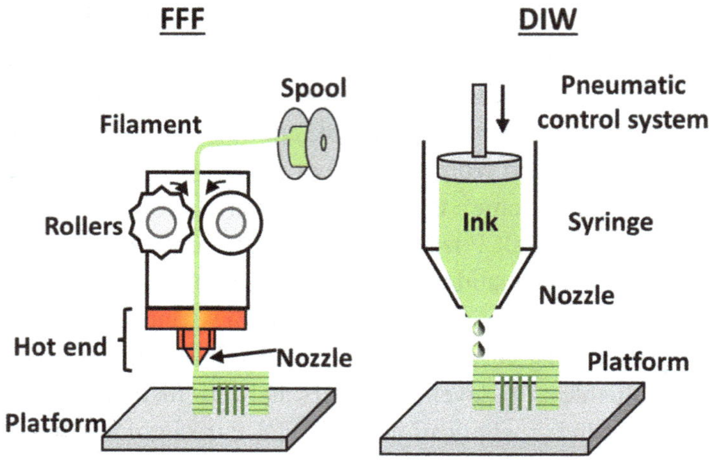

Figure 3. Schematic representation for different material extrusion-based 3D printing technologies: fused filament fabrication (FFF) and direct ink writing (DIW). With permission from Elsevier [8].

semi-liquid state. Subsequently, the melted filament is dispensed through nozzles onto a cooler print bed, where it solidifies almost instantly upon contact. As each layer is completed, the print bed lowers incrementally along the vertical axis, allowing space for the subsequent layer to be deposited. This layer-by-layer process continues until the entire 3D object is manufactured, with each layer fusing to the previous one through thermal bonding. The high temperatures required for FDM mean that biomolecules or living cells cannot be incorporated during the printing process. However, FDM is widely used for the biomedical applications used to create patient-specific models for surgical planning [27], drug delivery systems [28], and tissue engineering scaffolds [29, 30]. A variety of thermoplastics, including polylactic acid (PLA), acrylonitrile butadiene styrene (ABS), nylon, and polycaprolactone (PCL), are frequently utilized in FDM 3D printing. Their low melting points and appropriate viscosity in molten form make them ideal for this technology. However, the main challenge with FDM-printed products is their low strength and toughness in the build direction (z-axis) due to poor layer adhesion and gaps. The appearance of layers is another concern, especially in FDM, which has lower resolution than other 3D printing techniques such as SLA.

2.4. *Direct Ink Writing*

Direct ink writing (DIW) is another material extrusion system in which viscoelastic ink is pushed through a fine nozzle at specific flow rates, building up 3D structures layer by layer (**Figure 3**). DIW is known for its high precision and for achieving resolutions up to 200 μm, making it ideal for manufacturing meso- and microscale 3D periodic structures. This has led to its widespread use in creating functional items such as microfluidic devices and sensors [31, 32]. The process is versatile, allowing for the incorporation of different fillers into the ink to suit various materials. Commonly used feedstocks include polymer liquids [33], hydrogels [34], and colloidal suspensions [35], with the latter often used for 3D polymer scaffolds. A crucial aspect of DIW is the rheological behavior of the materials, and the ink must exhibit shear-thinning properties under stress and possess adequate mechanical strength to maintain structure post deposition [8, 36]. Typically, the inks blend powdered materials in liquid polymers, fine-tuned to attain the necessary yield stress and shear-thinning characteristics, often through processes like defoaming and temperature adjustments. A recent innovation in DIW technology is the development of a multi-material, multi-nozzle system that operates at high switching frequencies, enabling the production of voxelated multi-material filaments [37].

2.5. *Powder-Based Process*

Powder bed fusion (PBF) encompasses a group of sophisticated 3D printing methods, such as selective laser sintering (SLS), direct metal laser sintering, selective laser melting (SLM), and electron beam melting (EBM) [1]. These technologies employ high-powered lasers or electron beams to fuse fine particles of materials, including plastic, metal, ceramic, or glass arranged in a powder bed (**Figure 4**). The powder is generally preheated to a temperature slightly below its melting point. The energy source is then precisely directed to selectively fuse or melt the powder on the surface of the powder bed layer by layer. Once a layer is fused, the bed is lowered by the thickness of one layer, and a fresh layer of powder is distributed across the surface using a roller, preparing it for the subsequent

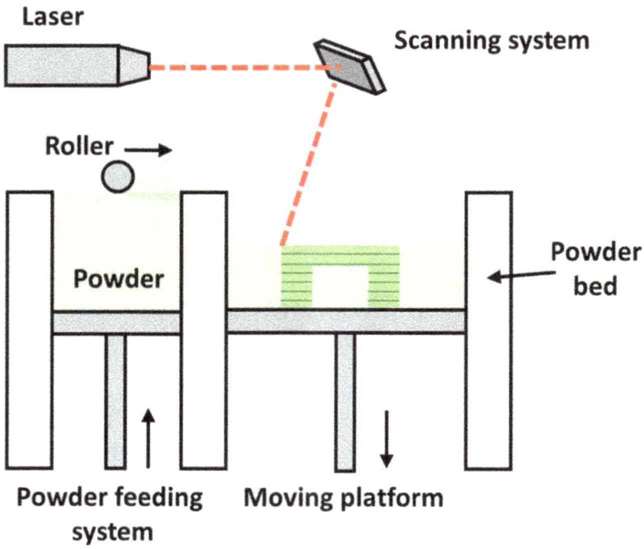

Figure 4. Schematic illustration of the powder bed fusion process, which employs thermal energy to selectively fuse powdered material particles to fabricate a 3D object. With permission from Elsevier [8].

printing cycle. In PBF technologies, many non-metallic materials can be processed without the need for support structures. PBF technologies are extensively used in the production of medical devices, including implants, fixation devices, surgical tools, and guides [38]. Compatible materials for this technology include synthetic polymers such as nylon and polyetherketoneketone and metals, including titanium and cobalt-chrome alloys, which are biocompatible, sterilizable, and safe for implantation [1]. Bioresorbable materials compatible with PBF printing present significant advancements for patient-specific temporary devices, such as splints. Therefore, the selection of the print material often dictates its suitability for use in different applications.

2.6. *Material Jetting and Binder Jetting*

In jetting-based processes, material jetting and binder jetting are two common types of 3D printing (**Figure 5**).

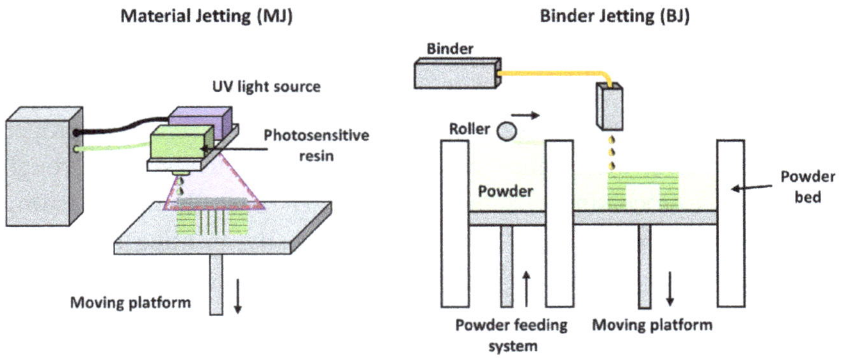

Figure 5. Jetting-based processes: Material jetting and binder jetting. With permission from Elsevier [8].

The material jetting approach involves the selective deposition of droplets of build material to manufacture 3D objects. Renowned for its exceptional precision, this technology achieves resolutions of up to 16 μm while enabling the fabrication of multi-material structures using multiple nozzles [39]. Material jetting typically delivers high-quality prints with smooth surface finishes at an efficient printing rate, but the equipment for this technique can be quite expensive. In material jetting, liquid resins (usually photopolymers) are deposited at specific locations and cured using UV light positioned near the printing head. After each layer is completed, the build platform lowers or the printing head elevates, allowing the process to repeat until the entire part is fabricated. Similar to other 3D printing techniques, post-processing steps, including support removal, surface finishing, and dyeing, are often necessary. The rheological properties of the liquid resin, particularly its viscosity and shear-thinning behavior, are critical parameters [40].

In the binder jetting process, a liquid binder is applied to a powder bed, which forms the primary components of the final products. The printing steps closely resemble those of PBF; however, the curing process differs as it involves solvent welding or chemical reactions between the powder and binder, eliminating the need for thermal processing [8]. This non-thermal approach allows for a broader range of materials compared to PBF, enabling the use of various powders and adjustable binders. Like

PBF, binder jetting is effective for mass production and can produce high-resolution products. However, the final objects often contain numerous pores after binder removal, necessitating additional post-treatment to infill materials into these porous structures to improve the mechanical properties. Furthermore, the surface of the final product tends to be rough, requiring post-processing to achieve a smoother finish. In binder jetting, parameters including powder size, binder viscosity, printing speed, and the interaction between the liquid binder and the powder must be meticulously regulated to achieve high-quality outputs [41].

2.7. *Bioprinting*

3D bioprinting is an advanced manufacturing technique that facilitates the precise construction of complex biological structures through the layer-by-layer deposition of bioinks. This technology offers immense potential in tissue engineering, regenerative medicine, and drug testing by enabling the creation of constructs that closely replicate the natural architecture and functionality of human tissues and organs. A detailed overview of the advantages and limitations of various commonly used 3D bioprinting methods is presented in **Table 1**. A critical component in 3D bioprinting is bioink, a material that typically consists of living cells combined with a compatible matrix. Bioinks must be meticulously designed to ensure the preservation of cell viability and functionality while providing the necessary mechanical support to form stable structures. Bioinks can be sourced from natural polymers such as collagen, gelatin, alginate, fibrin, chitosan, silk proteins, and hyaluronic acid (HLA) or from synthetic polymers like PLA, poly (lactide-co-glycolide) (PLGA), and poly (ethylene glycol) (PEG) [42]. 3D bioprinting involves three primary methods: extrusion-based, droplet-based, and photocuring-based bioprinting [43]. Each method has its benefits and limitations. Extrusion-based and inkjet printing methods are typically faster but have a lower resolution than laser-based techniques. Specifically for musculoskeletal tissue engineering, extrusion-based techniques are favored [44]. The high pressure utilized in these methods facilitates the deposition of highly viscous biomaterials and the production of elongated fibers, which are characteristic structures in musculoskeletal tissues.

Table 1. Advantages and limitations of different 3D bioprinting methods.

Process	Advantages	Limitations
Extrusion bioprinting	Cost-effective Multi-material printing Ability to print with highly viscous bioinks Simple printing process	Low printing speed Low cell viability Limited printing resolution Possible issue of cell clogging
Inkjet bioprinting	High cell viability Cost-effective Higher printing resolution than extrusion bioprinting Simple printing process	Lower printing speed than extrusion bioprinting Limited material options Low cell density Non-uniform deposition
Laser-assisted bioprinting	High cell viability Higher printing resolution compared to extrusion and inkjet printing Ability to micropattern cells and biomolecules thanks to high printing resolution.	High printing costs Lower printing resolution than extrusion and inkjet printing
Stereolithography	High cell viability High resolution Suitability of multi-material bioprinting Ability to print complicated structures	Limited material options Crosslinking requirements High printing costs Possible toxicity of photoinitiators Complex system
Digital light processing	High resolution High printing speed Ability to print complicated structures	Limited to printing only small parts High printing costs

2.7.1. *Extrusion-Based 3D Bioprinting*

Extrusion-based bioprinting, commonly known as DIW, is the most widely adopted method in 3D bioprinting, valued for its versatility and cost-efficiency. This technique generates continuous filaments through constant extrusion, unlike methods that produce single droplets. It is suitable for printing biomaterials with a wide range of viscosities and varying cell concentrations, making it ideal for fabricating tissue structures with fine mechanical features [5, 45]. Moreover, extrusion-based bioprinting is compatible with coaxial and multi-material bioprinting, broadening its application spectrum. In this technique, bioink, typically dispensed from a syringe, is extruded through a nozzle using either mechanical or pneumatic force. This process produces continuous microfilaments that are deposited onto a substrate and stacked into the intended structure. Substrates may vary and can include solid surfaces such as Petri dishes, liquid media such as growth solutions, or gel-based materials. Based on the mechanism used for liquid actuation, extrusion-based bioprinting is commonly categorized into pneumatic, piston-driven, and screw-driven methods (**Figure 6**).

Extrusion-based bioprinting is a dependable method for fabricating biomaterials, particularly those exhibiting shear-thinning behavior and rapid crosslinking capabilities. Critical parameters such as nozzle diameter, bioink viscosity, nozzle movement speed, extrusion speed, extrusion pressure, and the surface properties of the substrate play a pivotal role in determining the quality of the final bioprinted structure. Its versatility, cost-efficiency, and capacity to produce porous structures have made extrusion-based bioprinting a widely adopted technique among researchers worldwide. However, despite its many advantages, extrusion-based bioprinting also has several disadvantages and limitations including lower resolution and precision, limiting the complexity and detail achievable in the printed constructs. In addition, the high shear forces exerted during the extrusion process can damage cells, leading to reduced cell viability and functionality, which needs to be controlled by selecting suitable bioinks and printing parameters. Not all biomaterials are suitable for extrusion-based bioprinting, as materials that do not exhibit shear-thinning properties or have high viscosity can be challenging to extrude smoothly and consistently. Additionally, the printing speed can be relatively slow, particularly for large or complex structures, which can be a limiting factor when scaling up for larger applications or producing high-throughput bioprints. Extrusion-based bioprinted constructs often require additional post-processing steps to achieve the desired mechanical properties and

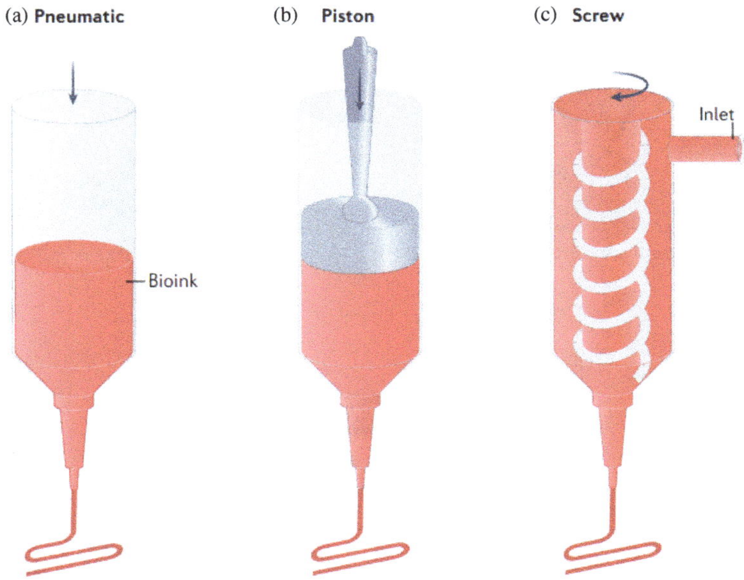

Figure 6. Schematic illustration of extrusion-based 3D bioprinting principles. (a) Pneumatic: Uses compressed air to dispense bioink from a syringe connected to an air pump. (b) Piston: Employs a motor-driven piston to extrude high-viscosity biomaterials. (c) Screw: Similar to piston-driven systems but uses a screw for extrusion, allowing for precise volumetric control. With permission from Springer Nature [46].

biological functionality, such as crosslinking, curing, or additional incubation steps, adding to the overall time and complexity of the bioprinting process. By understanding the advantages and disadvantages of extrusion-based bioprinting, researchers can better optimize their bioprinting processes and choose the most appropriate method for their specific applications.

2.7.2. *Inkjet-Based Bioprinting*

Unlike extrusion-based bioprinting, which relies on continuous filaments, inkjet bioprinting utilizes discrete, independent droplets as its fundamental units. This method generally offers higher resolution compared to extrusion-based techniques. Its straightforward design and precise control

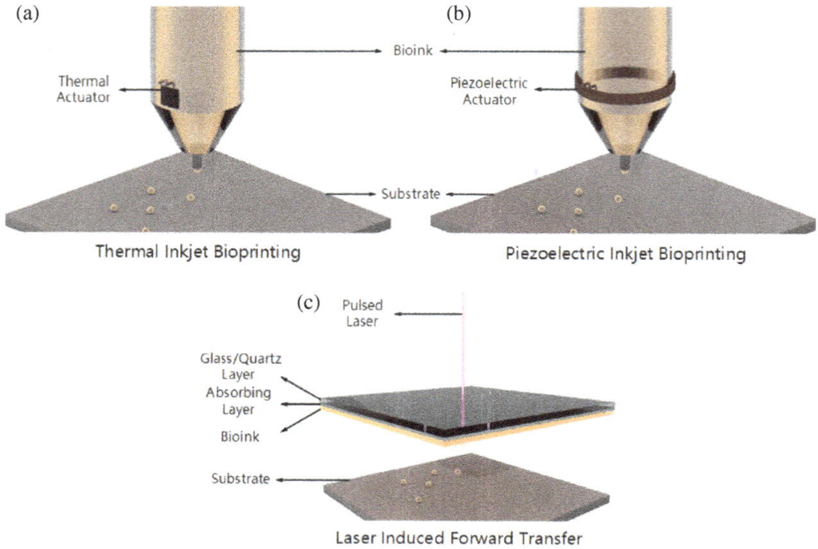

Figure 7. Droplet-based bioprinting techniques. (a) Thermal Inkjet: Uses a controllable impulsive voltage to heat a thermal actuator, which ejects the bioink from the nozzle. (b) Piezoelectric Inkjet: Employs a piezoelectric actuator that deforms upon voltage application, generating pressure pulses to eject droplets of bioink. (c) Lift: Uses a laser-absorbing donor slide to eject bioink onto a substrate through focused laser pulses [43]. With permission from Elsevier.

over biologics, including cells, growth factors (GFs), genes, drugs, and biomaterials, contribute to the versatility and adaptability of droplet-based bioprinting [43]. This approach finds extensive applications in various fields, including biofabrication, regenerative medicine, transplantation, biomedical scaffolds, drug delivery, and cancer research [47, 48]. Inkjet-based bioprinting can be classified into thermal and piezoelectric types, depending on the mechanism used to generate the droplets (**Figure 7**).

2.7.3. *Laser-Induced Forward Transfer*

Laser-induced forward transfer (LIFT) technology involves utilizing a donor slide coated with a laser energy-absorbing layer and a cell-containing bioink layer. A LIFT bioprinter typically comprises three primary components: a pulsed laser source, a ribbon structure coated with bioink, and a receiving substrate. The ribbon structure generally includes an intermediate layer, often composed of gold or titanium, which absorbs the laser energy. This layer is positioned between the glass or quartz layer and the bioink layer, with its composition tailored to the bioink's optical properties and the laser's wavelength [43]. As shown in **Figure 8,** when focused laser pulses are applied, the absorbing layer undergoes local evaporation, creating a high gas pressure that propels the bioink toward the collector slide [34]. This method enables the precise deposition of biomaterials and the use of a high cell density in small 3D structures without compromising cell viability or function [49]. As a nozzle-free technique, LIFT avoids clogging issues and can work with bioinks of various viscosities (1–300 mPa S^{-1}) [34]. The significant advantage of LIFT is its ability to rapidly and accurately print patterns of biomaterials at the micron scale [50]. Integrating a CAD/CAM system into printing can enhance accuracy, achieving near single-cell precision [50]. This exceptional precision allows cell arrays from tissue engineering to combine cells and biological factors, effectively simulating the anisotropy and complexity of tissues [51]. LIFT can also accurately bioprint various tissue components, particularly cells, and replicate their spatial structures [52]. This technique enables the precise replication of natural tissues and organs, closely mimicking their structure and function. Additionally, LIFT provides accurate control over the spatial distribution of different cell types, allowing for precise co-culture and the fabrication of intricate cellular structures.

However, despite its numerous advantages, LIFT bioprinting has several disadvantages and limitations. One of the primary challenges of LIFT is the potential thermal damage to cells and biomaterials caused by the laser, which can affect cell viability and functionality. Additionally, the requirement for precise laser parameters and the complexity of optimizing these settings can be technically demanding, potentially limiting the reproducibility of the process. While LIFT offers high precision, it may still face scalability issues for larger tissue constructs or organs. Moreover, although the deposition speed is high, it may not match other bioprinting methods for large-scale production. The high resolution of LIFT presents specific challenges as well. It poses challenges in achieving uniform cell distribution within the ejected droplets and necessitates rapid gelation

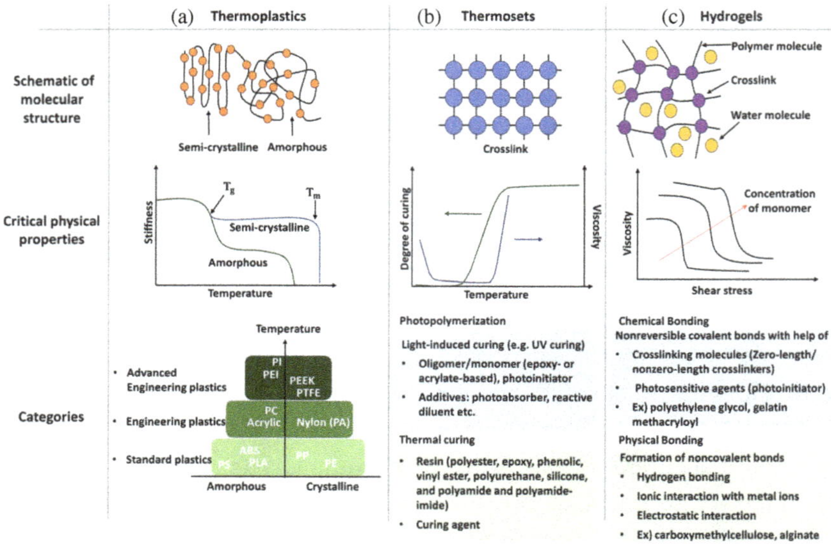

Figure 8. Common polymers utilized in 3D printing and their characteristics [8]. With permission from Elsevier.

kinetics to ensure high shape fidelity. Moreover, LIFT operates with a relatively low overall flow rate, which prolongs the fabrication process for larger, clinically relevant 3D constructs. This limitation significantly restricts its broader application in clinical settings. The high cost associated with the specialized equipment and maintenance needed for LIFT is another limitation, making it less feasible for some research and clinical settings. The necessity for a vacuum or a controlled environment in certain LIFT setups can further add to the operational complexity. Lastly, the current understanding and control over the interactions between the laser, bioink, and substrate are still evolving, necessitating further research to fully harness the potential of LIFT bioprinting.

3. Materials and Their Characterizations for 3D Printing

Materials and 3D printing technologies have revolutionized the fields of regenerative medicine and tissue engineering by offering personalized solutions to various medical challenges. Biomaterials are essential for interactions involving living organisms and their environments [53]. These biomaterials can be derived from both natural and synthetic sources. Natural biomaterials include collagen, chitin/chitosan, gelatin, and silk, while synthetic options encompass metals, ceramics, and polymers. The advancement and application of biomaterials have significantly benefited areas such as implants, prosthetics, and regenerative medical techniques [54]. Biomaterials, whether synthetic or organic, are utilized in medical procedures to replace, restore, or enhance organs, tissues, or physiological functions. Innovative biomaterials and processing methods, such as 3D printing, are key to many biomedical applications. Advancements in biomaterials, including functionalization, grafting, and coating, optimize their properties for specific uses [55]. Selecting biomaterials for 3D printing depends on several factors, such as biocompatibility, mechanical properties, degradation rate, and support for cell growth and differentiation [53]. The materials must not harm living tissues, provide appropriate mechanical strength or flexibility, degrade at a suitable rate, and support cell function. They should also endure sterilization without losing properties, be cost-effective, and gain regulatory approval for medical use. Additionally, the printability of biomaterials and their compatibility with the chosen printing method are crucial for producing high-quality bioprinted constructs. Ensuring the effective processing of these biomaterials is essential for maintaining structural integrity and preserving the biological activity of embedded cells. Therefore, a comprehensive understanding of these factors will enhance the development of innovative solutions in 3D bioprinting, leading to significant advancements in tissue engineering and regenerative medicine. Biomaterials sourced from nature closely mimic the biochemical and physical characteristics of the extracellular matrix (ECM). This similarity enables them to effectively support various cellular processes, including attachment, growth, movement, and specialization, leading to their high degree of biocompatibility. However, these natural materials often suffer from poor mechanical strength and face challenges in consistent production, despite their biological advantages [56]. On the other hand, synthetic materials offer distinct advantages in terms of reproducibility and customization, as they can be engineered to possess specific characteristics such as controlled degradation rates, enhanced mechanical properties, defined structures, and improved cell adhesion capabilities [57]. Various biomaterials used in 3D printing include synthetic polymers, hydrogel inks, metal alloys, ceramics, and composites. In the following, each of these materials will be briefly introduced regarding their applications in 3D printing.

3.1. *Polymers for 3D Printing*

The three primary types of polymers frequently utilized in 3D printing are thermoplastics, UV-curable thermosets (or photopolymers), and hydrogels. Thermoplastics and photopolymers are well-known for their versatility, while hydrogels consist of networks of hydrophilic polymer chains. The molecular structures, essential physical properties, and subcategories, including specific examples of these polymers, are detailed in **Figure 8**.

3.1.1. *Thermoplastic Polymers*

Thermoplastic polymers are widely utilized due to their ability to soften when heated, which allows them to be shaped and then harden upon cooling. They can be categorized into amorphous and semi-crystalline types based on their molecular structure, as depicted in **Figure 8a** [8]. Amorphous thermoplastics have a randomly organized molecular structure and do not have a defined melting point, making them easy to thermoform. In contrast, semi-crystalline thermoplastics have a highly ordered molecular structure with a distinct melting point; they transition from solid to liquid after absorbing a certain amount of heat. Semi-crystalline polymers boast strong mechanical properties due to their robust intermolecular forces. All thermoplastic polymers can be processed reversibly, making them ideal for extrusion-based 3D printing methods like FDM. In the printing process, the solid polymer (in the form of pellets or filaments) is heated until the polymer chains break and the material melts. After printing, the polymer cools and solidifies in the desired configuration, with the chains becoming interconnected and rigid again. Common thermoplastic feedstocks used in FDM include ABS, PLA, polyamide-nylon, polyethylene terephthalate glycol, and PCL and are selected for their low melting temperatures and suitable mechanical properties [8]. One particularly notable thermoplastic is PCL, a biodegradable polymer with a low melting point of ~60°C. PCL is valued for its biocompatibility and is often used in medical applications, such as in tissue engineering and drug delivery systems [58]. Its ease of processing and flexibility makes it a popular choice for 3D printing in the biomedical field.

3.1.2. *Thermoset Polymers*

Thermosetting polymers harden irreversibly through the curing of a viscous liquid prepolymer or resin. Unlike linear growth, the active sites within the polymer chains react with adjacent chains, creating a tightly interconnected polymer network. An increased crosslinking density in thermosets results in higher mechanical strength, hardness, and resistance to heat degradation and chemical attack. These polymers can be cured using heat or a suitable form of radiation, with the process further enhanced by high pressure and catalysts. **Figure 8b** illustrates the interconnected molecular structure of thermosets and the various components based on curing methods. Thermo-curing polymers undergo a curing reaction that accelerates with increasing temperature and then gradually slows as the system nears the glass transition point and proceeds until the resin achieves full cure. In contrast, photopolymers rely on UV radiation to initiate curing, utilizing its high-energy properties [59]. Among photopolymers, acrylate-based variants such as acrylate polyesters, acrylate silicones, and acrylate urethanes are extensively used due to their rapid polymerization rates driven by radical chain reactions. Photopolymer resins, predominantly epoxy- or acrylate-based, are widely employed in the VP process and droplet-based 3D printing methods, including inkjet printing. These resins undergo polymerization when exposed to UV light, typically within a wavelength range of 355 to 405 nm [8].

3.1.3. *Hydrogels*

Hydrogels are 3D crosslinked polymer networks capable of absorbing and retaining large amounts of water, often more than 90% of their total volume [60, 61]. The structural integrity of hydrogels is maintained through various intermolecular interactions, including hydrogen bonds, electrostatic interactions, hydrophobic interactions, water-mediated hydrogen bonds, van der Waals interactions, covalent cross-links, or a combination of these interactions (**Figure 8c**) [8, 62]. These materials are particularly well-suited for 3D bioprinting due to their biocompatibility, adjustable mechanical properties, and controlled degradability over time [63, 64]. They can incorporate bioactive cues, such as cell-adhesive peptides, nucleic acids, fatty acids, glycans, and GFs, to fabricate biomimetic supramolecular scaffolds [65]. Hydrogels can be classified into homopolymers (e.g., poly(hydroxyethyl methacrylate) (PHEMA) and PEG), copolymers (e.g., EG-PEGMA and carboxymethyl cellulose), and semi-interpenetrating networks based on their preparation methods [66]. Common solvents used in solution polymerization include water, ethanol, mixtures of water and ethanol, and benzyl alcohol [67]. The viscosity of hydrogels, as a key parameter in printing, is influenced by the monomer concentration and the macromolecule chain length. Higher monomer concentrations and longer chain lengths increase intermolecular attractions, resulting in higher viscosity. Hydrogels exhibit shear-thinning behavior as a result of a self-assembly process that carefully balances attractive forces, such as hydrogen bonding, ionic interactions, and electrostatic forces, with repulsive forces, such as electrostatic solvation. Despite the inherent weakness of individual noncovalent bonds, their combined interactions are sufficient to establish robust and stable network structures within the hydrogel. Under shear stress, these dynamic networks dissociate and reassemble, enabling shear-thinning behavior.

The swelling and mechanical properties of hydrogels are closely linked to their crosslinking density. A lower crosslinking density results in a higher swellability but reduced mechanical strength. Hydrogels can be crosslinked either chemically or physically, depending on the nature of the polymer backbone and their functional groups. Chemical crosslinking involves non-reversible covalent bonds between polymer chains, achieved by introducing crosslinkers (zero-length or non-zero-length) or through chemical reactions such as enzymatic crosslinking and UV exposure. On the other hand, physical crosslinking involves noncovalent bonds, including hydrogen bonding, ionic interactions with metal ions, and electrostatic

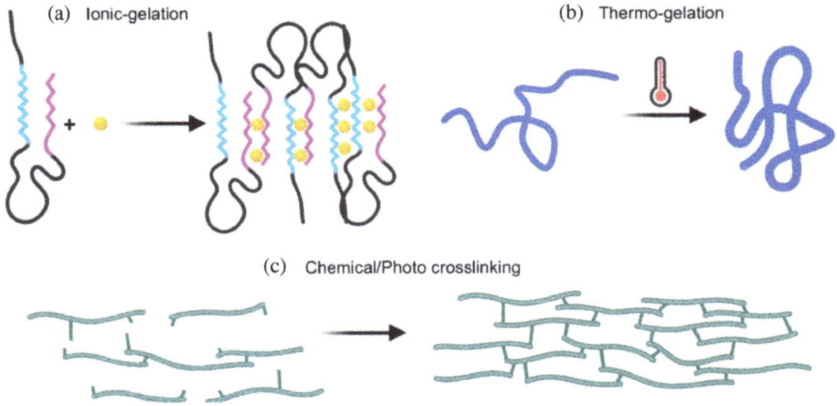

Figure 9. Typical hydrogel gelation methods: (a) ionic gelation, (b) thermal gelation, and (c) chemical/photo crosslinking [68]. With permission from Elsevier.

or hydrophobic interactions. Hydrogels formed through physical crosslinking are generally less durable than those created through chemical crosslinking. Additionally, the gelation process of hydrogels significantly influences both cell viability and print resolution. Gelation processes commonly involve ionic interactions, thermal mechanisms, enzymatic reactions, photo-crosslinking, or chemical crosslinking (**Figure 9**).

3.1.3.1. Hydrogel-Based Bioinks for 3D Bioprinting

Among the different polymers used, hydrogels have attracted much more attention in the development of a bioink. **Table 2** shows a library of hydrogels together with their rheological features, biological interactions, and gelation process. In bioprinting, hydrogel biomaterials are commonly employed as bioinks for cells and additive encapsulation. These hydrogels are preferred due to their advantageous characteristics, including high viscosity, shear-thinning behavior, and quick crosslinking abilities [69]. A frequently used component in both sacrificial and direct-write bioinks is gelatin, which exhibits temperature-dependent properties [70]. It undergoes a reversible transition to an alpha-helix structure at temperatures below 30°C and initiates physical crosslinking in aqueous solutions when heated above 40°C [71]. Gelatin inherently contains integrin-binding

Table 2. Typical hydrogel inks utilized in 3D bioprinting, along with their biological and physicochemical characteristics [68]. With permission from Elsevier.

Hydrogels	Molecule type	Shear-thinning	Biological interactions	Gelation process
Collagen	Protein	No	High cell adhesion	Thermal/ Enzymatic
Fibrin	Protein	No	High cell adhesion	Thermal/ Chemical/ Enzymatic
Gelatin	Protein	Yes	Medium cell adhesion	Thermal/ Chemical/ Enzymatic
Spider silk	Protein	Yes	Low cell adhesion	Self-assembly
Matrigel	Protein	Yes	High cell adhesion	Thermal
GelMA	Modified protein	Yes	Medium cell adhesion	Chemical/ Enzymatic
Self-assembling peptides	Protein	Yes	High cell adhesion	Self-assembly
Alginate	Polysaccharide	Yes	Low cell adhesion	Ionic/Chemical
Chitosan	Polysaccharide	No	Low cell adhesion	Ionic
Gellan gum	Polysaccharide	Yes	Low cell adhesion	Ionic/Chemical
Agarose	Polysaccharide	Yes	Low cell adhesion	Thermal
k-Carrageenan	Polysaccharide	Yes	Low cell adhesion	Ionic/Thermal
Methylcellulose	Polysaccharide	No	Low cell adhesion	Thermal

motifs, including vitronectin, fibronectin, and vimentin, which facilitate and enhance cell attachment. [71]. A popular gelatin derivative, gelatin methacryloyl (GelMA), is extensively utilized as a bioink owing to its rapid crosslinking capability when exposed to UV light (360–480 nm) in the presence of photoinitiators such as Irgacure 2959 [67]. GelMA is commonly incorporated with other materials or chemically tailored to design advanced bioinks for specialized applications [72].

Alginate-based hydrogels are also widely used as bioinks owing to their high viscosity, biocompatibility, and rapid crosslinking capabilities when exposed to multivalent cations such as Ca^{2+} or Ba^{2+} [72]. Despite these advantages, the primary limitation of alginate is its limited biological activity [73]. To enhance the biological functionality of alginate bioinks, various strategies have been explored mainly through combining it with other biomaterials (e.g., gelatin or collagen) and adjusting the molecular weight or degree of oxidation of the alginate [74, 75]. These advancements in the development of alginate bioink have expanded the potential applications of this material in the field of 3D bioprinting, enabling the fabrication of more complex and biologically relevant tissue constructs.

Bioinks offer a distinctive opportunity to integrate additional components, such as GFs, to enhance cell growth and differentiation within printed constructs. The subsequent sections will explore specific 3D bioprinting studies focusing on various types of musculoskeletal tissues.

3.2. *Metals for 3D Printing*

Metals have played a crucial role in load-bearing biomedical applications for a long time due to their favorable properties, including high mechanical properties, fatigue resistance, and fracture resistance. Some metals are particularly valued for their ductility, allowing them to endure multiple loading cycles through plastic deformation before significant crack propagation occurs [76]. Since the late 1920s, when steel was first used in vivo [77], advancements in "biometals" have led to the replacement of steel with titanium (Ti), tantalum (Ta), and zirconium (Zr) [78]. These newer metals are favored for their excellent wear resistance, biocompatibility, polarization resistance, and high corrosion resistance, enabling longer retention *in vivo* [77]. A critical aspect of metal research and development is alloying, which combines different elements to fabricate unique features. The most used alloys for biomedical applications are stainless steel and titanium alloys. Alloys can be directly fabricated into scaffolds for hard tissues or incorporated into polymer scaffolds or grafts for specific purposes [79]. Techniques like hot-dip aluminizing are utilized to apply metallic surface coatings that enhance the corrosion and oxidation resistance of implanted grafts, making them more resilient when in, for example, a challenging environment due to the presence of bodily fluids. For instance, Nover and colleagues fabricated tissue-engineered porous titanium-based osteochondral constructs to mimic biological bone structures, finding that the bone-like base supported the development of cartilage tissues [80]. Further, noble metal particles, including gold and silver, can be added into a hydrogel matrix to fabricate nanoparticle-hydrogel composite scaffolds with improved physical and biological characteristics [81]. Recently, scientists have engineered biodegradable or drug-delivering bioabsorbable temporary scaffolds to overcome the limitations associated with permanent ones. Magnesium and zinc alloys have gained particular interest due to their ability to gradually corrode, eliciting an appropriate host response, and completely degrading after supporting tissue healing [82, 83]. **Table 3** provides an overview of commonly used metals in musculoskeletal tissue engineering applications.

The traditional fabrication of metallic implants typically involves machining, which relies on high ductility to support subtractive manufacturing processes. However, creating porous metallic networks for tissue engineering applications poses significant challenges using these conventional methods. To overcome this, AM, particularly techniques such as PBF and directed energy deposition, have emerged as viable alternatives. These methods employ lasers or electron beams to selectively sinter or melt metal powders or filaments layer by layer, enabling the production of intricately designed parts tailored for specific applications [84].

3.3. *Ceramics for 3D Printing*

Ceramics are typically synthesized as solid, inorganic materials with a crystalline structure. In the context of biomedical applications, bioceramics refer to biocompatible ceramics that can be bioinert, bioactive, or bioresorbable [78]. Commonly used bioceramics include calcium phosphate, bioactive glasses, and glass ceramics, facilitating initial bone-implant contact and creating a strong bonding interface [92]. Given that the primary

Table 3. Metals frequently utilized in musculoskeletal tissue engineering [79]. With permission from Springer.

Metals	Applications	Fabrication method	Advantages	Reference
Titanium	Bone	Powder metallurgy with removed magnesium powder	High porosity enhanced cell proliferation	[85]
Titanium isopropoxide (TiO_2)	Bone	Sol-gel and salt-leaching	Enhanced osteoinductivity	[86]
Titanium alloy	Bone	SLM	Customized design and accurate manufacturing	[87]
Porous titanium	Cartilage and Bone	SLM	Improved mechanical and biochemical characteristics	[80]
Nitrocarburized stainless steel	Bone	Hydrogenated amorphous carbon deposition	Enhanced electrochemical performance and adhesion to the substrate	[88]
Gold nanoparticles	Bone	Composite hydrogel fabrication	Promoted cell proliferation, differentiation, and alkaline phosphatase activities	[89]
Gold and silver nanoparticles	Bone	Composite hydrogel fabrication	Enhanced antibacterial properties	[90]
Silver phosphate particles	Bone	*In situ* foaming	Improved antimicrobial activities	[91]

chemical component of bone is hydroxyapatite (HA), various calcium-phosphate (CaP) materials such as α-tricalcium phosphate (α-TCP), β-TCP, HA, and carbonate-based ceramics are extensively studied for bone regeneration [93, 94]. These CaP-based materials have gained popularity for use as resorbable and implantable devices [95–97]. Notably, most studies on 3D-printed ceramics focus on applications within the musculoskeletal system for orthopedic purposes. **Table 4** presents a summary of recent studies on the use of ceramics in 3D printing technology for orthopedic applications. Ceramic materials are widely favored for 3D printing applications demanding exceptional strength and durability, such as dental implants and bone scaffolds. These bioinks are formulated from biocompatible ceramics, such as HA and TCP, which are naturally occurring minerals in bones and teeth. The ceramics are converted into a printable ink by incorporating a binder or solvent and are subsequently subjected to high-temperature firing to achieve a dense, robust ceramic structure. 3D printing of ceramics has emerged as a promising method for creating scaffolds that mimic the natural structure of tissues such as bone. This AM approach allows for the production of geometrically stable devices, addressing the limitations of granular bioceramics, which often show randomized nucleation sites that hinder organized bone growth. The most promising techniques for 3D-printing ceramics currently include PBF and inkjet printing [98, 99]. The 3D printing of ceramics represents a significant advancement in the field of biomedical engineering. By leveraging the ability to produce complex, porous structures and tailoring material properties through various processing techniques, 3D-printed ceramics offer promising solutions for bone regeneration and other medical applications. Their inherent biocompatibility, potential antibacterial properties, and capacity for surface modification make them ideal candidates for next-generation implantable devices.

3.4. *Composites for 3D Printing*

Considering the advantages and limitations of different materials (polymers, metals, and ceramics), composite biomaterials for 3D printing are developed by combining these components to achieve the desired properties, making them suitable for a wide range of applications. These

Table 4. Summary of 3D printed ceramic studies investigated for orthopedic applications.

Materials	Printing method	Applications	Outcomes	Reference
13-93 Bioactive glass (BG)	SLS	Bone scaffolds	The 3D-printed scaffolds exhibited suitable pore interconnectivity, porosity, mechanical strength, and biocompatibility.	[100]
β-TCP/Poly(D, L)-lactide (PDLLA)	SLM	Bone implants	The 3D-printed scaffolds were biodegradable and demonstrated an adequate bending strength.	[101]
13-93 BG/alginate	Extrusion	Bone	The presence of 13-93 BG enhanced the mechanical properties, apatite mineralization, ion release, and porosity while reducing shrinkage.	[102]
Hydroxyapatite (HA)/chitosan, Alginate	Extrusion	Bone	The incorporation of HA in chitosan and alginate hydrogels enhanced cell viability, proliferation, and differentiation.	[103]
PEKK/calcium hydroxyapatite/ reduced graphene oxide	FDM	Hip implant	Enhanced osteogenesis	[104]
Biphasic calcium phosphate zirconia (ZrO_2)	FDM	Bone and cartilage	Fabrication of interconnected porous scaffolds with enhanced mechanical properties that elevated the expression of bone morphogenic protein	[105]

composite inks can be tailored to meet specific requirements, thereby enhancing their performance in biomedical engineering. They can be classified into synthetic polymer-based, hydrogel-based, ceramic-based, and metal-based composites. **Table 5** provides a summary of recent studies on the 3D printing of composites for musculoskeletal applications. Polymer-based composites are commonly employed in 3D printing, with PLA being a popular choice among polymeric inks. The addition of bioactive ceramics, such as calcium phosphate glass to PLA formulations, enhances bioactivity by improving cell adhesion and promoting the healing response. PCL is another widely used polymer, recognized for its controlled degradation properties, making it ideal for drug and GF delivery. To further enhance its physicochemical properties and osteogenic potential, PCL is often combined with materials such as HA particles or carbon nanomaterials, such as graphene oxide [106].

Hydrogel-based composites are characterized by their flexibility and the ability to undergo chemical cross-linking, which stabilizes the scaffold. The incorporation of bioactive glass is commonly employed to enhance both compressive strength and bioactivity. Hardy et al. pioneered the development of composite scaffolds made from poly(butylene terephthalate) or poly(butylene terephthalate-co-poly(alkylene glycol) terephthalate) combined with engineered spider silk protein, which showed improved biomineralization capabilities [107]. Scaffold properties can be enhanced by co-printing with stiffer polymers or by incorporating additives such as mesoporous bioactive glass and dexamethasone, which support cell attachment, proliferation, and ECM mineralization. However, hydrogels such as Pluronic are limited by their mechanical weakness, making them unsuitable for hard tissue scaffolds. To address this limitation, metal powders can be added to hydrogel-based bioinks, allowing for the production of stiffer and porous scaffold systems [108].

Ceramic-based composites typically utilize biphasic calcium phosphate (e.g., TCP and HA) powders to create scaffolds with enhanced cell viability and proliferation. Scaffold properties can be improved through coating with PLGA, although residual solvents may pose potential concerns. HA-poly (vinyl alcohol) composites offer improved mechanical strength and flexibility by decreasing sintering temperatures and increasing

Table 5. Summary of 3D printing composites investigated for musculoskeletal applications.

Composite material	Printing method	Applications	Findings	Reference
Wood-based cellulose nanofibril, alginate, gelatin	Extrusion	Bioinks for 3D bioprinting of bone	Cellulose nanofibrils modulated the flow behavior of the hydrogels, thus enhancing their printability. Suitable cytocompatibility.	[110]
GelMA, silicate nanoplatelets	Extrusion-based direct writing	Microstructured bone-like tissue constructs	Stability was preserved for 3 weeks of *in vitro* culture, facilitating osteogenesis and angiogenesis.	[111]
PCL, graphene oxide (GO)	Extrusion	Bone scaffolds	Incorporation of GO enhances scaffold wettability and biocompatibility.	[29]
Polyurethane, hyaluronic acid	DLP	Cartilage scaffolds	High cytocompatibility and differentiation into a chondrogenic phenotype.	[112]
GelMA, PCL, hyaluronic acid	Extrusion	Cartilage scaffolds	Scaffolds exhibited cartilage markers, including collagen type II and glycosaminoglycans, along with high cell viability in a bioink composed of 10% GelMA and hyaluronic acid.	[113]

(Continued)

Table 5. (*Continued*)

Composite material	Printing method	Applications	Findings	Reference
PEG-fibrinogen	Microfluidic Printing (like Extrusion)	Artificial skeletal muscle tissue	The method supports myogenic differentiation, resulting in aligned myotubes with enhanced functionality. In vivo implantation demonstrated the formation of organized muscle tissue, highlighting its potential for clinical applications.	[114]
ABS, collagen	Extrusion	Scaffold-fiber composites for tendon repair applications	Enhancing the strength and bioactivity of collagen scaffolds. Mechanical properties of scaffold-fiber composites can be modified by altering fiber geometry while maintaining collagen bioactivity.	[115]

layer-to-layer adhesion. Optimizing calcium phosphate concentration and exploring pore size and geometry can further enhance scaffold characteristics [109]. Composite materials have shown significant promise in promoting cell proliferation and differentiation, effectively mimicking natural tissues. Enhanced with natural additives including collagen, gelatin, and chitosan, as well as synthetic polymers such as PCL and PLA, composite bioceramics have been extensively researched for bone repair applications [79]. These composite biomaterials enable the creation of 3D-printed structures with tailored properties, combining the benefits of different materials to meet specific biomedical application requirements. By leveraging the unique characteristics of various materials, researchers can develop advanced scaffolds and implants that better mimic the complex nature of biological tissues, potentially improving outcomes in tissue engineering and regenerative medicine. Despite these advances, the fabrication processes for these scaffolds remain complex and require further refinement to enhance their efficiency and practicality for clinical application. By optimizing these processes, the practical utility and scalability of composite scaffolds in tissue engineering can be significantly improved.

4. Advances in 3D Printing for Musculoskeletal Applications

Recent advancements have led to innovative designs for implants, cell-supportive structures, and drug-delivery matrices tailored for musculoskeletal tissue repair [116–118]. As two of the most sophisticated methods for fabricating tissues, 3D printing and 3D bioprinting, the core AM and biofabrication technologies, provide alternative approaches for developing functional 3D tissue constructs with precise control over internal architecture and cell positioning. These methods enable the use of various biomaterials and bioinks to produce constructs with or without heterogeneous cell types and with tailored physical, mechanical, and biological properties [119, 120]. The ideal scaffold should replicate anatomically precise structures while also emulating the biological and mechanical properties of the native tissue. Musculoskeletal tissues, characterized by their hierarchical composition and dynamic loading situation, necessitate the construction of physiologically and mechanically functional constructs [121]. Therefore, several parameters must be considered when designing 3D-printed scaffolds for musculoskeletal tissue regeneration, including pore characteristics, biodegradability, scale, structural and compositional organization, and biomechanical properties, as well as its biological features [78, 122]. Due to the use of biomaterials as a cell-friendly environment and the combination of various biomaterials, 3D printing emerges as a promising strategy with advantageous approaches. These approaches pave the way for the development of functional tissue constructs that combine biological complexity with mechanical robustness, offering significant potential for regenerating musculoskeletal tissues such as bone, cartilage, skeletal muscle, tendons, and ligaments.

4.1. *3D Printing Approaches for Musculoskeletal Regeneration*

To date, numerous research groups have utilized 3D printing to fabricate 3D constructs with or without cells for musculoskeletal regeneration. The primary approaches in this field involve printing cell-free materials, cell-laden materials, or a combination of both to create efficient 3D constructs (**Figure 10**).

4.1.1. *Cell-Free Approach*

Cell-free approaches represent a promising frontier in tissue regeneration by offering a pathway to restore full functionality to injured musculoskeletal tissues. Central to this approach is the creation of scaffolds capable of attracting and recruiting endogenous stem and progenitor cells to the site of injury once it is implanted, hence facilitating natural tissue repair processes [124]. Among the aforementioned techniques, FDM, SLA, DLP, DIW, powder-based processes, material jetting, and binder jetting are particularly well-suited for musculoskeletal 3D printing. The absence of cells allows the use of more rigorous as well as harsh methods, enabling the creation of robust, biocompatible scaffolds with the necessary mechanical properties and intricate architectures essential for effective tissue repair. A critical step in the cell-free approach is appointing suitable biomaterials, which are utilized to create structural frameworks to support tissue regeneration. Synthetic biomaterials, noted for their robust mechanical properties, are predominantly employed in this regard [125, 126]. Recently, attention has been drawn to the use of thermoplastic composites and the creation of filaments or pellets for cell-free 3D printing scaffolds. Research has demonstrated the bioactivity of these 3D-printed composite scaffolds in musculoskeletal tissue engineering by incorporating bioceramics or natural biomaterials such as decellularized extracellular

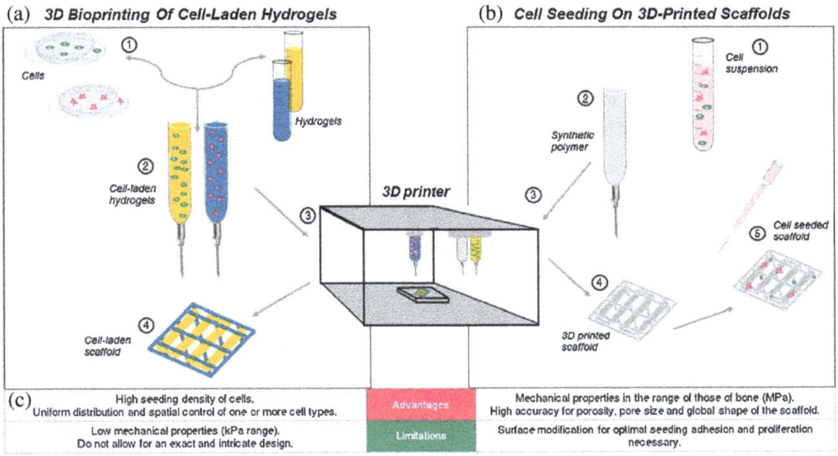

Figure 10. Strategies for the fabrication of 3D printed scaffolds. (a) a cell-laden strategy, in which a layer-by-layer deposition of bioink containing cells creates the 3D scaffold structure, and (b) a cell-free strategy, in which cell-free bioink is printed and cell seeding on the 3D printed structure is performed after printing [123].

matrix (dECM) into various composite filaments such as PCL, PLA, PLA/PCL, and PLGA [127–130]. For example, Goncalves et al. fabricated a PCL-nano bioceramic composite scaffold with an adjustable porosity (450–700 μm) and mechanical properties. This successful cell-free printing approach resulted in a scaffold with a compressive strength of 4 MPa, improved MG63 cell adhesion, and elicited favorable bioactivity, making it suitable for bone repair [131].

4.1.2. *Cell-Laden Approach*

The cell-laden approach in 3D printing integrates living cells directly into the bioink or biomaterial, typically hydrogels, during the printing process. This method aims to replicate the natural tissue environment from the beginning, promoting immediate cell-scaffold interactions and providing a conducive microenvironment for tissue regeneration at the implant site. Techniques such as DIW, inkjet-based bioprinting, extrusion-based 3D bioprinting, LIFT, and VP processes (including SLA and DLP) are frequently employed in this method. These approaches are chosen for their ability to precisely position cells and maintain their viability, which is critical for developing functional tissue constructs that integrate seamlessly with native tissues. The performance of cell-laden hydrogel matrices depends on the severity of crosslinking reactions and the cytotoxicity of byproducts and unreacted substances. Harmful monomers, initiators, and free radicals from photoinitiated polymerization using UV light can impair the efficacy of the 3D microenvironment both in vitro and *in vivo* [132]. Viscosity is a critical factor for the printability of hydrogels; high viscosity necessitates high pressure, potentially damaging cells with mechanical forces and shear stresses, while low viscosity may undermine structural integrity and resolution [133]. Additionally, the internal diameter of the nozzle impacts cell viability post-printing; larger nozzles require lower pressure, reducing shear stress and enhancing cell viability. Mechanical stability is also crucial, particularly in load-bearing applications, where hydrogels must remain stable until cells produce their functional ECM.

Compared to the cell-free approaches, the cell-laden strategy in the 3D printing of musculoskeletal tissue presents distinct advantages and disadvantages. Incorporating live cells into the printing process enhances biocompatibility and typically employs natural materials that closely mimic the ECM, thereby promoting cell proliferation, migration, and differentiation [134, 135]. However, cell-laden techniques often exhibit weaker mechanical strength and lower-resolution printing than cell-free methods [123, 136]. They also face challenges such as batch variability, higher costs, slower fabrication times, and reduced resistance to environmental stresses. Due to the accompaniment of cells with the process, the selection of 3D printing methods is also limited. Techniques involving harsh conditions (e.g., high temperature, high pressure, and high-energy radiation) are not suitable for cell-laden approaches.

4.1.3. *Hybrid Printing Approach*

Numerous 3D printers are designed to dispense both soft and stiff materials, in particular, hydrogels and thermoplastics, respectively. By utilizing these capabilities, complex geometries and composite scaffolds can be created, mimicking the very matrix, biophysical properties, bioactivity, and functions of various tissue types. This hybrid printing approach enables the fabrication of mechanically robust living tissue constructs featuring both rigid and flexible regions, as well as vascularized channels, thereby providing researchers with a golden opportunity to develop advanced tissue engineering solutions [137]. Importantly, one prominent strategy in this context is co-printing of synthetic biomaterials (stiff) with cell-laden natural biomaterials (soft) as a hybrid 3D-printed construction. This approach uses multi-nozzle bioprinting devices, since the stiff materials provide crucial support for the softer, cell-containing bioinks [118, 138]. Research has shown the practicality of co-printing thermoplastics such as PCL and PLGA with cell-seeded hydrogels such as gelatin methacrylate, alginate, and HLA, resulting in constructs with musculoskeletal tissue-like properties, angiogenic potential, mechanical stability, high cell viability, and strong cell differentiation [139–141]. For instance, Daly et al. employed multi-nozzle printing to fabricate a mechanically reinforced cartilaginous framework that replicated the geometry of a vertebral disk [142]. This involved printing a PCL framework, followed by the deposition of an RGD-alginate hydrogel containing adult stem cells. In this approach, developmental precursors of an adult organ were bioprinted, serving as a template for subsequent organogenesis *in vivo*. Upon implantation into a mouse model, the bioprinted construct facilitated the development of vascularized bone, featuring trabecular-like endochondral bone with a supportive marrow structure.

4.2. *Applications*

The future gold standard for producing 3D functional tissue equivalents that promote tissue regeneration is expected to be 3D printing. Presently, extensive research is conducted on cell-free 3D-printed ceramic, metallic, as well as polymeric structures, and cell-laden 3D bioprinted structures for musculoskeletal treatment. The studies discussed here first address 3D printers and then 3D bioprinters in the context of bone, cartilage, muscle, tendon, and ligament repair applications.

4.2.1. *Bone*

Bone, a dynamic tissue crucial for mechanical support, organ protection, and hemostasis, undergoes constant self-regeneration but faces challenges from various conditions such as aging, trauma, and failed arthroplasty [143–146]. Globally, around 2.2 million bone transplantation procedures are performed annually [147], highlighting the significant clinical need for effective treatment bone defects and fracture treatments. Repairing such defects involves a complex interplay of cells, ECM, and biochemical signals [148]. Various graft types (autografts, allografts, and xenografts) have been put forward but come with limitations, prompting the exploration of tissue engineering as a promising alternative [149]. Successful bone grafting hinges on osteoinductive properties, requiring mesenchymal stem cells (MSCs) to differentiate into osteoblasts, often facilitated by bone morphogenetic proteins (BMPs) [150]. Materials used for grafts include polymers (hydrogels and non-hydrogel polymers), metals, ceramics, and composites, sometimes combined with ECM components and cells [151]. Ideal bone graft materials should be fully resorbable, osteoinductive, osteoconductive, mimic native bone architecture, provide mechanical stability, and exhibit osteogenic potential [152, 153], posing a challenge for tissue engineering to meet all these criteria comprehensively. The advent of 3D printing offers precise control over scaffold shape, size, porosity, and mechanical properties, making it pivotal in current bone tissue engineering [154]. Metallic 3D-printed structures, tailored to patient-specific defects, provide implants with high mechanical strength [155]. Clinical trials have demonstrated the efficacy of Ti [156–158] and Ta alloys [159, 160] for various bone applications, including cancellous, cortical, and spinal implants, due to their suitable porosity that enhances compressive strength and modulus elasticity, mimicking human bone properties and minimizing the stress-shielding effect [161]. In a notable case study, Imanishi et al. [162] successfully implanted a 3D-printed Ti calcaneal prosthesis using EBM technology in a patient with chronic heel pain due to chondrosarcoma. Five months post-implantation, the patient achieved full weight-bearing without pain, demonstrating a positive clinical outcome (**Figure 11a**). Similarly, Faldini et al. [163] designed a customized 3D-printed ankle implant for a patient using cobalt-chromium-molybdenum

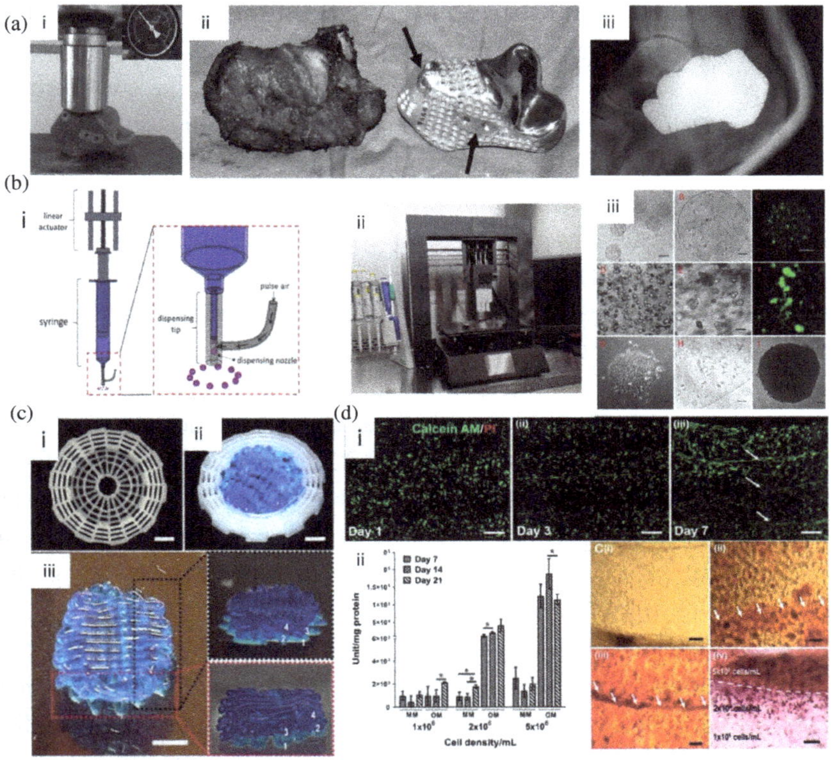

Figure 11. Advancements in the 3D printing of bone structures: (a) A 3D-printed titanium calcaneal prosthesis, (i) a prototype of the prosthesis demonstrating a load-bearing capacity exceeding 6 tons. (ii) Resected specimen alongside the prosthesis, (iii) a post-operative lateral radiograph. Adapted from Imanishi et al. [162] with permission from Elsevier. (b) Key features of the DVDOD 3D bioprinting technology. (i) Illustration of the dispensing mechanism, (ii) representative setup of a DVDOD 3D bioprinter, (iii) typical views of 143B human osteosarcoma cells. Adapted from Grottkau et al. [186] with permission from MDPI. (c) 3D printed hybrid structures. (i) PCL cage structure, (ii) PEG-based bioink bioprinted within the PCL cage, and (iii) multilayer bioprinting of the PEG-based bioink, (d) biocompatibility evaluation of the PEG-based bioink for hBMSCs. Adapted from Altunbek et al. [190] with permission from the American Chemical Society.

powders and biocompatible polyamide guidelines. With added porous coatings and an HA coating, the implant achieved an excellent clinical score 4 months after surgery, suggesting a promising future for 3D-printed implants in total ankle arthroplasty. Calcium silicate ceramics have been extensively researched for their ability to meet stringent scaffold requirements, including mechanical strength, biological compatibility, and osteoconductivity, due to their capacity to form HA upon exposure to physiological fluids [164, 165]. In a clinical trial that addressed zygomatic bone defects, Lee et al. [166] employed FDM to 3D print CaO-SiO_2-P_2O_5-B_2O_3 glass ceramic (BGS-7) implants, followed by a sintering process to enhance durability. Eight patients received these implants, and a CT scan at 6 months post-implantation revealed complete bone fusion without osteolytic signs, demonstrating the efficacy of 3D-printed constructs in zygomatic bone healing. Using the same material and bone defects in rabbits *via* an induced membrane approach, Cho et al. [167] utilized an extrusion-based 3D printing system to create a macro/microporous bioactive ceramic scaffold coated with rhBMP-2 for repairing femoral defects. Histological and morphological analyses indicated robust osseous bridging and extensive cortical bone formation along the scaffold, underscoring the successful reconstruction of critical-sized bone defects using this method.

Despite the high mechanical properties of individual synthetic and natural materials, their inappropriate physicochemical and biological properties limit their suitability for mimicking bone tissue. Recent studies have focused on composite biomaterials to optimize their properties for enhanced bone regeneration. For instance, incorporating osteoinductive ceramic nanopowders into these composites can potentially induce seeded cells to differentiate into osteoblasts [168]. Notably, Zhang et al. [169] utilized composite filaments of PLLA/nano-HA (nHA) to fabricate porous scaffolds for bone repair using FDM. The inclusion of high-loaded nHA enhanced scaffold hydrophilicity and achieved a compressive strength of 15 MPa, comparable to human cancellous bone (2–12 MPa). Although exhibiting brittle-like characteristics, the optimized scaffold demonstrated greater deformation tolerance before failure, improving mechanical compatibility. The scaffold exhibited favorable *in vitro* bioactivity, showing no cytotoxicity after rabbit MSCs were cultured for 5 days. In a 4-week *in vivo* trial in rabbits, the scaffold facilitated bone tissue formation within its pores, with the organized distribution of osteocytes, indicating mature bone tissue formation. This research presents a cost-effective, stable, and efficient method for personalized bone scaffold printing, supporting the advancement of personalized biomaterials in clinical applications. In another study, Jakus et al. [170] developed a hyperelastic bone (HB) ink by combining HA powder with either PCL or PLGA to bioprint elastic constructs for bone regeneration. The 3D printed HB constructs displayed remarkable elasticity, scalability, and ease of handling. Implantation in mouse subcutaneous, rat posterolateral spinal fusion, and macaque calvarial defect models demonstrated significant new bone formation with vascularization and rapid tissue integration. Moreover, Parupelli et al. [171] fabricated composite scaffolds using PCL and calcium magnesium phosphate (CMP) *via* 3D printing for bone tissue engineering. The addition of CMP resulted in a suitable rough-textured architecture and porosity, supporting the bioactivity and viability of fibroblast NIH/3T3 cells, making it a promising composite for bone tissue engineering applications.

In a critical development, it has been increasingly recognized that traditional synthetic polymers, despite their robust mechanical properties, frequently suffer from a crucial shortcoming: the lack of cell adhesion conductivity. This limitation severely hampers their effectiveness, as cell adhesion conductivity is vital for the successful integration and functionality of bone tissue [172]. Ensuring that cells can properly adhere and interact with the scaffold material is essential for promoting tissue regeneration and achieving optimal clinical outcomes. This challenge can be effectively tackled by integrating natural biomaterials and peptides with specific cell adhesion sequences into composite materials, thereby enhancing the bioactivity and cellular integration. Gao et al. [173] utilized DLP printing to develop a composite bone tissue engineering scaffold based on polyethylene glycol diacrylate, Pluronic F127 diacrylate, and GelMA. The inclusion of GelMA aimed to enhance cell adhesion and proliferation, leveraging its RGD sequence [174]. The scaffolds exhibited satisfactory mechanical properties and a degradation rate suitable for bone regeneration timelines. *In vitro* studies revealed that the scaffolds supported cell adhesion and proliferation while also enhancing the osteogenic differentiation of MSCs within an osteoinductive environment. Moreover, the scaffolds demonstrated excellent histocompatibility, guiding the growth of new bone tissue within defects when implanted *in vivo*. Recently, and owing to its tissue-specific composition, which replicates the native osteogenic microenvironment, the use of native bone decellularized extracellular matrix (bdECM) has emerged as a promising natural biomaterial [175, 176]. To assess the benefits of bdECM in mimicking the organic and inorganic bone microenvironment, La et al. [177] coated a 3D-printed PCL/PLGA/TCP scaffold with bdECM. *In vitro* analysis demonstrated enhanced osteoblast adhesion and alignment. To evaluate the bone defect healing potential, the scaffold was implanted in mice with calvarial defects. Compared to the collagen-coated PCL/PLGA/TCP control (PCL/PLGA/TCP/Col), the bdECM-coated scaffold (PCL/PLGA/TCP/bdECM) significantly enhanced bone defect healing. Micro-CT analysis revealed near complete new bone formation covering the implantation site, with histological analysis showing >85% new bone formation and 70% bone density within the PCL/PLGA/TCP/bdECM scaffold. Lee et al. utilized 3D bioprinting to develop a collagen-based SF scaffold with ECM-like properties and a nanoporous structure, creating an ideal environment for osteoblast differentiation during *in vitro* testing [178]. To overcome the mechanical weakness and enhance bone tissue engineering performance, using a hybrid printing approach, Ashrafnia Menarbazari et al. [179] 3D-printed PCL-based scaffolds modified with decellularized bone matrix (DBM)-oxidized sodium alginate (OA) containing tricalcium silicate (TCS). The addition of OA improved DBM viscosity, yielding a more stable hydrogel. The incorporation of TCS into the PCL-based scaffold increased both the compressive modulus (89.81 MPa) and toughness (359.31 $KJ.m^{-3}$). When seeded with placenta-derived MSCs, the modified PCL/TCS/DBM-OA scaffold exhibited enhanced alkaline phosphatase activity and demonstrated suitable biocompatibility. Likewise, incorporating bdECM into 3D-printed scaffolds enhanced scaffold bioactivity by replicating the bone-specific microenvironment, thereby significantly promoting osteogenic capacity both *in vitro* and *in vivo*. Despite the unique properties of 3D-printed metal-, bioceramic-, and polymer-based cell-free scaffolds in bone repair, their application in 3D bioprinting faces several challenges. These include insensitivity to light or high melting temperatures, which restrict their use. Moreover, these inks typically cannot encapsulate cells and may exhibit issues such as cytotoxicity, low degradation rates, and the stress shielding phenomenon. Additionally, the nonuniform distribution of cells within 3D-printed scaffolds seeded with cells poses a significant disadvantage [180].

Researchers are addressing these limitations using 3D bioprinting, an emerging biofabrication technology that utilizes cell-laden hydrogels as bioink. This approach holds promise for printing 3D structures directly into damaged or diseased bone tissue, facilitating controlled cell-based regeneration and remineralization [181]. Commonly used cells include MSCs, preosteoblasts, and human adipose-derived stem cells (hASCs), with induced pluripotent stem cells (iPSCs) also considered pending evaluation of their tumorigenic potential [175, 182, 183]. For example, 3D porous constructs were developed using hASCs-laden composites with β-TCP through an extrusion bioprinting process [184]. These mechanically stable collagen/cell-β-TCP constructs provided an environment conducive to enhancing the osteogenic activity of hASCs *in vitro* compared to the collagen bioink alone, indicating bioceramic-triggered osteogenic differentiation. In another approach, Gao et al. [185] employed inkjet bioprinting to co-print acrylated peptides and acrylated PEG embedded with marrow-derived human MSCs. This method allowed simultaneous cell delivery with minimal UV exposure. The resulting bioprinted bone-like scaffold exhibited significant amounts of calcified mineralized matrix and possessed mechanical properties suitable for bone constructs. Furthermore, the complex structure and increased mechanical stiffness (100.93% ± 2.55%) of the bioprinted cell-laden peptide-conjugated PEG scaffold promoted direct differentiation of MSCs toward the osteogenic lineage. Innovatively, Grottkau et al. [186] advanced traditional Drop-on-Demand (DOD) 3D bioprinting to direct-volumetric DOD (DVDOD) 3D bioprinting technology to overcome challenges such as low cell concentration and viability under high pressure **(Figure 11b)**. Their study successfully generated functional bone and iPSC loaded microtissues using an alginate hydrogel laden with 143B human osteosarcoma cells, preosteoblasts (MC3T3), and iPSCs separately. These DVDOD 3D bioprinted microtissues demonstrated suitability for orthopedic treatments by delivering microbone tissue to defect sites in a minimally invasive manner, offering large-scale tissue replication for developmental biology models. Furthermore, Demirtas et al. [103] successfully demonstrated the 3D bioprinting of a bone tissue construct comprised of osteoblast-laden chitosan/HA composites, which showed enhanced osteogenic differentiation compared to cell-free constructs, including alginate and chitosan with or without HA. However, the elastic modulus of these 3D (bio)printed constructs, ~15 kPa, was significantly lower than the elastic modulus of cancellous bone.

In most of the above-mentioned studies, however, the mechanical strength and compressive modulus of bioprinted constructs significantly fall short when compared to native human cancellous bone tissue, which typically has an elastic modulus ranging from 10.4 to 20.7 GPa and a compressive modulus of approximately 344 ± 2 MPa [44, 187, 188]. In a pioneering study, Kang et al. [189] utilized an integrated tissue-organ printer (ITOP) to fabricate human-scale tissue constructs. This multi-head extrusion bioprinter simultaneously deposited an 8 mm diameter, 1.2 mm thick disc-shaped framework of PCL/TCP for mechanical stability, along with human amniotic fluid-derived stem cell-laden composite hydrogels comprised of fibrinogen (FG), gelatin, glycerol, and HLA at optimized concentrations. Temporary sacrificial supports were incorporated into the printing process, dissolving after the tissue construct acquired sufficient rigidity to maintain its shape. Additionally, microchannels were integrated into the 3D pattern to facilitate nutrient and oxygen diffusion to the printed cells. *In vivo* implantation of these constructs in a rodent model with mandibular and calvarial bone defects over 5 months demonstrated mature bone formation and the development of a vascular network throughout the construct. These findings highlight the potential of bio-printed hybrid constructs as an effective substitute for promoting bone regeneration. In another approach, Altunbek et al. [190] employed a hybrid printing strategy to fabricate scaffolds that mimic segmental large bone defects. They utilized melt extrusion-based 3D printing to deposit a porous PCL cage (13 mm diameter, 3 mm thickness) with a zigzag/spiral pattern on the exterior. Meanwhile, microcapillary-based 3D printing was employed internally to bioprint an hBMSC-laden PEG bioink layer by layer. The zigzag/spiral PCL cage exhibited suitable mechanical strength and facilitated oxygen and nutrient diffusion. Moreover, the PEG-based hydrogel created a biocompatible environment conducive to hBMSC viability, differentiation, and mineralization, demonstrating potential for the development of personalized, functional implantable structures to address critical-size bone defects (**Figure 11c**).

Despite considerable advancements, the development of clinically relevant and functional bone substitutes remains challenging. Key obstacles include structural instability, constraints on construct size, insufficient mechanical strength, limited integration with host tissue, and short-lived osteogenic activity. Consequently, further clinical translation and *in vivo* studies of 3D bioprinted bone are essential. These efforts aim to develop methods to overcome these critical hurdles, paving the way for the widespread adoption of this technology. A summary of all the bone 3D printing studies discussed is presented in **Table 6**.

4.2.2. *Cartilage*

Human cartilage tissue plays a crucial role in supporting and facilitating joint movement. It can be classified into hyaline, elastic, and fibrocartilage, each serving distinct functions depending on its location and specialization [192]. Articular cartilage, a type of hyaline cartilage lining the articular joints, provides a smooth, lubricated surface and mechanical support by acting as a shock absorber and reducing friction between bones [193, 194]. Comprising an ECM with water, type II collagen (80%–90%), proteoglycans, non-collagenous proteins, glycoproteins, and highly specialized chondrocytes, articular cartilage forms four distinct zones: superficial, middle, deep, and calcified [195–198]. This avascular connective tissue, typically 2–7 mm thick, has limited intrinsic healing capacity due to the absence of blood flow. Consequently, untreated cartilage injuries tend to gradually progress toward osteoarthritis (OA) [199], for which no effective cure currently exists. A normal joint (cartilage–cartilage) tolerates compressive stresses ranging from 0.5 MPa to 5 MPa [200], necessitating scaffolds with adequate mechanical and biological properties for effective cartilaginous repair. Several grafting transplantation methods have been examined clinically for cartilage rehabilitation [201–203]. However, these methods present limitations such as short-term resolution, high procedural costs, poor biological compatibility, insufficient mimicry of natural tissues, and susceptibility to immune rejection [204, 205]. In these circumstances, tissue engineering, particularly 3D bioprinting, is featured as a promising option. Advancements in bioprinting cartilage

Table 6. A summary of studies that have investigated bone-related 3D printing approaches.

Printing technique	Materials	Cell type	Scaffold mechanical properties	*In-vitro/in-vivo* outcomes	Reference
EBM	Ti	–	The calcaneal prosthesis weighted 280 g with an ability to sustain a load of over 6 t	The patient achieved full weight-bearing without pain and demonstrated a positive clinical outcome 5 months post-implantation	[162]
FDM	CaO-SiO_2-P_2O_5-B_2O_3 ceramic	–	–	Complete bone fusion between the implant and the bone without signs of osteolysis	[166]
Extrusion	CaO-SiO_2-P_2O_5-B_2O_3 ceramic, rhBMP-2	-	-	100% healing rate after 8 weeks of implantation. Extensive cortical bone formation	[167]
FDM	PLLA, nano-HA,	rMSCs	Compressive strength: 15 MPa Elastic modulus: 45 MPa 15% mass lost after 12 days	Favorable *in vitro* bioactivity and cell viability Organized distribution of osteocytes and bone formation 4 weeks post-implantation	[169]

Extrusion	HA, PCL, PLGA	hMSC,	~32% to 67% strain to failure, ~4 to 11 MPa elastic modulus	Supported cell viability and proliferation. Induced osteogenic differentiation. Significant new bone formation with vascularization and rapid tissue integration after 4 weeks of implantation	[170]
DIW	PCL, CMP	NIH/3T3	Newtonian behavior, followed by non-Newtonian fluid characteristics at higher shear rates, indicating shear-thinning behavior	More than 100% cell viability with enhanced cell attachment and proliferation	[171]
DLP	PEGDA, Pluronic F127 diacrylate, GelMA	MSCs	Decreasing modulus from 127.4 ± 12 kPa to 92.34 ± 6.80 kPa by the addition of GelMA	Improved *in vivo* cell adhesion, proliferation, and osteogenic differentiation. Excellent *in vivo* histocompatibility and bone tissue growth	[173]

(*Continued*)

Table 6. *(Continued)*

Printing technique	Materials	Cell type	Scaffold mechanical properties	*In-vitro/in-vivo* outcomes	Reference
Extrusion	PCL, PLGA, TCP, bdECM	Calvarial osteoblasts	–	bdECM-enhanced osteoblast adhesion, aligned morphology, and osteogenic activity. Enhanced *in vivo* bone defect healing due to the bdECM	[177]
Extrusion	Collagen, dECM, silk-fibroin	MC3T3-E1	Compressive modulus: 0.03-0.04 MPa Compressive strength: 0.3 ± 0.04 MPa	Increased *in vitro* cell viability, bioactivity, cell attachment, migration, proliferation and differentiation in the CES scaffold compared to that of the pure collagen scaffold	[178]
Extrusion	PCL, decellularized bone matrix, oxidized sodium alginate, TCS	P MSCs	Compressive modulus: 89.81 MPa Toughness: 359.31 $KJ.m^{-3}$	Suitable biocompatibility. Enhanced bioactivity. Significantly promotes osteogenic activity both *in vitro* and *in vivo*	[179]
Extrusion	bTCP, collagen	MC3T3-E1, hASCs	–	Enhanced osteogenic activity of hASCs *in vitro*	[184]

Inkjet bioprinting	Acrylated peptides, acrylated PEG	MSCs	100.93 ± 2.55% increased mechanical stiffness	Excellent biocompatibility, with a cell viability of 87.9 ± 5.3%. Enhanced osteogenic and chondrogenic differentiation	[185]
Extrusion	Chitosan, HA	MC3T3-E1 pre-osteoblast	Elastic modulus: 15 kPa, softer than cancellous bone's elastic modulus	Suitable cell viability and proliferation after printing. Increased osteogenic differentiation and mineralization after 21 days of culture	[191]
Extrusion (multi-head)	PCL, TCP, gelatin, fibrinogen, hyaluronic acid, glycerol, Pluronic F-127	hAFSCs	–	Mature bone formation and development of a vascular network throughout the construct after 5 months of implantation *in vivo*	[189]
Extrusion	PCL, PEG	hBMSC	Compressive strength: 32.88 ± 1.82 MPa The structure showed plastic deformation	The PEG-based hydrogel created a biocompatible environment conducive to hBMSC viability, differentiation, and mineralization	[190]

tissue constructs focus on enhancing the mechanical strength of the hydrogels through the incorporation of synthetic polymers, replicating the intricate and heterogeneous zonal architecture of native cartilage, and fabricating osteochondral plugs that integrate both the cartilage and bone compartments [206, 207]. Furthermore, combining different cell types in the bioink, such as chondrocytes and MSCs, enhances the performance of bioprinted cartilage [208–212]. Notably, Golzar et al. [213] fabricated hydrophilic, UV-curable silicone-based inks for printing human articular cartilage (HAC) by combining aminosilicone, cellulose nanocrystal, and methacrylate anhydride (MA). Incorporating CNC and MA addressed the challenges of hydrophobicity, low viscosity, and the long curing time of the silicone elastomer. By varying the concentrations of CNC and MA, a multilayered structure with a gradual increase in compressive modulus from 0.25 to 1.32 MPa was successfully printed, mimicking the multizonal structure of HAC. The resultant constructs exhibited suitable hydrophilicity, rapid curing, shear thinning, mechanical stability, and biocompatibility, although overall stiffness and compressive strength require improvement. In another study, Costantini et al. [214] utilized a coaxial nozzle-based deposition system to 3D print biomimetic scaffolds for cartilage tissue engineering. Their bioink, comprising alginate, GelMA, chondroitin sulfate amino ethyl methacrylate (CS-AEMA), and hyaluronic acid methacrylate (HAMA), formed stable fibers during 3D printing, taking advantage of alginate with $CaCl_2$, and achieving a high printing resolution ($\approx$100 µm). Bone marrow-derived human MSCs seeded into the GelMA/CS-AEMA/HAMA bioink demonstrated a high cell density ($>10^7$ cells per mL^{-1}) and viability (85%–90%), promoting neocartilage formation through MSC differentiation. Moreover, using a novel combination of functional alginate and waterborne polyurethane (WBPU), Olmos-Juste et al. [215] developed 3D bioprinted scaffolds for articular cartilage regeneration (**Figure 12a**). The optimized WBPU scaffold exhibited suitable viscosity, viscoelasticity, structural integrity, and cell viability over 28 days of culture. These scaffolds maintained cell number and supported the synthesis of specialized ECM, producing up to 6 µg of glycosaminoglycans, indicating potential for the *in vitro* regeneration of articular cartilage tissue.

The current biomaterials used for cartilage repair face significant challenges, primarily due to limited cell–material interactions that often

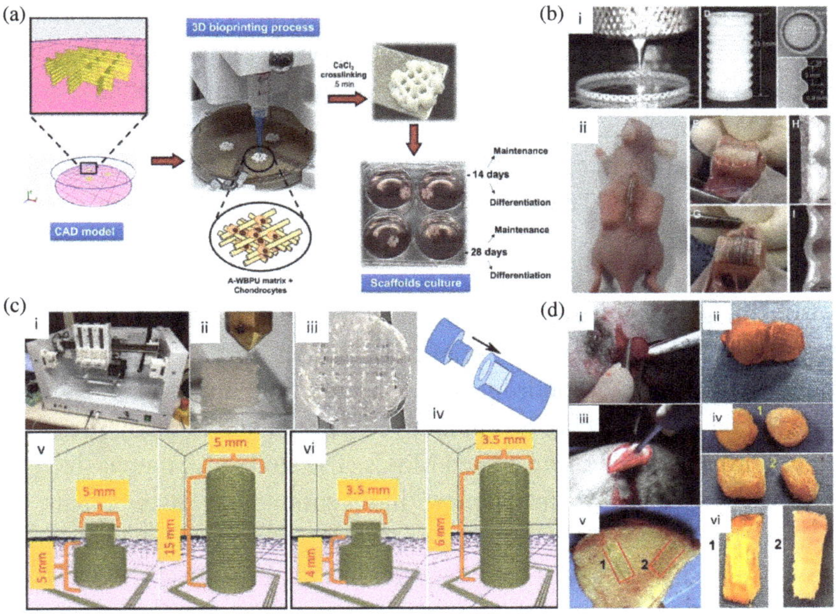

Figure 12. 3D printing of cartilage. (a) 3D bioprinting process of A3.2-WBPU and A6.4-WBPU formulations, starting from the computer-aided design (CAD) model to the creation of functional cell-laden scaffolds. Adapted from Olmos-Juste et al. [215] with permission from Elsevier. (b) (i) The extrusion-based printing process and the resulting porous bellows framework of a clinically relevant size. (ii) Subcutaneous implantation of trachea-mimetic constructs, both with and without sinusoidal-patterned tubular mesh wrapping. Adapted from Park et al. [222] with permission from Elsevier. (c) Scaffolding *via* 3D printing. (i) REGEMAT 3D bioprinting system (University of Granada, Spain). (ii) Side view of the printing process. (iii) Top view of the scaffolding process. (iv) Implant assembly outline. (v) Model for the lateral implant. (vi) Model for the external and inside joint implants. (d) Removal and lateral view of implants after 3 as well as 6 months. Adapted from Landa-Solís et al. [224] with permission from MDPI.

result in inferior tissue formation [216]. Additionally, these traditional biomaterials fail to mimic the complexity and intrinsic functions of the natural ECM. To overcome this challenge, recent research has demonstrated that integrating cartilage extracellular matrix (cECM) into scaffolds can enhance their mechanical and biological properties, thereby promoting chondrogenesis. Chen et al. [217] fabricated a 3D-printed dECM/FGelMa auxetic scaffold using meniscus-derived dECM laden with human chondrocytes (HCs) and fish GelMa. This study aimed to investigate the effects of 3D tensile stimulation on chondrocyte behavior. The inclusion of dECM was found to enhance the initial adhesion and proliferation of HCs. Moreover, increasing the dECM content led to higher proliferation rates of HCs and elevated expression of chondrogenesis-related markers. The findings also highlighted the critical role of tensile force in cartilage regeneration, with cyclic tensile stimulation promoting the production of chondrogenesis-related markers, such as collagen II and glycosaminoglycans. In another study, Rathan et al. [218] demonstrated the substantial benefits of adding cECM to an alginate bioink to enhance chondrogenesis. This combination significantly improved the bioink's chondro-inductive potential and robustly promoted the chondrogenesis of encapsulated MSCs. The study also emphasized the importance of external mechanical interventions in tissue repair. To mechanically reinforce the bioink, a porous 3D-printed PCL network with articular cartilage-like stiffness was fabricated, into which the cECM-functionalized bioink was deposited. This resulted in biomimetic constructs with compressive mechanical properties comparable to native articular cartilage. Similarly, using a dual-nozzle bioprinter, Yang et al. [219] reported the development of a bifunctional PCL/GelMA/dECM (DPGE) scaffold co-printed with aptamer-GE bioink. The PCL component featured large pores (~800–1,000 μm), providing the scaffold with the necessary mechanical strength and anatomical structure. The DPGE scaffold exhibited a compressive modulus of 24.62 ± 8.89 MPa, thereby capable of withstanding physiological compressive stresses. Despite numerous groundbreaking advancements in cartilage bioprinting, *in vivo* trials have remained relatively scarce and limited in scope. This scarcity is primarily due to the complex challenges of replicating the intricate structure and function of natural cartilage in a living organism. However, scientists have recently been making significant strides in overcoming these obstacles. Chen et al. [220] fabricated a 3D-printed electrospinning fiber-reinforced scaffold for cartilage regeneration using a composite of gelatin/PLGA fibers, dECM, and HLA. The inclusion of fibers not only enhanced the stiffness but also improved the toughness of the 3D-printed scaffolds. *In vivo* application of dECM-gelatin/PLGA composite scaffolds demonstrated biocompatibility and promoted the regeneration and remodeling of articular cartilage defects in rabbits 12 weeks post-surgery. In another *in vivo* study, a 3D-extrusion bioprinter was employed to fabricate nano-fibrillated cellulose-alginate scaffolds seeded with HCs and hMSCs. Apelgren et al. [221] implanted these scaffolds into the backs of 48 nude mice and explanted them after 30 and 60 days. The study assessed the proliferative capacity and cartilage formation ability of human cells. Results indicated chondrocyte proliferation within the scaffolds, and the co-culture method of hMSCs and chondrocytes demonstrated an additional proliferative effect, including the production of glycosaminoglycans and type II collagen. However, further examination of the mechanical properties of the printed scaffold is necessary. Park et al. [222], using extrusion-based 3D printing and a two-step printing approach, created a trachea-mimetic cellular construct of clinically relevant size. Initially, a PCL framework with inner and outer grooves was printed and treated with heat and oxygen plasma to enhance its mechanical properties. Collagen rings containing human nasal chondrocytes and human nasal turbinate stem cells were subsequently printed onto the grooves by a rotational printing process. After 8 weeks of subcutaneous implantation in nude mice, the significant infiltration of micro-vessels and the formation of mature chondrocytes and cartilage-like ECM were observed, indicating successful tissue integration (**Figure 12b**). Moreover, Wang et al. [223] developed a 3D-printed bioactive scaffold using poly(glycerol sebacate) (PGS) for cartilage regeneration. Through a super-swelling absorption modification process, gelatin (Gel) and chondroitin sulfate (CS) were absorbed into the micropores and secured within the molecular networks of the pre-printed PGS scaffold. This approach produced a chondrogenic-functionalized PGS-CS/Gel scaffold characterized by well-organized hierarchical structures, superior elasticity, enhanced hydrophilicity, and cartilaginous bioactivity. Following implantation in both nude mice and rabbit trochlear groove defect models, the scaffold promoted adhesion, proliferation, and migration of chondrocytes, leading to well-matched cartilage regeneration without residual scaffold material after only 4 weeks. Notably, in a novel approach, Landa-Solís et al. [224] developed an articular hybrid implant utilizing MSCs derived from sheep (**Figure 12c**). MSCs, pre-differentiated into chondrocytes, were seeded onto 3D-printed PLA scaffolds. Following 6 months of implantation within the femoral head and outside the joint capsule, significant expression of cartilage-specific markers, including SOX9, aggrecan, and COL2A1, were observed within the joint implant (**Figure 12d**). This study highlighted the critical role of pre-differentiated MSCs within the implants for inducing cartilage marker expression. Yan et al. [225] formulated a novel bioink using SF and hydroxypropyl cellulose methacrylate (HPCMA). The BMSC-laden SF-HPCMA scaffold, with a diameter of 6 mm and a thickness of 2 mm, exhibited a compressive modulus of 402 kPa, comparable to normal articular cartilage (200–2,000 kPa) [226]. Histological staining and micro-CT analysis after 12 weeks of implantation into rabbit knee cartilage defects revealed the high biocompatibility, proliferation, and chondrogenic differentiation of BMSCs, effectively repairing articular cartilage defects [225]. A summary of the discussed cartilage 3D printing studies is provided in **Table 7.**

4.2.3. *Skeletal Muscle*

Skeletal muscle plays an essential role in regulating breathing, maintaining energy balance, temperature regulation, facilitating locomotion, supporting the musculoskeletal framework, and protecting internal organs from external damage [227–229]. With increasing incidents of muscle injury due to trauma, sports, aging, and diseases such as myosarcoma or degenerative muscle disorders [230, 231], demand is steadily increasing for biocompatible muscle tissue substitutes that replicate the structure and function of native muscle tissue. Conservative treatments combining muscle stem cell therapy, nonsteroidal anti-inflammatory drugs, and physical therapy are effective for mild muscle injuries but inadequate for volumetric muscle loss (VML), defined as muscle loss exceeding 20% due to surgical resection or trauma, which lacks the ability to self-heal [232–235]. Due to the limited efficiency of VML current treatments, such as free muscle transfer, tissue engineering has emerged as a promising strategy for regenerating severely damaged muscle tissue [236]. Similar to anisotropic material, skeletal muscle scaffolds must facilitate unidirectional force transduction along the long axis of the fiber during contraction and relaxation [237, 238]. Considering the intricate structural organization of skeletal muscle, which includes muscle fibers, blood

Table 7. A summary of studies that have investigated cartilage-related 3D printing approaches.

Printing technique	Materials	Cell type	Scaffold properties	*In-vitro/in-vivo* outcomes	Reference
Extrusion	Aminosilicone, CNC, MA	NIH/3T3	Compressive modulus: ranging from 0.25 to 1.32 MPa. Enhancing shear-thinning property and the static viscosity	Favorable biocompatibility	[213]
Extrusion (two coaxial-needles system)	Alginate, GelMA, CS-AEMA, HAMA	BM-MSCs	Increasing viscosity from around 1 Pa s to 300 mPa s	The bioink facilitated a high cell density (>10^7 cells mL^{-1}) and viability (85%–90%), promoting neocartilage formation through MSC differentiation	[214]
Extrusion	Alginate, WBPU	ATDC5	Viscosities: 1,220 ± 54 Pa·s and 2,668 ± 2 Pa·s G′ values: increase from 770 ± 123 to 2,488 ± 122 Pa	Maintaining a cell density of 10^4 chondrocytes per scaffold after 28 days of *in vitro* cartilage formation, with the capability to synthesize up to 6 μg of GAG as part of the specialized ECM	[215]

(*Continued*)

Table 7. (*Continued*)

Printing technique	Materials	Cell type	Scaffold properties	*In-vitro/in-vivo* outcomes	Reference
Extrusion	Meniscus-derived dECM, FGelMa	HCs	Storage modulus: 33.24 ± 2.01 Pa Tensile strength: 21.8 ± 1.6 kPa Young's modulus: 81.9 ± 4.0 kPa	Enhances initial adhesion and proliferation of HCs and elevates the expression of chondrogenesis-related markers	[217]
Extrusion	cECM, Alginate, PCL, TGF-β3	MSCs	Enhanced viscosity and shear-thinning properties	Supported MSC viability postprinting and robust chondrogenesis *in vitro*	[218]
Extrusion	PCL, GelMA, dECM, Aptamer-GE	ADSCs	Compressive modulus: 24.62 ± 8.89 MPa	Favorable cell adhesion and proliferation, enhanced chondrogenesis, and significantly improved cartilage repair in rabbit full-thickness defects	[219]
Extrusion	Gelatin, PLGA, dECM, HA	Rabbit chondrocytes	Maximum stress value: 12.11 Kpa	Biocompatible and promoted the regeneration and remodeling of articular cartilage in defects in rabbits 12 weeks post-surgery	[220]

Extrusion	Cellulose, alginate	Human chondrocytes, MSCs	–	Chondrocyte proliferation within the scaffolds. Production of glycosaminoglycans and type II collagen	[221]
Extrusion	PCL, atelocollagen	hNCCs, hNTSCs	–	Formation of mature chondrocytes and cartilage-like ECM after 8 weeks of implantation	[222]
Extrusion	PGS, gelatin, chondroitin sulfate	Chondrocytes	Compression modulus: 0.162 ± 0.005–2.443 ± 0.071 MPa	Promoted *in vivo* cell adhesion, proliferation, and migration	[223]
Extrusion	PLA	MSCs	–	Significant expression of cartilage markers (SOX9, Aggrecan, and COL2A1) after 6 months of implantation within the femoral head and joint capsule in a sheep model	[224]
Extrusion	SF, HPCMA	BMSC	Compressive modulus of 402 kPa, comparable to normal articular cartilage (200–2,000 kPa)	High biocompatibility, proliferation, and chondrogenic differentiation of BMSCs effectively repaired articular cartilage defects after 12 weeks of implantation into rabbit knee cartilage defects	[225]

vessels, and neural networks, 3D bioprinting has proven to be an indispensable technology for developing anatomically and physiologically accurate muscle constructs [239, 240]. Using 3D bioprinting, researchers have been able to meticulously control fiber alignment and orientation, resulting in the fabrication of highly organized muscle scaffolds [241–243]. Additionally, native skeletal muscle is characterized by a relatively soft tissue stiffness of approximately 12 kPa, with an elastic modulus and shear modulus ranging between 5 and 170 kPa [187, 244]. Consequently, for muscle 3D bioprinting, replicating the native mechanical properties is less critical compared to other tissues. Instead, the primary challenges lie in achieving appropriate cellular density, organization, alignment, and intercellular connections. Ensuring synchronized contraction, effective nutrient circulation, and neurovascular integration are also essential [245]. Therefore, achieving properties like native muscle tissue stiffness and responsiveness to neurotransmitters and electrical stimulation is crucial in bioprinted muscle constructs. Hydrogel materials such as polyurethane, alginate, fibrin, collagen, gelatin, and muscle-derived extracellular matrix (mdECM) are favored for their natural softness and biocompatibility [134, 246–248]. However, the low mechanical strength of these bioinks often limits their printability. Various strategies, including using support materials such as PCL, polyvinyl alcohol (PVA), and PEG, employing sacrificial inks, and incorporating photo-polymerizable materials (e.g., GelMA, ColMA, PEGDMA, and GM-HA), have been developed to address these challenges [249–252]. Myoblasts, particularly mouse myoblast cells (C2C12) and muscle progenitors, are commonly used for skeletal muscle regeneration [235]. Moreover, unique stem cell populations capable of self-renewal and intercellular communication are being explored [253].

Multiple strategies have been adopted to bioprint muscle analogs that exhibit high cell alignment and synchronous contraction. A common technique involves leveraging the physical and chemical properties of biomaterials to modify their polymer chains, thereby enhancing specific attributes. For instance, photopolymerization is frequently employed in this context. Aiming to achieve higher uniaxial alignment of myogenic cells (C2C12 and hASCs), Hwangbo et al. [249] utilized a modified *in situ* crosslinking process of GelMA using a three-axis printing system with a dispensing system and dual UV exposure systems. C2C12-laden GelMA bioprinted using the ISC system demonstrated significant viability and alignment *in vitro*. The implantation of bioprinted muscle constructs laden with hASCs in C57BL/6 mice showed significant functional and volumetric restoration 2 weeks post-implantation, suggesting that stem cell-based therapies combined with modified bioprinting processes could effectively treat VML injuries. Similarly, Seyedmahmoud et al. [254] developed an optimized 10% (w/v) GelMA/8% (w/v) alginate 3D bioprinted construct crosslinked with UV and $CaCl_2$ for muscle tissue formation. C2C12-laden GelMA-alginate exhibited high cell viability and myotube formation. Incorporating calcium peroxide, as an oxygen-releasing particle technology, further enhanced cell viability, proliferation, and functional skeletal muscle tissue formation, particularly in thick tissue structures. Despite their ability to achieve well-aligned cell orientation, most photocurable hydrogels exhibit elastic properties and slow stress relaxation, which has been shown to limit cell proliferation and may even induce cellular apoptosis. Recent studies emphasize the preference for viscoelastic hydrogels. Addressing this, Li et al. [255] developed a tunable viscoelastic bioink by combining GelMA and FG, utilizing both photo-crosslinking and enzyme-crosslinking techniques (**Figures 13a–c**). They applied this bioink to create aligned skeletal muscle biomimetic scaffolds using a gel-in-gel strategy. This so-called supporting bath approach allows for the printing of hydrogel bioinks within a supported gel matrix, overcoming limitations in constructing multilayer structures and enhancing the controllability and complexity of biomimetic biostructures [256, 257]. The viscoelastic FG hydrogel, which exhibited stress relaxation, was 3D printed within a carbopol-supported gel matrix. *In vitro* studies demonstrated that cell-laden 3D constructs supported the alignment and elongation of C2C12 myoblasts due to their stress relaxation properties, effectively mimicking the native microenvironment and promoting myoblast proliferation and differentiation. Furthermore, *in vivo* studies with cell-free FG-aligned scaffolds demonstrated a conducive microenvironment that facilitated the recruitment of native cells, thereby promoting skeletal muscle regeneration following VML.

Additionally, efforts have been made by researchers to enhance scaffold orientation using various architectural strategies. One effective approach involves the use of an external sacrificial scaffold to impart alignment to

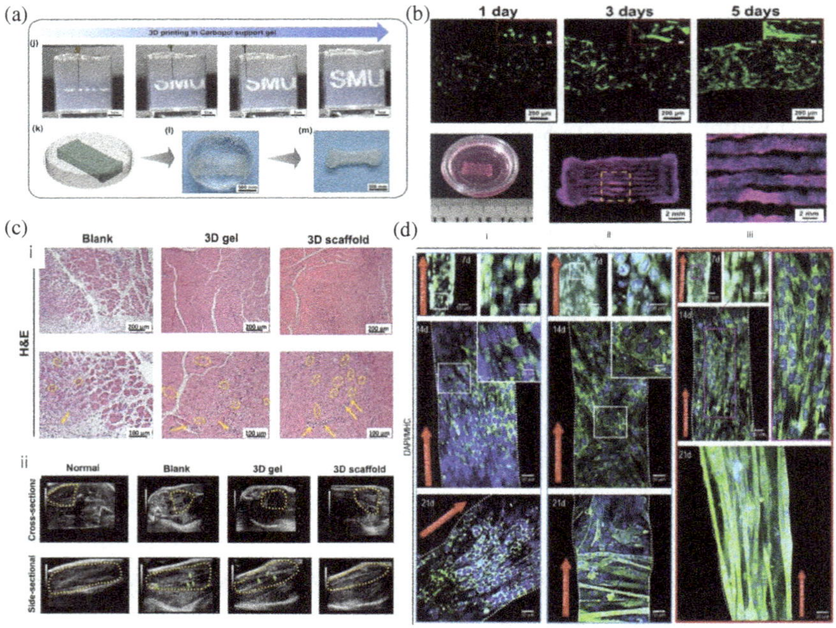

Figure 13. The 3D printing of skeletal muscle. (a–d) 3D printing and analysis of a fibrinogen (FG) and Interpenetrating Polymer Network (IPN) (FG IPN) hydrogel-based 3D bioprinted aligned scaffold. (a) Stress-relaxed FG IPN hydrogel being 3D printed in the carbopol-supported gel. (b) Live/dead staining, along with F-actin and DAPI imaging of C2C12 cells cultured within the 3D-aligned scaffolds. (c) (i) H&E-stained image of muscle regeneration 14 days post-surgery. (ii) Ultrasound imaging of regenerated muscle implanted with the 3D gel and 3D scaffold. Adapted from Li et al. [255] with permission from Elsevier. (d) DAPI (blue) and myosin heavy chain (MHC) (green) imaging of C2C12 cells within the (i) CON-1, (ii) CON-2, and (iii) dE-AS structures at 7, 14, and 21 days. Adapted from Kim et al. [274] with permission from Elsevier.

printed constructs. Kang et al. [189] introduced a multi-material 3D bioprinting technique that integrates multiple cell-laden bioink strands with a fugitive Pluronic F-127 hydrogel and supportive PCL pillars as external sacrificial scaffolds. Their method aimed to fabricate organized 3D muscle constructs using a composite bioink loaded with C2C12 cells, HLA, FG, gelatin, and glycerol. The engineered fiber bundle structures promoted muscle organization, with PCL pillars delivering mechanical cues essential for aligning cells along the longitudinal axis of the constructs. *In vitro* differentiation studies conducted over 7 days demonstrated high cell viability and the formation of muscle-like bundle structures featuring aligned myotubes. To evaluate the *in vivo* functionality, the bioprinted muscle constructs were implanted ectopically into nude rats with the common peroneal nerve positioned between them. Two weeks post-implantation, these constructs displayed highly aligned muscle-like fiber structures with clusters of acetylcholine receptors, demonstrating successful innervation in a mouse model after subcutaneous implantation. In another investigation, Kim and colleagues [258] developed a bioink composed of cell-loaded dECM-MA and a sacrificial fibrillating PVA component to achieve an *in situ* uniaxially aligned micro-topographical arrangement. During bioprinting, the fibrillar PVA component aligned at 20°C through a micro-nozzle, while the dECM component was cross-linked at 38°C to stabilize the scaffold properties. Post-printing, the aligned PVA phase was removed from the cell-laden structures through leaching, creating uniaxial topographical cues on dECM-MA-based bioinks. Myoblasts within these printed structures exhibited alignment and differentiation, resulting in a high degree of myotube formation, utilizing both skeletal muscle-specific biochemical signals and topographical guidance (**Figure 13d**). Topographical cues, such as contour-like staircases, are generally considered undesirable in most 3D-bioprinted scaffolds, except in the context of muscle tissue engineering, where they play a crucial role in aligning muscular cells [259–261]. Consequently, linear or rectilinear motions and meshline scaffolds are commonly employed in 3D-bioprinted muscle tissue engineering [245, 262]. In their study, Kim and colleagues [261] explored the clinical potential of bioprinted self-aligned skeletal muscle constructs derived from the dECM in treating extensive muscle defects in a rat model. They aimed to rapidly restore skeletal muscle function by fabricating biomimetic human skeletal muscle using a photo-crosslinkable mdECM-MA bioink combined with PVA seeded with human muscle progenitors. The self-alignment of cells within the constructs was achieved through the *in situ* creation of a uniaxially aligned micro-topographical structure, achieved by fibrillating and leaching PVA post-printing, without relying on external cues. The study demonstrated that these self-aligned muscle constructs provided both biochemical signals and topographical cues, enhancing integration with neural and vascular systems *in vivo*.

Skeletal muscle, as a highly organized tissue, requires the involvement of multiple cell types for complete structural and functional restoration. Studies have demonstrated enhanced myogenic differentiation when myoblasts are co-cultured with neural stem cells, fibroblasts, endothelial cells, or adipose cells [263–266]. Hwangbo et al. [249] employed *in situ* crosslinking techniques to bioprint uniaxially aligned constructs using cell-laden GelMA bioinks for skeletal muscle regeneration. By optimizing printing parameters and GelMA concentrations, they achieved >90% cell viability in the printed constructs. The implantation of these bioprinted muscle constructs, crosslinked *in situ* and loaded with C2C12 myoblasts and human adipose stem cells, into mice models with VML defects demonstrated a 1.4-fold increase in muscle fiber formation and reduced fibrosis during muscle recovery. This study highlights the potential of combining stem cell-based therapies with bioprinting to create biomimetic muscle constructs for VML repair. In another approach, Lian et al. [267] utilized DW bioprinting to construct muscle tissue using a blend of gelatin, alginate, and mouse myoblasts, followed by seeding of human umbilical vein endothelial cells (HUVECs) to promote vascularization. Following 3 weeks of implantation in nude mice, their prevascularized constructs showed more uniform vascular distribution and improved integration with host tissues. To achieve a more tissue-like response *in vitro*, bioprinted constructs often require maturation to ensure their suitability for *in vivo* implantation and their ability to exhibit an adult-like phenotype with regenerative capabilities [268]. Only a minority of the most recent studies have focused on applying external stimuli such as electrical, mechanical, and magnetic forces to enhance the functionality of 3D scaffolds. Electric fields applied during bioprinting can influence cellular behaviors including adhesion, migration, differentiation, alignment, and contraction [235, 269, 270]. Kim et al. [271] introduced an innovative approach called *in situ* E-field-assisted bioprinting, where hASCs laden with dECM-MA were subjected to electrical stimulation during printing. This method resulted in well-aligned cell structures. Subsequent implantation of these electronically stimulated structures in rats for 7 days demonstrated the formation of new myofibers in the injured muscle. Mechanical stimulation, specifically shear stress during bioprinting, has been explored by Distler et al., who used an oxidized alginate-gelatin bioink to create organized muscle constructs composed of C2C12 myoblasts [272]. By varying the nozzle size and extrusion pressure, they optimized the printing parameters to achieve proper cell alignment, viability, and cytocompatibility post-printing. The bioprinted constructs exhibited increased F-actin orientation, elevated wall shear stress (62.3 Pa), and enhanced myotube alignment after 15 days of *in vitro* culture. This promoted myogenesis, elongation, maturity, and differentiation. Additionally, Cedillo-Servin et al. [273] developed magnetically deformable microfiber meshes through melt electrowriting, incorporating magnetic reduced graphene nanoparticles into PCL. These structured magnetic PCL fiber scaffolds facilitated the organization of myotubes and served as a remotely controllable platform for the mechanical stimulation of myocyte cultures *in vitro*. Collagen/Matrigel hydrogels embedded with myoblasts were deposited on these magnetoactive scaffolds, which demonstrated suitable cell viability and differentiation performance under cyclic external magnetic fields (<300 mT). Over an 8-day period, the microfibers directed the development of 3D myotube architectures, showcasing the potential of centimeter-scale skeletal muscle constructs for reversible, continuous, and dynamic magneto-mechanical stimulation.

Despite significant advancements, creating clinically relevant 3D bioprinted skeletal muscle tissue remains difficult due to the need for complex neuronal and vascular networks. Understanding host immune responses to bioprinted implants is crucial for successful translation, as is the development of patient-specific implants using human cell sources such as patient-derived cells and iPSCs. More *in vivo* studies are essential to enhance muscle bioprinting techniques and the effectiveness of muscle repair technologies. An overview of the skeletal muscle 3D printing studies discussed is presented in **Table 8**.

4.2.4. *Ligaments and Tendons*

Tendons and ligaments are connective tissues optimized for maintaining joint stability and transmitting force between musculoskeletal tissues [275, 276]. This function relies on their high tensile strength (50–150 MPa) and elastic modulus (1–2 GPa) [277]. Tendons connect skeletal muscle to bone, facilitating movement by transmitting muscular force to

Table 8. A summary of studies that have investigated skeletal muscle-related 3D printing approaches.

Printing technique	Materials	Cell type	Scaffold properties	In vitro/in vivo outcomes	Reference
Extrusion	GelMA	C2C12, hASCs	Compressive moduli of CC and ISC: 17.22 and 21.05 kPa, respectively Tensile modulus of CC and ISC: 5.18 and 6.34 kPa, respectively	Significant *in vitro* cell viability and alignment. Significant functional and volumetric restoration 2 weeks post-implantation.	[249]
Extrusion	GelMA, alginate, CPO	C2C12	Alginate concentration and UV crosslinking resulted in significantly increasing the compressive modulus and viscosity	High cell viability and myotube formation Enhanced cell viability, proliferation, and functional skeletal muscle tissue formation by adding CPO.	[254]
Extrusion	GelMA, fibrinogen	C2C12	Suitable stress relaxation and rheological properties	*In vitro* cell alignment and elongation, as well as the promotion of myoblast proliferation and differentiation. *In vivo* cell-free FG-aligned scaffolds promoted skeletal muscle regeneration.	[255]
Extrusion	Pluronic F-127, PCL, gelatin, fibrinogen, hyaluronic acid, glycerol	C2C12	–	High *in vitro* cell viability and the formation of muscle-like bundle structures with oriented myotubes. Highly aligned muscle-like fiber structures with clusters of acetylcholine receptors after 2 weeks post-implantation.	[189]

Extrusion	dECM, MA, PVA	C2C12	–	High cell viability (>94%). Alignment and differentiation of myoblasts, resulting in a high degree of myotube formation.	[274]
Extrusion	Photo-crosslinkable mdECMMA, PVA	hMPC	–	Combined effects of tissue-specific biochemical signals and surface topography. Improved differentiation into muscle cells. Faster integration with neural networks and promotion of vascular growth *in vivo*	[261]
Extrusion	Oxidized alginate, gelatin	C2C12	–	Proper cell alignment, viability, and cytocompatibility post-printing. Enhanced myotube alignment after 15 days of *in vitro* culture. Promoted myogenesis, elongation, maturity, and differentiation	[272]
MEW	Graphene nanoparticles, PCL, collagen, matrigel	C2C12	PCL/rGNP@ –2%, 10%, and 20% bulk filaments showed significantly higher elastic moduli, 357 ± 16,369 ± 20, and 429 ± 23 MPa, respectively, when compared to PCL filaments, 316 ± 14 MPa	Suitable cell viability and differentiation. Reversible, continuous, and dynamic magneto-mechanical stimulation potential	[273]

bones without energy loss due to stretching [278]. Ligaments, on the other hand, though structurally similar to tendons, span joints and attach bones on either end, aiding joint stability [278]. However, due to their poor vascularity and complex structure, tendons and ligaments exhibit limited healing capabilities, making the development of biologically and mechanically robust tissues a significant challenge.

3D bioprinting offers a promising approach to address these challenges by creating customized scaffolds with appropriate porosity, geometry, and biological and mechanical properties similar to the native tissues. Various materials have been utilized for the 3D printing of tendons and ligaments, such as GelMA, SF, collagen, PCL, and PLA [275, 279–281]. These constructs generally involve seeding cells onto the structure post-printing rather than incorporating them into the bioink. However, other studies have utilized tendon and ligament dECM, nanofibrillar cellulose, and HA with cells included in the bioink before printing [148, 282–285]. Combining synthetic polymers for support scaffolds with natural hydrogels has been effective in creating complex scaffold systems for tendon, ligament, and interface engineering. In a study by Jiang et al. [286], a multilayered composite scaffold was developed using PLGA combined with a collagen-fibrin hydrogel, which encapsulated hASCs through 3D bioprinting. This construct aimed to balance biomechanical strength and biological functionality for tendon regeneration. The porous PLGA framework, fabricated using an extrusion method, was layered with an hASC-laden collagen-fibrin hydrogel, resulting in a composite scaffold with an elastic stiffness of 60 N mm^{-1} and an ultimate failure force of 17 N. Cultured in a tendon differentiation medium, these scaffolds supported hASC growth, proliferation, and tenogenic differentiation, with upregulated gene expression of tenomodulin, scleraxis, tenascin, and collagen type III. Subcutaneous implantation into BALB/cJ mice confirmed its *in vivo* biocompatibility and degradability. Chae et al. [287] investigated 3D cell-printed gradient constructs for rotator cuff (RC) regeneration in a rat model with chronic RC tears. Using an extrusion printer with six dispensing heads, they created stratified constructs with polyurethane/PCL frameworks and hMSCs-laden tendon-derived dECM bioinks. *In vitro* analyses demonstrated the scaffold's gradient delivered the capability for zone-specific tissue formation. After 4 weeks of *in vivo* implantation, real-time monitoring of tissue formation and regeneration, as well as the evaluation of walking gait to determine the effectiveness of treatment, indicated the effective restoration of shoulder function and tendon-bone interface healing. In another study that investigated interface construction, Laternser et al. [288] used an inkjet mode to produce 3D musculoskeletal-tendon-like tissues for drug screening using a novel microplate 3D bio-printing platform. Human primary muscle and rat tendon cells were printed within GelMA bioink layers to construct 3D muscle and tendon tissue models in a custom-designed 24-well plate. Tendon tissue was co-cultured around two posts, while muscle tissue differentiated between posts adjacent to the tendon tissue, demonstrating the feasibility of printing muscle/tendon co-cultures (**Figures 14a–b**). Moreover, Merceron and colleagues [289] developed a 3D bioprinted muscle-ligament unit using a 3D-based bioprinter. The design incorporated PCL and polyurethane as the polymeric base materials, with C2C12 and NIH/3T3 cells integrated into the bioink. For muscle development, polyurethane and C2C12 cells were utilized on the tissue side, while PCL and NIH/3T3 cells were employed on the tendon side to support delicate tendon formation. The printed structures showed improved muscle characteristics, with polyurethane providing elastomeric properties for muscle tissue and PCL supporting robust ligament structures. This study highlighted the potential of bioprinting to create differentiated tendon-producing cells for ECM transport.

Regarding ligament 3D printing, Raveendran and colleagues [290] optimized the microextrusion-based 3D bioprinting process using a GelMA bioink laden with periodontal ligament cells (PDLCs) for periodontal ligament tissue engineering. Parameters such as printing pressure, nozzle diameter, collector speed, photoinitiator type, polymer concentration and temperature, printing offset, and bioink viscosity were fine-tuned. The 3D bioprinted GelMA scaffolds exhibited minimal cytotoxicity, maintained high PDLC viability, and supported robust cellular proliferation within the constructs during 2 weeks of *in vitro* culture. In another study, Silva et al. [291] fabricated a 3D-printed ligament scaffold using PLA reinforced with chemically functionalized graphite nanoplatelets (f-EG) and silver (Ag) nanoparticles anchored on the surface (**Figure 14c**). The composite [PLA/(f-EG)/Ag)] scaffold exhibited a porosity range of 67%–71% and pore sizes from 484 to 496 μm, suitable for anterior

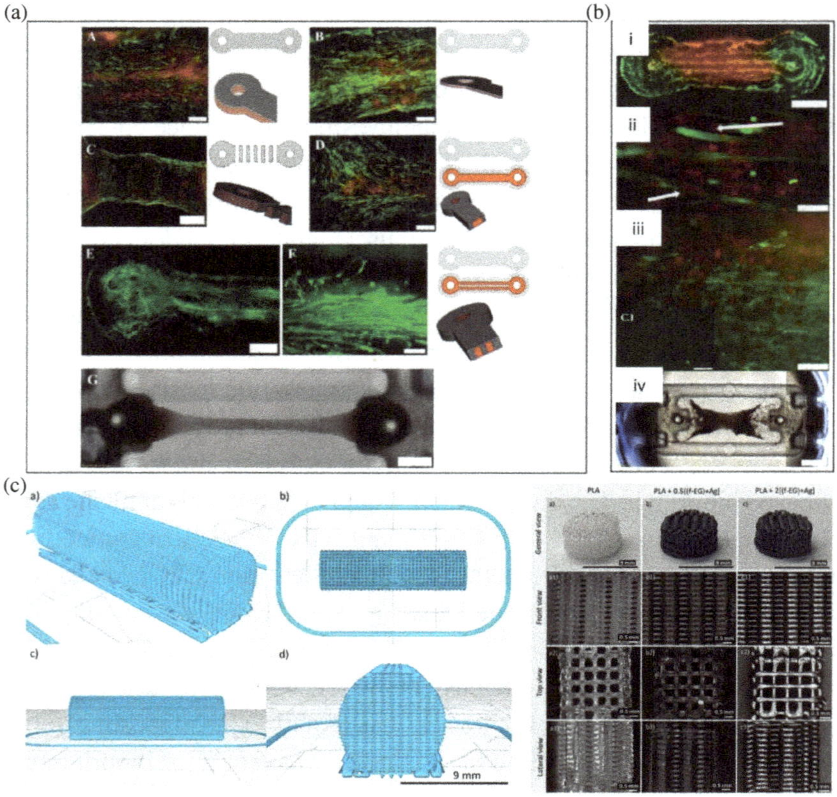

Figure 14. The 3D printing of tendons and ligaments. (a) The impact of different print forms on muscle tissue differentiation: Myoblasts were printed using various forms as illustrated, differentiated for 7 days, and analyzed histologically using MHC immunostaining (green) and propidium iodide nuclear staining (red). (b) A 3D-printed co-culture. Tenocytes were positioned around the posts, while myoblasts occupied the central portion of the dumbbell-shaped structure. Adapted from Laternser et al. [288]. (c) 3D-printed scaffolds composed of PLA, PLA+0.5[(f-EG)+Ag], and PLA+2[(f-EG)+Ag] viewed from front, top, and side perspectives. Adapted from Silva et al. [291] with permission from MDPI.

cruciate ligament (ACL) regeneration. Mechanical analysis revealed a storage modulus of 61.7 ± 9 MPa, comparable to ligaments and tendons under tension and compression. The study highlighted the reproducibility, speed, and simplicity of 3D printing in producing scaffolds suitable for ligament tissue engineering. Moreover, Gomez-Cerezo and colleagues [292] developed a 3D-printed polyethylene terephthalate (PET) scaffold designed as a bone-ligament-bone (BLB) structure for reconstructing the scapholunate interosseous ligament (SLIL). The BLB scaffold consisted of two bone compartments connected by aligned fibers, effectively replicating the architecture of the native tissue. The ligament portion demonstrated excellent tensile stiffness (260 ± 38 N/mm) and an ultimate load of 113 ± 13 N, thereby capable of withstanding physiological loads experienced by the native SLIL. To enhance scaffold biofunctionality, two approaches were employed: injecting GelMA solution containing hMSC spheroids to facilitate cell delivery, which resulted in suitable cell viability, migration, and elongated morphology, indicating topographical guidance by the scaffold's internal architecture; and seeding tendon-derived stem cells (TDSCs) followed by maturation in a bioreactor to enhance ECM formation before implantation. This method demonstrated the high resilience of the scaffold to cyclic deformation and the increased secretion of fibroblast-related proteins due to mechanical stimulation. Despite favorable gene expression and cellular properties, the mechanical properties of these scaffolds remain insufficient compared to native tendon and ligament tissues, rendering them unsuitable for preclinical evaluation. A summary of the 3D printing studies on ligaments and tendons is provided in **Table 9**.

5. Advanced Strategies Integrated with 3D Printing

5.1. *3D Printing Integrated with Controlled Delivery Systems*

Recent advancements in 3D printing technology have facilitated the integration of controlled delivery systems for bioactive cues within scaffolds, improving their functionality as structural templates for cell and tissue growth [293]. The incorporation of GFs, cytokines, and chemical compounds into these scaffolds has proven effective in promoting tissue regeneration by activating or stimulating resident and surrounding cells [294, 295]. Techniques for integrating bioactive cues include adsorption into hydrogels, surface coatings, and embedding within microspheres or particles. One approach involved infusing collagen and gelatin gels containing bone morphogenetic protein 2 (BMP-2) into a hollow cylinder

Table 9. A summary of studies that have investigated tendon- and ligament-related 3D printing approaches.

Printing technique	Materials	Cell type	Scaffold mechanical properties	*In-vitro/in-vivo* outcomes	Reference
Extrusion	PLGA, collagen, fibrin	hASCs	Elastic stiffness: 60 N mm^{-1}. Ultimate failure force: 17 N	hASC growth, proliferation, and tenogenic differentiation. *In vivo* biocompatibility and degradability	[286]
Extrusion (six dispensing heads)	PU, PCL, tendon-derived dECM	hBMMSCs	-	Effective restoration of shoulder function and tendon-bone interface healing after 4 weeks of *in vivo* implantation	[287]
Extrusion (four cartridges)	PCL, PU	C2C12, NIH/3T3	PU-C2C12 muscle side stiffness = 0.39 ± 0.05 MPa PCL-NIH/3T3 tendon side stiffness = 46.67 ± 2.67 MPa. Intermediate in the interface region stiffness = 1.03 ± 0.14 MPa	>80% cell viability at both 1- and 7-days post-printing, supporting initial tissue development and differentiation	[289]

Extrusion	GelMA	PDLCs	-	Negligible cytotoxicity, maintained high PDLC viability, and supported robust cellular proliferation over a 2-week *in vitro* period	[290]
Extrusion	PLA, functionalized graphite nanoplatelets (f-EG), Ag	-	Storage modulus: 61.7 ± 9 MPa, comparable to ligaments and tendons under tension and compression	-	[291]
Extrusion (dual extruder)	PET, GelMA	hMSCs, TDSCs	Tensile stiffness, ranging from 260 ± 38 N/mm, and an ultimate load of 113 ± 13 N, capable of withstanding physiological loads experienced by the native SLIL	Suitable cell viability, migration, and elongated morphology. Enhanced ECM formation in a bioreactor before implantation.	[292]

within a 3D-printed scaffold made from a PCL/PLGA composite [296]. These scaffolds exhibited an initial burst release of approximately 26%, followed by a cumulative release of around 47% of BMP-2 over a 28-day *in vitro* period, which subsequently improved bone healing *in vivo*. However, achieving controlled and sustained GF release from hydrogel-based systems over an extended period remains challenging. To address this issue, thin layers of bioactive cue-loaded coatings have been applied to 3D-printed scaffolds. These coatings facilitate controlled delivery while preserving the structural integrity of both the external and internal scaffold architecture. For instance, Lee et al. employed polydopamine chemistry to graft BMP-2 onto a 3D-printed PCL scaffold, which promoted osteogenic differentiation and may therefore be suitable for bone tissue engineering applications, such as treating bone defects, osteonecrosis, and joint replacements resulting from trauma, tumors, or infections [297]. The results demonstrated significantly enhanced cell proliferation and osteoconductivity, underscoring the potential of the scaffold in bone tissue engineering. However, ensuring a homogeneous and evenly distributed coating layer remains a significant challenge, particularly in anatomically shaped scaffolds with intricate contours and internal microstructures. To overcome these limitations, biodegradable microspheres have been integrated into 3D-printed scaffolds. Sun et al. [298] developed a one-step bioprinting process to create MSC-laden constructs with dual-factor release and gradient structures tailored for articular cartilage regeneration. The PCL framework featured a gradient structure with microchannels positioned between fibers. Microspheres loaded with transforming growth factor beta-3 (TGFβ3) and BMP-4 were strategically incorporated into specific construct layers to deliver zone-specific biochemical cues to the cells. When transplanted into a rabbit osteochondral defect model, the 3D bioprinted cartilage construct facilitated the spatiotemporal release of both cells and inductive proteins. In another study, We et al. [299] aimed to prevent tendon adhesion by loading TGF-β1 gene-silencing micro-RNA-based RNAi plasmids into polydopamine nanoparticles. These composite microspheres were then incorporated into a 3D-printed tendon scaffold, using PCL as the framework and a bioink composed of gelatin, HLA, and sodium alginate. The *in vivo* study on a chicken tendon defect model demonstrated that the loaded plasmids effectively prevented tendon adhesion and promoted functional tendon repair through TGF-β1 gene silencing.

5.2. *3D Printing of Scaffolds for Vascularized Musculoskeletal Regeneration*

Human tissues and organs are highly vascularized, enabling efficient gas exchange, nutrient diffusion, and waste removal [300]. In artificial constructs, the absence of angiogenesis severely restricts these processes due to the limited natural diffusion capacity of oxygen and nutrients in interstitial fluid. Therefore, incorporating a vascular network in engineered tissues is essential to mimic the functionality and viability of natural tissues. Bioprinting is a promising technique for revascularization due to its ability to create complex structures. Key components in vascular bioprinting include biomaterials, endothelial cells, and bioactive factors. Through 3D bioprinting, biomaterials, cells, and bioactive factors can be arranged in precise patterns, making this approach highly effective for generating structured macrovascular networks in engineered musculoskeletal tissues. Two primary methods are used in 3D bioprinting for vessel creation: indirect vessel formation using sacrificial hydrogels and direct endothelial cell printing [301, 302].

The concept of indirect vessel creation involves printing hydrogels such as gelatin and Pluronic F127 as sacrificial inks to form hollow, blood vessel-like structures, which are then removed by heating or cooling [235, 303]. These channels are subsequently seeded with endothelial cells to endothelialize the inner walls. However, this method has not yet been applied to create vascularized musculoskeletal constructs. Endothelial cells, which line blood vessels and capillaries, play a crucial role in revascularization after wound healing [304]. Various types of endothelial cells are utilized in tissue engineering, including those derived from the placenta, tissue-specific microvasculature, embryonic heart cells, and pluripotent stem cells, with HUVECs being the most commonly used due to their ease of isolation, abundance, and well-characterized properties. HUVEC cells can form endothelial networks *in vitro* [303, 305–307]. In a study by Ptiacco and colleagues [308], a 3D bio-printed cartilaginous framework was designed for the regeneration of large bone defects, aiming for rapid vascularization and bone remodeling. Human MSCs loaded in fibrin bioinks were printed within a PCL framework, and chondrogenic priming was performed to initiate bone mineralization and vessel formation. Results using an *in vivo* rabbit model demonstrated the template's capability for controlling the treatment of large bone defects with high regeneration efficiency. Nulty et al. [309] developed a fibrin bioink containing HUVEC/hBMSC cells, which was prevascularized *in vitro*. Following the successful vascularization observed in a nude mouse model within 14 days, the prevascularized 3D-printed PCL scaffolds were tested in a rat model and within critical-sized bone defects. Histological evaluations conducted 12 weeks post-implantation confirmed an enhanced regeneration potential and robust vascularization within the scaffolds.

The acellular matrix, enriched with tissue-specific vascular network skeletons and active cytokines, can be repopulated with endothelial cells to develop functional vascular channels [310]. Pretreatment with dECM bioink for vascularization has been found to prevent hypoxia and enhance *in vivo* muscle recovery [235]. Gao et al. [311] demonstrated that vascular dECM bioink provided endothelial progenitor cells with an optimal microenvironment, effectively promoting angiogenesis in a murine limb ischemia model. Additionally, Choi et al. [312] fabricated a pre-vascular muscle construct using coaxial nozzle printing with muscle and vascular dECM bioinks. Human skeletal muscle cells and HUVECs were incorporated into mdECM and vdECM bioinks, respectively, and coaxially bioprinted to mimic muscle structures encased by capillary networks. The *in vivo* application of these prevascularized muscle constructs significantly enhanced its regenerative capabilities, as evidenced by increased vascularization, innervation, and 85% functional recovery in a rat VML injury model.

Numerous *in vitro* studies have demonstrated the positive impact of bioactive factors, including GFs, cytokines, and signaling molecules, on musculoskeletal regeneration. These factors play a crucial role in mobilizing and activating transplanted cells while also recruiting native cells to the site. Vascular endothelial growth factor (VEGF) is particularly crucial for inducing angiogenesis and promoting musculoskeletal regeneration [313].

Park and colleagues [314] employed 3D printing to enable the dual delivery of BMPs and VEGF for the regeneration of large bone defects. The engineered structures were implanted into a mouse model, with the regeneration process observed over a 28-day *in vivo* period. The findings demonstrated significant micro-vessel formation within large bone defects and faster bone healing in prevascularized structures compared to their non-vascularized counterparts.

5.3. *Electrospinning Combined with 3D Printing*

Among traditional methods for fabricating tissue scaffolds, electrospun scaffolds have demonstrated notable efficacy in tissue regeneration. However, while electrospinning provides a promising approach for creating scaffolds with nanoscale topography and alignment, constructing a 3D architecture through this method alone can be time-intensive [315]. Conversely, 3D-printed scaffolds, though efficient in forming 3D structures, often lack the nanoscale features essential for cell elongation. Therefore, achieving the comprehensive set of properties required for musculoskeletal constructs, such as tissue-mimetic physical cues, hydrophilicity, conductivity, porosity, biocompatibility, and stability, presents a significant challenge when relying on a single fabrication technique. Combining 3D printing and electrospinning emerges as the most advantageous strategy to address the limitations inherent in each method and to produce scaffolds with enhanced biomedical applicability [316]. This integrated approach holds promise for creating musculoskeletal constructs with superior mechanical properties, improved interconnectivity, high porosity, and enhanced cell attachment. Various methods have been employed to merge electrospinning and 3D printing techniques for biomedical applications, including those aimed at musculoskeletal tissue repair. One of the simplest methods involves directly electrospinning nanofibers onto the surface of 3D-printed structures [317]. This approach offers several benefits, including straightforward manufacturing and processing, the ability to create scaffolds with intricate 3D geometries and customized structures, and improved mechanical performance of the resulting scaffolds [318]. Using FDM 3D printing, Saniei et al. [319] successfully fabricated PLA screws with smooth, flawless surfaces. These screws were then coated with PVA-nHA nanofibers at varying concentrations of nHA using an electrospinning technique to enhance bioactivity and cell affinity **(Figure 15a)**. The PVA-nHA nanofibers, which were uniform, solid, and bead-free, had diameters ranging from 263.1 nm ± 45 nm to 326.3 nm ± 40 nm. This nanostructure engineered onto the screw surface effectively mimicked an ECM, which has the potential to improve tissue regeneration. The findings indicated that the optimized PVA-nHA nanofibers created an ideal environment for MC3T3-E1 cell adhesion and proliferation, highlighting their promising potential as a coating for the surface modification of 3D-printed bioabsorbable screws. Similarly, Farsi et al. [320] utilized FDM to fabricate PLA scaffolds intended for cartilage applications, which were subsequently coated with PVA and HLA fibers. This electrospun coating significantly enhanced the mechanical properties of the scaffolds, increasing the elastic modulus to 19.25 ± 0.38 MPa and tensile strength to 6.56 ± 0.14 MPa. The addition of PVA/HLA fibers also imparted hydrophilicity to the porous scaffold without introducing toxicity. Furthermore, the scaffold demonstrated strong chondrocyte adhesion, with cells exhibiting a broad, spindle-shaped, and regular morphology. Therefore, the porous PLA/PVA/HLA scaffold shows promising potential for use in cartilage regeneration. However, this technique has certain limitations, including the uneven distribution of electrospun fibers on complex scaffolds and the difficulty in achieving strong adhesion between the electrospun fibers and the 3D-printed structure. An alternative approach involves the development of hybrid scaffolds through the sequential application of 3D printing and electrospinning techniques **(Figure 15b)** [321]. This method begins with the creation of a base layer using 3D printing, followed by the deposition of electrospun nanofibers on top. The process of layering through alternating 3D printing and electrospinning is repeated to combine these layers effectively. The primary advantages of this approach include the fabrication of scaffolds that mimic the internal structure of the ECM, precise cell placement within the scaffolds, the ability to use multiple materials and scales in manufacturing, and the production of scaffolds with improved mechanical properties [316, 318]. In a study conducted by Liy et al. [322], an innovative hybrid bi-layer scaffold was developed utilizing both electrospinning and 3D printing techniques. The

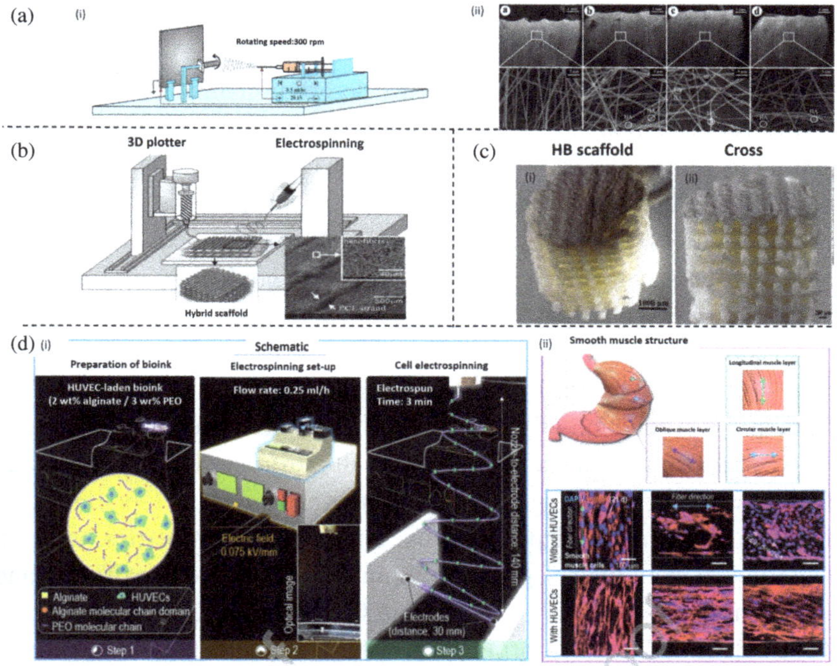

Figure 15. Techniques to combine electrospun fibers with 3D-printed structures. (a) (i) Schematic representation of the coating process, illustrating the electrospinning of nanofibers onto the surface of 3D-printed structures. (ii) Scanning electron microscopy images of coated screws with PVA and PVA-nHA nanofibers in different formulations (from left to right: P10, P10-259 nHA0.1, P10-nHA0.5, and P10-nHA1). Adapted from Saniei et al. [319] with permission from Elsevier. (b) A schematic of the hybrid process. Adapted from Kim et al. [325]. (c) Stereoscopic images of the hybrid bi-layer (HB) scaffold, including cross-sectional views (i, ii). Adapted from Liu et al. [322] with permission from Elsevier. (d) (i) A schematic of the cell electrospinning process using HUVECs. (ii) A schematic and fluorescence images of smooth muscle cells. Adapted from Yeo et al. [324] with permission from Elsevier.

upper layer of the scaffold comprised a heparin-conjugated PCL/Gel nanofiber membrane, which was fabricated through electrospinning. The lower layer was formed by 3D printing a PCL/Gel/n-HA (PGH) scaffold (**Figure 15c**). *In vitro* assessments revealed that both layers effectively supported L929 fibroblast adhesion and proliferation, largely due to the properties of the heparin-conjugated PCL/Gel fibrous membrane. Additionally, the PGH lower layer significantly enhanced the osteogenic differentiation of BMSCs. After 20 weeks of implantation, the hybrid scaffold demonstrated successful *in vivo* bone repair and regeneration, resulting in substantial new bone tissue formation in a rabbit bone defect model. Although the alternating use of 3D printing and electrospinning techniques offers several advantages, it is also accompanied by challenges, particularly in the complexity involved in producing scaffolds with diverse and intricate shapes.

An additional combinatorial technique involves the utilization of electrospun nanofibers as ink in the 3D printing process [323]. This method results in the production of scaffolds with improved mechanical strength, precise dimensions, and a well-defined microstructure. This approach offers several key advantages, including the capability to fabricate scaffolds with customized shapes, improved mechanical properties, uniform integration of nanofiber segments within the 3D-printed scaffolds, and strong adhesion between the electrospun fibers and the printed structures [316, 318]. To achieve uniform cell distribution, precise micro/nanoscale topographical guidance, and desirable mechanical properties, Yeo et al. [324] utilized PCL/collagen as a mechanical support, incorporating HUVEC-laden alginate bioink through uniaxial electrospinning (**Figure 15d**). Subsequently, C2C12 cells were cultured on this vascularized HUVEC-laden scaffold. The resulting co-cultured structure demonstrated the pronounced presence of the myosin heavy chain, which exhibited striated patterns and the enhanced expression of myogenic-specific genes. Electrospun fibers used as inks in 3D printing are challenged by issues such as uncontrolled fiber arrangement and nozzle blockages. To address these limitations, a novel study involved processing a cartilage decellularized matrix (CDM) into a powder and mixing it with an HLA solution to create an ink [220]. Additionally, gelatin/PLGA fibers were produced through electrospinning and then processed into short, dry fibers. It was hypothesized that these dry short gelatin/PLGA fibers could serve as reinforcements to mitigate the softness and mechanical instability of 3D-printed CDM scaffolds. The nanofibers were subsequently blended with the CDM and HLA mixture and used to print a 3D structure. The incorporation of electrospun fibers did not affect the printability of the CDM-based inks.

Instead, it enhanced both the stiffness and toughness of the 3D-printed CDM-based scaffolds. The CDM-fiber scaffolds, reinforced with electrospun fibers, demonstrated commendable biocompatibility *in vitro* and *in vivo* and showed potential for improving the repair of articular cartilage defects in rabbits.

6. Conclusions and Future Perspectives

Despite substantial progress in the 3D bioprinting of musculoskeletal tissues, considerable challenges and limitations persist, hindering the effectiveness of printed constructs both *in vivo* and in their translation to real-world applications. One major challenge is improving materials to achieve a balance between well-defined cell viability and appropriate mechanical properties. Although various materials have been employed to ensure suitable mechanical properties for musculoskeletal tissues, achieving an equilibrium between mechanical strength and cell viability remains elusive. Natural polymers, while conducive to cell viability, often lack the necessary mechanical strength, whereas synthetic polymers, despite their robustness, fail to support adequate cell viability. For instance, scaffolds made from PCL have demonstrated high mechanical strength but only moderate cell viability. Conversely, GelMA scaffolds, while promoting excellent cell viability, often suffer from insufficient mechanical properties. While the combination of these materials has shown promise, further studies are needed to optimize this balance.

Another significant challenge is the maturation of 3D-printed tissues to prepare them for clinical trials. Although 3D printing enables the creation of constructs with specific shapes and sizes, integrating various cell types to form functional tissues, these constructs require maturation through mechanical, electrical, and biological stimuli to be suitable for *in vitro* and clinical applications. Studies have shown that mechanical stimulation can enhance the differentiation of stem cells within bioprinted constructs, while electrical stimulation can improve the alignment and functionality of muscle tissues. Insufficient vascularization further hampers the development of mature tissue by restricting the transport of essential nutrients and waste to and from cells. Although advancements have been made in the vascularization techniques used, the creation of a fully functional vascular network continues to be a major challenge in bioprinting. For example, even with advancements in bioprinting VEGF-laden bioinks, achieving consistent and functional vascularization throughout large constructs remains challenging. Addressing these challenges is crucial for establishing 3D bioprinting as the gold standard for musculoskeletal defect regeneration. Despite significant advancements, 3D bioprinting technology for musculoskeletal tissue repair has yet to reach clinical practice. Key challenges include mismatched mechanical properties of bioink materials, unexamined material degradation during tissue remodeling, and uncertain effects on cartilage lubrication. Continued progress in this field could lead to anatomically precise and mechanically compatible tissue constructs suitable for clinical implantation. Currently, no bioprinting method can produce structures with mechanical properties that meet these clinical standards in terms of size, shape, and structural integrity. Despite these challenges, hybrid printing approaches have shown promise in enhancing mechanical properties while maintaining high cell viability and promoting osteogenic differentiation.

In summary, recent advancements in 3D bioprinting present a promising avenue for the development of musculoskeletal tissues in translational regenerative medicine. This chapter offers an in-depth review of the latest 3D printing strategies and the critical requirements for designing regenerative implants. Despite the difficulties, the collaborative efforts of researchers, including chemists, biologists, engineers, clinicians, and policymakers worldwide, bring musculoskeletal bioprinting closer to clinical practice. Continued interdisciplinary research and innovation will be pivotal in overcoming the existing limitations and unlocking the full potential of 3D bioprinting for musculoskeletal tissue engineering.

References

1. Liacouras PC, Huo E, Mitsouras D. 3D Printing technologies and materials. In: Rybicki FJ, Morris JM, Grant GT. (eds). *3D Printing at Hospitals and Medical Centers: A Practical Guide for Medical Professionals*. Cham: Springer International Publishing, 2024. p. 47–69.

2. Ryan KR, Down MP, Hurst NJ, Keefe EM, Banks CE. Additive manufacturing (3D printing) of electrically conductive polymers and polymer nanocomposites and their applications. *EScience*. 2022;2(4):365–81.
3. Ho G, Kubušová V, Irabien C, Li V, Weinstein A, Weinstein Sh, et al. Multiscale design of cell-free biologically active architectural structures. *Front. Bioeng. Biotechnol.* 2023;11:1125156.
4. Van Eck CF, Chen AF, Klatt BA, D'Antonio J, Fu F. The classification of implants: Class I, II, III. *J. Long Term Eff. Med. Implants*. 2009;19(3): 185–93.
5. Decante G, Costa JB, Silva-Correia J, Collins MN, Reis RL, Oliveira JM. Engineering bioinks for 3D bioprinting. *Biofabrication*. 2021;13(3):032001.
6. Hull CW. Apparatus for production of three-dimensional objects by stereolithography. United States Patent, Appl., No. 638905, Filed, 1984.
7. Bozkurt Y, Karayel E. 3D printing technology; methods, biomedical applications, future opportunities and trends. *J. Mater. Res. Technol.* 2021;14: 1430–50.
8. Park S, Shou W, Makatura L, Matusik W, Fu K. 3D printing of polymer composites: Materials, processes, and applications. *Matter*. 2022;5(1): 43–76.
9. Surmen HK, Ortes F, Arslan YZ. Fundamentals of 3D printing and its applications in biomedical engineering. In: Singh S, Prakash C, Singh R. (eds) *3D Printing in Biomedical Engineering*. Singapore: Springer, 2020. p. 23–41.
10. Asaoka K, Kuwayama N, Okuno O, Miura I. Mechanical properties and biomechanical compatibility of porous titanium for dental implants. *J. Biomed. Mater. Res.* 1985;19(6):699–713.
11. Bandyopadhyay A, Bose S, Das S. 3D printing of biomaterials. *MRS Bull.* 2015;40(2):108–15.
12. Ni R, Qian B, Liu C, Liu X, Qiu J. A cross-linking strategy with moderated pre-polymerization of resin for stereolithography. *RSC Adv.* 2018;8(52): 29583–88.
13. Bagheri A, Jin J. Photopolymerization in 3D printing. *ACS Appl. Polym. Mater.* 2019;1(4):593–611.
14. Peng S, Li Y, Wu L, Zhong J, Weng Z, Zheng L, et al. 3D printing mechanically robust and transparent polyurethane elastomers for stretchable electronic sensors. *ACS Appl. Mater. Interfaces*. 2020;12(5):6479–88.
15. Chaput C, Chartier T. Fabrication of ceramics by stereolithography. *RTe J.* 2007.

16. Melchels FP, Feijen J, Grijpma DW. A review on stereolithography and its applications in biomedical engineering. *Biomaterials*. 2010;31(24):6121–30.
17. Lai J, Wang C, Wang M. 3D printing in biomedical engineering: Processes, materials, and applications. *Appl. Phys. Rev*. 2021;8(2): 021322.
18. Vaezi M, Seitz H, Yang S. A review on 3D micro-additive manufacturing technologies. *Int. J. Adv. Manuf. Tech*. 2013;67:1721–54.
19. Sahafnejad-Mohammadi I, Karamimoghadam M, Zolfagharian A, Akrami M, Bodaghi M. 4D printing technology in medical engineering: A narrative review. *J. Braz. Soc. Mech. Sci. Eng*. 2022;44(6):233.
20. Ligon SC, Liska R, Stampfl J, Gurr M, Mülhaupt R. Polymers for 3D printing and customized additive manufacturing. *Chem. Rev*. 2017;117(15): 10212–290.
21. Hong H, Seo YB, Kim DY, Lee JS, Lee YJ, Lee H, et al. Digital light processing 3D printed silk fibroin hydrogel for cartilage tissue engineering. *Biomaterials*. 2020;232:119679.
22. Mott EJ, Busso M, Luo X, Dolder C, Wang MO, Fisher JP, et al. Digital micromirror device (DMD)-based 3D printing of poly (propylene fumarate) scaffolds. *Mater. Sci. Eng: C*. 2016;61:301–11.
23. Li X, Xie B, Jin J, Chai Y, Chen Y. 3D printing temporary crown and bridge by temperature controlled mask image projection stereolithography. *Proc. Manuf*. 2018;26:1023–33.
24. Sultan MT, Lee OJ, Lee JS, Park CH. Three-dimensional digital light-processing bioprinting using silk fibroin-based bio-ink: Recent advancements in biomedical applications. *Biomedicines*. 2022;10(12):3224.
25. Masood S. Advances in fused deposition modeling. In: *Comprehensive Materials Processing*. 2014;10:69–91.
26. Kazmer D. Three-dimensional printing of plastics. In: *Applied Plastics Engineering Handbook*. Elsevier, 2017. p. 617–34.
27. Kamio T, Hayashi K, Onda T, Takaki T, Shibahara T, Yakushiji T, et al. Utilizing a low-cost desktop 3D printer to develop a "one-stop 3D printing lab" for oral and maxillofacial surgery and dentistry fields. *3D Print. Med*. 2018;4:1–7.
28. Goyanes A, Wang J, Buanz A, Martínez-Pacheco R, Telford R, Gaisford S, et al. 3D printing of medicines: Engineering novel oral devices with unique design and drug release characteristics. *Mol. Pharm*. 2015;12(11):4077–84.
29. Sahafnejad-Mohammadi I, Rahmati S, Najmoddin N, Bodaghi M. Biomimetic polycaprolactone-graphene oxide composites for 3D printing bone scaffolds. *Macromol. Mater. Eng*. 2023;308(5):2200558.

30. Entezari M, Mozafari M, Bakhtiyari M, Moradi F, Bagher Z, Soleimani M. Three-dimensional-printed polycaprolactone/polypyrrole conducting scaffolds for differentiation of human olfactory ecto-mesenchymal stem cells into Schwann cell-like phenotypes and promotion of neurite outgrowth. *J. Biomed. Mater. Res. A*. 2022;110(5):1134–46.
31. Ching T, Li Y, Karyappa R, Ohno A, Toh Y-C, Hashimoto M. Fabrication of integrated microfluidic devices by direct ink writing (DIW) 3D printing. *Sens. Actuat. B: Chem.* 2019;297:126609.
32. Guo SZ, Qiu K, Meng F, Park SH, McAlpine MC. 3D printed stretchable tactile sensors. *Adv. Mater*. 2017;29(27):1701218.
33. Hinton TJ, Jallerat Q, Palchesko RN, Park JH, Grodzicki MS, Shue HJ, et al. Three-dimensional printing of complex biological structures by freeform reversible embedding of suspended hydrogels. *Sci. Adv*. 2015;1(9):e1500758.
34. Malda J, Visser J, Melchels FP, Jüngst T, Hennink WE, Dhert WJA, et al. 25th anniversary article: Engineering hydrogels for biofabrication. *Adv. Mater*. 2013;25(36):5011–28.
35. Xie B, Parkhill RL, Warren WL, Smay JE. Direct writing of three-dimensional polymer scaffolds using colloidal gels. *Adv. Funct. Mater*. 2006; 16(13):1685–93.
36. Lewis JA. Direct ink writing of 3D functional materials. *Adv. Funct. Mater*. 2006;16(17):2193–2204.
37. Skylar-Scott MA, Mueller J, Visser CW, Lewis JA. Voxelated soft matter via multimaterial multinozzle 3D printing. *Nature*. 2019;575(7782):330–5.
38. Joshua RJN, Raj SA, Sultan MTH, Łukaszewicz A, Józwik J, Oksiuta Z, et al. Powder bed fusion 3D printing in precision manufacturing for biomedical applications: A comprehensive review. *Materials*. 2024;17(3):769.
39. Gibson I, Rosen D, Stucker B, Khorasani A. *Additive Manufacturing Technologies*. Vol. 17. Berlin: Springer, 2021.
40. Truby RL, Lewis JA. Printing soft matter in three dimensions. *Nature*. 2016;540(7633):371–378.
41. Utela B, Storti D, Anderson R, Ganter M. A review of process development steps for new material systems in three dimensional printing (3DP). *J. Manuf. Process*. 2008;10(2):96–104.
42. Ma X, Liu J, Zhu W, Tang M, Lawrence N, Yu C, et al. 3D bioprinting of functional tissue models for personalized drug screening and in vitro disease modeling. *Adv. Drug Deliv. Rev*. 2018;132:235–51.
43. Gu Z, Fu J, Lin H, He Y. Development of 3D bioprinting: From printing methods to biomedical applications. *Asian J. Pharm. Sci*. 2020;15(5):529–557.

44. Potyondy T, Uquillas JA, Tebon PJ, Byambaa B, Hasan A, Tavafoghi M, et al. Recent advances in 3D bioprinting of musculoskeletal tissues. *Biofabrication*. 2021;13(2):022001.
45. Ozbolat IT, Hospodiuk M. Current advances and future perspectives in extrusion-based bioprinting. *Biomaterials*. 2016;76:321–343.
46. Zhang YS, Haghiashtiani G, Hübscher T, Kelly DJ, Lee JM, Lutolf M, et al. 3D extrusion bioprinting. *Nat. Rev. Methods Prim*. 2021;1(1):75.
47. Cheng C, Williamson EJ, Chiu GTC, Han B. Engineering biomaterials by inkjet printing of hydrogels with functional particulates. *Med-x*. 2024;2(1): 1–20.
48. Park JA, Lee Y, Jung S. Inkjet-based bioprinting for tissue engineering. *Organoid*. 2023;3:e12.
49. Guillotin B, Guillemot F. Cell patterning technologies for organotypic tissue fabrication. *Trends Biotechnol*. 2011;29(4):183–90.
50. Kryou C, Zergioti I. Laser-induced forward transfer on regenerative medicine applications. *Biomed. Mater. Devices*. 2023;1(1):5–20.
51. Barron JA, Krizman DB, Ringeisen BR. Laser printing of single cells: statistical analysis, cell viability, and stress. *Ann. Biomed. Eng*. 2005;33:121–30.
52. Guillemot F, Souquet A, Catros S, Guillotin B. Laser-assisted cell printing: Principle, physical parameters versus cell fate and perspectives in tissue engineering. *Nanomedicine*. 2010;5(3):507–15.
53. Bhatti S, Singh J. 3D printing of biomaterials for biomedical applications: A review. *Int. J. Interact. Des. Manuf*. 2023:1–22.
54. Al-Shalawi FD, Ariff AHM, Jung D-W, Ariffin MKAM, Kim CLS, Brabazon D, et al. Biomaterials as implants in the orthopedic field for regenerative medicine: Metal versus synthetic polymers. *Polymers*. 2023; 15(12):2601.
55. Williams D. The continuing evolution of biomaterials. *Biomaterials*. 2011;32:1–2.
56. Tavafoghi M, Sheikhi A, Tutar R, Jahangiry J, Baidya A, Haghniaz R, et al. Engineering tough, injectable, naturally derived, bioadhesive composite hydrogels. *Adv. Healthc. Mater*. 2020;9(10):1901722.
57. Chimene D, Lennox KK, Kaunas RR, Gaharwar AK. Advanced bioinks for 3D printing: A materials science perspective. *Ann. Biomed. Eng*. 2016; 44:2090–102.
58. Zare P, Pezeshki-Modaress M, Davachi SM, Chahsetareh H, Simorgh S, Asgari N, et al. An additive manufacturing-based 3D printed poly ε-caprolactone/alginate sulfate/extracellular matrix construct for nasal cartilage regeneration. *J. Biomed. Mater. Res. A*. 2022;110(6):1199–1209.

59. Shirai M. Photoinitiated Polymerization. In: Kobayashi S, Müllen K (eds). *Encyclopedia of Polymeric Nanomaterials*. Berlin: Springer. 2015:1579–85.
60. Zhang YS, Khademhosseini A. Advances in engineering hydrogels. *Science*. 2017;356(6337):eaaf3627.
61. Annabi N, Tamayol A, Uquillas JA, Akbari M, Bertassoni LE, Cha C, et al. 25th anniversary article: Rational design and applications of hydrogels in regenerative medicine. *Adv. Mater*. 2014;26(1):85–124.
62. Guan X, Avci-Adali M, Alarçin E, Cheng H, Kashaf SS, Li Y, et al. Development of hydrogels for regenerative engineering. *Biotechnol. J*. 2017;12(5):1600394.
63. Ding X, Fan L, Wang L, Zhou M, Wang Y, Zhao Y. Designing self-healing hydrogels for biomedical applications. *Mater. Horiz*. 2023;10:3929–47.
64. Yoon J, Han H, Jang J. Nanomaterials-incorporated hydrogels for 3D bio-printing technology. *Nano Convergence*. 2023;10(1):52.
65. Prince E, Kumacheva E. Design and applications of man-made biomimetic fibrillar hydrogels. *Nat. Rev. Mater.* 2019;4(2):99–115.
66. Bahram M, Mohseni N, Moghtader M. An introduction to hydrogels and some recent applications. In: Majee SB (eds). *Emerging Concepts in Analysis and Applications of Hydrogels*. IntechOpen. 2016.
67. Ahmed EM. Hydrogel: Preparation, characterization, and applications: A review. *J. Adv. Res*. 2015;6(2):105–21.
68. Pugliese R, Beltrami B, Regondi S, Lunetta C. Polymeric biomaterials for 3D printing in medicine: An overview. *Ann. 3D Printed Med.* 2021;2:100011.
69. Kesti M, Müller M, Becher J, Schnabelrauch M, D'Este M, Eglin D, et al. A versatile bioink for three-dimensional printing of cellular scaffolds based on thermally and photo-triggered tandem gelation. *Acta Biomater*. 2015;11: 162–72.
70. Yang J, He HM, Li D, Zhang Q, Xu LZ, Ruan CS. Advanced strategies in the application of gelatin-based bioink for extrusion bioprinting. *Bio-Des. Manuf.* 2023;6(5):586–608.
71. Gomes S, Leonor IB, Mano JF, Reis RL, Kaplan DL Natural and genetically engineered proteins for tissue engineering. *Prog. Polym. Sci*. 2012;37(1): 1–17.
72. Bertassoni LE, Cecconi M, Manoharan V, Nikkhah M, Hjortnaes J, Cristino AL, et al. Hydrogel bioprinted microchannel networks for vascularization of tissue engineering constructs. *Lab Chip*. 2014;14(13):2202–11.
73. Ashammakhi N, Hasan A, Kaarela O, Byambaa B, Sheikhi A, Gaharwar AK, et al. Advancing frontiers in bone bioprinting. *Adv. Healthc. Mater.* 2019;8(7):1801048.

74. Freeman FE, Kelly DJ. Tuning alginate bioink stiffness and composition for controlled growth factor delivery and to spatially direct MSC fate within bioprinted tissues. *Sci. Rep.* 2017;7(1):17042.
75. Gonzalez-Fernandez T, Tenorio AJ, Campbell KT, Silva EA, Leach JK. Alginate-based bioinks for 3D bioprinting and fabrication of anatomically accurate bone grafts. *Tissue Eng. Part A.* 2021;27(17-18):1168–81.
76. Peralta P, Laird C. Fatigue of metals. In: *Physical Metallurgy*. Elsevier. 2014:1765–1880.
77. Niinomi M. Recent metallic materials for biomedical applications. *Metall. Mater. Trans. A.* 2002;33:477–86.
78. Rodriguez Colon R, Nayak VV, Parente PEL, Leucht P, Tovar N, Lin CC, et al. The presence of 3D printing in orthopedics: A clinical and material review. *J. Orthop. Res.* 2023;41(3):601–613.
79. Zhou Y, Sooriyaarachchi D, Liu D, Ta GZ. Biomimetic strategies for fabricating musculoskeletal tissue scaffolds: A review. *Int. J. Adv. Manuf. Technol.* 2021;112:1211–29.
80. Nover AB, Lee SL, Georgescu MS, Howard DR, Saunders RA, Yu WT, et al. Porous titanium bases for osteochondral tissue engineering. *Acta Biomaterialia.* 2015;27:286–93.
81. Tan H-L, Teow S-Y, Pushpamalar J. Application of metal nanoparticle–hydrogel composites in tissue regeneration. *Bioengineering.* 2019;6(1):17.
82. Wei L, Gao Z. Recent research advances on corrosion mechanism and protection, and novel coating materials of magnesium alloys: A review. *RSC Adv.* 2023;13(12):8427–63.
83. Hu Y, Guo X, Qiao Y, Wang X, Lin Q. Preparation of medical Mg–Zn alloys and the effect of different zinc contents on the alloy. *J. Mater. Sci.: Mater. Med.* 2022;33(1):9.
84. Wang Z, Wang C, Li C, Qin Y, Zhong L, Chen B, et al. Analysis of factors influencing bone ingrowth into three-dimensional printed porous metal scaffolds: A review. *J. Alloys Compd.* 2017;717:271–85.
85. Chen Y, Frith JE, Dehghan-Manshadi A, Attar H, Kent D, Soro NDM, et al. Mechanical properties and biocompatibility of porous titanium scaffolds for bone tissue engineering. *J. Mech. Behav. Biomed. Mater.* 2017;75:169–74.
86. Kim J-H, Kim D-K, Lee OJ, Ju HW, Lee JM, Moon BM, et al. Osteoinductive silk fibroin/titanium dioxide/hydroxyapatite hybrid scaffold for bone tissue engineering. *Int. J. Biol. Macromol.* 2016;82:160–67.

87. Zhao L, Pei X, Jiang L, Hu C, Sun J, Xing F, et al. Bionic design and 3D printing of porous titanium alloy scaffolds for bone tissue repair. *Compos. Part B: Eng.* 2019;162:154–61.
88. Derakhshandeh SMR, Hadavi SMM, Eshraghi MJ, Javaheri M, Mozafari M. Improved electrochemical performance of nitrocarburised stainless steel by hydrogenated amorphous carbon thin films for bone tissue engineering. *IET Nanobiotechnol.* 2017;11(6):656–60.
89. Heo DN, Ko W-K, Bae MS, Lee JB, Lee D-W, Byun W, et al. Enhanced bone regeneration with a gold nanoparticle–hydrogel complex. *J. Mater. Chem. B.* 2014;2(11):1584–93.
90. Ribeiro M, Ferraz MP, Monteiro FJ, Fernandes MH, Beppu MM, Mantione D, et al. Antibacterial silk fibroin/nanohydroxyapatite hydrogels with silver and gold nanoparticles for bone regeneration. *Nanomed: Nanotechnol. Biol. Med.* 2017;13(1):231–39.
91. Jiang J, Li L, Li K, Li G, You F, Zuo Y, et al. Antibacterial nanohydroxyapatite/polyurethane composite scaffolds with silver phosphate particles for bone regeneration. *J. Biomater. Sci. Polym. Ed.* 2016;27(16):1584–98.
92. Seidenstuecker M, Kerr L, Bernstein A, Mayr HO, Suedkamp NP, Gadow R, et al. 3D powder printed bioglass and β-tricalcium phosphate bone scaffolds. *Materials.* 2017;11(1):13.
93. Tovar N, Witek L, Atria P, Sobieraj M, Bowers M, Lopez CD, et al. Form and functional repair of long bone using 3D-printed bioactive scaffolds. *J. Tissue Eng. Regen. Med.* 2018;12(9):1986–99.
94. Kim WJ, Yun H-S, Kim GH. An innovative cell-laden α-TCP/collagen scaffold fabricated using a two-step printing process for potential application in regenerating hard tissues. *Sci. Rep.* 2017;**7**(1):3181.
95. Dawood A, Marti Marti B, Sauret-Jackson V, Darwood A. 3D printing in dentistry. *Br. Dent. J.* 2015;219(11):521–29.
96. Koeneman J, Lemons J, Ducheyne P, Lacefield W, Magee F, Calahan T, et al. Workshop on characterization of calcium phosphate materials. *J. Appl. Biomater.* 1990;1(1):79–90.
97. Duheyne P, Beight J, Cuckler J, Evans B, Radin S. Effect of calcium phosphate coating characteristics on early post-operative bone tissue ingrowth. *Biomaterials.* 1990;11(8):531–40.
98. Punj S, Singh J, Singh K. Ceramic biomaterials: Properties, state of the art and future prospectives. *Ceram. Int.*. 2021;47(20):28059–074.
99. Zafar MJ, Zhu D, Zhang Z. 3D printing of bioceramics for bone tissue engineering. *Materials.* 2019;12(20):3361.

100. Kolan KC, Leu MC, Hilmas GE, Brown RF, Velez M. Fabrication of 13–93 bioactive glass scaffolds for bone tissue engineering using indirect selective laser sintering. *Biofabrication.* 2011;3(2):025004.
101. Lindner M, Hoeges S, Meiners W, Wissenbach K, Smeets R, Telle R, et al. Manufacturing of individual biodegradable bone substitute implants using selective laser melting technique. *J. Biomed. Mater. Res. A.* 2011;97(4): 466–71.
102. Luo G, Ma Y, Cui X, Jiang L, Wu M, Hu Y, et al. 13-93 bioactive glass/alginate composite scaffolds 3D printed under mild conditions for bone regeneration. *RSC Adv.* 2017;7(20):11880–9.
103. Demirtaş TT, Irmak G., Gümüşderelioğlu M. A bioprintable form of chitosan hydrogel for bone tissue engineering. *Biofabrication.* 2017;9(3):035003.
104. Oladapo BI, Zahedi SA, Ismail SO. Mechanical performances of hip implant design and fabrication with PEEK composite. *Polymer.* 2021; 227:123865.
105. Sa MW, Nguyen B-NB, Moriarty RA, Kamalitdinov T, Fisher JP, Kim JY. Fabrication and evaluation of 3D printed BCP scaffolds reinforced with ZrO2 for bone tissue applications. *Biotechnol. Bioeng.* 2018;115(4): 989–99.
106. Murphy C, Kolan K, Li W, Semon J, Day D, Leu M. 3D bioprinting of stem cells and polymer/bioactive glass composite scaffolds for bone tissue engineering. *Int. J. Bioprint.* 2017;3(1):005.
107. Hardy JG, Torres-Rendon JG, Leal-Egaña A, Walther A, Schlaad H, Cölfen H, et al. Biomineralization of engineered spider silk protein-based composite materials for bone tissue engineering. *Materials.* 2016;9(7):560.
108. Luo Y, Zhai D, Huan Z, Zhu H, Xia L, Chang J, et al. Three-dimensional printing of hollow-struts-packed bioceramic scaffolds for bone regeneration. *ACS Appl. Mater. Interfaces.* 2015;**7**(43):24377–83.
109. Cox SC, Thornby JA, Gibbons GJ, Williams MA, Mallick KK. 3D printing of porous hydroxyapatite scaffolds intended for use in bone tissue engineering applications. *Mater. Sci. Eng: C.* 2015;47:237–47.
110. Ojansivu M, Rashad A, Ahlinder A, Massera J, Mishra A, Syverud K, et al. Wood-based nanocellulose and bioactive glass modified gelatin–alginate bioinks for 3D bioprinting of bone cells. *Biofabrication.* 2019;11(3):035010.
111. Byambaa B, Annabi N, Yue K, Trujillo-de Santiago G, Alvarez MM, Jia W, et al. Bioprinted osteogenic and vasculogenic patterns for engineering 3D bone tissue. *Adv. Healthc. Mater.* 2017;6(16):1700015.
112. Shie M-Y, Chang W-C, Wei L-J, Huang Y-H, Chen C-H, Shih C-T, et al. 3D printing of cytocompatible water-based light-cured polyurethane with

hyaluronic acid for cartilage tissue engineering applications. *Materials*. 2017;10(2):136.
113. Schuurman W, Levett PA, Pot MW, van Weeren PR, Dhert WJA, Hutmacher DW, et al. Gelatin-methacrylamide hydrogels as potential biomaterials for fabrication of tissue-engineered cartilage constructs. *Macromol. Biosci*. 2013;13(5):551–61.
114. Costantini M, Testa S, Mozetic P, Barbetta A, Fuoco C, Fornetti E, et al. Microfluidic-enhanced 3D bioprinting of aligned myoblast-laden hydrogels leads to functionally organized myofibers in vitro and in vivo. *Biomaterials*. 2017;131:98–110.
115. Mozdzen LC, Rodgers R, Banks JM, Bailey RC, Harley BAC. Increasing the strength and bioactivity of collagen scaffolds using customizable arrays of 3D-printed polymer fibers. *Acta Biomater*. 2016;33:25–33.
116. Akoury E, Weber MH, Rosenzweig DH. 3D-Printed nanoporous scaffolds impregnated with zoledronate for the treatment of spinal bone metastases. *MRS Adv*. 2019;4(21):1245–51.
117. Lim SH, Kathuria H, Tan JJY, Kang L. 3D printed drug delivery and testing systems — a passing fad or the future? *Adv. Drug Deliv. Rev*. 2018;132:139–68.
118. Haglund L, Ahangar P, Rosenzweig DH. Advancements in 3D printed scaffolds to mimic matrix complexities for musculoskeletal repair. *Curr. Opin. Biomed. Eng*. 2019;10:142–48.
119. Zennifer A, Manivannan S, Sethuraman S, Kumbar SG, Sundaramurthi D. 3D bioprinting and photocrosslinking: emerging strategies & future perspectives. *Biomater. Adv*. 2022;134:112576.
120. Arif ZU, Khalid MY, Noroozi R, Hossain M, Shi HTH, Tariq A, et al. Additive manufacturing of sustainable biomaterials for biomedical applications. *Asian J. Pharm. Sci*. 2023;18:100812.
121. Li J, Kim C, Pan C-C, Babian A, Lui E, Young JL, et al. Hybprinting for musculoskeletal tissue engineering. *Iscience*. 2022;25(5):104229.
122. Mondal D, Willett TL. Three-dimensional printable nanocomposite biomaterials as bone scaffolds and grafts. In: *Smart Multifunctional Nano-inks*. Elsevier, 2023:579–94.
123. Piard CM, Chen Y, Fisher JP. Cell-laden 3D printed scaffolds for bone tissue engineering. *Clinical Reviews in Bone and Mineral Metabolism*. 2015;13:245–55.
124. Deng S, Cao H, Cui X, Fan Y, Wang Q, Zhang X. Optimization of exosome-based cell-free strategies to enhance endogenous cell functions in tissue regeneration. *Acta Biomaterialia*. 2023:171:68–84.

125. Shen Z, Sun F, Shan Y, Lu Y, Wu C, Zhang B, et al. Construction of a novel cell-free tracheal scaffold promoting vascularization for repairing tracheal defects. *Mater. Today Bio*. 2023;23:100841.
126. Liu Y, Zheng K, Meng Z, Wang L, Liu X, Guo B, et al. A cell-free tissue-engineered tracheal substitute with sequential cytokine release maintained airway opening in a rabbit tracheal full circumferential defect model. *Biomaterials*. 2023;300:122208.
127. Oladapo BI, Zahedi S, Adeoye A. 3D printing of bone scaffolds with hybrid biomaterials. *Compos. Part B: Eng*. 2019;158:428–36.
128. Bruyas A, Lou F, Stahl AM, Gardner M, Maloney W, Goodman S, et al. Systematic characterization of 3D-printed PCL/β-TCP scaffolds for biomedical devices and bone tissue engineering: Influence of composition and porosity. *J. Mater. Res*. 2018;33(14):1948–59.
129. Long J, Yao Z, Zhang W, Liu B, Chen K, Li L, et al. Regulation of osteoimmune microenvironment and osteogenesis by 3D-printed PLAG/black phosphorus scaffolds for bone regeneration. *Adv. Sci*. 2023;10(28):2302539.
130. Costa CPL. *PLA-PCL Textile Reinforced Composites for Connective Tissues Applications*. Getafe: Universidad Carlos III de Madrid, 2024.
131. Goncalves EM, Oliveira FJ, Silva RF, Neto MA, Fernandes MH, Amaral M, et al. Three-dimensional printed PCL-hydroxyapatite scaffolds filled with CNT s for bone cell growth stimulation. *J. Biomed. Mater. Res. Part B: Appl. Biomater.* 2016;104(6):1210–19.
132. Unagolla JM, Jayasuriya AC. Hydrogel-based 3D bioprinting: A comprehensive review on cell-laden hydrogels, bioink formulations, and future perspectives. *Appl. Mater. Today*. 2020;18:100479.
133. Berg J, Hiller T, Kissner MS, Qazi TH, Duda GN, Hocke AC, et al. Optimization of cell-laden bioinks for 3D bioprinting and efficient infection with influenza A virus. *Sci. Rep*. 2018;8(1):13877.
134. Li C, Cui W. 3D bioprinting of cell-laden constructs for regenerative medicine. *Eng. Regen*. 2021;2:195–205.
135. Swetha S, Lavanya K, Sruthia R, Selvamurugan N. An insight into cell-laden 3D-printed constructs for bone tissue engineering. *J. Mater. Chem. B*. 2020;8(43):9836–62.
136. Billiet T, Gevaert E, De Schryver T, Cornelissen M, Dubruel P. The 3D printing of gelatin methacrylamide cell-laden tissue-engineered constructs with high cell viability. *Biomaterials*. 2014;35(1):49–62.
137. Piard C, Baker H, Kamalitdinov T, Fisher J. Bioprinted osteon-like scaffolds enhance in vivo neovascularization. *Biofabrication*. 2019;11(2):025013.

138. Mir TA, Nakamura M. Three-dimensional bioprinting: toward the era of manufacturing human organs as spare parts for healthcare and medicine. *Tissue Eng. Part B: Rev*. 2017;23(3):245–56.
139. Chen YW, Shen Y-F, Ho C-C, Yu J, Wu Y-HA, Wang K, et al. Osteogenic and angiogenic potentials of the cell-laden hydrogel/mussel-inspired calcium silicate complex hierarchical porous scaffold fabricated by 3D bioprinting. *Mater. Sci. Eng: C*. 2018;91:679–687.
140. Stichler S, Böck T, Paxton N, Bertlein S, Levato R, Schill V, et al. Double printing of hyaluronic acid/poly (glycidol) hybrid hydrogels with poly (ε-caprolactone)forMSCchondrogenesis.*Biofabrication*.2017;9(4):044108.
141. Datta P, Dhawan A, Yu Y, Hayes D, Gudapati H, Ozbolat IT. Bioprinting of osteochondral tissues: A perspective on current gaps and future trends. *Int. J. Bioprint.* 2017;3(2):007.
142. Daly AC, Cunniffe GM, Sathy BN, Jeon O, Alsberg E, Kelly DJ. 3D bioprinting of developmentally inspired templates for whole bone organ engineering. *Adv. Healthc. Mater*. 2016;5(18):2353–62.
143. García-Gareta E, Coathup MJ, Blunn GW. Osteoinduction of bone grafting materials for bone repair and regeneration. *Bone*. 2015;81:112–121.
144. Wang H, Cui J, Li S, Tao A, Du S, Kan Z. Fabrication of functional and biodegradable scaffolds using nucleated poly (4-hydroxybutyrate) via 3D printing for bone tissue engineering. *Polym. Test*. 2023;118:107881.
145. Esmaeili S, Aghdam HA, Motififard M, Saber-Samandari S, Montazeran AH, Bigonah M, et al. A porous polymeric–hydroxyapatite scaffold used for femur fractures treatment: fabrication, analysis, and simulation. *Eur. J. Orthop. Surg. Traumatol*. 2020;30:123–31.
146. Paek K, Kim S, Tak S, Kim MK, Park J, Chung S, et al. A high-throughput biomimetic bone-on-a-chip platform with artificial intelligence-assisted image analysis for osteoporosis drug testing. *Bioeng. Transl. Med.* 2023; 8(1):e10313.
147. Shahrezaie M, Zamanian A, Sahranavard M, Shahrezaee MH. A critical review on the 3D bioprinting in large bone defects regeneration. *Bioprinting*. 2023;37:e00327.
148. Chae S, Sun Y, Choi Y-J, Ha D-H, Jeon I, Cho D-W. 3D cell-printing of tendon-bone interface using tissue-derived extracellular matrix bioinks for chronic rotator cuff repair. *Biofabrication*. 2021;13(3):035005.
149. Amini Z, Lari R. A systematic review of decellularized allograft and xenograft–derived scaffolds in bone tissue regeneration. *Tissue and Cell.* 2021; 69:101494.

150. Genova T, Roato I, Carossa M, Motta C, Cavagnetto D, Mussano F. Advances on bone substitutes through 3D bioprinting. *Int. J. Mol. Sci.* 2020; 21(19):7012.
151. Zhang Z, Jin Y, Yin J, Xu C, Xiong R, Christensen K, et al. Evaluation of bioink printability for bioprinting applications. *Appl. Phys. Rev*. 2018;5(4): 041304.
152. Valtanen RS, Yang YP, Gurtner GC, Maloney WJ, Lowenberg DW. Synthetic and Bone tissue engineering graft substitutes: What is the future? *Injury*. 2021;52:S72–S77.
153. Wickramasinghe ML, Dias GJ, Premadasa KMGP. A novel classification of bone graft materials. *J. Biomed. Mater. Res. Part B: Appl. Biomater*. 2022; 110(7):1724–49.
154. Ejnisman L, Gobbato B, de França Camargo AF, Zancul E. Three-dimensional printing in orthopedics: From the basics to surgical applications. *Curr. Rev. Musculoskelet. Med*. 2021;14:1–8.
155. Velásquez-García LF, Kornbluth Y. Biomedical applications of metal 3D printing. *Ann. Rev. Biomed. Eng*. 2021;23:307–38.
156. Li J, Li Z, Shi Y, Wang H, Li R, Tu J, et al. In vitro and in vivo comparisons of the porous Ti6Al4V alloys fabricated by the selective laser melting technique and a new sintering technique. *J. Mech. Behav. Biomed. Mater*. 2019; 91:149–58.
157. Przekora A, Kazimierczak P, Wojcik M, Chodorski E, Kropiwnicki J. Mesh Ti6Al4V material manufactured by selective laser melting (SLM) as a promising intervertebral fusion cage. *Int. J. Mol. Sci*. 2022;23(7):3985.
158. Zhang Y, Zhang L, Sun R, Jia Y, Chen X, Liu Y, et al. A new 3D printed titanium metal trabecular bone reconstruction system for early osteonecrosis of the femoral head. *Medicine*. 2018;97(26):e11088.
159. Liu B, Ma Z, Li J, Xie H, Wei X, Wang B, et al. Experimental study of a 3D printed permanent implantable porous Ta-coated bone plate for fracture fixation. *Bioact. Mater*. 2022;10:269–80.
160. Bandyopadhyay A, Mitra I, Shivaram A, Dasgupta N, Bose S. Direct comparison of additively manufactured porous titanium and tantalum implants towards in vivo osseointegration. *Addit. Manuf*. 2019;28:259–66.
161. Jain K, Shukla R, Yadav A, Ujjwal RR, Flora SJS. 3D printing in development of nanomedicines. *Nanomaterials*. 2021;11(2):420.
162. Imanishi J, Choong PF. Three-dimensional printed calcaneal prosthesis following total calcanectomy. *Int. J. Surg. Case Rep*. 2015;10:83–87.
163. Faldini C, Mazzotti A, Belvedere C, Durastanti G, Panciera A, Geraci G, et al. A new ligament-compatible patient-specific 3D-printed implant and

instrumentation for total ankle arthroplasty: From biomechanical studies to clinical cases. *J. Orthop. Traumatol.* 2020;21:1–9.

164. Díaz-Pérez M, Grima L, Moshtaghioun BM, Peña JI. CaO–MgO–SiO2–P2O5-based multiphase bio-ceramics fabricated by directional solidification: Microstructure features and in vitro bioactivity studies. *Ceram. Int.* 2021;47(12):17041–048.
165. Namdar A, Salahinejad E. Advances in ion-doping of Ca-Mg silicate bioceramics for bone tissue engineering. *Coord. Chem. Rev.* 2023;478:215001.
166. Lee U-L, Lim J-Y, Park S-N, Choi B-H, Kang H, Choi W-C. A clinical trial to evaluate the efficacy and safety of 3D printed bioceramic implants for the reconstruction of zygomatic bone defects. *Materials.* 2020;13(20): 4515.
167. Cho JW, Kim B-S, Yeo D-H, Lim EJ, Sakong S, Lim J, et al. 3D-printed, bioactive ceramic scaffold with rhBMP-2 in treating critical femoral bone defects in rabbits using the induced membrane technique. *J. Orthop. Res.* 2021;39(12):2671–80.
168. Beheshtizadeh N, Farzin A, Rezvantalab S, Pazhouhnia Z, Lotfibakhshaiesh N, Ai J, et al. 3D printing of complicated GelMA-coated Alginate/Tricalcium silicate scaffold for accelerated bone regeneration. *Int. J. Biol. Macromol.* 2023;229:636–53.
169. Zhang B, Wang L, Song P, Pei X, Sun H, Wu L, et al. 3D printed bone tissue regenerative PLA/HA scaffolds with comprehensive performance optimizations. *Mater. Design.* 2021;201:109490.
170. Jakus AE, Rutz AL, Jordan SW, Kannan A, Mitchell SM, Yun C, et al. Hyperelastic “bone”: A highly versatile, growth factor–free, osteoregenerative, scalable, and surgically friendly biomaterial. *Sci. Transl. Med.* 2016;8(358):358ra127–358ra127.
171. Parupelli SK, Saudi S, Bhattarai N, Desai S. 3D printing of PCL-ceramic composite scaffolds for bone tissue engineering applications. *Int. J. Bioprint.* 2023;9(2):0196.
172. Mahnavi A, Shahriari-Khalaji M, Hosseinpour B, Ahangarian M, Aidun A, Bungau S, et al. Evaluation of cell adhesion and osteoconductivity in bone substitutes modified by polydopamine. *Front. Bioeng. Biotechnol.* 2023; 10:1057699.
173. Gao J, Li M, Cheng J, Liu X, Liu Z, Liu J, et al. 3D-Printed GelMA/PEGDA/F127DA scaffolds for bone regeneration. *J. Funct. Biomater.* 2023; 14(2):96.
174. Zhai X, Wu Y, Tan H. Gelatin-based targeted delivery systems for tissue engineering. *Curr. Drug Targets.* 2023;24(8):673–87.

175. De Santis MM, Alsafadi HN, Tas S, Bölükbas DA, Prithiviraj S, Da Silva IAN, et al. Extracellular-matrix-reinforced bioinks for 3D bioprinting human tissue. *Adv. Mater*. 2021;33(3):2005476.
176. Wan H, Xiang J, Mao G, Pan S, Li B, Lu Y. Recent advances in the application of 3D-printing bioinks based on decellularized extracellular matrix in tissue engineering. *ACS Omega*. 2024;9:24219–235.
177. La W-G, Jang J, Kim BS, Lee MS, Cho D-W, Yang HS. Systemically replicated organic and inorganic bony microenvironment for new bone formation generated by a 3D printing technology. *RSC Adv*. 2016;6(14):11546–53.
178. Lee H, Yang GH, Kim M, Lee JY, Huh JT, Kim GH. Fabrication of micro/nanoporous collagen/dECM/silk-fibroin biocomposite scaffolds using a low temperature 3D printing process for bone tissue regeneration. *Mater. Sci. Eng: C*. 2018;84:140–7.
179. Menarbazari AA, Mansoori-Kermani A, Mashayekhan S, Soleimani A. 3D-printed polycaprolactone/tricalcium silicate scaffolds modified with decellularized bone ECM-oxidized alginate for bone tissue engineering. *Int. J. Biol. Macromol*. 2024;265:130827.
180. Bendtsen ST, Quinnell SP, Wei M. Development of a novel alginate-polyvinyl alcohol-hydroxyapatite hydrogel for 3D bioprinting bone tissue engineered scaffolds. *J. Biomed. Mater. Res. A*. 2017;105(5):1457–68.
181. Yang S, Zhu B, Yin P, Zhao L, Wang Y, Fu Z, et al. Integration of human umbilical cord mesenchymal stem cells-derived exosomes with hydroxyapatite-embedded hyaluronic acid-alginate hydrogel for bone regeneration. *ACS Biomater. Sci. Eng*. 2020;6(3):1590–1602.
182. Yang WS, Kim WJ, Ahn JY, Lee JU, Ko DW, Park S, et al. New bioink derived from neonatal chicken bone marrow cells and its 3D-bioprinted niche for osteogenic stimulators. *ACS Appl. Mater. Interfaces*. 2020;12(44):49386–397.
183. Ruiz-Alonso S, et al. 3D Bioprinting for musculoskeletal applications. In: Muñoz JLP, del Burgo Martínez LS, Ochoa GP, Sesma JZ (eds). *3D Printing and Bioprinting for Pharmaceutical and Medical Applications*. CRC Press, 2023. 147–68.
184. Kim W, Kim G. Collagen/bioceramic-based composite bioink to fabricate a porous 3D hASCs-laden structure for bone tissue regeneration. *Biofabrication*. 2019;12(1):015007.
185. Gao G, Yonezawa T, Hubbell K, Dai G, Cui X. Inkjet-bioprinted acrylated peptides and PEG hydrogel with human mesenchymal stem cells promote robust bone and cartilage formation with minimal printhead clogging. *Biotechnol. J*. 2015;10(10):1568–77.

186. Grottkau BE, Hui Z, Pang Y. A novel 3D bioprinter using direct-volumetric drop-on-demand technology for fabricating micro-tissues and drug-delivery. *Int. J. Mol. Sci.* 2020;21(10):3482.
187. Guimarães CF, Gasperini L, Marques AP, Reis RL. The stiffness of living tissues and its implications for tissue engineering. *Nat. Rev. Mater.* 2020;5(5):351–70.
188. Kim JH, Seol Y-J, Ko IK, Kang H-W, Lee YK, Yoo JJ, et al. 3D bioprinted human skeletal muscle constructs for muscle function restoration. *Sci. Rep.* 2018;8(1):12307.
189. Kang H-W, Lee SJ, Ko IK, Kengla C, Yoo JJ, Atala A. A 3D bioprinting system to produce human-scale tissue constructs with structural integrity. *Nat. Biotechnol.* 2016;34(3):312–19.
190. Altunbek M, Afghah SF, Fallah A, Acar AA, Koc B. Design and 3D printing of personalized hybrid and gradient structures for critical size bone defects. *ACS Appl. Bio Mater.* 2023;6(5):1873–85.
191. Demirtaş T, Irmak G, Gümüşderelioğlu M. A bioprintable form of chitosan hydrogel for bone tissue engineering. *Biofabrication.* 2017;9:035003.
192. Vaca-González JJ, Culma JJS, Nova LMH, Garzón-Alvarado DA. Anatomy, molecular structures, and hyaluronic acid–Gelatin injectable hydrogels as a therapeutic alternative for hyaline cartilage recovery: A review. *J. Biomed. Mater. Res. B: Appl. Biomater.* 2023;111(9):1705–22.
193. Loeser RF, Goldring SR, Scanzello CR, Goldring MB. Osteoarthritis: A disease of the joint as an organ. *Arthritis Rheum.* 2012;64(6):1697.
194. Zhou J, Li Q, Tian Z, Yao Q, Zhang M. Recent advances in 3D bioprinted cartilage-mimicking constructs for applications in tissue engineering. *Mater. Today Bio.* 2023;23:100870.
195. Sophia Fox AJ, Bedi A, Rodeo SA. The basic science of articular cartilage: structure, composition, and function. *Sports Health.* 2009;1(6):461–8.
196. Wang M, et al. From materials to clinical: Advances in 3D-printed scaffolds for cartilage tissue engineering. *Phys. Chem. Chem. Phys.* 2023.
197. Trengove A, Di Bella C, O'Connor AJ. The challenge of cartilage integration: Understanding a major barrier to chondral repair. *Tissue Eng. Part B: Rev.* 2022;28(1):114–28.
198. Elhadad AA, Alcudia A, Begines B, Pérez-Soriano EM, Torres Y. A multidisciplinary perspective on the latest trends in artificial cartilage fabrication to mimic real tissue. *Appl. Mater. Today.* 2022;29:101603.
199. HuysseWC, Van Den Berghe T, Verstraete KL. Internal derangement of the knee: Cartilage and osteochondral injuries. In: *Musculoskeletal Imaging.* Springer, 2023:1–27.

200. Arokoski JPA, Jurvelin JS, Väätäinen U, Helminen HJ. Normal and pathological adaptations of articular cartilage to joint loading. *Scand. J. Med. Sci. Sports.* 2000;10(4):186–98.
201. Marom N, Bugbee W, Williams III RJ. Osteochondral grafts failures. *Oper. Tech. Sports Med.* 2020;28(1):150712.
202. Wang M, Wu Y, Li G, Lin Q, Zhang W, Liu H, et al. Articular cartilage repair biomaterials: Strategies and applications. *Mater. Today Bio.* 2024;24: 100948.
203. Wang X, Ren Z, Liu Y, Ma Y, Huang L, Song W, et al. Characteristics and clinical outcomes after osteochondral allograft transplantation for treating articular cartilage defects: Systematic review and single-arm meta-analysis of studies from 2001 to 2020. *Orthop. J. Sports Med.* 2023;11(9):23259671 231199418.
204. Di Piazza E, Harman T, Rosenberg JE, Guo Y, Hussain LR, Fowler EF, et al. Bioprinting technology in skin, heart, pancreas and cartilage tissues: Progress and challenges in clinical practice. *Int. J. Environ. Res. Public Health.* 2021;18(20):10806.
205. Guo X, Wang Y, Qin L, Shen B, Cheng L, Duan C, et al. Progress and prospect of technical and regulatory challenges on tissue-engineered cartilage as therapeutic combination product. *Bioact. Mater.* 2023;20:501–18.
206. Mok S-W, Nizak R, Fu SC, Ho KWK, Qin L, Saris DBF, et al. From the printer: Potential of three-dimensional printing for orthopaedic applications. *J. Orthop. Transl.* 2016;6:42–49.
207. Ren X, Wang F, Chen C, Gong X, Yin L, Yang L. Engineering zonal cartilage through bioprinting collagen type II hydrogel constructs with biomimetic chondrocyte density gradient. *BMC Musculoskelet. Disord.* 2016;17:301.
208. Murphy SV, De Coppi P, Atala A. Opportunities and challenges of translational 3D bioprinting. *Nat. Biomed. Eng.* 2020 Apr;4(4):370–80.
209. Dong X, Premaratne ID, Bernstein JL, Samadi A, Lin AJ, Toyoda Y, et al. Three-dimensional-printed external scaffolds mitigate loss of volume and topography in engineered elastic cartilage constructs. *Cartilage.* 2021;13(2 Suppl):1780S–1789S.
210. Xie X, Wu S, Mou S, Guo N, Wang Z, Sun J. Microtissue-based bioink as a chondrocyte microshelter for DLP bioprinting. *Adv. Healthc. Mater.* 2022;11(22):2201877.
211. Liu Y, Peng L, Li L, Huang C, Shi K, Meng X, et al. 3D-bioprinted BMSC-laden biomimetic multiphasic scaffolds for efficient repair of osteochondral defects in an osteoarthritic rat model. *Biomaterials.* 2021;279:121216.

212. Jones EA, English A, Henshaw K, Kinsey SE, Markham AF, Emery P, et al. Enumeration and phenotypic characterization of synovial fluid multipotential mesenchymal progenitor cells in inflammatory and degenerative arthritis. *Arthritis Rheum.* 2004;50(3):817–27.
213. Golzar H, Wu Y, Ganguly S, Tang X. Micro-extrusion 3D printing of articular cartilage substitutes with a multizonal structure using hydrophilic and rapidly curing silicone-based ink materials. *Addit. Manuf.* 2023;73: 103691.
214. Costantini M, Idaszek J, Szöke K, Jaroszewicz J, Dentini M, Barbetta A, et al. 3D bioprinting of BM-MSCs-loaded ECM biomimetic hydrogels for in vitro neocartilage formation. *Biofabrication* 2016;8(3):035002.
215. Olmos-Juste R, Larrañaga-Jaurrieta G, Larraza I, Ramos-Diez S, Camarero-Espinosa S, Gabilondo N, et al. Alginate-waterborne polyurethane 3D bioprinted scaffolds for articular cartilage tissue engineering. *Int. J. Biol. Macromol.* 2023;253:127070.
216. Pati F, Jang J, Ha DH, Won Kim S, Rhie JW, Shim JH, et al. Printing three-dimensional tissue analogues with decellularized extracellular matrix bioink. *Nat. Commun.* 2014;5(1):3935.
217. Chen Y-W, Lin Y-H, Lin T-L, Alvin Lee K-X, Yu M-H, Shie M-Y. 3D-biofabricated chondrocyte-laden decellularized extracellular matrix-contained gelatin methacrylate auxetic scaffolds under cyclic tensile stimulation for cartilage regeneration. *Biofabrication.* 2023;15(4):045007.
218. Rathan S, Dejob L, Schipani R, Haffner B, Möbius ME, Kelly DJ. Fiber reinforced cartilage ECM functionalized bioinks for functional cartilage tissue engineering. *Adv. Healthc. Mater.* 2019;8(7):1801501.
219. Yang Z, Zhao T, Guo C, Cao F, Li H, Liao Z, et al. 3D-bioprinted difunctional scaffold for in situ cartilage regeneration based on aptamer-directed cell recruitment and growth factor-enhanced cell chondrogenesis. *ACS Appl. Mater. Interfaces.* 2021;13(20):23369–83.
220. Chen W, Xu Y, Li Y, Jia L, Mo X, Jiang G, et al. 3D printing electrospinning fiber-reinforced decellularized extracellular matrix for cartilage regeneration. *Chem. Eng. J.* 2020;382:122986.
221. Apelgren P, Amoroso M, Lindahl A, Brantsing C, Rotter N, Gatenholm P, et al. Chondrocytes and stem cells in 3D-bioprinted structures create human cartilage in vivo. *PLoS One* 2017;12(12):e0189428.
222. Park JH, Ahn M, Park SH, Kim H, Bae M, Park W, et al. 3D bioprinting of a trachea-mimetic cellular construct of a clinically relevant size. *Biomaterials.* 2021;279:121246.

223. Wang S, Luo B, Bai B, Wang Q, Chen H, Tan X, et al. 3D printed chondrogenic functionalized PGS bioactive scaffold for cartilage regeneration. *Adv. Healthc. Mater.* 2023;12(27):e2301006.
224. Landa-Solís C, Ibarra C, Salinas-Rojas A, Ortega-Sánchez C, Luna-Angulo AB, del Rocío Aguilar-Gaytán M, et al. An osteocartilaginous 3D printing implant using a biocompatible polymer and pre-differentiated mesenchymal stem cells in sheep. *Appl. Sci.* 2023;13(18):10177.
225. Yan K, Zhang X, Liu Y, Cheng J, Zhai C, Shen K, et al. 3D-bioprinted silk fibroin-hydroxypropyl cellulose methacrylate porous scaffold with optimized performance for repairing articular cartilage defects. *Mater. Des.* 2023;225:111531.
226. Zhang X, Liu Y, Luo C, Zhai C, Li Z, Zhang Y, et al. Crosslinker-free silk/decellularized extracellular matrix porous bioink for 3D bioprinting-based cartilage tissue engineering. *Mater. Sci. Eng. C.* 2021;118:111388.
227. Yelin E, Weinstein S, King T. The burden of musculoskeletal diseases in the United States. *Semin. Arthritis Rheum.* 2016;46:259–60.
228. Alarcin E, Bal-Öztürk A, Avci H, Ghorbanpoor H, Guzel FD, Akpek A, et al. Current strategies for the regeneration of skeletal muscle tissue. *Int. J. Mol. Sci.* 2021;22(11):5929.
229. Espino-Gonzalez E, Dalbram E, Mounier R, Gondin J, Farup J, Jessen N, et al. Impaired skeletal muscle regeneration in diabetes: From cellular and molecular mechanisms to novel treatments. *Cell Metab.* 2024;36:1204–1236.
230. Suzuki K, Matsumoto M, Katoh Y, Liu L, Ochiai K, Aizawa Y, et al. Bach1 promotes muscle regeneration through repressing Smad-mediated inhibition of myoblast differentiation. *PLoS One.* 2020;15(8):e0236781.
231. Wan R, Liu S, Feng C, Luo W, Zhang H, Wu Y, et al. The revolution of exosomes: From biological functions to therapeutic applications in skeletal muscle diseases. *J. Orthop. Transl.* 2024;45:132–39.
232. Ronzoni FL, Giarratana N, Crippa S, Quattrocelli M, Cassano M, Ceccarelli G, et al. Guide cells support muscle regeneration and affect neuro-muscular junction organization. *Int. J. Mol. Sci.* 2021;22(4):1939.
233. Feige P, Brun CE, Ritso M, Rudnicki MA. Orienting muscle stem cells for regeneration in homeostasis, aging, and disease. *Cell Stem Cell.* 2018;23(5):653–64.
234. Pagano C, Latterini L, Di Michele A, Luzi F, Puglia D, Ricci M, et al. Polymeric bioadhesive patch based on ketoprofen-hydrotalcite hybrid for local treatments. *Pharmaceutics.* 2020;12(8):733.

235. Ma H, Xing F, Yu P, Xu J, Wu X, Luo R, et al. Integrated design and fabrication strategies based on bioprinting for skeletal muscle regeneration: Current status and future perspectives. *Mater. Des.* 2023;225:111591.
236. Jammalamadaka U, Tappa K. Recent advances in biomaterials for 3D printing and tissue engineering. *J. Funct. Biomater.* 2018;9(1):22.
237. Luo W, Zhang H, Wan R, Cai Y, Liu Y, Wu Y, et al. Biomaterials-based technologies in skeletal muscle tissue engineering. *Adv. Healthc. Mater.* 2024;13:2304196.
238. Oppen D, Grossmann L, Weiss J. Insights into characterizing and producing anisotropic food structures. *Crit. Rev. Food Sci. Nutr.* 2024;64(4):1158–76.
239. Kakarla AB, Kong I, Turek I, Kong C, Irving H. Printable gelatin, alginate and boron nitride nanotubes hydrogel-based ink for 3D bioprinting and tissue engineering applications. *Mater. Des.* 2022;213:110362.
240. Zhang Y, Kumar P, Lv S, Xiong D, Zhao H, Cai Z, et al. Recent advances in 3D bioprinting of vascularized tissues. *Mater. Des.* 2021;199:109398.
241. Kim K, Jin S, Shin M. Effect of 3D-printable anisotropic fibrous hydrogels on fabricating artificial skeletal muscle constructs. *Adv. Ther.* 2024;7(1):2300170.
242. Spedicati M, Zoso A, Mortati L, Chiono V, Marcello E, Carmagnola I. Three-dimensional microfibrous scaffold with aligned topography produced via a combination of melt-extrusion additive manufacturing and porogen leaching for in vitro skeletal muscle modeling. *Bioengineering* 2024;11(4):332.
243. Wu J, Yun Z, Song W, Yu T, Xue W, Liu Q, et al. Highly oriented hydrogels for tissue regeneration: Design strategies, cellular mechanisms, and biomedical applications. *Theranostics* 2024;14(5):1982–2035.
244. Vogt C, Tahtinen M, Zhao F. Engineering approaches for creating skeletal muscle. In: Shi D, Liu Q (eds). *Tissue Engineering and Nanotheranostics.* World Scientific, 2018:1–27.
245. Popov A, Malferrari S, Kalaskar D. 3D bioprinting for musculoskeletal applications. *J. 3D Print. Med.* 2017;1(3):191–211.
246. Samandari M, Quint J, Rodríguez-delaRosa A, Sinha I, Pourquie O, Tamayol A. Bioinks and bioprinting strategies for skeletal muscle tissue engineering. *Adv. Mater.* 2022;34(12):e2105883.
247. Park W, Gao G, Cho D-W. Tissue-specific decellularized extracellular matrix bioinks for musculoskeletal tissue regeneration and modeling using 3D bioprinting technology. *Int. J. Mol. Sci.* 2021;22(15):7837.

248. Gokyer S, Yilgor E, Yilgor I, Berber E, Vrana E, Orhan K, et al. 3D printed biodegradable polyurethaneurea elastomer recapitulates skeletal muscle structure and function. *ACS Biomater. Sci. Eng.* 2021;7(11):5189–205.
249. Hwangbo H, Lee H, Jin E-J, Lee JY, Jo Y, Ryu D, et al. Bio-printing of aligned GelMA-based cell-laden structure for muscle tissue regeneration. *Bioact. Mater.* 2022;8:57–70.
250. Yeo M, Kim G. Electrohydrodynamic-direct-printed cell-laden microfibrous structure using alginate-based bioink for effective myotube formation. *Carbohydr. Polym.* 2021;272:118444.
251. Kim JH, Kim I, Seol Y-J, Ko IK, Yoo JJ, Atala A, et al. Neural cell integration into 3D bioprinted skeletal muscle constructs accelerates restoration of muscle function. *Nat. Commun.* 2020;11(1):1025.
252. Kim JH, Ko IK, Jeon MJ, Kim I, Vanschaayk MM, Atala A, et al. Pelvic floor muscle function recovery using biofabricated tissue constructs with neuromuscular junctions. *Acta Biomater.* 2021;121:237–49.
253. Sun J, Xing F, Zou M, Gong M, Li L, Xiang Z. Comparison of chondrogenesis-related biological behaviors between human urine-derived stem cells and human bone marrow mesenchymal stem cells from the same individual. *Stem Cell Res. Ther.* 2021;12:366.
254. Seyedmahmoud R, Çelebi-Saltik B, Barros N, Nasiri R, Banton E, Shamloo A, et al. Three-dimensional bioprinting of functional skeletal muscle tissue using gelatin methacryloyl-alginate bioinks. *Micromachines* 2019;10(10): 679.
255. Li T, Hou J, Wang L, Zeng G, Wang Z, Yu L, et al. Bioprinted anisotropic scaffolds with fast stress relaxation bioink for engineering 3D skeletal muscle and repairing volumetric muscle loss. *Acta Biomater.* 2023;156:21–36.
256. Compaan AM, Song K, Huang Y. Gellan fluid gel as a versatile support bath material for fluid extrusion bioprinting. *ACS Appl. Mater. Interfaces.* 2019;11(6):5714–26.
257. Fan D, Diller S, Mansi S, Wang C, Mela P, Özkale B. A multi-functional 3D-printable gel-in-gel system for the delivery of probiotics to the intestine. *Food Hydrocoll.* 2024;156:110267.
258. Wei X, Huang B, Chen K, Fan Z, Wang L, Xu M. Dot extrusion bioprinting of spatially controlled heterogenous tumor models. *Mater. Des.* 2022;223: 111152.
259. Urciuolo A, Poli I, Brandolino L, Raffa P, Scattolini V, Laterza C, et al. Intravital three-dimensional bioprinting. *Nat. Biomed. Eng.* 2020;4(9): 901–15.

260. Fan T, Wang S, Jiang Z, Ji S, Cao W, Liu W, et al. Controllable assembly of skeletal muscle-like bundles through 3D bioprinting. *Biofabrication* 2021;14(1):015009.
261. Lee H, Kim WJ, Lee JU, Park KS, Yoo JJ, Atala A, et al. Self-aligned myofibers in 3D bioprinted extracellular matrix-based construct accelerate skeletal muscle function restoration. *Appl. Phys. Rev.* 2021;8(2):021405.
262. Miao S, Nowicki M, Cui H, Lee S-J, Zhou X, Mills DK, et al. 4D anisotropic skeletal muscle tissue constructs fabricated by staircase effect strategy. *Biofabrication* 2019;11(3):035030.
263. Zhang C, Wang G, Lin H, Shang Y, Liu N, Zhen Y, et al. Cartilage 3D bioprinting for rhinoplasty using adipose-derived stem cells as seed cells: Review and recent advances. *Cell Prolif.* 2023;56(4):e13417.
264. Krieger J, Park B-W, Lambert CR, Malcuit C. 3D skeletal muscle fascicle engineering is improved with TGF-β1 treatment of myogenic cells and their co-culture with myofibroblasts. *PeerJ.* 2018;6:e4939.
265. Bechshøft CJL, Schjerling P, Kjaer M, Mackey AL. The influence of direct and indirect fibroblast cell contact on human myogenic cell behavior and gene expression in vitro. *J. Appl. Physiol.* 2019;127(2):342–55.
266. Ronzoni FL, Aliberti F, Scocozza F, Benedetti L, Auricchio F, Sampaolesi M, et al. Myoblast 3D bioprinting to burst in vitro skeletal muscle differentiation. *J. Tissue Eng. Regen. Med.* 2022;16(5):484–95.
267. Lian Q, et al. Direct-writing process and in vivo evaluation of prevascularized composite constructs for muscle tissue engineering application. *J. Bionic Eng.* 2020;17:457–68.
268. Sabetkish S, Currie P, Meagher L. Recent trends in 3D bioprinting technology for skeletal muscle regeneration. *Acta Biomater.* 2024;181:46–66.
269. Tsai H-F, IJspeert C, Shen AQ. Voltage-gated ion channels mediate the electrotaxis of glioblastoma cells in a hybrid PMMA/PDMS microdevice. *APL Bioeng.* 2020;4(3):036102.
270. Rems L, Kasimova MA, Testa I, Delemotte L. Pulsed electric fields can create pores in the voltage sensors of voltage-gated ion channels. *Biophys. J.* 2020;119(1):190–205.
271. Kim W, Lee H, Lee CK, Kyung JW, An SB, Han I-B, et al. A bioprinting process supplemented with in situ electrical stimulation directly induces significant myotube formation and myogenesis. *Adv. Funct. Mater.* 2021;31(51):2105170.
272. Distler T, Solisito AA, Schneidereit D, Friedrich O, Detsch R, Boccaccini AR. 3D printed oxidized alginate-gelatin bioink provides guidance for

C2C12 muscle precursor cell orientation and differentiation via shear stress during bioprinting. *Biofabrication* 2020;12(4):045005.

273. Cedillo-Servin G, Dahri O, Meneses J, van Duijn J, Moon H, Sage F, et al. 3D printed magneto-active microfiber scaffolds for remote stimulation and guided organization of 3D in vitro skeletal muscle models. *Small.* 2024; 20(12):e2307178.
274. Kim WJ, Lee H, Lee JU, Atala A, Yoo JJ, Lee SJ, et al. Efficient myotube formation in 3D bioprinted tissue construct by biochemical and topographical cues. *Biomaterials.* 2020;230:119632.
275. Chae S, Choi Y-J, Cho D-W. Mechanically and biologically promoted cell-laden constructs generated using tissue-specific bioinks for tendon/ligament tissue engineering applications. *Biofabrication.* 2022;14(2):025013.
276. Leong NL, Kator JL, Clemens TL, James A, Enamoto-Iwamoto M, Jiang J. Tendon and ligament healing and current approaches to tendon and ligament regeneration. *J. Orthop. Res.* 2020;38(1):7–12.
277. Martin RB, Burr DB, Sharkey NA, Fyhrie DP. Mechanical properties of ligament and tendon. In: *Skeletal Tissue Mechanics.* 2015:175–225.
278. Heidari BS, Ruan R, Vahabli E, Chen P, De-Juan-Pardo EM, Zheng M, et al. Natural, synthetic and commercially-available biopolymers used to regenerate tendons and ligaments. *Bioact. Mater.* 2023;19:179–97.
279. Chae S, Cho D-W. Biomaterial-based 3D bioprinting strategy for orthopedic tissue engineering. *Acta Biomater.* 2023;156:4–20.
280. Xue Y, Kim H-J, Lee J, Liu Y, Hoffman T, Chen Y, et al. Co-electrospun silk fibroin and gelatin methacryloyl sheet seeded with mesenchymal stem cells for tendon regeneration. *Small.* 2022;18(21):e2107714.
281. Zsidai B, Horvath A, Winkler PW, Narup E, Kaarre J, Svantesson E, et al. Different injury patterns exist among patients undergoing operative treatment of isolated PCL, combined PCL/ACL, and isolated ACL injuries: A study from the Swedish national knee ligament registry. *Knee Surg. Sports Traumatol. Arthrosc.* 2022;30(10):3451–60.
282. Toprakhisar B, Nadernezhad A, Bakirci E, Khani N, Skvortsov GA, Koc B. Development of bioink from decellularized tendon extracellular matrix for 3D bioprinting. *Macromol. Biosci.* 2018;18(10):e1800024.
283. Zhang Y, Lei T, Tang C, Chen Y, Liao Y, Ju W, et al. 3D printing of chemical-empowered tendon stem/progenitor cells for functional tissue repair. *Biomaterials.* 2021;271:120722.
284. Diaz F, Zimmermann L, Dale TP, Forsyth NR, Boccaccini AR. Tuning the properties of all natural polymeric scaffolds for tendon repair with cellulose microfibers. *Carbohydr. Polym. Technol. Appl.* 2024;7:100447.

285. Uehlin AF, Vines JB, Feldman DS, Dean D, Thomas V. Inkjet printing of nanohydroxyapatite gradients on fibrous scaffold for bone–ligament enthesis. *JOM.* 2022;74(9):3336–48.
286. Jiang X, Wu S, Kuss M, Kong Y, Shi W, Streubel PN, et al. 3D printing of multilayered scaffolds for rotator cuff tendon regeneration. *Bioact. Mater.* 2020;5(3):636–43.
287. Chae S, Yong U, Park W, Choi Y-m, Jeon I-H, Kang H, et al. 3D cell-printing of gradient multi-tissue interfaces for rotator cuff regeneration. *Bioact. Mater.* 2023;19:611–25.
288. Laternser S, Keller H, Leupin O, Rausch M, Graf-Hausner U, Rimann M. A novel microplate 3D bioprinting platform for the engineering of muscle and tendon tissues. *SLAS Technol.* 2018;23(6):599–613.
289. Merceron TK, Burt M, Seol YJ, Kang HW, Lee SJ, Yoo JJ, et al. A 3D bioprinted complex structure for engineering the muscle–tendon unit. *Biofabrication* 2015;7(3):035003.
290. Raveendran NT, Vaquette C, Meinert C, Ipe DS, Ivanovski S. Optimization of 3D bioprinting of periodontal ligament cells. *Dent. Mater.* 2019;35(12):1683–94.
291. Silva M, Pinho I, Gonçalves H, Vale AC, Paiva MC, Alves NM, et al. Engineering ligament scaffolds based on PLA/graphite nanoplatelet composites by 3D printing or braiding. *J. Compos. Sci.* 2023;7(3):104.
292. Gomez-Cerezo MN, Perevoshchikova N, Ruan R, Moerman KM, Bindra R, Lloyd DG, et al. Additively manufactured polyethylene terephthalate scaffolds for scapholunate interosseous ligament reconstruction. *Biomater. Adv.* 2023;149:213397.
293. Tarafder S, Lee CH. 3D printing integrated with controlled delivery for musculoskeletal tissue engineering. *J. 3D Print. Med.* 2017;1(3):181–89.
294. Poerio A, Mano JF, Cleymand F. Advanced 3D printing strategies for the controlled delivery of growth factors. *ACS Biomater. Sci. Eng.* 2023;9(12):6531–47.
295. Zhang Y, Wang C. Recent advances in 3D printing hydrogel for topical drug delivery. *MedComm — Biomater. Appl.* 2022;1(1).
296. Shim J-H, Kim SE, Park JY, Kundu J, Kim SW, Kang SS, et al. Three-dimensional printing of rhBMP-2-loaded scaffolds with long-term delivery for enhanced bone regeneration in a rabbit diaphyseal defect. *Tissue Eng. Part A.* 2014;20(13–14):1980–92.
297. Lee SJ, Lee D, Yoon TR, Kim HK, Jo HH, Park JS, et al. Surface modification of 3D-printed porous scaffolds via mussel-inspired polydopamine and

effective immobilization of rhBMP-2 to promote osteogenic differentiation for bone tissue engineering. *Acta Biomater.* 2016;40:182–91.

298. Sun Y, You Y, Jiang W, Wang B, Wu Q, Dai K. 3D bioprinting dual-factor releasing and gradient-structured constructs ready to implant for anisotropic cartilage regeneration. *Sci. Adv.* 2020;6(37):eaay1422.
299. Wu G, Sun B, Zhao C, Wang Z, Teng S, Yang M, et al. Three-dimensional tendon scaffold loaded with TGF-β1 gene silencing plasmid prevents tendon adhesion and promotes tendon repair. *ACS Biomater. Sci. Eng.* 2021; 7(12):5739–48.
300. Tomasina C, Bodet T, Mota C, Moroni L, Camarero-Espinosa S. Bioprinting vasculature: Materials, cells and emergent techniques. *Materials.* 2019; 12(17):2701.
301. Datta P, Ayan B, Ozbolat IT. Bioprinting for vascular and vascularized tissue biofabrication. *Acta Biomater.* 2017;51:1–20.
302. Ostrovidov S, Salehi S, Costantini M, Suthiwanich K, Ebrahimi M, Sadeghian RB, et al. 3D bioprinting in skeletal muscle tissue engineering. *Small.* 2019;15(24):1805530.
303. Gholobova D, Terrie L, Gerard M, Declercq H, Thorrez L. Vascularization of tissue-engineered skeletal muscle constructs. *Biomaterials.* 2020;235: 119708.
304. Cheng B, Fu X. The role of stem cell on wound healing after revascularization: Healing following revascularization: Unlocking skin potential. *Int. J. Low. Extrem. Wounds.* 2024;23(1):63–69.
305. Levenberg S, Rouwkema J, Macdonald M, Garfein ES, Kohane DS, Darland DC, et al. Engineering vascularized skeletal muscle tissue. *Nat. Biotechnol.* 2005;23(7):879–84.
306. Cai Q, Liao W, Xue F, Wang X, Zhou W, Li Y, et al. Selection of different endothelialization modes and different seed cells for tissue-engineered vascular graft. *Bioact. Mater.* 2021;6(8):2557–68.
307. Mir A, Lee E, Shih W, Koljaka S, Wang A, Jorgensen C, et al. 3D bioprinting for vascularization. *Bioengineering.* 2023;10(5):606.
308. Pitacco P, Sadowska JM, O'Brien FJ, Kelly DJ. 3D bioprinting of cartilaginous templates for large bone defect healing. *Acta Biomater.* 2023; 156:61–74.
309. Nulty J, Freeman FE, Browe DC, Burdis R, Ahern DP, Pitacco P, et al. 3D bioprinting of prevascularised implants for the repair of critically-sized bone defects. *Acta Biomater.* 2021;126:154–69.

310. Li B, Shu Y, Ma H, Cao K, Cheng YY, Jia Z, et al. Three-dimensional printing and decellularized-extracellular-matrix based methods for advances in artificial blood vessel fabrication: A review. *Tissue Cell.* 2024;87:102304.
311. Gao G, Lee JH, Jang J, Lee DH, Kong J-S, Kim BS, et al. Tissue engineered bio-blood-vessels constructed using a tissue-specific bioink and 3D coaxial cell printing technique: A novel therapy for ischemic disease. *Adv. Funct. Mater.* 2017;27(33):1700798.
312. Choi Y-J, Jun YJ, Kim DY, Yi HG, Chae SH, Kang J, et al. A 3D cell printed muscle construct with tissue-derived bioink for the treatment of volumetric muscle loss. *Biomaterials* 2019;206:160–69.
313. Borselli C, Storrie H, Benesch-Lee F, Shvartsman D, Cezar C, Lichtman JW, et al. Functional muscle regeneration with combined delivery of angiogenesis and myogenesis factors. *Proc. Natl. Acad. Sci. U. S. A.* 2010;107(8): 3287–92.
314. Park JY, Shim J-H, Choi S-A, Jang J, Kim M, Lee SH, et al. 3D printing technology to control BMP-2 and VEGF delivery spatially and temporally to promote large-volume bone regeneration. *J. Mater. Chem. B* 2015;3(27): 5415–25.
315. Thangadurai M, Ajith A, Budharaju H, Sethuraman S, Sundaramurthi D. Advances in electrospinning and 3D bioprinting strategies to enhance functional regeneration of skeletal muscle tissue. *Biomater. Adv.* 2022;142:213135.
316. Yang DL, Faraz F, Wang J-X, Radacsi N. Combination of 3D printing and electrospinning techniques for biofabrication. *Adv. Mater. Technol.* 2022; 7(7):2101309.
317. Rajzer I, Kurowska A, Jabłoński A, Jatteau S, Śliwka M, Ziąbka M, et al. Layered gelatin/PLLA scaffolds fabricated by electrospinning and 3D printing-for nasal cartilages and subchondral bone reconstruction. *Mater. Des.* 2018;155:297–306.
318. Ghosh A, Orasugh JT, Ray SS, Chattopadhyay D. Integration of 3D printing--coelectrospinning: Concept shifting in biomedical applications. *ACS Omega.* 2023;8(31):28002–25.
319. Saniei H, Mousavi S. Surface modification of PLA 3D-printed implants by electrospinning with enhanced bioactivity and cell affinity. *Polymer.* 2020; 196:122467.
320. Farsi M, Asefnejad A, Baharifar H. A hyaluronic acid/PVA electrospun coating on 3D printed PLA scaffold for orthopedic application. *Prog. Biomater.* 2022;11(1):67–77.

321. Gonzalez-Pujana A, Carranza T, Santos-Vizcaino E, Igartua M, Guerrero P, Hernandez RM, et al. Hybrid 3D printed and electrospun multi-scale hierarchical polycaprolactone scaffolds to induce bone differentiation. *Pharmaceutics* 2022;14(12):2843.
322. Liu J, Zou Q, Wang C, Lin M, Li Y, Zhang R, et al. Electrospinning and 3D printed hybrid bi-layer scaffold for guided bone regeneration. *Mater. Des.* 2021;210:110047.
323. Smith JA, Mele E. Electrospinning and additive manufacturing: Adding three-dimensionality to electrospun scaffolds for tissue engineering. *Front. Bioeng. Biotechnol.* 2021;9:674738.
324. Yeo M, Kim G. Micro/nano-hierarchical scaffold fabricated using a cell electrospinning/3D printing process for co-culturing myoblasts and HUVECs to induce myoblast alignment and differentiation. *Acta Biomater.* 2020;107:102–14.
325. Kim GH, Son JG, Park S, Kim WD. Hybrid process for fabricating 3D hierarchical scaffolds combining rapid prototyping and electrospinning. *Macromol. Rapid Commun.* 2008;29(19):1577–81.

© 2026 World Scientific Publishing Company
https://doi.org/10.1142/9789819819645_0008

Chapter 8

Nanotechnology and Bone Regeneration

Pedram Sotoudehbagha[1], Samira Farjaminejad[2], Haaris Ali Syed[3], Sun Latt[1,4], Thomas Hartmann[5], Tara Menon Pattilachan[4], Nadia Aboutalebianarki[1,6], Melanie Coathup[1], Mehdi Razavi[1,6,7,*]

[1]*Biionix (Bionic Materials, Implants & Interfaces) Cluster, Department of Medicine, University of Central Florida College of Medicine, Orlando, FL 32827, USA*
[2]*School of Health and Medical Sciences, City St George's, University of London, London EC1V 0HB, UK*
[3]*College of Osteopathic Medicine, Kansas City University, Kansas City, Missouri, USA*
[4]*Burnett School of Biomedical Sciences, University of Central Florida College of Medicine, Orlando, FL 32827, USA*
[5]*University of Central Florida College of Medicine, Orlando, FL 32827, USA*
[6]*Department of Materials Science and Engineering, University of Central Florida, Orlando, FL 32816, USA*
[7]*Biomedical Engineering Program, Department of Mechanical and Aerospace Engineering, University of Central Florida, Orlando, FL 32816, USA*

***Corresponding author:** Mehdi Razavi, 6900 Lake Nona Blvd Orlando, FL 32827. Email: Mehdi.Razavi@ucf.edu

Chapter Outline

Abstract

Nanotechnology has emerged as a powerful tool in bone tissue engineering, offering innovative strategies to overcome the limitations of conventional regenerative approaches. By leveraging nanoscale design, materials can be engineered to better replicate the architecture and function of native bone while also enabling controlled interactions with cells, biomolecules, and the extracellular matrix. This chapter provides a comprehensive overview of how nanostructured materials are being applied to enhance bone regeneration. Five major categories are explored: nanoparticles, advanced nanostructures, nanostructured implants, nanocomposite scaffolds, and nanostructures for drug delivery. For each category, we examine the underlying principles, state-of-the-art applications, synthesis techniques, and characterization methods. Together, these advances highlight how nanoscale control over structure and properties can improve mechanical performance, biocompatibility, and osteoinductivity, ultimately paving the way for next-generation therapies for critical bone defects.

1. Introduction

Bone, also called osseous tissue, consists of cellular components encapsulated within a vast, mineralized extracellular matrix (ECM). In the ECM, 40% comprises organic compounds, and 60% comprises inorganic compounds, of which hydroxyapatite (HA) is the primary mineral in the inorganic component [1, 2]. These scaffolds are essential for bone regeneration due to their ability to maintain sustained release of osteoinductive factors and to provide a nidus point where new bone-forming cells can proliferate and grow. Despite bone's innate ability to self-heal, there are many instances where this process is too slow, such as in cases of advanced age, obesity, anemia, diabetes, malnutrition, smoking, and a variety of other conditions [3]. Moreover, some bone injuries may result in nonunion fractures because of excessively large defects or infection [4]. Therefore, much research has gone into finding therapies to solve these acute and difficult-to-treat cases. Nanostructured materials offer superior bone regeneration compared to their microscale and macroscale counterparts. This nanoscale advantage results from the ability to have more precise control when working at submicron resolutions, allowing for a greater mimicry of natural bone [5]. For instance, nanoscale surface roughness induced greater osteoblastic cell adhesion and alkaline phosphatase activity compared to microscale surface roughness [5]. More broadly, nanostructured scaffolds can enhance mechanical properties, biocompatibility, and osteoinductivity. Through incorporating nanoparticles (NPs) into metals, for example, grain refinement can occur, leading to improvements in grain boundaries and subsequent mechanical properties [6]. A material's biocompatibility depends on a variety of tunable features, such as size, shape, composition, surface charge, and surface functionalization [7]. Nanostructured materials hold an advantage over microstructured materials because their properties can be tuned more precisely, allowing for greater control over biocompatibility [8]. Moreover, precise modification of nanomaterial surfaces can lead to interactions with growth factors and the ECM to induce an osteoinductive microenvironment [9]. In this chapter, five categories of nanostructured materials with potential applications in bone regeneration are reviewed: NPs, advanced nanostructures, nanostructured implants, nanocomposite scaffolds, and nanostructures for drug delivery. For each category, we provide background information along with common applications, synthesis strategies, and characterization methods.

2. Nanoparticles

2.1. *Introduction*

NPs can be produced from materials such as ceramics, metals, and natural or synthetic polymers, each offering specific advantages including strong penetration ability and a large, adaptable surface area [10]. These properties make NPs valuable in tissue engineering and regenerative medicine, where they have been used to enhance imaging technologies, strengthen materials, improve bioinks, and deliver antimicrobial or bioactive agents. This flexibility emphasizes their important role in advancing tissue engineering and regenerative medicine technologies [11]. NPs are also applied in advanced drug delivery systems that enable the controlled release of bioactive molecules, such as growth factors or anticancer drugs, to improve treatment results. In addition, they are being studied for use in gene therapy applications [12]. This section focuses on how NPs have been utilized

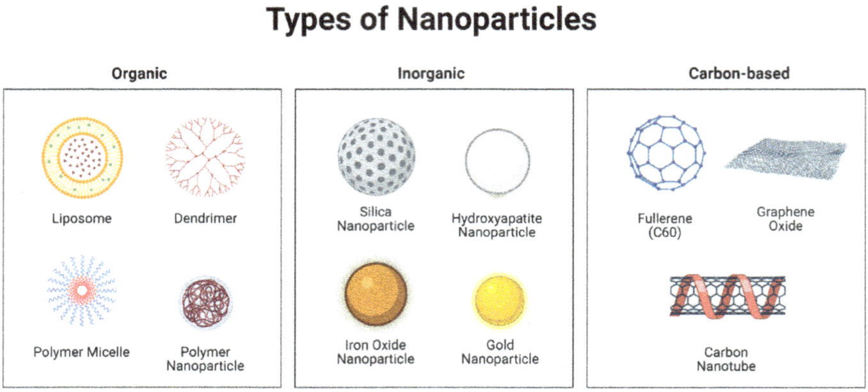

Figure 1. Types of nanoparticles with examples categorized by origin: inorganic, organic, and carbon-based (created with BioRender.com).

to modulate the function and activity of bone cells and their role in bone tissue regeneration. **Figure 1** presents various NP types, with representative examples from inorganic, organic, and carbon-based classes.

2.2. *Types of Nanoparticles*

2.2.1. *Inorganic nanoparticles*

Inorganic NPs are a class of nanomaterials that do not contain carbon in their structure [13]. They are generally more chemically stable than organic NPs and are often hydrophilic, biocompatible, and less toxic to biological systems. Due to these properties, they have been widely investigated for medical and tissue engineering applications [14]. Common categories of inorganic NPs include ceramic NPs (e.g., silica, HA, and zirconia) and metal NPs (e.g., gold, silver, and copper). Each group exhibits unique physicochemical and biological properties, making them suitable for diverse applications in bone regeneration and beyond [15].

2.2.1.1. Ceramic Nanoparticles

Ceramic NPs are widely studied in bone tissue engineering due to their similarity to the mineral phase of natural bone. They are biocompatible, bioactive, and mechanically strong, providing essential support for bone repair and regeneration. At the nanoscale, their high surface area enhances protein adsorption and cell attachment, stimulating osteoblast activity and improving implant integration [15]. Nano-hydroxyapatite (nano-HA) is the most common, mimicking bone structure to improve osteoconductivity, osteoinductivity, and protein adsorption, thereby promoting new bone formation [16]. Titanium oxide nanotubes also enhance the bioactivity of implant surfaces by supporting osteoblast proliferation and serving as carrier vehicles for controlled release of drugs and growth factors [17]. Nanosilica, particularly mesoporous silica NPs, shows high biocompatibility and a porous structure that supports cell attachment and bone formation. Its ability to act as a carrier for bioactive molecules makes it especially useful in tissue engineering [18]. Nanoclays, including montmorillonite, halloysite, and synthetic laponite, reinforce scaffolds, release bioactive ions, and support osteogenic differentiation. Their ability to strengthen materials and enable the controlled release of therapeutic molecules makes them promising candidates for bone regeneration [15, 19].

2.2.1.2. Metal Nanoparticles

Metal NPs can be synthesized through both top-down and bottom-up methods using metals, such as gold, silver, iron, copper, zirconium, aluminum, and nickel. At the nanoscale, they display unique optical, electrical, catalytic, and antibacterial properties, arising from their large surface-to-volume ratio and quantum effects, which are not observed in bulk metals [13, 15]. Their size and shape strongly influence conductivity, magnetic behavior, and interactions with biological systems, making them useful in catalysis, sensing, imaging, and biomedical applications [20]. Gold NPs and copper NPs (CuNPs) promote the osteogenic differentiation of stem cells, a process essential for new bone tissue formation, and they also enhance cell proliferation to accelerate bone repair [21]. Gold NPs are particularly valuable due to their low toxicity, antibacterial activity, and high biocompatibility, supporting bone regeneration through signaling pathways, such as Wnt/β-catenin, extracellular signal–regulated kinase pathway/mitogen-activated protein kinase (MAPK), and p38/MAPK [21]. CuNPs play a dual role by promoting osteogenesis and angiogenesis while also offering antibacterial effects. Notably, surface modification techniques have been shown to improve their stability and reduce toxicity [21]. As mentioned, CuNPs support angiogenesis, ensuring nutrient and oxygen supply for regenerating tissues [22]. Zirconium NPs enhance osteoblast activity through bone morphogenetic protein (BMP)/SMAD signaling and contribute to scaffold strength and biocompatibility [23]. Aluminum (Al) NPs, especially in oxidized forms such as Al_2O_3, reinforce scaffolds, improve cell adhesion and proliferation, and support long-term implant integration [15]. Moreover, these NPs improve the mechanical properties of the scaffold, providing strength and stability to withstand physiological loads during regeneration [24]. Silver NPs are widely applied in scaffolds and coatings for their potent antimicrobial activity, though their effectiveness requires careful control to avoid cytotoxicity [25]. Iron NPs (FeNPs) improve scaffold strength and porosity and, when combined with magnetic fields, enhance stem cell proliferation and osteogenesis, where alloying strategies further optimize degradation and reduce toxicity [26]. Nickel (Ni) NPs and Ni-doped HA promote osteoblastic differentiation *via* Ca^{2+}-dependent Wnt5 signaling, while Ni-based scaffolds provide resilience, angiogenic potential, and favorable conditions for vascularization and nutrient supply [27]. Some metal NPs also serve as drug carriers, enabling controlled delivery of growth factors or antibiotics directly to the regeneration site, which enhances treatment outcomes [15].

A notable subgroup of metal NPs are magnetic NPs (MNPs), particularly the iron oxides such as Fe_3O_4 and γ-Fe_2O_3; these exhibit superparamagnetism, responding to external magnetic fields without retaining permanent magnetization. Their stability, biocompatibility, and controlled magnetic behavior make them attractive for drug delivery, imaging [28], cancer therapy, and bone tissue engineering [29]. In the human body, FeNPs integrate naturally with iron metabolism, releasing ions through endosomal and lysosomal pathways to maintain homeostasis [30]. When incorporated into scaffolds, they enhance osteogenic differentiation, improve mechanical strength, and support bone repair when under magnetic stimulation [31, 32].

2.2.2. *Organic Nanoparticles*

Organic NPs are nanoscale materials, typically less than 100 nm in size, synthesized from organic molecules [33]. These include systems such as micelles, dendrimers, liposomes, nanogels, polymeric NPs, and layered biopolymers. Some, such as micelles and liposomes, are hollow spherical structures that are biodegradable and nontoxic. They can naturally break down in the body, making them safe for biomedical use. The term also refers to nanocapsules, which are very sensitive to light and heat. Because of these features, organic NPs are widely used in drug delivery, helping to carry medicines directly to target sites [34, 35].

2.2.2.1. Liposomes

Liposomes are artificial, membrane-like vesicles that were the first nano-delivery systems tested in clinical trials and remain among the most successful drug carriers to date [36]. Structurally, they are double-layered vesicles formed when phospholipids and additives self-assemble in water. In this arrangement, the hydrophilic heads of the phospholipids interact with water, while the hydrophobic tails cluster together, forming a stable bilayer structure [37]. Liposomes are widely used as drug carriers because of their biocompatibility, biodegradability, and ability to improve drug stability [38]. Their performance depends on several factors such as composition, size, charge, and preparation method, and they can be engineered to respond to stimuli or environmental conditions such as pH, enzymes, or light [39]. Both hydrophilic and hydrophobic drugs can be loaded, with some formulations where, for instance, the cationic cholesterol derivative, DC-Chol (3β-[N-(N',N'-dimethylaminoethane)-carbamoyl]cholesterol), or the amphiphile dimethyldioctadecylammonium, also known as DDA, has already been applied in cancer immunotherapy [36]. In bone tissue engineering, targeted liposomes with phosphorylated cholesterol or specific ligands are currently being developed to accelerate fracture healing and promote osteogenic differentiation [40].

2.2.2.2. Polymeric Nanoparticles

Polymers are organic materials composed of long chains of atoms connected by covalent bonds. Both natural and synthetic polymers are widely used in bone tissue engineering. Natural options include collagen and gelatin, which serve as key structural proteins in bone, while synthetic polymers such as poly (lactic-co-glycolic acid) (PLGA) provide greater flexibility for chemical modification and molecular design. Polymeric NPs have been developed in various forms, such as nanofibers, micelles, and scaffold composites; synthetic types such as polylactic acid (PLA), PLGA, polyethylene glycol (PEG), poly(ε-caprolactone) (PCL), and polyglycolic acid (PGA) have shown particular promise for bone regeneration approaches [15]. The dimensions of a polymeric NP can be tailored to specific applications to improve efficiency and targeting. As mentioned, these NPs can be fabricated in different forms, including nanofibers, nanocapsules, and polymeric micelles [37, 41]. Their main advantages include excellent biocompatibility, ease of functionalization, flexible synthesis routes, and the ability to carry diverse types of molecules. Because of these features, polymeric NPs show significant promise for applications ranging from drug delivery to the treatment of various diseases [36]. Polymeric NPs are widely applied in bone tissue engineering for the localized and sustained delivery of therapeutic molecules [36]. For example, PLGA NPs enable the controlled release of osteogenic growth factors such as BMP-2, while PEGylation enhances their circulation time and biocompatibility. Composites that combine polymers with HA improve osteoconductivity and mechanical strength, thereby supporting bone repair [15]. Beyond drug delivery, polymeric NPs are currently being explored for gene transfer applications, immunomodulation, and angiogenesis, all of which are essential to effective bone regeneration. Despite challenges such as variable drug-loading efficiency and potential toxic by-products, ongoing advances in polymer chemistry and nanofabrication continue to expand their clinical potential in bone tissue engineering [36].

2.2.2.3. Dendrimers

Dendrimers are a class of polymeric NPs characterized by a nanosized, radially symmetric, tree-like structure. They are built from a central core that branches out into successive layers, ending with multiple functional groups on the surface [42]. This unique structure provides high uniformity (monodispersity), controllable size, and a large number of reactive end groups, distinguishing dendrimers from conventional polymeric NPs [43]. Because of their unique structure, dendrimers have been widely studied for biomedical applications, particularly in nanomedicine, diagnostics, and drug or gene delivery [44]. Two main strategies are employed for drug delivery using dendrimers: (1) encapsulating drugs inside the dendrimer through non-covalent interactions (formulation approach), or (2) covalently linking drugs to the dendrimer surface (nanostructure approach). Their high drug-loading capacity, good targeting potential, and tunable release behavior make them promising carriers. However, they also face challenges such as size-dependent toxicity (especially cationic dendrimers) and limited drug retention. Despite these issues, dendrimers remain attractive for exploring how polymer size, charge, and structure influence biological performance, including cytotoxicity, biodistribution, and circulation time [43].

2.2.3. *Carbon-Based Nanoparticles*

Carbon-based NPs represent a diverse class of nanomaterials derived from different carbon allotropes, including fullerenes, graphene, graphene oxide (GO), carbon nanotubes (CNTs), carbon nanofibers (CNFs), and activated carbon. Their unique atomic arrangements, ranging from spherical cages (C_{60}), two-dimensional (2D) graphene sheets, cylindrical nanotubes, fibrous morphologies, to highly porous activated carbon, give them exceptional mechanical, electrical, thermal, and chemical properties. These characteristics, along with high stability, tunable surface chemistry, and versatile synthesis methods, make carbon nanostructures essential building blocks in nanotechnology and advanced material applications [45]. However, there are concerns about their toxicity, biocompatibility, and biodegradability.

Carbon-based NPs are employed across multiple disciplines, including energy storage, electronics, catalysis, and biomedical engineering. Fullerenes (e.g., C_{60}) show unique electron-accepting and catalytic properties, making them useful in materials science and environmental remediation [46]. Compared to other carbon nanomaterials, fullerenes generally exhibit lower toxicity compared to other carbon-based NPs with higher aspect ratios [47]. Their enhanced biocompatibility, combined with intrinsic antioxidant properties resulting from an abundance of conjugated carbon double bonds, positions fullerenes as attractive candidates for bone tissue engineering applications [48]. Cheng et al. reported that the fullerene functionalization of zirconia and titanium implant surfaces provided antibacterial and anti-inflammatory properties, though no significant promotion of osteogenic differentiation in MC3T3-E1 osteoblast precursors was observed [49]. In a fullerene derivative, Yang et al. found that polyhydroxylated fullerene induced no significant cytotoxicity, significantly reduced intracellular reactive oxygen species (ROS) levels, and significantly upregulated the expression of osteogenic markers — osteocalcin, alkaline phosphatase, and Runt-related transcription factor 2 (RUNX2) — when cultured with human adipose-derived stem cells [50]. More recently, Yang et al. demonstrated that polyhydroxylated fullerene inhibited osteoclast formation from RAW264.7 macrophages in media supplemented with receptor activator of nuclear factor kappa-B ligand (RANKL) — a potent driver of osteoclastogenesis [51]. Graphene and GO are frequently incorporated into polymer composites to enhance strength and conductivity. Their hydrophilic, functionalized surfaces make them suitable for drug delivery, biosensing, and protective coatings [52]. CNTs, with their remarkable tensile strength and conductivity, are applied in composite reinforcement, biosensors, drug carriers, hydrogen storage, and electronic devices [53]. Huang et al. used the conductive properties of CNTs to create a CNT/carboxymethyl chitosan smart scaffold capable of promoting osteogenic differentiation and enabling noninvasive monitoring of bone regeneration [54]. As mineralization of the scaffold progressed, the scaffold's conductivity decreased, thereby providing an indirect indicator of bone healing [54]. CNFs provide a cost-effective alternative to CNTs with applications in electrical and mechanical composites, benefiting from their tunable nanostructure and wide availability [55]. Samadian et al. investigated an electrospun CNF nanocomposite scaffold containing HA, engineered to mimic the mineralized ECM of bone [56]. In a 6-mm femoral defect model, this biomimetic scaffold induced healthy bone tissue formation, as evaluated by computed tomography (CT) imaging and histological analysis, while the negative control exhibited no new bone formation [56]. In addition, activated carbon and its nanoporous derivatives are extensively used in adsorption, separation, and purification processes, including water treatment, gas storage, and pollutant removal [57]. Collectively, these carbon nanostructures offer multifunctionality, making them valuable across regenerative medicine, environmental applications, and industrial sectors. Additional information on the nanotubes can be found in Section 3.2.2.

2.3. *Synthesis Methods*

NPs can be produced using two main ways: the bottom-up and the top-down methods. In the bottom-up method, particles are built step by step starting from atoms and molecules, while in the top-down method, larger materials are broken down into smaller pieces until they reach the nanoscale [13].

2.3.1. *Bottom-Up Methods*

The bottom-up approach relies on chemical and physical forces that allow atoms or molecules to self-assemble into NPs. This strategy is inspired by natural systems, which use simple building blocks to form complex structures [13]. Some of the common techniques are discussed here.

2.3.1.1. The Sol–Gel Process

The sol–gel method is a versatile chemical process used to produce metal oxides, ceramics, and glasses. Starting from metal salts or alkoxides, a sol (liquid) is formed, which then transforms into a gel (solid). By drying and heating this gel, NPs with controlled size, porosity, and purity can be obtained. The process operates at relatively low temperatures and is widely applied in coatings, thin films, and porous ceramics [13].

2.3.1.2. The Spinning Method

This method uses a rapidly rotating disc to efficiently mix liquid reagents. The high surface area and thin liquid film on the disc allow for very fast reactions and NP nucleation. It is simple, scalable, and safer compared to traditional reactors [58].

2.3.1.3. Chemical Vapor Deposition

In this process, volatile precursors in the gas phase react and deposit a thin solid layer onto a surface. Variants include thermal chemical vapor deposition (CVD), plasma-enhanced CVD, and photo-induced CVD, each suited to different coating materials. Although effective, it may involve hazardous gases [59].

2.3.1.4. Pyrolysis

Pyrolysis is a high-temperature method where precursors are decomposed in the absence of oxygen to form NPs. This technique is commonly used for large-scale production but often faces challenges related to particle aggregation [60].

2.3.1.5. Biosynthesis

Biosynthesis is a green approach that uses living organisms — such as bacteria, fungi, yeast, algae, or viruses — to produce NPs in an environmentally safe way. This method is attractive as it avoids the use of toxic chemicals and allows for improved control over the NP properties. The process works *via* microorganisms absorbing metal ions from their surroundings and reducing them to elemental NPs, either inside or outside of the cell. For example, bacteria and microalgae can produce nanomaterials such as exopolysaccharides, nanocellulose, and nanowires [61].

2.3.2. *Top-Down Methods*

The top-down approach involves breaking down bulk materials into NPs. While these methods are more accessible, they may have limitations in controlling particle size and shape [12]. Examples of these methods include:

2.3.2.1. Mechanical Milling

Ball milling is one of the most widely used and cost-effective top-down methods for NP synthesis. In this process, powdered material is placed inside a rotating stainless-steel or zirconia vial containing hard balls made of iron, hardened steel, zirconia, silicon carbide, or tungsten carbide. As the vial rotates, repeated collisions between the balls and the powder transfer kinetic energy, causing mechanical attrition that reduces particle size to the nanoscale [12, 62]. This method is versatile and can produce NPs from different materials and alloys. It also induces crystallite refinement, structural defects, surface modification, and sometimes metastable phase formation [13]. However, its limitations include possible contamination from the milling media, sensitivity to the milling environment, long processing times for achieving very small particles (<20 nm), and noise or environmental disruption during operation [63].

2.3.2.2. Nanolithography

Nanolithography is a fabrication technique used to produce structures at the nanometer scale, typically with at least one dimension ranging from 1 to 100 nm. It is considered a powerful tool for creating precise nanoscale patterns and well-defined 2D arrays, such as metal structures, with controlled shape, size, and spacing. The process generally involves multiple steps, beginning with printing a desired design onto a light-sensitive material, followed by the selective removal of exposed regions to generate the intended structure. Several nanolithographic approaches have been developed, including optical, electron-beam, multiphoton, nanoimprint, and scanning probe lithography [64]. The main advantage of this technique is its capacity to mass-produce NPs with uniform size and morphology. However, it requires sophisticated instrumentation and carries high costs, which remain significant limitations [65].

2.3.2.3. Laser Ablation

Laser ablation is a method for producing NPs by irradiating a metal target in liquid and creating a plasma plume that condenses into NPs [66]. It is a rapid and versatile technique for generating metal, semiconductor, polymer, and alloy NPs without hazardous precursors, high temperatures, or pressures, yielding ultrapure colloidal solutions suitable for biomedical use [67]. This method is considered a "green" synthesis method, although long-term ablation can reduce efficiency as increasing NP concentrations block the laser path [68].

2.3.2.4. Thermal Decomposition

Thermal decomposition is a practical method for synthesizing stable, monodispersed metal NPs by breaking chemical bonds through the application of heat at precise decomposition temperatures [69]. This endothermic process allows for improved control over NP size and shape and is influenced by factors such as reaction time, temperature, reactant concentration, and surfactant type. Solvent-free approaches have been reported as simple and effective, enabling large-scale production compared to biological methods. However, challenges remain, including difficulties with certain metal compositions, limited control over film properties, and restrictions in source material availability [13].

3. Advanced Nanostructured Materials

3.1. *Introduction*

Nanostructured materials have emerged as highly promising tools for bone regeneration, offering unique properties that can enhance cell–material interactions and tissue repair. Among these, nanowires, nanotubes, and nanocoatings have been widely explored, while emerging materials such as black phosphorus nanosheets and MXenes have recently attracted significant attention due to their novel physicochemical characteristics. Other innovative nanomaterials, including metal–organic frameworks, self-assembling peptide nanofibers, 2D MoS_2 nanosheets, and quantum dots, also hold potential but are not discussed in detail here. This section provides an overview of the background, synthesis techniques, characterization methods, and current and potential translational applications of these nanomaterials in bone tissue engineering and regenerative medicine.

3.2. *Types of Nanostructured Materials*

3.2.1. *Nanowires*

Nanowires are cylindrically shaped structures with a cross-sectional diameter of approximately 1 nm [70]. In current practice, the most prevalent use for nanowires has been in electronics. Due to their nanoscale size and excellent conductive abilities, electronic manufacturers fabricate numerous nanowire transistors into a single microprocessor, leading to a drastic increase in processing speeds. Through recent research, the unique electron properties of nanowires matched with their miniscule size have made them of particular interest in many other fields, including in bone regeneration. With their nanometer-scale diameter, nanowires have shown promise in detecting pathogens and biochemical species, which can serve a protective role in bone scaffolding [71]. In addition, similar to their use in electronics, the excellent electron and charge-carrying capacity of nanowires *via* their metallic associations make them more useful in bone regeneration compared to other nanomaterials. Of the many types of nanowires that exist, the main ones include superconducting, metallic, semiconducting, and insulating.

The characterization of nanowire morphology and nanostructure is typically performed using scanning electron microscopy (SEM), transmission electron microscopy (TEM), and atomic force microscopy (AFM) [72–74]. Surface chemical characterization is also conducted using Fourier transform infrared spectroscopy (FTIR), X-ray photoelectron spectroscopy (XPS), and time-of-flight secondary ion mass spectrometry [74]. Nanowires can be synthesized and grown using multiple different processes, with one of the most common techniques being the vapor–liquid–solid (VLS) method, which is primarily used to form semiconductor nanowires. A characteristic feature of this synthesis method is the presence of a catalytic particle, most commonly some form of ionic metal (i.e., Si, Au), to mediate nanowire growth. This unique feature allows for direct control over nanowire composition and morphology. During the VLS process, the catalytic particle becomes supersaturated following the degradation of its gas precursors, such as $SiCl_4$ or SiH_4. Crystallization on the particle–nanowire interface allows for the growth of the semiconductor nanostructure [75]. The classic VLS mechanism relies on the principle that an ideal liquid surface captures all impinging metal source atoms, while a solid surface of the same metal rejects almost all atoms at sufficiently high temperature.

Another method for nanowire synthesis is laser-assisted growth [76], which is particularly useful for forming nanowires with features such as ultrathin diameters, high melting temperatures, or multiple elemental components. A unique feature of this technique over other growth technologies is the ability to form complex chemical compositions. The reason for this is that, unlike other techniques, it is unnecessary to prepare the source materials in a crystalline form before preparation, regardless of the number of elements involved. The laser-assisted method works by ablating the source materials into their vapor phases, which can then easily be transferred and congealed for nanowire growth. Two other synthetic techniques for nanowire formation include thermal evaporation [77] and solution-based methods [78]. Thermal evaporation of solid source materials is performed by creating a temperature gradient under vacuum conditions, allowing the evaporation of commercial metal oxide powders, and then nanowire production when the vaporized powders enter the low-temperature regions of the chamber. This process is also called vapor–solid growth because it skips the liquid phase seen in the VLS method. Solution-based methods offer advantages by yielding significant amounts of product at low cost with easy setup. Solution-based methods have been shown to have excellent control of the shape and composition of the nanowires. Specific solution-based methods used for nanowires include metal-catalyzed solution–liquid–solid growth from metal seeds, self-assembly attachment growth, and anisotropic growth of crystals by thermodynamic or kinetic control. In addition to techniques used for nanowire growth, multiple mechanisms and mediums help promote nanowire synthesis. One popular growth mechanism is the use of metal catalysts, such as in the VLS growth technique. Other growth mechanisms include oxide-assisted, external electric field, and even self-catalytic growth. Regarding bone regeneration, nanowires have been shown to have many promising applications. One application is the use of substrate-bound PCL nanowires in managing critical-sized bone defects. A major goal is to create an engineered scaffold that incites the natural healing process within bone defects by stimulating cycles of osteoinduction and osteoconduction. However, when the defect is large, these processes are not self-stimulated and, therefore, require a catalytic agent to induce bone regeneration. In this respect, research has shown that fabricating uniform arrays of PCL-coated nanowires stimulates bone growth in these critical-sized bone defects [79]. Results showed that PCL nanowires supported increased cell adhesion, increased levels of alkaline phosphatase, and accelerated calcium phosphate (CaP) mineralization compared to control surfaces. In addition, increased levels of the bone-forming proteins, osteocalcin and osteopontin, were measured both intracellularly and extracellularly. Another potential application for nanowires in the treatment of bone regeneration involves using zinc, chitosan, and the solvothermal synthesis method. In this study, zinc was catalytically attached to an HA nanowire surface, and then, chitosan was incorporated *via* a freeze-drying process to form the complete nanocomposite structure [80]. The final nanostructure displayed features of high flexibility, a vast surface area, and improved mechanical properties secondary to its excellent water retention capacity and highly porous structure. Furthermore, the nanocomposite structure was investigated *in vitro*, where the scaffold was shown to promote the osteogenic differentiation of rat bone marrow–derived mesenchymal stem cells while also facilitating bone regeneration *in vivo* (**Figure 2**) [80]. Modifying the surface topography of nanowire-based scaffolds during fabrication with biodegradable polymers, along with functionalizing nanowires using biomolecules such as enzymes, antibodies, and nucleic acids, can enhance their biomedical potential [81]. In addition, incorporating angiogenic growth factors, such as vascular endothelial growth factor, within the nanowire scaffold has been shown to facilitate vasculogenesis pre- or post-transplantation, thereby improving tissue regeneration and integration [82].

In addition to bone formation, nanowires have also been shown to deliver antibacterial activity to the scaffold environment during bone regeneration. This was shown *via* the use of a silver nanowire, chitosan, and HA composite [83]. *In vitro*, this nanostructured scaffold was shown to deliver antibacterial activities against both Gram-positive and Gram-negative bacteria and prevent biofilm formation in the presence of more virulent strains. In addition to decreasing the risk of infection, the scaffolding nanostructure did not impair bone regeneration but enhanced the mechanical strength and calcium salt deposition. This dual functionality was also reported following investigation in a preclinical model of periodontitis — an inflammatory disease of the tooth periosteum that can lead to significant nerve pain and potential tooth loss [84]. Guided tissue regeneration followed by the deposition of an osteoinductive material is the mainstay of treatment for periodontitis; however, there is a significant risk of infection and re-bleeding after the procedure. In a study [85],

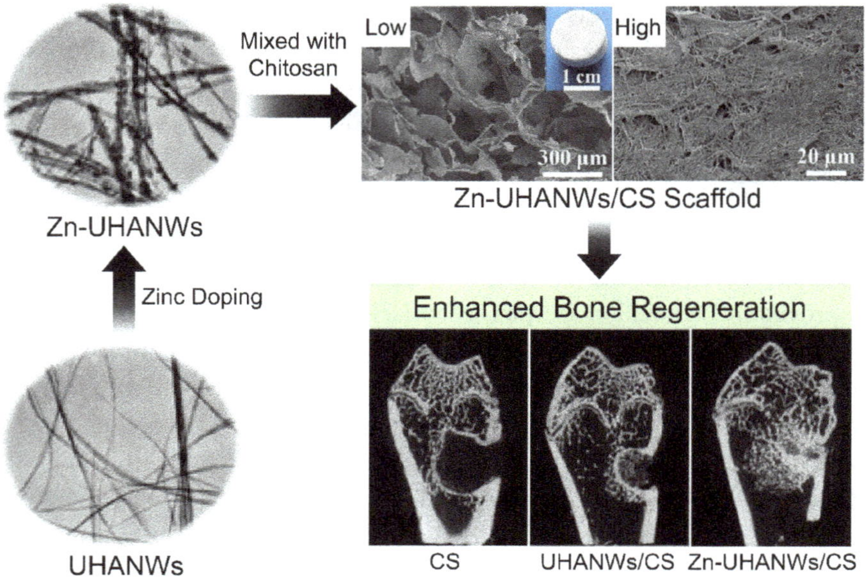

Figure 2. Zinc-containing nanoparticle-decorated hydroxyapatite nanowires (Zn-UHANWs) and a biomimetic Zn-UHANWs/chitosan (CS) (Zn-UHANWs/CS) composite porous scaffold are synthesized. The scaffold exhibits enhanced mechanical properties, an excellent water-retention capacity, and good biodegradability and promotes *in vivo* bone regeneration (reprinted from ref. [80] with permission from John Wiley and Sons).

researchers synthesized a nanostructure composed of HA nanowires combined with a PLA membrane. When investigated in a rat mandibular defect model, this physiochemically modified nanostructure was shown to promote the expression of more bone-related growth markers. Furthermore, the newly formed bone was of improved quality, and the scaffold was successful in providing a protective antibacterial environment, thereby facilitating bone regeneration. This study illustrates the promise of this dual-functioning biomaterial as both an environmental barrier against infection and a promoter of bone formation.

3.2.2. *Nanotubes*

Nanotubes are hollow, tubular-shaped nanostructures with nanometer-range diameters and unrestricted lengths. Despite structural similarities to nanowires, nanotubes can be differentiated due to differences in their aspect ratios, calculated as the length-to-diameter ratio. While the aspect ratio of nanowires tends to approach or slightly surpass 1:1,000 [86, 87], nanotubes have a much higher aspect ratio. Wang et al. reported the creation of nanotubes with an aspect ratio of up to 1:132,000,000 [88]. Due to their unique structure, nanotubes demonstrate a high Young's modulus and tensile strength, leading to their use in applications that require improved mechanical properties. In addition, they provide high electrical and thermal conductivity, elasticity, flexibility, and low thermal expansion coefficient [89]. With these features, the most common industrial uses for nanotubes include energy storage, the automotive industry, and electronics. The most common type of nanotube is carbon-based, with other types including metallic-based and oxide-based [90]. CNTs are unique compared to other nanotubes due to their lightweight carbon-based frame, with their density one-sixth that of steel. They are typically categorized based on the number of rolled sheets they possess, i.e., single-walled, double-walled, or multiwalled [91].

The synthesis of nanotubes can occur through a variety of different methods depending on the material used to form the structure. CNTs, the most well-studied type, are primarily synthesized by one of three methods: CVD, laser ablation, or carbon arc discharge. CVD uses the decomposition of carbon-containing gases to grow carbon atoms on a transition metal catalyst [92, 93]. Laser ablation uses the laser vaporization of carbon and transition metals that eventually form into CNTs as the vapors cool [94]. Carbon arc discharge uses an electrical arc to generate plasma that sublimates a carbon precursor [95]. The carbon vapor aggregates and cools to form CNTs. All three techniques have similar yield rates and can synthesize both single-walled nanotubes and multiwalled nanotubes (MWNTs). As the current standard for CNT production, the advantage of the CVD technique is due to its simplicity, use in larger-scale production, and high purity. The method works by using a catalyst or substrate to cleave a carbon atom-containing gas on its surface. At elevated temperatures, the catalyst decomposes the carbon source and simultaneously transforms it into a tubular nanostructure [96]. Regarding laser ablation, one of its main advantages compared to CVD and arc-discharge techniques is that it can be performed at room temperature. However, its disadvantages include the need for additional purification steps of the crude product following synthesis. Finally, arc discharge is both simple and inexpensive to perform but, compared to other synthesis techniques, can increase the occurrence of tangled nanotubes [97]. Aside from CNTs, other synthetic methods for forming nanotubes include more specialized processes, such as the dynamic hydrothermal process for titanium dioxide nanotubes [98]. Characterization of nanotubes involves SEM, TEM, Raman spectroscopy, and reciprocal space analysis. SEM is used to determine the morphology and length of nanotubes, while Raman spectroscopy and TEM are typically applied to determine the electronic properties and morphology of the nanotube structure. Finally, reciprocal space analysis provides detailed quantitative information on the 3D nanotube structure [99].

Nanotubes have shown promise in bone regeneration, as many of their structural properties make them viable scaffolding agents — an important step in reforming bone defects. For instance, CNTs have shown promise in many clinical applications due to their excellent strength, inert chemical stability, and overall fibrinous structure [100]. An example of this utility is MWNTs paired with bacterial cellulose, which can support osteoblast viability, adhesion, and proliferation at a greater rate compared to control cultures [101, 102]. In addition, it was found that carbon MWNTs did not affect cellular viability but instead also enhanced osteoblast adhesion [102]. Another study demonstrated the ability of CNTs to promote bone defect repair [103]. In this study, a 3D block composed entirely of MWNTs and the protein, human rhBMP-2, was implanted into murine muscle. Results showed that ectopic bone formed with a density and maximum compression strength comparable to that of native cortical bone [103]. Aside from CNTs, TiO_2 nanotubes also have a growing body of data that supports their use in stimulating bone regeneration. Titanium and its related alloys are effective following bone implantation due to their relatively bioinert and non-immunogenic *in vivo* properties compared to other metals. The surface layer of TiO_2 provides some resistance to post-implant corrosion and increases biocompatibility with native human tissue. Electrochemical anodization is a method used to synthesize titanium oxide/nanotube nanocomposites, which have shown enhanced growth and accelerated osteo-differentiation of mesenchymal stem cells [104]. To this end, BMP-2 and macrophage-derived exosomes were incorporated into titanium nanotubes to create a more targeted bone regeneration strategy, thereby minimizing unwanted systemic side effects. Results showed that this functionalized nanotube significantly increased the expression of osteoblast growth markers, indicating that the biomaterial had an osteogenic effect (**Figure 3a**) [105]. The unique ability to modulate the cellular response of bone-forming cells through nanostructured materials, such as titanium nanotubes, has broadened potential therapies for bone defects [106].

Nanotubes have previously been shown to possess bone regenerative and antimicrobial properties when paired with other minerals, such as halloysite, a nanoclay composed of aluminosilicate [$Al_2Si_2O_5(OH)_4$]. A study reported that halloysite nanotubes were incorporated into gelatin methacrylate using a photopolymerization technique. The results showed that the halloysite nanotubes were cytocompatible in rats *in vivo* and induced bone regeneration by increasing alkaline phosphatase activity and upregulating osteogenic differentiation-related genes, such as COL-1, RUNX2, BMP-4, and BSP (**Figure 3b**) [107]. Further, halloysite nanotubes fabricated with a nanosilver and gelatin methacrylate hybrid hydrogel displayed anti-inflammatory properties and improved modulation of the osteoimmune microenvironment [108]. The hydrogel also showed comparable biocompatibility with human periodontal ligament stem cells and stimulated bone repair through the osteogenic differentiation of mesenchymal stem cells (**Figure 3c**) [108].

3.2.3. *Nanocoatings*

Nanocoatings are films with nanoscale thickness that can be applied to surfaces as a protective mechanism or to improve a material's functionality. The functional properties of nanocoatings depend on the material used to synthesize the nanomaterial but can include features such as abrasion and corrosion resistance, hydrophobic/hydrophilic properties, antibacterial properties, friction reduction, and heat resistance [109]. Based on these properties, the most intuitive uses of nanocoatings are to protect machinery and equipment from wear, thereby improving product lifetime, as well as in self-cleaning surfaces and thermal insulation [110–112]. Due to their versatility and proven clinical benefits in other medical applications,

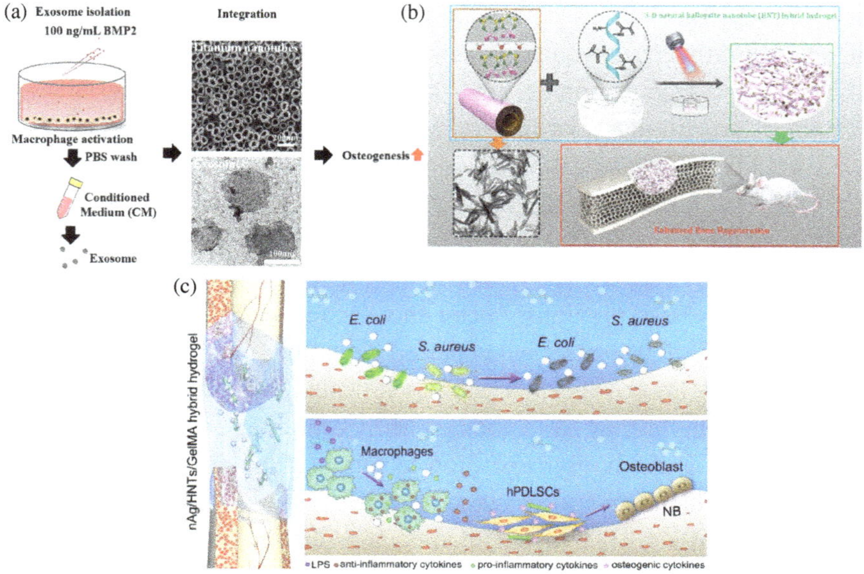

Figure 3. (a) Fabrication of BMP-2/macrophage-derived exosomes and their incorporation in titanium oxide nanotubes (reprinted from ref. [105] with permission from John Wiley and Sons), (b) halloysite nanotube-based scaffold for enhanced bone regeneration in rats (reprinted from ref. [107] with permission from the American Chemical Society), (c) nanosilver-incorporated halloysite nanotubes/gelatin methacrylate hybrid hydrogel with osteoimmunomodulatory and antibacterial activity for bone regeneration (reprinted from ref. [108] with permission from Elsevier).

nanocoatings have begun to show promise in enhancing bone regeneration, especially as an adjunct to other therapies [110, 113]. Superhydrophobic TiO_2–oleic acid nanocomposite coatings were fabricated using a vacuum cold spray process, wherein the TiO_2 NPs were synthesized *via* a sol–gel method (**Figure 4a**) [110]. The resulting surfaces exhibited superhydrophobicity, with potential applications in antifouling, anticorrosion, anti-icing, oil/water separation, and drag reduction. **Figure 4b** shows a nanocoating applied to titanium mini-screw dental implants, with subsequent X-ray imaging used to confirm successful implantation and assess postoperative outcomes.

The size, layer thickness, and distribution of the particles in the coating, as well as the surface properties of the substrate used to form a nanocoating, have a crucial effect on its final properties. Multiple mechanisms

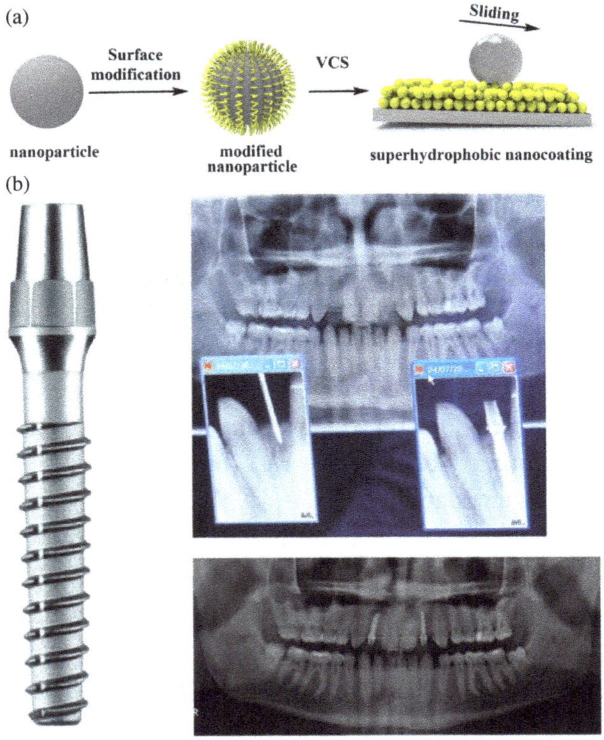

Figure 4. (a) The formation of a hydrophobic nanocoating (reprinted from ref. [110] with permission from Elsevier) and (b) a nanocoated titanium mini-screw dental implant with X-ray images taken post-surgery. A control image of implant incorporation. Reprinted from ref. [113] with permission from Elsevier).

are available to develop nanocoatings depending on their function. Some of the most common techniques used include CVD, physical vapor deposition, spray coating, sol–gel, and electrospinning [111]. CVD and physical vapor deposition can be used to form nanocoatings through a comparable process to nanotube formation. The technique occurs through the evaporation of the coating material by a high-energy source, the transfer of evaporated molecules to the substrate, and finally, a chemical reaction that allows deposition onto the substrate. Another method used to form nanocoatings is spray coating. In this process, the coating material is first formed into a liquid, molten, or particle form and then transferred through a nozzle onto the target substrate. Next, the sol–gel process forms nanocoatings at low temperatures *via* a chemical reaction. The technique begins with the dispersion of colloidal particles into a liquid form, followed by deposition of a liquid solution onto the substrate, and finally, ends with polymerization and final heat treatment to form a crystalline coating. The last technique discussed here is electrospinning, which utilizes an external electric field. This process operates by entering charged polymeric solutions into a high-voltage environment. The desirable nanocoating structure is formed *via* an external electric field from a nozzle that shapes the nanocoating into its final form. Common techniques for the characterization of nanocoatings involve SEM, FTIR, and contact angle measurement [114–116]. SEM provides details of the nanostructure and surface topography, while FTIR provides information about the functional groups present in the nanocoating. Contact angle measurement quantifies the surface wettability of the nanocoating.

Nanocoatings can enhance bone regeneration through a variety of methods. An example of this versatility is the use of iron scaffolds to stimulate osteoinduction. Pure iron has load-bearing and mechanical properties that are desirable for facilitating new bone formation. However, previous manufacturing techniques offered poor control over the macropore structure and surface nanostructure of iron scaffolds, restricting their use in clinical applications. Yang et al. utilized 3D printing to achieve finer control over the structure of iron scaffolds, and their bioactivity was improved by applying an HA nanocoating. The HA-nanocoated iron scaffolds greatly enhanced the viability and alkaline phosphatase activity of rabbit bone marrow mesenchymal stem cells and improved bone growth [117]. Another method for biomimicking an osteoinductive scaffold is the use of a layer-by-layer nanocoating approach. Here, researchers utilized electrospun PCL fibers and ionic mineralization to formulate an artificial bone scaffold. The ionic mineralization consisted of cationic type-I collagen and anionic chondroitin sulfate, which mimic the native bone scaffold components. The PCL fibers were nanocoated with multiple layers to induce bone regeneration. Through the layer-by-layer technique, both the number of layers and the duration of mineralization could be adjusted for optimization. It was found that the optimal combination consisted of 10 nanobilayers of type-I collagen and chondroitin sulfate, followed by 1 day of mineralization. Following implantation in mice, *in vivo* results indicated that the artificial scaffold promoted adhesion, proliferation, and osteogenic differentiation of bone-forming cells [115]. Dentistry, particularly bone–enamel repair, is another promising area for nanocoating applications. The primary cause of dental implant failure is contamination and inflammation, which hinder tissue healing and integration. One of the major determinants in defining a successful dental implant is its osseointegration with the alveolar bone and surrounding tissue. The integration of foreign tissue during any surgery or implantation is a significant concern, and its success relies on the cellular response of the surrounding tissues to the implant. Nanocoatings have shown promise in addressing multiple adverse effects associated with dental implants. For instance, dental implants coated with phyto-bioactive-treated rayon/polyester nanocoatings were reported. Results showed that the nanocoatings were resistant to the adhesion of *Candida albicans* — a common oral inhabitant — and subsequent biofilm formation. Another example is the use of nanocoatings on the dental screws used to anchor an implant into the patient's gumline. Titanium is commonly used to manufacture these screws due to its high resistance to body fluids, tensile strength, and corrosion resistance. Titanium mini-screws coated with nanoclay-reinforced magnesium-substituted β-tricalcium phosphate (TCP) have been investigated for the anchoring step. In this study, it was found that the specialized nanocoating delivered enhanced stability to the mini-screw *via* its natural nanoporosity and the surface features applied to the titanium surface [111].

3.2.4. *Emerging Nanomaterials*

Black phosphorous is an allotrope of phosphorous that, like graphene, exhibits a layered structure [118]. Unlike graphene, however, the layers of black phosphorous nanosheets are puckered and arranged in a hexagonal lattice, allowing for distinct properties such as anisotropic charge transport and a tunable bandgap [119, 120]. Although first identified nearly a century ago, black phosphorous, particularly as 2D nanosheets, has only recently emerged as a focus of nanomaterial research, driven by advances in modern synthesis and characterization techniques [118]. The formation of black phosphorous nanosheets can be conducted through a top-down approach, using mechanical exfoliation, liquid exfoliation, or electrochemical exfoliation, or through a bottom-up approach, using pulsed laser deposition, solvothermal synthesis, or CVD methods [119, 121]. Of the top-down approaches, mechanical exfoliation presents the most facile and commonly used technique, though it limits large-scale synthesis [119]. Current bottom-up synthesis methods have encountered similar limitations, producing black phosphorous nanosheets on the scale of a few centimeters or millimeters [121]. The characterization of black phosphorous nanosheets is commonly conducted using X-ray diffraction (XRD), XPS, SEM, TEM, and Raman spectroscopy [118, 122]. Broadly, black phosphorus has been commonly used for energy storage, electronic, and optoelectronic applications [123]. However, its biomedical applications are increasingly being explored due to its conductivity, biocompatibility, and biodegradability [124]. Applications in bone tissue regeneration are particularly interesting, as phosphorus is a natural component of bone. However, controlled degradation is required to prevent harmful effects from local excessive phosphate release. Notably, recent studies have reported black phosphorus to exhibit osteoimmunomodulatory, antimicrobial, and osteogenic effects. Qiu et al. reported that loading of 3D-printed PCL scaffolds with black phosphorous nanosheets promoted the osteogenic differentiation of bone marrow mesenchymal stem cells through osteoimmunomodulation [125]. Li et al. showed promising photothermal antibacterial activity in hydrogels incorporating black phosphorous nanosheets [126]. Chen et al. found that incorporating black phosphorous nanosheets into a poly(propylene fumarate) bone cement enhanced pre-osteoblast differentiation and adhesion [127].

MXenes are a family of 2D transition metal carbides, nitrides, and carbonitrides [128]. They are described by the general formula of $M_{n+1}X_nT_x$, where M is a transition metal, X is a carbon or nitrogen, and T_x refers to the surface termination groups, typically O, OH, or F [129]. The quantity n refers to the number of atomic layers. MXenes are commonly synthesized through a top-down approach involving wet chemical etching and subsequent delamination of MAX phases [130]. MAX phases are multilayered 3D precursors to MXenes and characterized by a similar general formula, $M_{n+1}AX_n$, in which layers of an early transition metal bonded to carbon and/or nitrogen are interleaved with an A-layer element from the main group [131]. As the bonding of the A-layer is relatively weaker than the *MX* layer, the *A*-layer can be selectively removed through chemical etching to yield MXenes [129]. Common techniques used to characterize MXenes include XRD to verify the conversion from MAX to MXene, SEM to assess surface morphology, AFM to quantify flake thickness, and nuclear magnetic resonance to determine the nature of surface functional groups [132, 133]. MXenes were originally investigated for applications in fields including catalysis, energy storage, and electronics due to their large surface area, tunable surface chemistry, electrical conductivity, and hydrophilicity [134–136]. These same attributes, particularly their excellent electronic properties, also make MXenes highly attractive for biosensing applications including the detection of pathogens or biomolecules [130]. Within the scope of bone regeneration, MXenes offer functionalizable surfaces to promote osteoblast adhesion and osteoimmunomodulation. To this end, Jang et al. found that Ti_3C_2 MXene particles promoted osteogenic differentiation [137]. Huang et al. reported that decorating Ti_3C_2 nanosheets onto β-TCP-based scaffolds allowed for spatiotemporal osteoimmunomodulation through the use of near-infrared irradiation [138].

4. Nanostructured Implants and Nanocomposite Scaffolds

4.1. *Introduction*

When dealing with fractures or severe injuries, orthopedic surgeons may opt for invasive methods such as bone implants or bone grafting procedures. However, given the innate reactivity of the human body, careful consideration must be given to the materials used to create the implants, so they integrate with native tissue while maintaining integrity for the required duration [139]. Traditionally, most bone fixation and repair devices have been fabricated using metals such as stainless steel, titanium, or their alloys. These metals are not biodegradable and thus can elevate the chance of infection and other tissue complications that limit optimal integration [140]. To promote improved results, utilizing a treatment approach, such as a nanostructured bone implant and nanocomposite scaffold, may be preferential for encouraging desirable implant–tissue interactions. In this section, the promising applications of nanograined implants and nanocomposite scaffolds will be reviewed by first providing a background on the material classifications, followed by a closer look at the synthetic and characterization methods. The utility and limitations for their use in industrial applications will subsequently be provided.

4.2. *Classification of the Material*

Both nanostructured implants and nanocomposite scaffolds are useful integrations within regenerative medicine and tissue engineering. Since the long-term efficiency of orthopedic implants also correlates with their surface characteristics and interactions with the biological environment [141], it is crucial to focus on surface properties, as well as bulk material properties.

4.2.1. *Nanostructured Implants*

4.2.1.1. Metals

Metallic materials are used for fabricating orthopedic implants because of their high strength, decent biocompatibility, fine corrosion properties, and fatigue resistance. However, the release of metallic ions in the body poses potential issues for healing and increases the risk of implant rejection. Thus, corrosion-resistant, i.e., inert, metals such as stainless steel, titanium alloys, and cobalt–chromium alloys were developed. The mechanical and functional properties of these metallic materials can be enhanced through severe plastic deformation (SPD), which enables the production of ultrafine-grained metals with nanograin structures or nanometric precipitated phases. These SPD methods can aid in refining the grain structure, thereby improving mechanical properties and thus expanding their use in biomedical implant applications [142]. Nanograins provide a unique combination of high strength and ductility while also enhancing biological performance by influencing protein adsorption and regulating interactions with osteoblasts and osteoclasts. Their increased surface area further promotes higher surface reactivity, thereby offering additional functional benefits [142]. For example, it was observed that immobilizing lysine–arginine–serine–arginine onto nanostructured Ti increased osteoblast adhesion compared to micron-structured Ti alone [143]. Besides improved functionalization, changes in the morphology of the oxide film on the nanograined Ti surface made it a favorable attachment site for cells [144]. Although these alloys are not toxic, their higher elastic modulus results in stress shielding and bone resorption due to reduced transfer of loads to bone across the bone–implant interface. Hence, bioabsorbable metals such as Fe alloys [145], Mg alloys [146], and Zn alloys [147] were developed. These alloys support mechanical strength during the initial healing process but are subsequently resorbed within body fluids, without causing a foreign body reaction, by corrosion mechanisms. Thus, as the implant degrades, there is a gradual and increasing transfer of mechanical load borne by the bone structure, thereby facilitating healthy tissue function. There are various surface modification methods used to control the degradation rate of bioabsorbable metals. For instance, a nanostructured zinc phosphate coating on a Zn alloy surface decreased Zn^{2+} release, improved biocompatibility and osteogenic properties, decreased the corrosion rate, promoted HA deposition, and improved the proliferation of pre-osteoblasts [148]. Plasma ion implantation is another method used to control degradation. Nitrogen plasma immersion ion implantation results in the formation of nanocrystalline oxides and nitrides, as well as the development of nanograins on the surface of Fe-based alloys. This coating was shown to reduce the corrosion rate when measured in Hank's modified balanced salt solution [112]. Metal matrix nanocomposites are a method for producing bulk bioactive metallic implants. Incorporating bioactive glass–ceramic NPs in molten Mg, followed by hot rolling, results in the homogeneous dispersion of NPs in the Mg matrix [149]. The release of ions from the NPs, including magnesium and silicon, enhanced osteogenesis and angiogenesis, thereby improving biocompatibility [150].

4.2.1.1.1. Synthesis of Nanostructured Metals

There are two known methods used to produce metals with reduced grain size: (a) the bottom-up approach and (b) the top-down approach [151, 152]. Bottom-up methods assemble polycrystalline metals into nanograined materials beginning at the atomic scale [153]. For example, bottom-up methods include inert gas condensation, CVD, and high-energy ball milling. These methods are suitable for scaffold fabrication and coatings due to the high porosity they formed. The second method, i.e., the "top-down" approach, involves the refinement of coarse grains into ultrafine grains and is processed using SPD [152, 153]. Using this approach simultaneously improves the degree of grain refinement and decreases grain size to <100 nm, along with increasing the amount of high-angle grain boundaries [152, 153]. In the following sections, the most practical methods to obtain nanograins are explained in more detail.

4.2.1.1.1.1. *High-Energy Ball Milling*

High-energy ball milling is one method for preparing nanostructured metal powders that can be used as feedstock. Notably, the spark plasma sintering (SPS) method was recently reported to significantly improve the density and decrease the porosity of samples prepared using the ball milling technique. Extensive studies have been conducted to optimize the preparation of metallic implants using the ball milling approach, and it is pertinent to incorporate different grain structures to control degradation rates and improve biocompatibility [154–157]. In this way, bimodal Fe-based alloys have been prepared and have been shown to consist of both nano- and micro-structured grains. The nanostructured grains increase mechanical strength, while the microstructured grains improve ductility. Moreover, it was observed that the combination of nano- and micro-structured alloys is a suitable method for controlling the degradation of Fe-based alloys (**Figure 5**). Further, silver can be added to Fe-based alloys to deliver antibacterial properties and inactivate platelet adhesion, thereby decreasing blood clot formation on the implant surface.

4.2.1.1.1.2. *Equal Channel Angular Pressing*

Equal channel angular pressing (ECAP) is a processing method where a metal undergoes intense plastic straining through simple shear without any cross-sectional sample reduction to produce ultrafine-grained materials [142, 158]. In this process, the metallic materials are pressed into a die through a rectangular or circular channel, and the intensity of

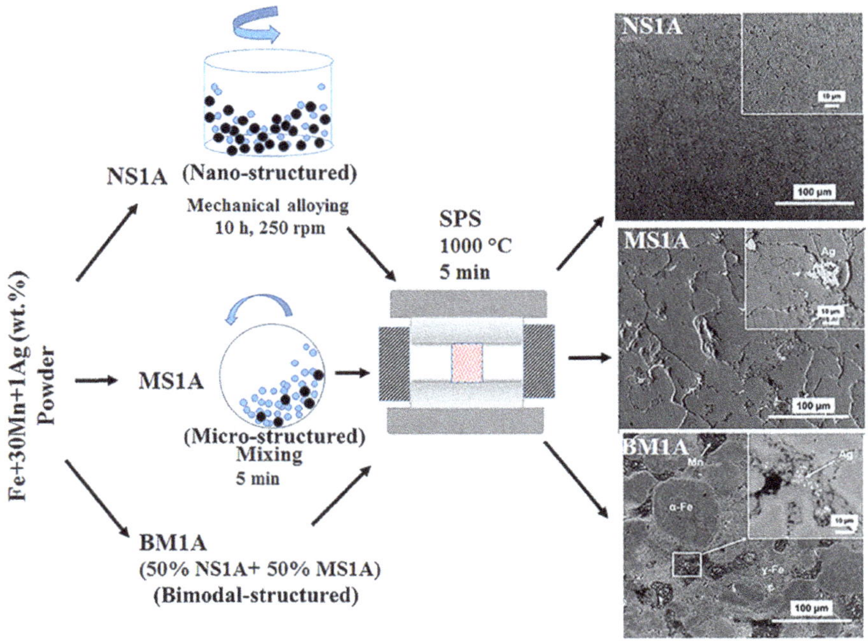

Figure 5. The ball milling process to produce bioabsorbable Fe–Mn–Ag alloys. Micrographs show SEM images of nanostructured (NS1A), microstructured (MS1A), and bimodal structured (BM1A) samples after spark plasma sintering (SPS) consolidation (reprinted from ref. [154] with permission from Elsevier).

the plastic deformation depends on the bending angle of the channel [142]. The strain produced during ECAP depends on the angle between the two channel segments and the outer arc of curvature where they intersect [158].

4.2.1.1.1.3. *High-Pressure Torsion*

High-pressure torsion (HPT) is a method in which samples are exposed to torsional shear strain while under high pressure. In this method, a thin layer of material is placed between two large anvils that apply pressure, and then the material is torsionally strained through the rotation of one or both anvils. However, it is challenging to scale up samples using this method due to slow process speeds and high-energy demand. Moreover, this method can only be applied to thin, small, disc-shaped samples in the range of 10 to 20 mm in diameter and 0.2 to 2 mm in thickness [153, 159].

4.2.1.1.1.4. *Hydrostatic Extrusion*

Hydrostatic extrusion is an extrusion method in which the billet and surrounding operating chamber are filled with oil. Movement of the piston causes compression of the medium, which induces hydrostatic pressure within the chamber [142, 160]. Exceeding the stress in the billet above the material's yield strength initiates plastic deformation. This method can be applied to higher material volumes compared to other SPD methods, such as HPT and ECAP. Moreover, due to material compacting during the process, the production of microcracks within the material is restricted. However, several limitations restrict this approach. For example, restrained high plastic deformation due to a reduction in the diameter of the sample, the high-energy consumption needed to press the medium, the time- and energy-consuming processes of fluid injection, the need for fluid removal after each extrusion cycle, a limited process temperature, and the high requirement for a sealed system [160].

4.2.1.1.1.5. *Ultrasonic Shot Peening*

Ultrasonic shot peening is a cold-working surface treatment that uses sonotrodes vibrating at ultrasonic frequencies to accelerate small, spherical shot media, which then bombard a surface. Shots with specific kinetic energy hit the surface, thereby changing its microstructure [142, 161]. Using this method, for example, several spherical steel balls can be vibrated by a generator that produces vibrations (50 Hz to 20 kHz), leading to the production of shots [162].

4.2.1.1.1.6. *Cryo-Rolling*

Cryo-rolling (CR) uses liquid nitrogen to provide an ultra-cold environment that decreases grain size by suppressing dynamic recovery. Compared to other SPD methods, CR is a continuous and efficient method capable of being scaled up to produce many thin sheets containing an inherent nanostructure [142]. Moreover, this method can also increase hardness and strength. However, low ductility and formability restrict the use of this application in industrial applications.

4.2.1.1.1.7. *Constrained Groove Pressing*

Constrained groove pressing (CGP) is a method that uses grooves subject to repetitive shear deformation at different strain levels using a combination of grooved and flat dies. This process could be applied at both high and low temperatures to change the microstructure of metals [142]. The CGP method enhances the hardness, fatigue, and strength of metals by reducing the grain size without altering the sample's direction.

4.2.1.2. Ceramics

Since CaP makes up a large portion of bone, it is a suitable synthetic material for use in bone regeneration. In this respect, many CaP ceramics such as HA [163], TCP [164], and bioglass (BG) [165] have been studied. CaP scaffolds are useful due to their osteoconductivity, osteoinductivity, and bioactivity, but they lack rigidity. Compared to conventional ceramics, nanostructured ceramics possess increased mechanical strength, biodegradability, and bioactivity. Cell–material interactions, such as those between osteoblast progenitors and ceramics, are greatly influenced by surface morphology. Importantly, the specific nanotopography of the material surface directly influences stem cell behavior and differentiation, primarily through integrin-mediated focal adhesion signaling and the degree of actin polymerization [166]. Therefore, improved control of the nanostructure of material surfaces can confer improved control over the osteogenic differentiation of stem cells. In one study, Zhang et al. observed improved cell adhesion and the upregulation of osteogenic markers, including alkaline phosphatase, osteocalcin, osteopontin, and RUNX2, in a β-TCP scaffold with a finer nanostructure and increased surface roughness [167]. Ergun et al. studied osteoblast adhesion to nanograined HA and TCP composites containing $CaTiO_3$, and results showed nearly 4.5 times more adhesion compared to pure HA [168]. Mesoporous bioactive glass with highly oriented nanostructured pores is a robust choice for the delivery of bioactive molecules such as growth factors. The increased specific surface area and pore volume provide an adaptable structure for optimized cargo delivery [169].

4.2.1.2.1. Synthesis of Ceramics

Nanoceramics can be synthesized using both top-down and bottom-up approaches. However, due to the limitations of top-down methods, most nanoceramics are typically fabricated using bottom-up strategies. Common examples include sol–gel processing, spray pyrolysis (SP), hydrothermal synthesis, and self-propagating high-temperature synthesis (SHS) [170].

4.2.1.2.1.1. *Sol–Gel*

The sol–gel method is a versatile chemical route for synthesizing dense and homogeneous ceramic and vitreous materials at relatively low temperatures. This process typically uses metal alkoxide precursors, which readily react with water to form metal–oxygen bonds, making the technique especially suitable for producing metal oxides, hydroxides, and related ceramic materials [171]. The synthesis proceeds in several stages. First, hydrolysis and condensation reactions occur in a colloidal solution containing the precursors, catalyst, water, and sometimes a co-solvent. These reactions lead to polymerization and the formation of a 3D network. In the second stage, this network evolves into a gelled, porous solid structure filled with liquid. Depending on the drying process, the gel can yield different products. This includes supercritical drying which produces aerogels with extremely low density, while slow evaporation yields xerogels, which are fragile solids. Finally, sintering of the xerogel produces dense, pore-free ceramics. Overall, sol–gel processing provides a flexible pathway for fabricating a wide variety of inorganic materials, including ceramic NPs and quantum-confined oxide particles.

4.2.1.2.1.2. *Spray Pyrolysis*

SP is a cost-effective and scalable technique for producing nanomaterials and thin films by atomizing a precursor solution or suspension into a heated environment, where droplets undergo evaporation, decomposition, and phase transitions to form solid particles or uniform coatings on a substrate [172]. This method enables the fabrication of metals, semiconductors, and ceramics with high purity and controlled morphology, making it suitable for both laboratory and industrial applications. However, challenges such as nozzle deterioration, fluctuations in solution concentration, and droplet variability can affect particle size distribution, film uniformity, and overall material quality. Despite these limitations, SP remains a versatile, single-step process for creating dense ceramic powders and thin films with broad technological applications.

4.2.1.2.1.3. *Hydrothermal Synthesis*

Hydrothermal synthesis is an environmentally friendly and cost-effective method that uses water as the reaction medium instead of organic solvents. In this process, precursors containing the desired cations and anions are reacted in an autoclave at elevated temperatures (typically ~160°C). The dissolved species migrate under temperature gradients, leading to supersaturation, nucleation, and subsequent crystal growth through adsorption, decomposition, and incorporation at the growth interface [173–175]. The resulting precipitates are filtered, washed to remove by-products and prevent agglomeration, and then dried (often at ~110°C) to obtain the final product. This method enables controlled nucleation and grain growth, making it highly effective for producing nanostructured ceramics with tailored microstructures and properties.

4.2.1.2.1.4. *Self-Propagating High-Temperature Synthesis*

SHS is an exothermic, self-sustaining process that enables the rapid production of advanced materials such as ceramics, nitrides, borides, carbides, oxides, and intermetallic compounds. Once the reactants are ignited, the heat released propagates as a combustion wave through the mixture, eliminating the need for continuous external heating [176]. This allows powders or bulk materials to be synthesized and even sintered in a single step (SHS-sintering), bypassing the conventional multistage process of powder production, milling, and sintering. The unique advantage of SHS lies in its ability to achieve extremely high temperatures in very short timescales, promoting phase formation, mass transfer, and densification. For non-oxide ceramics, where covalent bonding restricts atomic mobility and slows solid-state sintering, SHS facilitates consolidation either through liquid-phase sintering with additives or *via* reaction bonding. Additional benefits include self-purification, structural uniformity, and predictable control over particle size and morphology, making SHS an efficient and versatile route for producing high-performance materials [177].

4.2.2. *Nanocomposite Scaffolds*

Nanocomposites are defined as the combination of multiple materials or phases such that the resulting composite has at least one dimension in the nanoscale range. Nanocomposite scaffolds are widely used within the fields of tissue engineering and regenerative medicine due to their ability to mimic natural biological properties and their flexibility for modification to meet the functional needs of specific tissue types or bone regions. Scaffolds, by nature, are support structures; thus, nanocomposite scaffolds aim to guide cellular processes toward regeneration, proliferation, and differentiation [178]. Similar to nanostructured metals and ceramics, nanocomposite scaffolds will ideally be biodegradable and biocompatible with the host, with sufficient mechanical and physical characteristics (e.g., a high elastic modulus) for their usage. Pores, at a cellular level, are critical for cell permeation and movement as well as nutrient delivery. Thus, the porosity of nanocomposite scaffolds promotes cell spreading and the transport of oxygen, waste, nutrients, and growth factors, extends the degradation time, and facilitates the regeneration and development of bone tissue [179]. Although metal- and ceramic-based composites exist, this section focuses on polymer-based composites.

4.2.2.1. Natural-Based Polymeric Scaffolds

Natural polymers are gaining popularity for their use in nanocomposite scaffolds due to their innate, biocompatible nature, biomineralization capabilities, and potential ligands that can interact with cell surface receptors to enhance osteogenesis [180]. Due to their high integration within the bone ECM, proteins, such as collagen and its denatured form gelatin, are favored as natural-based materials. Fibrous proteins such as collagen are found in bone, cartilage, and blood vessel walls, attesting to their noncytotoxic, biocompatible, and biodegradable properties. The downside of collagen includes its low mechanical strength, limited elasticity, and poor dimensional stability *in vivo* due to swelling [181]. In this respect, gelatin may be more preferential, having higher solubility, improved plane strain modulus, fracture toughness, and lower cost [181]. Another class of protein of interest is silk, which is composed of fibroin and sericin. Silk fibroin scaffolds have been reported to be fabricated onto nanosized CaP scaffolds, and the results demonstrated new bone growth directly on the surface of the implants, attesting to their osteoconductive and anti-inflammatory properties [182].

Polysaccharides, such as chitosan (CS), gelatin gum derivatives, and alginate, are also being investigated as materials for nanocomposite scaffolding. Chitin and CS are derived from the organic matrix of arthropod exoskeletons and mollusk endoskeletons. They are also essential components of fungal and algal cell walls; however, CS derived from exoskeletons or endoskeletons is often easier to isolate and incorporate [183]. As a cationic polymer, CS engages electrostatically with negatively charged biomolecules and receptors. It shows promising properties such as biocompatibility, support for cell ingrowth, and a uniquely intrinsic antibacterial nature, but it is not by itself osteoconductive and has low mechanical strength [184]. When combined in a nanocomposite scaffolding approach, CS may be useful in bone regeneration. Zhang et al. utilized 3D porous CS/HA scaffolds that showed a higher degree of cell proliferation and cell adhesion, along with a 33.1% increase in compressive strength and six times more alkaline phosphatase activity compared to pure CS scaffolds [185]. Alginate, an anionic and hydrophilic polysaccharide, is another scaffolding option derived from bacteria and brown seaweed. Alginate also shares strong biocompatibility and biodegradability, along with other common characteristics common to proteins and polysaccharides [186]. Due to its hydrophilic and water-soluble properties, alginate is mostly incorporated in hydrogels, which are 3D cross-linked network polymers of high water content.

Injectable hydrogels are particularly useful in minimally invasive applications in surgery, which can prove useful in surgical orthopedic settings. Nanocomposite hydrogels may serve as a targeted, flexible, natural-based material and may be combined with other biomimetic nanocomposites of glycosaminoglycans, such as hyaluronic acid or CaP. Hyaluronic acid is also innately part of the bone ECM with a strong water-binding ability and viscoelasticity [181]. It can be chemically modified, and its incorporation into cross-linked networks promotes neocartilage formation [187].

4.2.2.2. Synthetic-Based Polymeric Scaffolds

Although natural-based materials may have advantages due to their innate biodegradable and biocompatible properties, synthetic polymers are growing nanocomposite materials of interest. This is largely due to their customizable degradation kinetics and mechanical properties [188]. Synthetic polymers of interest include PCL, PLA, and PLGA. PCL, for example, is a thermoplastic material, which means it can be softened and/or melted by an increase in temperature or heat. Alone, these properties are of limited use in orthopedic applications, but when integrated into a scaffold, such as a PCL/TiO_2 composite, they reportedly show improved mechanical properties, pore structure, and increasing trend for enhanced cell viability and differentiation, leading to ECM mineralization [189]. Both synthetic- and natural-based polymers may be conjugated with metallic or ceramic nanocomposite scaffolds. Combining CaP within composite scaffolds can help deflect their shortcomings. These composite scaffolds have been shown to exhibit strong osteogenesis, stiffness, and potential as a preferable tool for bone defect repair [190]. BG, on the other hand, is an amorphous, silicate-based material that has previously received approval from the U.S. Food and Drug Administration (FDA) for use as a bone filler in periodontal disease treatments, as well as for bone implants used in middle ear surgery [191]. It is famously efficient in drug delivery, attributed to its porous structure, surface area, biodegradability, and biocompatibility [188]. However, it still suffers from drawbacks such as low mechanical strength and limited flexibility, which can be overcome by combining it with other biomaterials, for example, through the use of nanocomposite scaffolds.

Additive manufacturing, more popularly known as 3D printing, may also be a promising avenue of interest for biopolymer/ceramic-based nanocomposite scaffolding, particularly in drug delivery [188]. This technique combines a natural/synthetic polymer solution with ceramic powder, thus incorporating nanocomposites such as polymer–nanoceramics, NPs, and nanofibers. 3D printing is not limited to a specific material type, as long as the ideal material is in abundance and can effectively undergo computer-aided reconstruction of a model [192]. This is currently of high interest within nanocomposite scaffold research, as it can aid in the reduction of material costs and allow for effective control, flexibility, and accessibility as per the patient's clinical needs (**Figure 6**).

MNPs can also be used to enhance the properties of composite scaffolds by providing local mechano-activation, reducing intracellular H_2O_2, and promoting osteogenic signaling [193–195]. As a result, MNP-functionalized scaffolds have been reported to improve cell growth and significantly enhance bone regeneration *in vitro* and *in vivo*. Banafsheh et al. studied a biofunctional magnetic scaffold that utilized MNPs and phosphorylated PCL combined with gelatin. Human dental pulp stem cells showed no cytotoxicity after integration within the magnetic scaffold. The use of MNPs allowed for greater alkaline phosphatase activity, which is significant given its role during stem cell differentiation into osteoblast phenotypes, and for the increased expression of osteogenic biomarkers such as RUNX2 and BMP-2 [196].

4.2.2.3. Synthesis of Nanocomposites

4.2.2.3.1. Electrospinning

Electrospinning has been extensively investigated and is a simple method for producing porous nanofibers. The fabricated polymeric nanofibers provide a large surface area with increased mechanical properties and appropriate structures for cell attachment, thereby making them favorable for use in biomedical and tissue engineering [197]. The application of an electrical field between two electrodes — one placed in the polymer solution and the other on the collector — causes the liquid to become charged. At the critical point of liquid stream eruption, the electrostatic repulsion

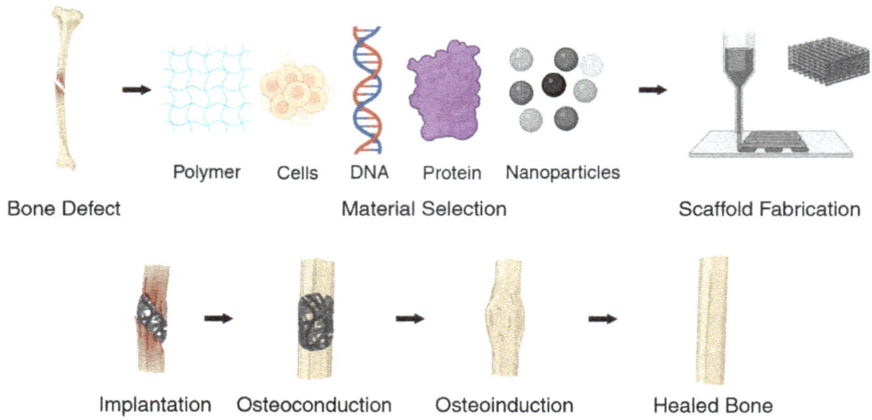

Figure 6. The process of bone tissue engineering using 3D printing and 3D bioprinting. To fill a bone defect, the appropriate materials must be selected to create a composite scaffold. Such materials include, but are not limited to, polymers, metals, ceramics, cells, RNA, proteins, and various NPs. Following the material selection, the scaffold is fabricated using a variety of 3D bioprinting methods. In this figure, extrusion-based bioprinting is depicted. Then, the scaffold is implanted to occupy the void of the bone defect. With the help of the scaffold, osteoconduction and osteoinduction will help populate the defect over time to completely heal the bone (created with BioRender.com).

overcomes the surface tension, and the polymer solution held at the needle tip by surface tension is ejected from the nozzle, producing the fibers [197]. The properties of the fabricated nanofibers vary based on the solution type and processing parameters such as electrical field intensity, polymer concentration, and flow rate. Electrospinning of nanofiber-based scaffolds is efficient, simple, and enforces the required characteristics for biomedical applications [197]. For example, Patel et al. synthesized a PLA and cellulose nanocrystal nanocomposite scaffold using the electrospinning technique for bone tissue repair [198]. The nanocomposite scaffold exhibited higher thermal stability, excellent proliferation, superior biocompatibility, higher mineralization, and increased expression of osteogenic gene markers compared to pure polymer scaffolds. In addition, a rat calvarial defect model was used to monitor the bone regeneration potential of the fabricated nanocomposite scaffold. The results confirmed excellent biocompatibility and superior osteoinductivity compared to control animals [198]. Recently, drug-eluting nanofibrous scaffolds fabricated using

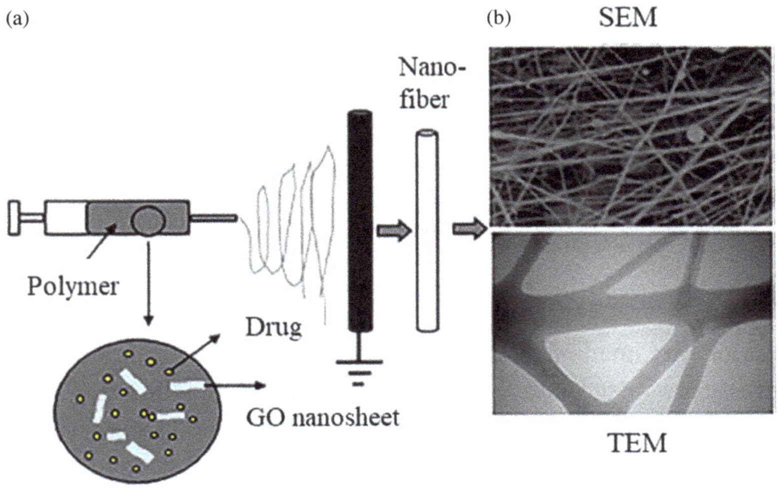

Figure 7. (a) A schematic of the nanofiber production process and the development of a scaffold composed of PCL and GO. (b) SEM and TEM images of the synthesized nanofibers (reprinted from ref. [199] with permission from Elsevier).

electrospinning technology have gained considerable interest for biomimicking the ECM in regenerative medicine. For instance, Rostami et al. synthesized an electrospun nanocomposite scaffold composed of PCL, GO nanosheets, and an osteogenic drug (dexamethasone) (**Figure 7**) [199]. Their study showed that the addition of GO and dexamethasone improved the hydrophilicity, cell viability, osteogenic differentiation, and biomineralization of the scaffold compared with PCL-only scaffolds [199].

4.2.2.3.2. Solvent/Solution Casting

Solvent casting is a method in which a dissolved polymer in a suitable solvent is mixed with NPs and then cast into a mold, followed by solvent evaporation. This method has been widely used because it is simple with no need for equipment and can offer the desired properties for bone regeneration [200]. Mohan et al. synthesized polyhydroxy butyrate (PHB)-based nanocomposites using nano-clay with modified montmorillonite (MMT) *via* the solvent-casting technique [201]. The results revealed that the loading percentage of MMT affected the matrix structure. The dispersed MMT

NPs supported pore formation on the surface of the polymer, and the pore size was proportional to the weight percentage of MMT. The PHB/MMT nanocomposite displayed enhanced thermal stability, improved porosity, a non-immunogenic nature, and strong biocompatibility compared to the pure polymer. This suggests the promising potential of this nanocomposite in bone tissue engineering applications [201].

4.2.2.3.3. Infiltration

Infiltration is a method of nanocomposite fabrication in which NPs or nanofibers are mixed in a molten matrix metal. In this method, NPs fill the spaces between the dispersed phase inclusions and change the matrix structure [202]. External pressure such as mechanical, centrifugal, or ultrasonic can be applied to obtain a homogeneous dispersion of NPs in the molten metal matrix [202]. Parande et al. fabricated a Mg-based alloy/HA nanocomposite using this technique [203]. Their evaluation showed that the addition of HA resulted in significant grain refinement of the Mg alloy matrix. The results revealed that adding HA enhanced the yield strength, Young's modulus, ductility, and corrosion resistance under compression loading in the nanocomposite compared to the Mg alloy alone. In addition, incorporating HA enhanced the hydrophilicity of the Mg alloy, leading to increased cell attachment without inducing cytotoxicity. Hence, Mg alloy–based HA nanocomposites may be a new candidate for bone repair applications [203].

4.2.2.3.4. Electrophoretic Deposition

Electrophoretic deposition (EPD) is a simple method for producing composite coatings. During EPD, charged NPs are dispersed in a stable solvent under an electric field between two electrodes and deposited onto a conductive substrate of opposite charge [204, 205]. The main driving force in the EPD method is the electrophoretic movement of charged particles in the solvent under the influence of the applied electric field [205, 206]. EPD as a coating methodology for biomaterials has numerous advantages, such as the need for simple equipment, no limitation on substrate shape, the possibility to deposit temperature-sensitive biomaterials at room temperature, and homogeneous, high-purity coatings [204–206]. Singh et al. fabricated a BG and Fe_3O_4 nanocomposite coating to improve the bioactivity and antibacterial properties of CS [206]. The nanocomposite coating was embedded in a CS matrix using the EPD method. SEM/energy-dispersive X-ray analysis (EDX) and XRD, respectively, confirmed the coating. In terms of their antibacterial properties, results showed that after adding the Fe_3O_4 NPs, microorganism growth was reduced significantly. Further, the evaluation of scaffold bioactivity confirmed improved bone bonding of the nanocomposite compared to the pure polymer. Moreover, the corrosion resistance of the BG–1% Fe_3O_4 nanocomposite coating showed superior corrosion resistance compared to other formulations investigated [207] (**Figure 8**).

EPD offers easy control of the thickness and morphology of a deposited film through simple adjustments of the suspension, such as particle size, dielectric constant of liquid, conductivity of suspension, viscosity of the suspension, zeta potential, and stability of the suspension. Moreover, parameters related to the EPD process can simply control the nanocomposite characteristics. For example, this includes alteration of the deposition time, applied voltage, NP concentration in the suspension, and substrate conductivity.

4.2.2.4. Characterization

The toxicity of nanostructured implants and nanocomposites is a crucial factor that needs to be considered. Hence, a comprehensive investigation of these materials is required to enable their use in biomedical applications [208]. A 3-(4,5-dimethylthiazol-2-yl)-2,5-diphenyltetrazolium bromide assay and live-dead assay are methods used to measure alterations in cell viability and cell proliferation when cells are subjected to fabricated nanocomposites [209, 210]. Other biological tests are performed based on the specific nanocomposite application. For example, related gene expression, osteogenesis (alkaline phosphatase activity or alizarin red staining), angiogenesis (tube formation or scratch test), and antibacterial (disc diffusion) evaluation can also provide vital information to prove the usefulness of fabricated nanocomposites and their applicability in bone regeneration [210–212]. Surface and chemical analyses of nanostructured implants and

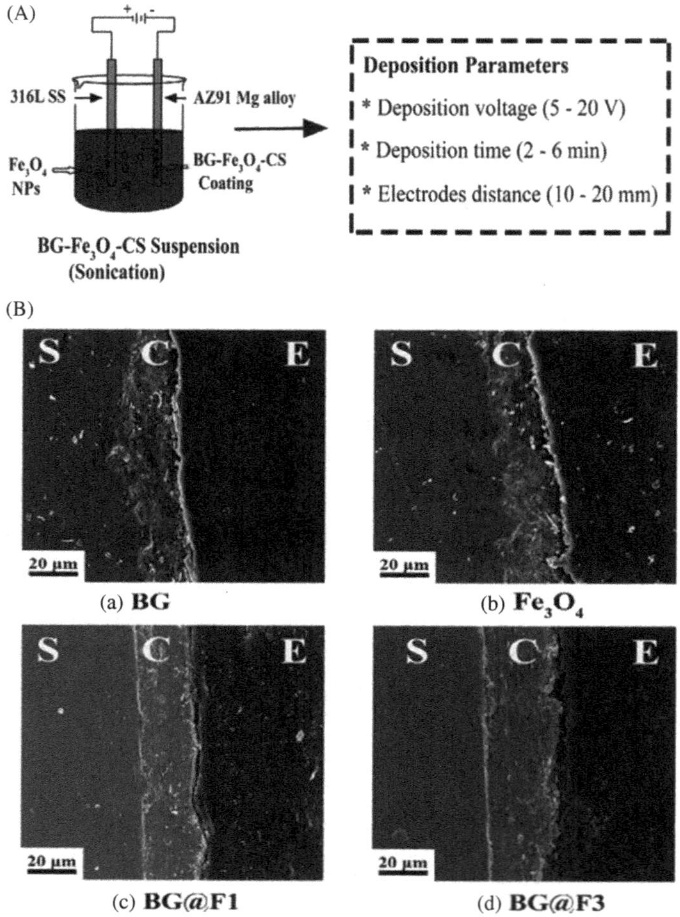

Figure 8. (A) The synthesis process of a bioglass (BG)–iron oxide (Fe_3O_4)–chitosan (CS) nanocomposite BG–Fe_3O_4–CS coating on an AZ91 Mg alloy *via* the EPD method. (B) SEM images of electrophoretically deposited: (a) BG, (b) Fe_3O_4, (c) BG–1 wt.% Fe_3O_4, (BG@F1), (d) BG–3 wt.% Fe_3O_4 (BG@F3) (reprinted from ref. [207] with permission from Elsevier).

nanocomposites are beneficial by providing information on the chemical composition of nanocomposites and types of chemical bonds present on the surface [213]. FTIR, Raman spectroscopy, and SEM/EDX are frequently used for surface characterization [214, 215]. In addition, performing glow discharge spectrometry and inductively coupled plasma spectroscopy can aid in characterizing the concentration of the deposited layer on the nanocomposite surface and ion release from the implants. Mechanical characterization of nanostructured implants and nanocomposites is also necessary to determine mechanical durability [213]. The most common mechanical tests used to study these properties are compression tests, tensile tests, hardness tests, failure analysis, and dynamic mechanical analysis [213, 216, 217]. Mechanical characterization of a fabricated nanocomposite can give us insight into the performance of a nanocomposite when subjected to operational and physiological loads.

5. Nanostructures for Drug Delivery

5.1. *Introduction*

Ceramic, metallic, and polymeric 3D scaffolds can be used to mechanically support load-bearing bone as well as act as a delivery method for nanotherapeutics. Much research continues to be done on the use of scaffolds loaded with NPs and nanotherapeutics, such as drug delivery systems. This is because scaffolds can be designed to precisely imitate the complex structure of bone tissue, restoring mechanical stability to load-bearing bone tissue while delivering regenerative therapeutics [44]. In some cases, nanoencapsulation of therapeutics or biomolecules can increase their delivery efficiency through avoidance of early-stage degradation (**Figure 9**). This section focuses on nanotechnology-based drug delivery for bone regeneration, including inorganic, organic, and composite systems.

5.2. *Classification*

5.2.1. *Inorganic Nanostructure Systems*

Ceramics have been a commonly used drug delivery method for bone repair and regeneration, particularly because of their osteoconductive nature. The most common types of ceramics are particle-based HA, CaP, or TCP. Modifying ceramics by changing their surface roughness or topography can influence the absorption of therapeutic molecules.

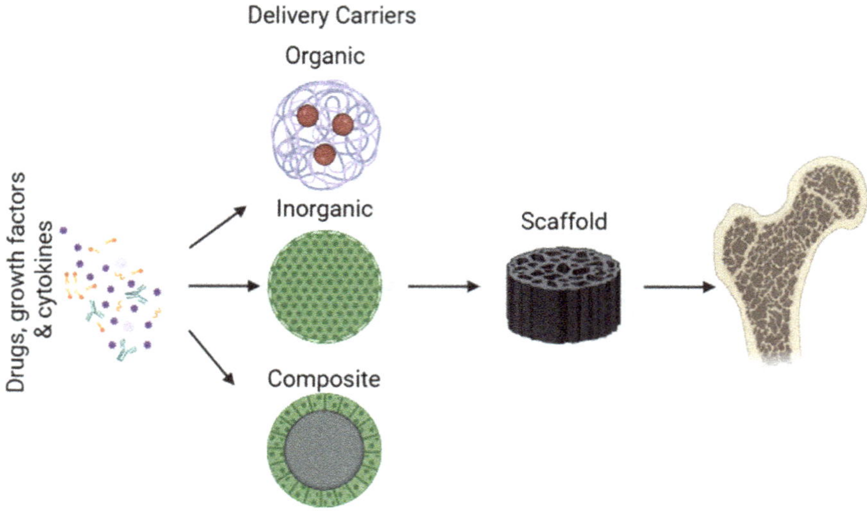

Figure 9. A schematic illustration of organic, inorganic, and composite nanotherapeutic delivery methods to a scaffold (created with BioRender.com).

Nanotherapeutic delivery methods may allow more controlled release of smaller quantities of rhBMP-2 or other drugs, potentially minimizing their adverse effects. rhBMP-2 is an FDA-approved treatment for clinical use in bone healing and repair. One potential downside to this treatment is that there is an increased relative dosage of growth factors required in human models compared to rat models. However, high doses of rhBMP-2 increase the risk for edema [44, 218]. Huang et al. demonstrated improved bioactivity of rhBMP-2 on a rougher, crystal-coated polished surface of HA compared to a non-polished, crystal-coated surface and a sintered, crystal-coated surface [219]. Surface functionalization can further enhance bone healing. One clinical application involved surface functionalization of HA-based ceramics to increase the binding affinity for rhBMP-2, allowing for its more sustained release [220]. A primary concern with ceramic-based NP delivery systems is poor biodegradation [5]. There are still key challenges for the nano-HA-based drug delivery systems, including biocompatibility, safety assessment, and regulatory approval. Besides, scalability remains a challenge due to the need for cost-effective, reproducible large-scale production [221].

Metallic oxide compounds in the form of tubules are another example of inorganic nanostructured delivery systems. These tubules may be made of silica (SiO_2), TiO_2, or other metalloid oxides, each possessing its distinct properties. Similar to ceramic-based materials, SiO_2-based tubules can be functionalized to bind specific molecules to facilitate their sustained release. In addition, SiO_2-based tubules can promote cell adhesion and differentiation. Studies have shown that TiO_2 shares many of these same beneficial qualities but can lead to dose-dependent cytotoxicity. The mechanism of this is not fully understood at this time, though it is postulated that metallic compounds can induce apoptosis of osteoblasts due to their high affinity to adhere together [5]. Other inorganic NPs for bone healing, including zirconia, bioactive glass, metals, and carbon-based NPs, have been previously and extensively reviewed [15].

5.2.2. *Organic Nanostructure Systems*

As an alternative to inorganic nanostructure delivery systems, research is also being conducted using organic nanoscale polymers for drug delivery. Organic nanoscaled polymers harness similar advantages to other nanomedicines and over their larger counterparts, such as high effective surface area and enhanced cell permeability, which increase drug delivery [222, 223]. Of key importance, organic nanoscale polymers have great stability and easily functionalized surfaces, which are immensely beneficial for improving drug targeting capabilities and preventing NP agglomeration [223]. These polymers can be synthetic or natural, each with slightly different qualities. Common examples of synthetic polymers include PEG, PLGA, PCL, PLA, PGA, and poly(propylene fumarate) [224]. Research has demonstrated both the benefits and disadvantages of using these different synthetic polymers to deliver drugs such as BMP-2, steroids, and antibiotics. PEG, PCL, and PLGA are synthetic polymers reported to have the greatest biocompatibility. Of these, PLGA is favored due to FDA approval and its structure and degradation rates. Unfortunately, degradation products of many of these polymers can be cytotoxic, and therefore, their degradation should be controlled accordingly [5]. Growth factors, such as BMP, can be encapsulated in PLGA and PEG NPs and released sustainably over time to enhance bone regeneration [225]. Lipids are another organic nanostructure capable of delivering both hydrophobic and hydrophilic compounds by encapsulation. However, they require a modification to be thermodynamically stabilized against physicochemical and mechanical tensions [226]. The encapsulation strategy protects bioactive ingredients by preventing premature leakage and enabling controlled release. Lipid-based matrices include solid lipid NPs, nanostructured lipid carriers, and nanoemulsions [226]. Perfluorocarbons (PFCs) are safe, biocompatible compounds that play a key role in advanced medical imaging by more effectively detecting physiological and pathological changes [227]. Beyond imaging, PFC-based NPs and nanodroplets have been developed as innovative gene and drug delivery treatments [228]. An ultrasound-responsive nanobubble (NB) carrier with a PFC gas core was recently studied as a novel method to treat osteoporosis. The NBs were loaded with gene-silencing cathepsin K siRNA and cerium oxide NPS and delivered with the goal of targeting and strengthening bone [112]. *In vitro* analysis showed enhanced osteogenic activity and the inhibition of osteoclastogenesis. Notably, an *in vivo* study conducted in mice showed successful bone targeting, improved bone microarchitecture, reduced bone resorption, and no signs of toxicity [228].

5.2.3. *Composite Nanostructure Systems*

Although there are a variety of materials available for nanotherapeutic delivery, each one often comes with its distinct advantages and disadvantages. Composite delivery systems allow us to overcome the limitations of individual materials. By combining multiple materials into a single delivery system, their synergistic interactions can yield enhanced performance compared to the individual components alone. As a result, the benefits of each material can be maximized while mitigating potential drawbacks from individual materials; this can be leveraged in a way that allows for better overall functionality. Compared to larger composites, nanoscale composites allow for several improved physicochemical properties, including improved solution dispersion, drug release characteristics, and drug penetration [229]. Research is currently being carried out on different combinations of composites using individual materials, such as ceramics, metallic compounds, and polymers. Polymers are well-known components in composite systems for their ability to be linked together and functionalized. As previously described, ceramics can also be used in composite delivery systems due to their high osteoconductivity [230]. Some of these composite delivery systems have well-controlled drug release rates, good bioavailability, and osteogenic and osteoconductive properties. Several combinations of polymer and HA composite materials have been researched for delivering BMP-2 in a controlled and sustained fashion. Su et al. produced a nanocomposite scaffold from PLGA, PCL, and nano-HA that demonstrated improved BMP-2 release [231]. The development of optimized, biocompatible composite drug delivery systems capable of releasing drugs in response to external forces — such as physical, chemical, or ultrasound stimuli — could be groundbreaking in bone healing and regeneration, ensuring both efficacy and safety [5] (**Figure 10**). Physical

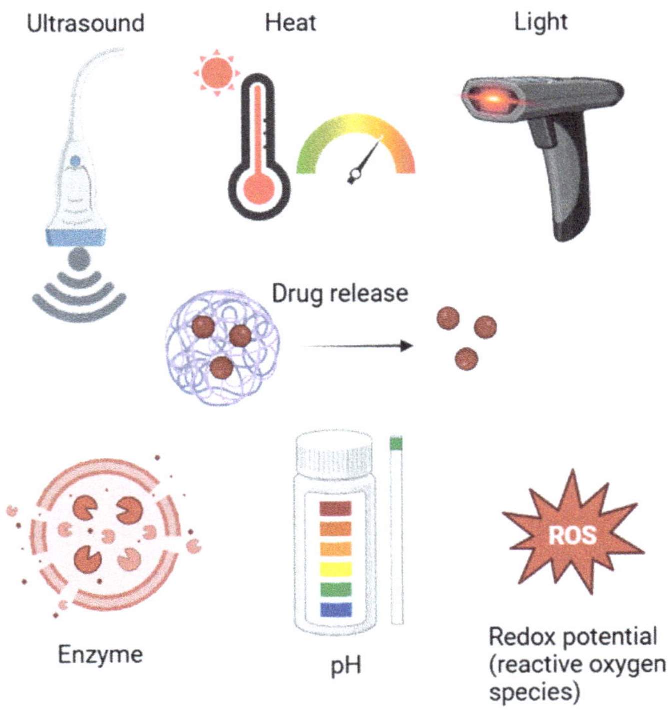

Figure 10. Enhanced drug delivery by the combination of physical, chemical, and ultrasound stimulation (created with BioRender.com).

stimuli include heat- and light-responsive systems. For example, antibacterial peptides can be encapsulated in poly(N-isopropylacrylamide) at lower temperatures and released by increasing the temperature to 33°C [232]. In the case of chemical stimulation, pH adjustment, redox potential, and enzyme activity have been studied over the years. For instance, CS NPs loaded with tamoxifen can be utilized for targeted drug delivery in tumor treatment [233]. The release of tamoxifen was found to be more efficient at pH levels 4 and 6 compared to pH 7 and above. Ultrasound can be utilized for targeted and controlled drug delivery by triggering the expansion of drug-loaded NPs when exposed to ultrasonic energy, thereby facilitating drug release. For instance, in a study, tetrodotoxin and protoporphyrin IX were encapsulated in micrometric liposomes, and ultrasound exposure generated ROS. These ROS interacted with the liposome membrane, causing instability and subsequent release of tetrodotoxin [234].

6. Conclusions

The purpose of this chapter was to discuss nanotechnology in bone regeneration. The advancement of nanotechnology in recent years has attracted the scientific community to focus on its merits for bone regeneration and orthopedic challenges. NPs, advanced nanomaterials, nanostructured implants, nanocomposites, and nanostructures for drug delivery were discussed. Significant progress has been made to address the potential challenges associated with using advanced nanomaterials. As the clinical presence of these novel materials continues to rise, physicians and the medical community should consider adapting to these revolutionary alternative treatments. However, currently, most of this technology remains in the developmental stage, and although the present research has been promising, once optimized, future pursuits should aim to add more clarity through specifying therapeutic indications, identifying potential side effects, and ultimately conducting clinical trials.

The variable use of nanostructured implants and nanocomposite scaffolds in the context of orthopedics and bone regeneration was discussed, with a focus on the range of materials used, their synthetic methods, characterization methods, and their applications in industry and clinical settings.

As nanotechnology in orthopedics is a relatively novel field, more combinations and approaches within nanostructured implants and nanocomposites still need to be explored. However, given the demonstrated biocompatible, biodegradable, and long-lasting effects and results within the bone ECM, the use of these technologies should be given serious consideration by physicians and researchers as well. Systemic nanotherapeutic strategies that deliver growth factors, cytokines, and drugs have been used for a wide range of medical applications. Indeed, many of these delivery systems show highly efficacious results, with some having gained FDA approval for the treatment of cancer and infectious diseases. Thus, nanotherapeutics have the potential to play an important role in the future treatment of bone-related pathologies. Although a significant amount of research has already been conducted within the field of bone regeneration, the development and use of systemic nanotherapeutics as a whole is still in its infancy. Nonetheless, nanotherapeutic delivery systems show promise, but their real clinical applications outside of novel experimentation are yet to be determined within the orthopedic arena. It is possible that the right nanotherapeutic drug coupled with an optimal delivery system could be the breakthrough needed to treat debilitating bone diseases. Given the increasing global relevance of our aging population as well as space travel, research into regenerative bone therapeutics to address age- and microgravity-related bone loss will become a priority in biomedical research. Nanotechnology demonstrates significant potential for improving the precision of bone regenerative therapeutics and enhancing bone defect repair, leading to improved clinical outcomes.

References

1. Mohamed AM. An overview of bone cells and their regulating factors of differentiation. *Malays. J. Med. Sci.* 2008;15(1):4.
2. Lin X, Patil S, Gao Y-G, Qian A. The bone extracellular matrix in bone formation and regeneration. *Front. Pharmacol.* 2020;11:757.
3. Sheen JR, Mabrouk A, Garla VV. Fracture Healing Overview. In: StatPearls [Internet]. StatPearls Publishing; 2023.
4. Li Y, Chen S-K, Li L, Qin L, Wang X-L, Lai Y-X. Bone defect animal models for testing efficacy of bone substitute biomaterials. *J. Orthop. Translat.* 2015;3(3):95–104.

5. Lyons JG, Plantz Ma, Hsu WK, Hsu EL, Minardi S. Nanostructured biomaterials for bone regeneration. *Front. Bioeng. Biotechnol.* 2020;8:922.
6. Wu Q, Miao W-S, Zhang Y-D, Gao H-J, Hui D. Mechanical properties of nanomaterials: A review. *Nanotechnol. Rev.* 2020;9(1):259–73.
7. Kyriakides TR, Raj A, Tseng TH, Xiao H, Nguyen R, Mohammed FS, et al. Biocompatibility of nanomaterials and their immunological properties, *Biomed. Mater.* 2021;16(4):042005.
8. Baig N, Kammakakam I, Falath W. Nanomaterials: A review of synthesis methods, properties, recent progress, and challenges. *Mate. Adv.* 2021;2(6):1821–71.
9. Gou Y, Qi K, Wei Y, Gu Z, Xie H. Advances of calcium phosphate nanoceramics for the osteoinductive potential and mechanistic pathways in maxillofacial bone defect repair. *Nano TransMed.* 2024;3:100033.
10. Abbasi R, Shineh G, Mobaraki M, Doughty S, Tayebi L. Structural parameters of nanoparticles affecting their toxicity for biomedical applications: A review. *J. Nanopart. Res.* 2023;25(3):43.
11. Das KK, Basu B, Maiti P, Dubey AK. Interplay of piezoelectricity and electrical stimulation in tissue engineering and regenerative medicine. *Appl. Mater. Today* 2024;39:102332.
12. Tautzenberger A, Kovtun A, Ignatius A. Nanoparticles and their potential for application in bone. *Int. J. Nanomed.* 2012:4545–57.
13. Khan Y, Sadia H, Ali Shah SZ, Khan MN, Shah AA, Ullah N, et al. Classification, synthetic, and characterization approaches to nanoparticles, and their applications in various fields of nanotechnology: A review. *Catalysts* 2022;12(11):1386.
14. Alshammari BH, Lashin MM, Mahmood MA, Al-Mubaddel FS, Ilyas N, Rahman N, et al. Organic and inorganic nanomaterials: Fabrication, properties and applications. *RSC Adv.* 2023;13(20):13735–85.
15. Farjaminejad S, Farjaminejad R, Garcia-Godoy F. Nanoparticles in bone regeneration: A narrative review of current advances and future directions in tissue engineering. *J. Funct. Biomater.* 2024;15(9):241.
16. Farjaminejad S, Hasani M, Farjaminejad R, Foroozandeh A, Abdouss M, Hasanzadeh M. Hydroxyapatites and nano-hydroxyapatites as scaffolds in drug delivery towards efficient bone regeneration: A review. *Carbohydr. Polym. Technol. App.* 2025;9:100692.
17. Wang B, Wu Z, Wang S, Ang S, Niu Q, Wu Y, et al. Mg/Cu-doped TiO2 nanotube array: A novel dual-function system with self-antibacterial activity and excellent cell compatibility. *Mater. Sci. Eng.C* 2021;128:112322.

18. Shadjou N, Hasanzadeh M. Silica-based mesoporous nanobiomaterials as promoter of bone regeneration process. *J. Biomed. Mater. Res. A* 2015; 103(11):3703–16.
19. Nisha A, Bhardwaj R, Verma M, Acharya A. Functionalized nanoclays in bioactive materials. *Compos. Interfaces* 2024;31(7):857–81.
20. Cheung H-Y, Yip S, Han N, Dong G, Fang M, Yang Z-X, et al. Modulating electrical properties of InAs nanowires via molecular monolayers. *ACS Nano* 2015;9(7):7545–52.
21. Giljohann DA, Seferos DS, Daniel WL, Massich MD, Patel PC, Mirkin CA. Gold nanoparticles for biology and medicine. *Spher. Nucl. Acids* 2020: 55–90.
22. Yoshida YG, Yan S, Xu H, Yang J. Novel metal nanomaterials to promote angiogenesis in tissue regeneration. *Eng. Regen.* 2023;4(3):265–76.
23. Khan MM, Deen KM, Haider W. Combinatorial development and assessment of a Zr-based metallic glass for prospective biomedical applications. *J. Non-Cryst. Solids* 2019;523:119544.
24. Polo-Corrales L, Latorre-Esteves M, Ramirez-Vick JE. Scaffold design for bone regeneration. *J. Nanosci. Nanotechnol.* 2014;14(1):15–56.
25. Akturk A, Erol Taygun M, Goller G. Optimization of the electrospinning process variables for gelatin/silver nanoparticles/bioactive glass nanocomposites for bone tissue engineering. *Polym. Comp.* 2020;41(6): 2411–25.
26. Md Yusop AH, Ulum MF, Al Sakkaf A, Hartanto D, Nur H. Insight into the bioabsorption of Fe-based materials and their current developments in bone applications. *Biotechnol. J.* 2021;16(12): 2100255.
27. Priya BA, Senthilguru K, Agarwal T, Narayana SGH, Giri S, Pramanik K, et al. Nickel doped nanohydroxyapatite: Vascular endothelial growth factor inducing biomaterial for bone tissue engineering. *RSC Adv.* 2015;5(89): 72515–28.
28. Farjaminejad S, Farjaminejad R, Sotoudehbagha P, Razavi M. Non-invasive medical imaging in the evaluation of composite scaffolds in tissue engineering: Methods, challenges, and future directions. *J. Compos. Sci.* 2025;9(8):400.
29. Berry CC. Possible exploitation of magnetic nanoparticle–cell interaction for biomedical applications. *J. Mater. Chem.* 2005;15(5):543–7.
30. Arami H, Khandhar A, Liggitt D, Krishnan KM. In vivo delivery, pharmacokinetics, biodistribution and toxicity of iron oxide nanoparticles. *Chem. Soc. Rev.* 2015;44(23):8576–8607.
31. Li Y, Ye D, Li M, Ma M, Gu N. Adaptive materials based on iron oxide nanoparticles for bone regeneration. *ChemPhysChem.* 2018;19(16):1965–79.

32. Friedrich RP, Cicha I, Alexiou C. Iron oxide nanoparticles in regenerative medicine and tissue engineering. *Nanomaterials* 2021;11(9):2337.
33. Qi H, Zhang C. Organic nanoparticles for electrogenerated chemiluminescence assay. *Curr Opin Electrochem* 2022;34:101023.
34. Rao JP, Geckeler KE. Polymer nanoparticles: Preparation techniques and size-control parameters. *Prog. Polym. Sci.* 2011;36(7):887–913.
35. Chenthamara D, Subramaniam S, Ramakrishnan SG, Krishnaswamy S, Essa MM, Lin F-H, et al. Therapeutic efficacy of nanoparticles and routes of administration. *Biomater. Res.* 2019;23(1):20.
36. Zhang G, Zhen C, Yang J, Wang J, Wang S, Fang Y, et al. Recent advances of nanoparticles on bone tissue engineering and bone cells. *Nanoscale Adv.* 2024;6(8):1957–73.
37. Vieira S, Vial S, Reis RL, Oliveira JM. Nanoparticles for bone tissue engineering. *Biotechnol. Prog.* 2017;33(3):590–611.
38. Bozzuto G, Molinari A. Liposomes as nanomedical devices. *Int. J. Nanomed.* 2015:975–99.
39. Yuba E, Tajima N, Yoshizaki Y, Harada A, Hayashi H, Kono K. Dextran derivative-based pH-sensitive liposomes for cancer immunotherapy. *Biomaterials* 2014;35(9):3091–101.
40. Kang M, Lee C-S, Lee M. Bioactive scaffolds integrated with liposomal or extracellular vesicles for bone regeneration. *Bioengineering* 2021;8(10):137.
41. Carreiró F, Oliveira FM, Neves A, Pires B, Nagasamy Venkatesh D, Durazzo A, et al. Polymeric nanoparticles: Production, characterization, toxicology and ecotoxicology. *Molecules* 2020;25:3731.
42. Kim Y, Park EJ, Na EH. Recent progress in dendrimer-based nanomedicine development. *Arch. Pharm. Res.* 2018;41(6):571–82.
43. Chauhan AS. Dendrimers for drug delivery. *Molecules* 2018;23(4):938.
44. Hajiali H, Ouyang L, Llopis-Hernandez V, Dobre O, Rose FR. Review of emerging nanotechnology in bone regeneration: Progress, challenges, and perspectives. *Nanoscale* 2021;13(23):10266–80.
45. Ayanda OS, Mmuoegbulam AO, Okezie O, Durumin Iya NI, Mohammed SAE, James PH, et al. Recent progress in carbon-based nanomaterials: critical review. *J. Nanopart. Res.* 2024;26(5):106.
46. Coro J, Suarez M, Silva LS, Eguiluz KI, Salazar-Banda GR. Fullerene applications in fuel cells: A review. *Int. J. Hydrogen Energy* 2016;41(40):17944–59.
47. Khorsandi Z, Borjian-Boroujeni M, Yekani R, Varma RS. Carbon nanomaterials with chitosan: A winning combination for drug delivery systems. *J Drug Deliv. Sci. Technol.* 2021;66:102847.

48. Chen Y, Li X. The utilization of carbon-based nanomaterials in bone tissue regeneration and engineering: Respective featured applications and future prospects. *Med. Novel Technol. Dev.* 2022;16:100168.
49. Cheng J, Dorner-Reisel A, Wang T, Freiberger E, Ritter U, Moje J, et al. Biological characterization of the osteogenic, antibacterial and anti-inflammatory properties of fullerene-modified zirconia and titanium alloy implant surfaces. *Diam. Relat. Mater.* 2025;155:112339.
50. Yang X, Li C-J, Wan Y, Smith P, Shang G, Cui Q. Antioxidative fullerol promotes osteogenesis of human adipose-derived stem cells. *Int. J. Nanomed.* 2014;9:4023–31.
51. Yang X, Costello A, Shang G, Liu H, Wang W, Ren C, et al. Antioxidative fullerol prevents bone loss due to its anti-osteoclastogenic and pro-osteogenic activities. *Nanomedicine.* 2025;68:102847.
52. Ghauri FA, Raza MA, Baig MS, Ibrahim S. Corrosion study of the graphene oxide and reduced graphene oxide-based epoxy coatings. *Mater. Res. Exp.* 2017;4(12):125601.
53. Kaur R, Vatta P, Kaur M. Carbon nanotubes: A review article. *Int. J. Res. Appl. Sci. Eng. Technol.* 2018;6(4):5075–7.
54. Shar A, Shar A, Joung D. Carbon nanotube nanocomposite scaffolds: Advances in fabrication and applications for tissue regeneration and cancer therapy. *Front. Bioeng. Biotechnol.* 2023;11:1299166.
55. Feng L, Xie N, Zhong J. Carbon nanofibers and their composites: A review of synthesizing, properties and applications. *Materials* 2014;7(5):3919–45.
56. Samadian H, Mobasheri H, Azami M, Faridi-Majidi R. Osteoconductive and electroactive carbon nanofibers/hydroxyapatite nanocomposite tailored for bone tissue engineering: In vitro and in vivo studies. *Sci. Rep.* 2020;10(1):14853.
57. Mestre AS, Carvalho AP. Nanoporous carbon synthesis: An old story with exciting new chapters. In: Ghrib T, editor. *Porosity*. London: IntechOpen; 2018. p. 37–68.
58. Hassellöv M, Readman JW, Ranville JF, Tiede K. Nanoparticle analysis and characterization methodologies in environmental risk assessment of engineered nanoparticles. *Ecotoxicology* 2008;17(5):344–61.
59. Dion CD, Tavares JR. Photo-initiated chemical vapor deposition as a scalable particle functionalization technology (a practical review). *Powder Technol.* 2013;239:484–91.
60. Dhand C, Dwivedi N, Loh XJ, Ying ANJ, Verma NK, Beuerman RW, et al. Methods and strategies for the synthesis of diverse nanoparticles and their applications: A comprehensive overview. *Rsc Adv.* 2015;5(127):105003–7.

61. Kuppusamy P, Yusoff MM, Maniam GP, Govindan N. Biosynthesis of metallic nanoparticles using plant derivatives and their new avenues in pharmacological applications–An updated report. *Saudi Pharm. J.* 2016;24(4):473–84.
62. Zhang D. Processing of advanced materials using high-energy mechanical milling. *Prog. Mater. Sci.* 2004;49(3–4):537–60.
63. Tavakoli A, Sohrabi M, Kargari A. A review of methods for synthesis of nanostructured metals with emphasis on iron compounds. *Chem. Papers* 2007;61(3):151–70.
64. Pimpin A, Srituravanich W. Review on micro-and nanolithography techniques and their applications. *Eng. J.* 2012;16(1):37–56.
65. Hulteen JC, Treichel DA, Smith MT, Duval ML, Jensen TR, Van Duyne RP. Nanosphere lithography: Size-tunable silver nanoparticle and surface cluster arrays. *J. Phys. Chem. B* 1999;103(19):3854–63.
66. Amendola V, Meneghetti M. Laser ablation synthesis in solution and size manipulation of noble metal nanoparticles. *Phys. Chem. Chem. Phys.* 2009; 11(20):3805–21.
67. Makarov GN. Laser applications in nanotechnology: Nanofabrication using laser ablation and laser nanolithography. *Phys.-Uspekhi* 2013;56(7):643.
68. Ghorbani HR. A review of methods for synthesis of Al nanoparticles, Orient. *J. Chem.* 2014;30(4):1941–9.
69. Palacios-Hernández T, Hirata-Flores GA, Contreras-López OE, Mendoza-Sánchez ME, Valeriano-Arreola I, González-Vergara E, et al. Synthesis of Cu and Co metal oxide nanoparticles from thermal decomposition of tartrate complexes. *Inorganica Chim Acta* 2012;392:277–82.
70. Rahong S, Yasui T, Kaji N, Baba Y. Recent developments in nanowires for bio-applications from molecular to cellular levels. *Lab Chip* 2016;16(7): 1126–38.
71. Nuzaihan MNM, Hashim U, Md Arshad MK, Kasjoo SR, Rahman SF, Ruslinda AR, et. Electrical detection of dengue virus (DENV) DNA oligomer using silicon nanowire biosensor with novel molecular gate control. *Biosens. Bioelectron.* 2016;83:106–14.
72. Kashyap V, Pawar H, Kumar C, Chaudhary N, Saxena K. Analysis of synthesized doped vertical silicon nanowire arrays for effective sensing of nitrogen dioxide: As gas sensors. *Front. Mater.* 2022;9:1022317.
73. Proenca MP, Sousa CT, Ventura J, Vazquez M, Araujo JP. Distinguishing nanowire and nanotube formation by the deposition current transients. *Nanoscale Res. Lett.* 2012;7:1–9.

74. Ahoulou S, Perret E, Nedelec J-M. Functionalization and characterization of silicon nanowires for sensing applications: A Review. *Nanomaterials* 2021;11(4):999.
75. Wang H, Zepeda-Ruiz LA, Gilmer Gh, Upmanyu M. Atomistics of vapour–liquid–solid nanowire growth. *Nat. Commun.* 2013;4(1):1956.
76. Grigoropoulos CP. Laser synthesis and functionalization of nanostructures. *Int. J. Extreme Manuf.* 2019;1(1):012002.
77. Abdallah B, Kakhia M, Zetoun W, Alkafri N. PbS doped ZnO nanowires films synthesis by thermal evaporation method: Morphological, structural and optical properties, *Microelectron. J.* 2021;111:105045.
78. Kumar A, Shaikh MO, Chuang CH. Silver nanowire synthesis and strategies for fabricating transparent conducting electrodes. *Nanomaterials (Basel)* 2021;11(3):693.
79. Porter JR, Henson A, Popat KC. Biodegradable poly(ε-caprolactone) nanowires for bone tissue engineering applications. *Biomaterials* 2009; 30(5):780–8.
80. Sun, T-W, Yu W-L, Zhu Y-J, Chen F, Zhang Y-G, Jiang Y-Y, et al. Porous nanocomposite comprising ultralong hydroxyapatite Nanowires decorated with zinc-containing nanoparticles and chitosan: Synthesis and application in bone defect repair. *Chem. Eur. J.* 2018;24(35):8809–21.
81. Inal O, Badilli U, Ozkan AS, Mollarasouli F. Chapter 11 — Bioactive hybrid nanowires for drug delivery. In: Kesharwani P, Jain NK, editors. *Hybrid Nanomaterials for Drug Delivery*. Woodhead Publishing; 2022. p. 269–301.
82. Lavanya K, Abinaya S, Selvamurugan N. Recent advances in one-dimensional nanowire-incorporated bone tissue engineering scaffolds. *Mater. Today Commun.* 2022;33:104229.
83. De Mori A, Hafidh M, Mele N, Yusuf R, Cerri G, Gavini E, et al. Sustained release from injectable composite gels loaded with silver nanowires designed to combat bacterial resistance in bone regeneration applications. *Pharmaceutics* 2019;11(3):116.
84. Neville BW, Damm DD, Allen CM, Chi AC. 4 — Periodontal pathology. In: Neville BW, Damm DD, Allen CM, Chi AC, editors. *Color Atlas of Oral and Maxillofacial Diseases*. Philadelphia: Elsevier; 2019. p. 93–107.
85. Han J, Ma B, Liu H, Wang T, Wang F, Xie C, et al. Hydroxyapatite nanowires modified polylactic acid membrane plays barrier/osteoinduction dual roles and promotes bone regeneration in a rat mandible defect model. *J. Biomed. Mater. Res. A* 2018;106(12):3099–110.

86. Li J, Duan Y, Hu H, Zhao Y, Wang Q. Flexible NWs sensors in polymer, metal oxide and semiconductor materials for chemical and biological detection. *Sens. Actuators, B* 2015;219:65–82.
87. Ran Y, He W, Wang K, Ji S, Ye C. A one-step route to Ag nanowires with a diameter below 40 nm and an aspect ratio above 1000. *Chem. Commun.* 2014;50(94):14877–80.
88. Graver JE, Hartung EJ, Williams A. Resonance structures and aromaticity in capped carbon nanotubes. *Carbon* 2021;173:1082–92.
89. Popov VN. Carbon nanotubes: Properties and application. *Mater. Sci. Eng. R* 2004;43(3):61–102.
90. Du GH, Chen Q, Che RC, Yuan ZY, Peng L-M. Preparation and structure analysis of titanium oxide nanotubes. *Appl Phys. Lett.* 2001;79(22):3702–4.
91. Maruyama T. Chapter 6 — Carbon nanotubes. In: Thomas S, Sarathchandran C, Ilangovan SA, Moreno-Piraján JC, editors. *Handbook of Carbon-Based Nanomaterials*. Elsevier; 2021. p. 299–319.
92. Shah KA, Tali BA. Synthesis of carbon nanotubes by catalytic chemical vapour deposition: A review on carbon sources, catalysts and substrates. *Mater. Sci. Semicond. Proc.* 2016;41:67–82.
93. Nessim GD. Properties, synthesis, and growth mechanisms of carbon nanotubes with special focus on thermal chemical vapor deposition. *Nanoscale* 2010;2(8):1306–23.
94. Baddour CE, Briens C. Carbon nanotube synthesis: A review. *Int. J. Chem. React. Eng.* 2005;3(1).
95. Arora N, Sharma N. Arc discharge synthesis of carbon nanotubes: Comprehensive review. *Diamond Relat. Mater.* 2014;50:135–50.
96. Yahyazadeh A, Khoshandam B. Carbon nanotube synthesis via the catalytic chemical vapor deposition of methane in the presence of iron, molybdenum, and iron–molybdenum alloy thin layer catalysts. *Results Phys.* 2017;7:3826–37.
97. Eatemadi A, Daraee H, Karimkhanloo H, Kouhi M, Zarghami N, Akbarzadeh A, et al. Carbon nanotubes: Properties, synthesis, purification, and medical applications, *Nanoscale Res. Lett.* 2014;9(1):393.
98. Vu THT, Au HT, Tran LT, Nguyen TMT, Tran TTT, Pham MT, et al. Synthesis of titanium dioxide nanotubes via one-step dynamic hydrothermal process. *J. Mater. Sci.* 2014;49(16):5617–25.
99. Belin T, Epron F. Characterization methods of carbon nanotubes: A review. *Mater. Sci. Eng. B* 2005;119(2):105–18.

100. Tanaka M, Aoki K, Haniu H, Kamanaka T, Takizawa T, Sobajima A, et al. Applications of carbon nanotubes in bone regenerative medicine. *Nanomaterials (Basel)* 2020;10(4):659.
101. Pei B, Wang W, Dunne N, Li X. Applications of carbon nanotubes in bone tissue regeneration and engineering: Superiority, concerns, current advancements, and prospects. *Nanomaterials* 2019;9(10):1501.
102. Gutiérrez-Hernández JM, Escobar-García DM, Escalante A, Flores H, González FJ, Gatenholm P, Toriz G. In vitro evaluation of osteoblastic cells on bacterial cellulose modified with multi-walled carbon nanotubes as scaffold for bone regeneration. *Mater. Sci. Eng. C* 2017;75:445–53.
103. Tanaka M, Sato Y, Haniu H, Nomura H, Kobayashi S, Takanashi S, et al. A three-dimensional block structure consisting exclusively of carbon nanotubes serving as bone regeneration scaffold and as bone defect filler. *PLOS One* 2017;12(2):e0172601.
104. Brammer KS, Frandsen CJ, Jin S. TiO2 nanotubes for bone regeneration. *Trends Biotechnol.* 2012;30(6):315–22.
105. Wei F, Li M, Crawford R, Zhou Y, Xiao Y. Exosome-integrated titanium oxide nanotubes for targeted bone regeneration. *Acta Biomater* 2019;86:480–92.
106. Kubota S, Johkura K, Asanuma K, Okouchi Y, Ogiwara N, Sasaki K, Kasuga T. Titanium oxide nanotubes for bone regeneration. *J. Mater. Sci. Mater. Med.* 2004;15(9):1031–35.
107. Huang K, Ou Q, Xie Y, Chen X, Fang Y, Huang C, et al. Halloysite nanotube based scaffold for enhanced bone regeneration. *ACS Biomater. Sci. Eng.* 2019;5(8):4037–47.
108. Ou Q, Huang K, Fu C, Huang C, Fang Y, Gu Z, et al. Nanosilver-incorporated halloysite nanotubes/gelatin methacrylate hybrid hydrogel with osteoimmunomodulatory and antibacterial activity for bone regeneration. *Chem. Eng. J.* 2020;382:123019.
109. Abdeen DH, El Hachach M, Koc M, Atieh MA. A review on the corrosion behaviour of nanocoatings on metallic substrates. *Materials (Basel)* 2019; 12(2):210.
110. Wang Z, Chen X, Gong Y, Zhang B, Li H. Superhydrophobic nanocoatings prepared by a novel vacuum cold spray process. *Surf. Coat. Technol.* 2017; 325:52–7.
111. Yilmaz O, Yorgancioglu A. Chapter 8 — Nanocoatings: Preparation, properties, and biomedical applications. In: Vasile C, editor. *Polymeric Nanomaterials in Nanotherapeutics*. Elsevier; 2019. p. 299–331.

112. Sotoudeh Bagha P, Paternoster C, Khakbiz M, Sheibani S, Gholami N, Mantovani D. Surface modification of an absorbable bimodal Fe-Mn-Ag alloy by nitrogen plasma immersion ion implantation. *Materials* 2023;16(3):1048.
113. Mishnaevsky L, Levashov E, Valiev RZ, Segurado J, Sabirov I, Enikeev N, et al. Nanostructured titanium-based materials for medical implants: Modeling and development. *Mater. Sci. Eng. R* 2014;81:1–19.
114. Guo L, Li H. Fabrication and characterization of thin nano-hydroxyapatite coatings on titanium. *Surf. Coat. Technol.* 2004;185(2–3):268–74.
115. Zheng J, Rahman N, Li L, Zhang J, Tan H, Xue Y, et al. Biofunctionalization of electrospun fiber membranes by LbL-collagen/chondroitin sulfate nanocoating followed by mineralization for bone regeneration. *Mater. Sci. Eng. C* 2021;128:112295.
116. Li D, Dai D, Wang J, Zhang C. Honeycomb bionic graphene oxide quantum dot/layered double hydroxide composite nanocoating promotes osteoporotic bone regeneration via activating mitophagy. *Small* 2024;20(50):2403907.
117. Yang C, Huan Z, Wang X, Wu C, Chang J. 3D printed Fe Scaffolds with HA nanocoating for bone regeneration. *ACS Biomater. Sci. Eng.* 2018;4(2): 608–16.
118. Eswaraiah V, Zeng Q, Long Y, Liu Z. Black phosphorus nanosheets: Synthesis, characterization and applications. *Small* 2016;12(26):3480–502.
119. Mishra SR, Gadore V, Chavda V, Panda S, Roy S, Sahoo P, et al. Ahmaruzzaman, black phosphorene: A versatile allotrope revolutionizing environmental, energy, and biomedical applications. *Coord. Chem. Rev.* 2025;524:216345.
120. Qu G, Liu W, Zhao Y, Gao J, Xia T, Shi J, et al. Improved biocompatibility of black phosphorus nanosheets by chemical modification. *Angew. Chem.* 2017;129(46):14680–5.
121. Goren AY, Gungormus E, Vatanpour V, Yoon Y, Khataee A. Recent progress on synthesis and properties of black phosphorus and phosphorene as new-age nanomaterials for water decontamination. *ACS Appl. Mater. Interfaces* 2024;16(16):20055–78.
122. Lu Q, Li X, Chen H, Jia Y, Liu T, Liu X, et al. Study on black phosphorus characteristics using a two-step thinning method. *Materials* 2022;15(2):615.
123. Choi JR, Yong KW, Choi JY, Nilghaz A, Lin Y, Xu J, et al. Black phosphorus and its biomedical applications. *Theranostics* 2018;8(4):1005.
124. Jing X, Xiong Z, Lin Z, Sun T. The application of black phosphorus nanomaterials in bone tissue engineering. *Pharmaceutics* 2022;14(12):2634.

125. Qiu M, Tulufu N, Tang G, Ye W, Qi J, Deng L, et al. Black phosphorus accelerates bone regeneration based on immunoregulation, *Adv. Sci.* 2024; 11(1):2304824.
126. Li Q, Wang R, Xue J, Wang R, Zhang S, Kang H, et al. ZIF-8-modified black phosphorus nanosheets incorporated into injectable dual-component hydrogels for enhanced photothermal antibacterial and osteogenic activities. *ACS Appl. Mater. Interfaces* 2024;16(25):32058–77.
127. Chen J, Huang X, Wang J, Chen W, Teng Y, Yin D. Incorporation of black phosphorus nanosheets into poly (propylene fumarate) biodegradable bone cement to enhance bioactivity and osteogenesis. *J. Orthop. Surg. Res.* 2024; 19(1):98.
128. Gogotsi Y, Anasori B. The rise of MXenes. In: *MXenes*. Jenny Stanford Publishing; 2023. p. 3–11.
129. Anayee M, Wang RJ, Downes M, Ippolito S, Gogotsi Y. Layer-by-layer mechanism of the MAX phase to MXene transformation. *Matter* 2025;8(6): 102092.
130. Saxena A, Tyagi A, Vats S, Gupta I, Gupta A, Kaur R, et al. Mxene-integrated composites for biomedical applications: Synthesis, cancer diagnosis, and emerging frontiers. *Small Sci.* 2025;5(4):2400492.
131. Dahlqvist M, Barsoum MW, Rosen J. MAX phases–past, present, and future. *Mater. Today* 2024;72:1–24.
132. Hope MA, Forse AC, Griffith KJ, Lukatskaya MR, Ghidiu M, Gogotsi Y, et al. NMR reveals the surface functionalisation of Ti 3 C 2 MXene. *Phys. Chem. Chem. Phys.* 2016;18(7):5099–102.
133. Sarkar S, Hossain SA, Chakraborty P, Ghosh S, Bhattacharya S, Mukherjee S. MXene: Recent advances in synthesis, characterization and emerging applications in energy, biomedical and environmental remediation. *Surf. Interfaces* 2024;51:104628.
134. Ali R, Islam M, Shafi M, Ali S, Wang HE. Developments and prospects of MXenes for energy storage and environmental sustainability. *Coord. Chem. Rev.* 2025;540:216797.
135. Abraham AM, George SC. A review of MXene's retroactive development in energy storage applications. *ChemistrySelect* 2025;10(30):e02846.
136. Mishra RK, Avinashi SK, Fatima Z, Singh R, Gautam C. Fabrication, surface morphology, and energy storage performance of MXene-based materials for metal-ion batteries: A Review. *ACS Appl. Energy Mater.* 2025;8(16): 11813–63.

137. Jang JH, Lee EJ. Influence of MXene particles with a stacked-lamellar structure on osteogenic differentiation of human mesenchymal stem cells. *Materials (Basel)* 2021;14(16):4453.
138. Huang B, Li S, Dai S, Lu X, Wang P, Li X, et al. $Ti_3C_2T_x$ MXene-Decorated 3D-printed ceramic scaffolds for enhancing osteogenesis by spatiotemporally orchestrating inflammatory and bone repair responses. *Adv. Sci.* 2024;11(34):2400229.
139. Kim T, See CW, Li X, Zhu D. Orthopedic implants and devices for bone fractures and defects: Past, present and perspective. *Eng. Regen.* 2020;1:6–18.
140. Sheikh Z, Najeeb S, Khurshid Z, Verma V, Rashid H, Glogauer M. Biodegradable materials for bone repair and tissue engineering applications. *Materials (Basel)* 2015;8(9):5744–94.
141. Shayan M, Moradi M, Plakseychuk AY, Shankar R, Chun Y. Osteoblast cell response to oxide films formed on nanograin 316L stainless steel obtained by two-dimensional linear plane-strain machining. *Mater. Lett.* 2016;177: 94–8.
142. Kalantari K, Saleh B, Webster TJ. Biological applications of severely plastically deformed nano-grained medical devices: A review. *Nanomaterials (Basel)* 2021;11(3):748.
143. Balasundaram G, Webster TJ. Increased osteoblast adhesion on nanograined Ti modified with KRSR. *J. Biomed. Mater. Res. A* 2007;80(3):602–11.
144. Estrin Y, Lapovok R, Medvedev AE, Kasper C, Ivanova E, Lowe TC. 4.4 — Mechanical performance and cell response of pure titanium with ultrafine-grained structure produced by severe plastic deformation. In: Froes FH, Qian M, editors. *Titanium in Medical and Dental Applications*. Woodhead Publishing; 2018. p. 419–54.
145. Sotoudehbagha P, Sheibani S, Khakbiz M, Ebrahimi-Barough S, Hermawan H. Novel antibacterial biodegradable Fe-Mn-Ag alloys produced by mechanical alloying. *Mater. Sci. Eng. C* 2018;88:88–94.
146. Razavi M, Huang Y. A magnesium-based nanobiocomposite processed by a novel technique combining high shear solidification and hot extrusion. *Recent Pat. Nanotechnol.* 2019;13(1):38–48.
147. Sotoudeh Bagha P, Khaleghpanah S, Sheibani S, Khakbiz M, Zakeri A. Characterization of nanostructured biodegradable Zn-Mn alloy synthesized by mechanical alloying. *J. Alloys Comp.* 2018;735:1319–27.
148. Qian J, Chen Y, Zhang W, Mo X, Zou D, Soliman H, et al. Micro/nano-structured metal–organic/inorganic hybrid coatings on biodegradable Zn for osteogenic and biocompatible improvement. *Adv. Mater. Interfaces* 2022; 9(6):2101852.

149. Larraza A, Burke S, Sotoudehbagha P, Razavi M. Fabrication and processing of magnesium-based metal matrix nanocomposites for bioabsorbable implants. *Metals* 2024;14(12):1318.
150. Latt S, Sotoudehbagha P, Cardenas V, Larraza A, Razavi M. Diopside-based bioactive glass-ceramic nanoparticles for osteoimmunomodulation. *Ceram. Int.* 2025;51:36947–60.
151. Varghese RJ, Parani S, Thomas S, Oluwafemi OS, Wu J. Introduction to nanomaterials: Synthesis and applications. In: *Nanomaterials for Solar Cell Applications*. Elsevier; 2019. p. 75–95.
152. Ka UB, Panemangalorea DB, Bhat S. Equal channel angular processing — a modern deforming technique for quality products. *Adv. Weld. Deform.* 2021;381.
153. Huang Y, Langdon TG. Advances in ultrafine-grained materials. *Mater. Today* 2013;16(3):85–93.
154. Sotoudeh Bagha P, Khakbiz M, Sheibani S, Hermawan H. Design and characterization of nano and bimodal structured biodegradable Fe-Mn-Ag alloy with accelerated corrosion rate. *J. Alloys Comp.* 2018;767:955–65.
155. Sotoudeh Bagha P, Khakbiz M, Safaie N, Sheibani S, Ebrahimi-Barough S. Effect of high energy ball milling on the properties of biodegradable nanostructured Fe-35 wt.%Mn alloy. *J. Alloys Comp.* 2018;768:166–75.
156. Safaie N, Khakbiz M, Sheibani S, SotoudehBagha P. Synthesizing of nanostructured Fe-Mn alloys by mechanical alloying process. *Procedia Mater. Sci.* 2015;11:381–5.
157. Bagha PS, Khakbiz M, Sheibani S, Ebrahimi-Barough S, Hermawan H. In vitro degradation, hemocompatibility, and cytocompatibility of nanostructured absorbable Fe–Mn–Ag alloys for biomedical application. *ACS Biomater. Sci. Eng.* 2020;6(4):2094–106.
158. Srinivasan R, Chaudhury PK, Cherukuri B, Han Q, Swenson D, Gros P. *Continuous Severe Plastic Deformation Processing of Aluminum Alloys*. Dayton: Wright State University; 2006.
159. Zhilyaev AP, Langdon TG. Using high-pressure torsion for metal processing: Fundamentals and applications. *Prog. Mater. Sci.* 2008;53(6):893–979.
160. Garbacz H, Topolski K, Motyka M. Hydrostatic extrusion. In: *Nanocrystalline Titanium*. Elsevier; 2019. p. 37–53.
161. Li N-B, Sun S-J, Bai H-Y, Xu W-H, Xiao G-Y, Zhang Y-L, et al. Evolution of nano/submicro-scale oxide structures on Ti6Al4V achieved by an ultrasonic shot peening-induction heating approach for high-performance surface design of bone implants. *J Alloys Compd.* 2020;831:154876.

162. Jindal S, Bansal R, Singh BP, Pandey R, Narayanan S, Wani MR, Singh V. Enhanced osteoblast proliferation and corrosion resistance of commercially pure titanium through surface nanostructuring by ultrasonic shot peening and stress relieving. *J. Oral Implant.* 2014;40(S1):347–55.
163. Zofkova I, Nemcikova P, Matucha P. Trace elements and bone health. *Clin. Chem. Lab Med.* 2013;51(8):1555–61.
164. Sergi R, Bellucci D, Candidato RT, Lusvarghi L, Bolelli G, Pawlowski L, et al. Bioactive Zn-doped hydroxyapatite coatings and their antibacterial efficacy against Escherichia coli and Staphylococcus aureus. *Surf. Coat. Technol.* 2018;352:84–91.
165. Mancuso E, Bretcanu OA, Marshall M, Birch MA, McCaskie AW, Dalgarno KW. Novel bioglasses for bone tissue repair and regeneration: Effect of glass design on sintering ability, ion release and biocompatibility. *Mater. Des.* 2017;129:239–48.
166. Kong Y, Duan J, Liu F, Han L, Li G, Sun C, et al. Regulation of stem cell fate using nanostructure-mediated physical signals. *Chem. Soc. Rev.* 2021; 50(22):12828–72.
167. Zhang H, Zhang H, Xiong Y, Dong L, Li X. Development of hierarchical porous bioceramic scaffolds with controlled micro/nano surface topography for accelerating bone regeneration. *Mater. Sci. Eng. C* 2021;130: 112437.
168. Ergun C, Liu H, Halloran JW, Webster TJ. Increased osteoblast adhesion on nanograined hydroxyapatite and tricalcium phosphate containing calcium titanate. *J. Biomed. Mater. Res. A* 2007;80(4):990–7.
169. Lalzawmliana V, Anand A, Roy M, Kundu B, Nandi SK. Mesoporous bioactive glasses for bone healing and biomolecules delivery. *Mater. Sci. Eng. C. Mater. Biol. Appl.* 2020;106:110180.
170. Singh N, Guin M, Tomar R. Nanostructured ceramics. In: *Ceramic Science and Engineering*. Elsevier; 2022. p. 545–73.
171. Fernández-Hernán JP, Torres B, López AJ, Rams J. The role of the sol-gel synthesis process in the biomedical field and its use to enhance the performance of bioabsorbable magnesium implants. *Gels* 2022;8(7):426.
172. Paramasivam G, Palem VV, Sundaram T, Sundaram V, Kishore SC, Bellucci S. Nanomaterials: Synthesis and applications in theranostics. *Nanomaterials* 2021;11(12):3228.
173. Yang G, Park S-J. Conventional and microwave hydrothermal synthesis and application of functional materials: A review. *Materials* 2019;12(7): 1177.

174. Piticescu RM, Piticescu R, Taloi D, Badilita V. Hydrothermal synthesis of ceramic nanomaterials for functional applications. *Nanotechnology* 2003; 14(2):312–7.
175. Suchanek WL, Lencka MM, Riman RE. Hydrothermal synthesis of ceramic materials. In: *Aqueous Systems at Elevated Temperatures and Pressures*. Elsevier; 2004. p. 717–44.
176. Hublikar LV, Ganachari SV, Yaradoddi JS, Mokashi AU. Zinc and cobalt nano ferrites and their potential applications in environmental sustainability. 2020.
177. Levashov E, Mukasyan A, Rogachev A, Shtansky D. Self-propagating high-temperature synthesis of advanced materials and coatings. *Int. Mater. Rev.* 2017;62(4):203–39.
178. Wahid F, Khan T, Hussain Z, Ullah H. 30 — Nanocomposite scaffolds for tissue engineering: Properties, preparation, and applications. In: Inamuddin, Asiri AM, Mohammad A, editors. *Applications of Nanocomposite Materials in Drug Delivery*. Woodhead Publishing; 2018. p. 701–35.
179. Christy PN, Basha SK, Kumari VS, Bashir AKH, Maaza M, Kaviyarasu K, et al. Biopolymeric nanocomposite scaffolds for bone tissue engineering applications — A review. *J. Drug Deliv. Sci. Technol.* 2020;55:101452.
180. Kavya KC, Jayakumar R, Nair S, Chennazhi KP. Fabrication and characterization of chitosan/gelatin/nSiO_2 composite scaffold for bone tissue engineering. *Int. J. Biol. Macromol.* 2013;59:255–63.
181. Pina S, Oliveira JM, Reis RL. Natural-based nanocomposites for bone tissue engineering and regenerative medicine: A review. *Adv. Mater.* 2015;27(7): 1143–69.
182. Yan L-P, Salgado AJ, Oliveira JM, Oliveira AL, Reis RL. De novo bone formation on macro/microporous silk and silk/nano-sized calcium phosphate scaffolds. *J. Bioact. Compat. Polym.* 2013;28(5):439–52.
183. Silva TH, Alves A, Ferreira BM, Oliveira JM, Reys LL, Ferreira RJF, et al. Materials of marine origin: A review on polymers and ceramics of biomedical interest. *Int. Mater. Rev* 2012;57(5):276–306.
184. Di Martino A, Sittinger M, Risbud MV. Chitosan: A versatile biopolymer for orthopaedic tissue-engineering. *Biomaterials* 2005;26(30):5983–90.
185. Zhang J, Nie J, Zhang Q, Li Y, Wang Z, Hu Q. Preparation and characterization of bionic bone structure chitosan/hydroxyapatite scaffold for bone tissue engineering. *J. Biomater. Sci. Polym. Ed.* 2014;25(1):61–74.
186. Sun J, Tan J. Alginate-based biomaterials for regenerative medicine applications. *Materials (Basel)* 2103;6(4):1285–309.

187. Li L, Duan X, Fan Z, Chen L, Xing F, Xu Z, et al. Mesenchymal stem cells in combination with hyaluronic acid for articular cartilage defects. *Sci. Rep.* 2018;8(1):9900.
188. Lavanya K, Swetha S, Selvamurugan N. Biopolymers/ceramic-based nanocomposite scaffolds for drug delivery in bone tissue engineering. In: Hasnain MS, Nayak AK, Alkahtani S, editors. *Polymeric and Natural Composites: Materials, Manufacturing and Biomedical Applications*. Springer International Publishing; 2022. p. 337–76.
189. Khoshroo K, Jafarzadeh Kashi TS, Moztarzadeh F, Tahriri M, Jazayeri HE, Tayebi L. Development of 3D PCL microsphere/TiO2 nanotube composite scaffolds for bone tissue engineering. *Mater. Sci. Eng. C. Mater. Biol. Appl.* 2017;70(Pt 1):586–98.
190. Sun H, Yang HL. Calcium phosphate scaffolds combined with bone morphogenetic proteins or mesenchymal stem cells in bone tissue engineering. *Chin. Med. J. (Engl)* 2015;128(8):1121–7.
191. Erol-Taygun M, Unalan I, Idris MIB, Mano JF, Boccaccini AR. Bioactive glass-polymer nanocomposites for bone tissue regeneration applications: A review. *Adv. Eng. Mater.* 2019;21(8):1900287.
192. Seo C, Zhang C, Liu H. Chapter 8 — A review on the 3D printing of composite scaffolds for bone tissue engineering. In: Chen Y, editor. *Musculoskeletal Tissue Engineering*. Elsevier; 2022. p. 201–41.
193. Jaalouk DE, Lammerding J. Mechanotransduction gone awry. *Nat. Rev. Mol. Cell Biol.* 2009;10(1):63–73.
194. Huang D-M, Hsiao J-K, Chen Y-C, Chien L-Y, Yao M, Chen Y-K, et al. The promotion of human mesenchymal stem cell proliferation by superparamagnetic iron oxide nanoparticles. *Biomaterials*. 2009;30(22):3645–51.
195. Hu S, Zhou Y, Zhao Y, Xu Y, Zhang F, Gu N, et al. Enhanced bone regeneration and visual monitoring via superparamagnetic iron oxide nanoparticle scaffold in rats. *J. Tissue Eng. Regen. Med.* 2018;12(4):e2085–98.
196. Safari B, Aghanejad A, Kadkhoda J, Aghazade M, Roshangar L, Davaran S. Biofunctional phosphorylated magnetic scaffold for bone tissue engineering. *Colloids Surf B*. 2022;211:112284.
197. Davoodi P, Gill EL, Wang W, Huang YYS. Advances and innovations in electrospinning technology. In: *Biomedical Applications of Electrospinning and Electrospraying*. Elsevier; 2021. p. 45–81.
198. Patel DK, Dutta SD, Hexiu J, Ganguly K, Lim K-T. Bioactive electrospun nanocomposite scaffolds of poly (lactic acid)/cellulose nanocrystals for bone tissue engineering. *Int. J. Biol. Macromol.* 2020;162:1429–41.

199. Rostami F, Tamjid E, Behmanesh M. Drug-eluting PCL/graphene oxide nanocomposite scaffolds for enhanced osteogenic differentiation of mesenchymal stem cells. *Mater. Sci. Eng. C* 2020;115:111102.
200. Pazourková L, Martynková G, Plachá D. Preparation and mechanical properties of polymeric nanocomposites with hydroxyapatite and hydroxyapatite, clay mineral fillers-review. *J. Nanotechnol. Nanomed. Nanobiotechnol.* 2015;2(007):1–8.
201. Mohan A, Girdhar M, Kumar R, Chaturvedi HS, Vadhel A, Solanki PR, et al. Polyhydroxybutyrate-based nanocomposites for bone tissue engineering. *Pharmaceuticals* 2021;14(11):1163.
202. Rane AV, Kanny K, Abitha V, Thomas S. Methods for synthesis of nanoparticles and fabrication of nanocomposites. In: *Synthesis of Inorganic Nanomaterials*. Elsevier; 2018. p. 121–139.
203. Parande G, Manakari V, Prasadh S, Chauhan D, Rahate S, Wong R, et al. Strength retention, corrosion control and biocompatibility of Mg–Zn–Si/HA nanocomposites. *J. Mech. Behav. Biomed. Mater.* 2020;103:103584.
204. Besra L, Liu M. A review on fundamentals and applications of electrophoretic deposition (EPD). *Prog. Mater. Sci.* 2007;52(1):1–61.
205. Avcu E, Baştan FE, Abdullah HZ, Rehman MAU, Avcu YY, Boccaccini AR. Electrophoretic deposition of chitosan-based composite coatings for biomedical applications: A review. *Prog. Mater. Sci.* 2019;103:69–108.
206. Sikkema R, Baker K, Zhitomirsky I. Electrophoretic deposition of polymers and proteins for biomedical applications. *Adv. Colloid Interface Sci.* 2020;284:102272.
207. Singh S, Singh G, Bala N, Aggarwal K. Characterization and preparation of Fe3O4 nanoparticles loaded bioglass-chitosan nanocomposite coating on Mg alloy and in vitro bioactivity assessment. *Int. J. Biol. Macromol.* 2020; 151:519–28.
208. Love SA, Maurer-Jones MA, Thompson JW, Lin Y-S, Haynes CL. Assessing nanoparticle toxicity. *Ann. Rev. Analyt. Chem.* 2012;5:181–205.
209. Schlagenhauf L, Buerki-Thurnherr T, Kuo Y-Y, Wichser A, Nüesch F, Wick P, et al. Carbon nanotubes released from an epoxy-based nanocomposite: Quantification and particle toxicity. *Environ. Sci. Technol.* 2015;49(17):10616–23.
210. Purohit SD, Singh H, Bhaskar R, Yadav I, Chou C-F, Gupta MK, et al. Gelatin — alginate — cerium oxide nanocomposite scaffold for bone regeneration. *Mater. Sci. Eng. C* 2020;116:111111.
211. Zhang X, Zhang C, Lin Y, Hu P, Shen Y, Wang K, et al. Nanocomposite membranes enhance bone regeneration through restoring physiological electric microenvironment. *ACS Nano* 2016;10(8):7279–86.

212. Zare M, Namratha K, Alghamdi S, Mohammad YHE, Hezam A, Zare M, et al. Novel green biomimetic approach for synthesis of ZnO-Ag nanocomposite; antimicrobial activity against food-borne pathogen, biocompatibility and solar photocatalysis. *Sci. Rep.* 2019;9(1):1–15.
213. Vinyas M, Athul S, Harursampath D, Loja M, Thoi TN. A comprehensive review on analysis of nanocomposites: From manufacturing to properties characterization. *Mater. Res. Exp.* 2019;6(9):092002.
214. Mourdikoudis S, Pallares RM, Thanh NT. Characterization techniques for nanoparticles: Comparison and complementarity upon studying nanoparticle properties. *Nanoscale* 2018;10(27):12871–934.
215. Plou J, Molina-Martínez B, García-Astrain C, Langer J, García I, Ercilla A, et al. Nanocomposite scaffolds for monitoring of drug diffusion in three-dimensional cell environments by surface-enhanced Raman spectroscopy. *Nano Lett.* 20201;21(20):8785–93.
216. Hejazi F, Bagheri-Khoulenjani S, Olov N, Zeini D, Solouk A, Mirzadeh H. Fabrication of nanocomposite/nanofibrous functionally graded biomimetic scaffolds for osteochondral tissue regeneration. *J. Biomed. Mater. Res. A* 2021;109(9):1657–69.
217. Kavlak S, Can HK. An emphasis on dynamic mechanical properties of novel stilbene containing copolymer/organo-MMT nanocomposites fabricated via in situ interlamellar copolymerization. *J. Appl. Polym. Sci.* 2022;139(1):51417.
218. Ramly EP, Alfonso AR, Kantar RS, Wang MM, Siso JRD, Ibrahim A, et al. Flores, safety and efficacy of recombinant human bone morphogenetic protein-2 (rhBMP-2) in craniofacial surgery. *Plast. Reconstr. Surg–Global Open* 2019;7(8):e2347.
219. Huang B, Yuan Y, Ding S, Li J, Ren J, Feng B, et al. Nanostructured hydroxyapatite surfaces-mediated adsorption alters recognition of BMP receptor IA and bioactivity of bone morphogenetic protein-2. *Acta Biomater.* 2015; 27:275–85.
220. Zhou P, Wu J, Xia Y, Yuan Y, Zhang H, Xu S, et al. Loading BMP-2 on nanostructured hydroxyapatite microspheres for rapid bone regeneration. *Int. J. Nanomed.* 2018:4083–92.
221. Farjaminejad S, Hasani M, Farjaminejad R, Foroozandeh A, Abdouss M, Hasanzadeh M. The critical role of nano-hydroxyapatites as an advanced scaffold in drug delivery towards efficient bone regeneration: Recent progress and challenges. *Carbohydr. Polym. Technol. Appl.* 2025:100692.
222. Gagliardi A, Giuliano E, Venkateswararao E, Fresta M, Bulotta S, Awasthi V, et al. Biodegradable polymeric nanoparticles for drug delivery to solid tumors. *Front. Pharmacol.* 2021;12:601626.

223. Elmowafy M, Shalaby K, Elkomy MH, Alsaidan OA, Gomaa HA, Abdelgawad MA, et al. Polymeric nanoparticles for delivery of natural bioactive agents: Recent advances and challenges. *Polymers* 2023;15(5):1123.
224. Farjaminejad S, Farjaminejad R, Hasani M, Garcia-Godoy F, Abdouss M, Marya A, et al. Advances and challenges in polymer-based scaffolds for bone tissue engineering: A path towards personalized regenerative medicine. *Polymers* 2024;16(23):3303.
225. Walmsley GG, McArdle A, Tevlin R, Momeni A, Atashroo D, Hu MS, et al. Nanotechnology in bone tissue engineering. *Nanomed.: Nanotechnol. Biol. Med.* 2015;11(5):1253–63.
226. Safaeian Laein S, Katouzian I, Mozafari M, Farnudiyan-Habibi A, Akbarbaglu Z, Shadan MR, et al. Biological and thermodynamic stabilization of lipid-based delivery systems through natural biopolymers; controlled release and molecular dynamics simulations. *Crit. Rev. Food Sci. Nutr.* 2024;64(22):7728–47.
227. Kakaei N, Amirian R, Azadi M, Mohammadi G, Izadi Z. Perfluorocarbons: A perspective of theranostic applications and challenges. *Front. Bioeng. Biotechnol.* 2023;11:1115254.
228. Sotoudehbagha P, Flores AC, Hartmann T, Pattilachan T, Razavi M. Bone-targeted ultrasound-responsive nanobubbles for siRNA delivery to treat osteoporosis in mice. *Biomater. Adv.* 2025;166:214078.
229. Kumari PVK, Rao YS, Akhila S. Role of nanocomposites in drug delivery. GSC *Biol. Pharm. Sci.* 2019;8(3):094–103.
230. Yuan H, Fernandes H, Habibovic P, De Boer J, Barradas AM, De Ruiter A, et al. Osteoinductive ceramics as a synthetic alternative to autologous bone grafting. *Proc. Natl. Acad. Sci.* 2010;107(31):13614–19.
231. Su J, Xu H, Sun J, Gong X, Zhao H. Dual delivery of BMP-2 and bFGF from a new nano-composite scaffold, loaded with vascular stents for large-size mandibular defect regeneration. *Int. J. Mol Sci.* 2013;14(6): 12714–28.
232. Cao M, Wang Y, Hu X, Gong H, Li R, Cox H, et al. Reversible thermoresponsive peptide–PNIPAM hydrogels for controlled drug delivery. *Biomacromolecules* 2019;20(9):3601–10.
233. Vivek R, Babu VN, Thangam R, Subramanian K, Kannan K. pH-responsive drug delivery of chitosan nanoparticles as Tamoxifen carriers for effective anti-tumor activity in breast cancer cells. *Colloids Surf, B* 2013;111:117–23.
234. Couvreur P. Ultrasound-triggered pain relief. *Nat. Biomed. Eng.* 2017;1(8): 625–26.

https://doi.org/10.1142/9789819819645_0009

Chapter 9

Artificial Intelligence–Enabled Technology and Health: Improving Diagnostic and Therapeutic Efficacy

Bahadir Balkanli[1], Hakan Sesen[2,*]

[1]*Department of Orthopaedics and Traumatology, Şişli Etfal Education and Research Hospital, İstanbul, Turkey*
[2]*Department of Orthopaedics and Traumatology, Atatürk Sanatoryum Education and Research Hospital, Ankara, Turkey*

Chapter Outline

* **Corresponding author:** Hakan Sesen, Department of Orthopaedics and Traumatology, Atatürk Sanatoryum Education and Research Hospital, Ankara, Turkey. Email: hakansesen73@yahoo.com

Abstract

Artificial intelligence (AI) systems are designed to perform tasks that typically require human intelligence and can imitate human cognitive functions. The advent of the Fourth Industrial Revolution has ushered in a new era known as Health 4.0, which aims to significantly enhance efficiency in diagnosis, treatment, and patient care within health systems. The advancements of AI in both physical and virtual realms have been shown to substantially improve patient diagnosis and treatment processes. Deep learning (DL) and machine learning (ML) — based AI algorithms can analyze patient health data to support clinical decision-making. These AI algorithms can play a remarkable role in disease diagnosis through image classification and analysis using X-ray, computed tomography (CT), and magnetic resonance imaging (MRI). When integrated with clinical decision support systems (CDSSs), AI algorithms can increase diagnostic accuracy and facilitate personalized treatment plans. Furthermore, AI-supported models, including ML-based CDSSs that analyze large datasets from electronic health records (EHRs), have the potential to reduce medical errors and improve patient outcomes. In robotic joint arthroplasty, AI algorithms offer personalized treatment approaches. These algorithms have been shown to contribute to reducing preoperative planning time, surgery time, hospital stay, and complication rates, thereby increasing patient satisfaction. Due to the sheer size and diversity of data generated by health systems, rapid evaluation using traditional methods is often impossible. However, evaluating this data using AI-supported systems may lead to cost reductions, enhanced quality of service, and increased productivity within healthcare institutions. This chapter highlights the crucial role of AI algorithms in health care and their importance in improving patient outcomes through advanced diagnoses and treatment processes. AI possesses tremendous transformative potential in healthcare. Nevertheless, challenges such as data privacy and ethical issues require more detailed attention.

1. Introduction

Artificial intelligence (AI) is a rapidly evolving technology that is driving fundamental changes across many scientific disciplines, including modern medicine. The current period, often termed "the digital revolution," marks a significant turning point where various technologies converge [1]. The Fourth Industrial Revolution (Industry 4.0) has brought about substantial transformations in health care, mirroring its impact on the manufacturing sector, thereby initiating a new era known as Health 4.0. John McCarthy [2] and Alan Turing [3] are credited with coining the phrase "AI." AI was officially defined in 1956 as a field of science and engineering dedicated to creating intelligent machines. As predicted by Pang *et al.*, this revolution has contributed to the continuous development and enhanced effectiveness of healthcare services [1].

1.1 *Artificial Intelligence and the Fourth Industrial Revolution (Health 4.0)*

The primary goal of AI is to develop "smart" systems capable of performing functions that typically require human intelligence. AI has assumed a significant role in numerous aspects of modern life, including health, communications, and security. In healthcare services, it is particularly used to boost the productivity of diagnosis, treatment, and patient care processes [4, 5]. However, the widespread adoption of AI technology in routine clinical practice is currently limited due to its nascent maturity and associated risks. AI is a general term and can be defined as the use of computers that model intelligent behaviors with minimal human intervention and requirements [6]. Modern AI originated in 1956 at Dartmouth College [7] and is focused on automating intellectual tasks performed by humans.

1.2. *Virtual and Physical Applications of Artificial Intelligence in Health Care*

In medicine, AI applications are broadly categorized into two main areas: virtual and physical [8]. Virtual AI is an expansive domain that includes DL, information management, and healthcare management systems. These systems support physicians in diagnosis and treatment processes by analyzing patient health data. Physical AI, on the other hand, encompasses tangible applications such as targeted drug delivery systems and robots employed in surgical procedures [6]. Advances in DL techniques, coupled with the increased availability of large datasets and greater computational power, have considerably improved success in areas such as object recognition, speech recognition, drug discovery, and genomic analysis through AI [9, 10]. Concrete examples of these advancements include breast cancer screening using mammography, the diagnosis of skin lesions, the diagnosis of prostate cancer using prostate magnetic resonance imaging (MRI), and the use of radiographic evaluations to determine bone age [9, 11–13]. Despite these successes, the full potential of AI in surgery remains largely untapped. Factors such as the dynamic and variable nature of surgical procedures, sudden changes in patient data, and the difficulty of transferring surgical experience are the primary limitations to the adoption of AI in surgery [14]. This section will delve into the historical development of AI, its applications in the healthcare sector, and how this technology has advanced diagnosis and treatment processes. As described previously, the application of AI in medicine is divided into two categories: virtual and physical. The virtual branch includes patient health record systems, physician decision support systems, and health management systems, while the physical branch includes robots used by surgeons and nanorobots employed for drug delivery [6].

2. Artificial Intelligence in Diagnosis and Imaging

2.1. *Machine Learning and Deep Learning in Medicine*

ML was first defined as a subset of AI in 2015 [15]. While AI is a general term for computer programs that can imitate human thought and behavior, ML combines data input with various algorithms, enabling machines to learn without explicit programming [16]. It includes algorithms that identify data through iterative training and improvement [17]. This encompasses supervised, unsupervised, and reinforcement learning [18]. With advancements in AI models, classifying and organizing data has become possible. The term "deep learning" was popularized by Igor Aizenberg *et al.* DL is a subset of ML which itself is a subset of AI (AI > ML > DL) [16]. DL mimics the human brain but requires a substantial amount of data for the system to function effectively [19]. DL, through supervised, unsupervised, and reinforcement ML, utilizes artificial neural networks with multiple processing layers [20]. Artificial neural networks are an ML algorithm that mimics synapses in neurons [21]. Excellent results can be achieved in complex tasks such as processing large-sized and high-volume datasets [18].

2.2. *Applications in Radiological Imaging*

Significant progress has been made in radiology with the integration of technologies, including AI and ML, following the evolution that began with Wilhelm Röntgen's discovery of radiation in 1895. Radiology now plays an indispensable role in the current diagnosis and treatment of diseases. Ultrasound, which provides simultaneous imaging using high-frequency sound waves, has simplified bedside evaluations and clinical diagnoses [22]. The advancement of imaging systems such as computed tomography (CT) and MRI has enabled three-dimensional (3D) imaging in medicine [23, 24]. Nuclear medicine methods such as positron emission tomography and single-photon emission CT allow for the evaluation of metabolic activities within tissues [25, 26]. These developments have led to the growth of less invasive and more reliable diagnostic methods, such as biopsies performed under imaging guidance [27]. All these technological advancements have contributed to earlier disease diagnosis, personalization of treatment processes, and improved patient outcomes [28]. The use of Picture Archiving and Communication Systems and the widespread adoption of digital radiography have facilitated access to and sharing of radiological images. The concept of AI emerged in the 1940s and was officially defined in 1956 [29]. ML, and especially DL, developed by drawing inspiration from the human brain's working mechanisms, have created a significant leap forward in the field of image processing [10]. The increase in medical imaging data was accelerated by the widespread use of electronic health records (EHRs) and medical imaging archives. This has provided a substantial data source for the development of AI algorithms. AI was primarily designed to imitate human mental functions and can be categorized into two main types: narrow AI and broad AI. Narrow AI performs specific functions such as speech recognition, whereas broad AI aims to mimic more general human intelligence characteristics, such as problem-solving and decision-making [30]. As mentioned previously, ML, as a subcluster of AI, focuses on developing software that can make decisions autonomously by learning from data. DL is a subbranch of ML and has achieved results exceeding human performance in tasks such as image recognition [10]. Image classification has become automated due to DL, and errors have been significantly reduced. Hybrid DL is an approach that combines more than one DL model to achieve an improved performance, with successful applications particularly in health care [31]. By analyzing large amounts of medical image data, DL algorithms can diagnose diseases early and identify subtle details that may be imperceptible to the human eye. AI algorithms support radiologists in better interpreting medical images, thereby accelerating the diagnosis process [32]. Radiology is one of the areas where AI applications are most prevalent. A European study reported that over 100 commercially available AI-supported radiology software programs were commonly used in neuroradiology and thoracic radiology [33]. These programs are compatible with various imaging methods, such as CT, MRI, and X-rays.

2.3. *Diagnostic Accuracy in X-Ray, Computed Tomography, and Magnetic Resonance Imaging*

AI has brought about a significant transformation in the field of radiology. In routine examinations, particularly for pulmonary radiographs, AI algorithms have reduced the workload for radiologists and assisted in making quicker and more accurate diagnoses. For example, an AI-based system detected abnormalities from chest radiographs with a 94% positive predictive value. The AI system allowed abnormal chest radiographs with critical findings to reach the radiologist's opinion earlier, by an average of 2.7 days [33]. In mammograms used for breast cancer screening, the performance of AI systems has approached that of radiologists in cancer detection and risk prediction, although gaps exist in clinical assessment due to the inability to optimize DL [34]. The accuracy rate of AI-supported systems in chest radiography for detecting pulmonary nodules in lung cancers was found to be similar to that of radiologists [35]. AI plays a significant role in imaging methods such as CT. With the increased use of CT, especially in acute trauma patients, AI systems help reduce the workload for radiologists and assist in making quicker and more accurate diagnoses [36, 37]. AI applications have also become more widespread in areas beyond orthopedics and traumatology. AI-supported algorithms are used in diverse fields such as neuroradiology, thoracic radiology, and cardiovascular imaging [38, 39]. In cardiovascular imaging, AI systems undertake tasks such as identifying the formation of high-risk plaque and determining its relationship with cardiovascular events. The importance of MRI in modern musculoskeletal imaging is undeniable, but its use is restricted by availability and patient tolerance of lengthy procedures. Lin *et al.* demonstrated that DL-based image reconstruction enabled faster MRI acquisition without compromising image quality [40]. With DL-AI-supported systems, turbo spin echo MRI applications have been accelerated tenfold, reducing MRI processing time to 2–3 min. A multicenter study in China involving 70,000 MRI images reported that AI improved the MR signal-to-noise ratio, yielding successful results in preliminary screening [41]. Successful results have also been reported in osteosarcoma prescreening, offering an alternative in developing countries where access to medical facilities is challenging. In various disciplines such as breast radiology, cardiac MRI, neuroradiology, and prostate MRI, the use of AI-supported systems has become more widespread [12, 42–45].

2.4. *Artificial Intelligence in Musculoskeletal Radiology and Trauma*

A convolutional neural network (CNN)-based AI model demonstrated 76% sensitivity and 92% specificity in detecting scaphoid fractures *via* radiography [46]. A deep convolutional neural network (DCNN)-based image recognition model reported 86% accuracy in the radiographic assessment of vertebral fractures [47]. For detecting various pathologies such as primary bone tumors, a multitask DL model achieved 80.2% accuracy, 62.9% sensitivity, and 88.2% specificity in classifying bone tumors as either malignant or benign [48]. Age determination from pediatric hand radiographs has been developed using DL-based AI-supported systems, but further developments are required [49, 50]. Although many AI algorithms have been developed for radiology applications involving the musculoskeletal system, such as fracture determination, osteoarthritis, and bone density measurement, the number of applications with Food and Drug Administration (FDA) approval is still limited [51, 52]. With the development of AI-ML systems, in the future, bone mineral density measurements will likely be possible using MRI without exposing individuals to radiation. In addition, the combination of ML and dual-energy X-ray absorptiometry has significantly improved fracture risk prediction. With continued success, it is estimated that this could considerably reduce costs while enabling clinicians to offer precautionary treatment to patients before fractures develop. A study by Regnard *et al.* showed that AI algorithms could detect various pathologies, including extremity and pelvic fractures, with higher sensitivity than radiologists [53]. This has the potential to detect overlooked pathologies and reduce misdiagnosis rates.

AI-ML-supported systems have also been utilized to aid decision-making in surgical procedures such as arthroplasty [54]. By optimizing patient selection for arthroplasty, these systems have the potential to predict patient satisfaction, complications, and costs. AI algorithms have also proven effective in specific tasks, including scoliosis measurements on spinal radiographs [55]. Cobb angle measurements are time-consuming for clinicians and radiologists. Measurements made using AI-supported systems may offer time savings, reduce error rates, and offer advantages in tracking consecutive measurements. The literature describes the use of AI-supported systems in various traumatic conditions, including pelvic, femoral, calcaneus, cervical, and rib fractures [56–61]. These systems have successfully identified and classified fractures and even determined the fracture region. AI-DL systems, when planned and implemented with an appropriate methodology, can perform on par with or even surpass healthcare professionals in fracture detection and classification using radiographs and CT. Radiomics is created by extracting features from quantitative data within a radiological image that are imperceptible to the naked eye. DL, combined with radiomics, is an emerging area of high interest, as this technology offers the possibility for AI to learn from the entire image. However, AI is not limited to fracture determination; it has also been employed to improve CT image quality. By enhancing image quality on low-dose CT scans, it has become possible to reduce radiation exposure to patients [62]. AI-supported predictive models have been developed not only to differentiate between benign soft tissue tumors and soft tissue sarcomas but also to predict factors such as histological grade, response to neoadjuvant chemotherapy and/or radiotherapy, patient survival, and the probability of distant metastasis [63]. Roblot *et al.* showed that CNN-based AI systems were successful in detecting knee ligament injuries and meniscus tears on MRI scans [64]. DL holds great promise for the future of knee MRI interpretation [65]. In another study evaluating abnormal torsion of the lower extremities, a DL-based AI system was capable of automatically evaluating femoral and tibial torsion [66]. Finally, AI-supported systems based on ML and DL have shown encouraging results in predicting osteoporosis and the risk of fragility fracture [67, 68].

3. Clinical Decision Support Systems

3.1. *Role and Function of Artificial Intelligence-Based Clinical Decision Support Systems*

The integration of AI with decision support systems has been a long-standing topic of discussion [69]. Clinical decision support systems (CDSSs) are information systems that utilize AI algorithms to assist healthcare professionals in patient care decision-making [70]. The large volume of data generated through EHRs and medical devices has necessitated advanced analytical methods such as ML [71]. In this context, ML-based CDSSs have the potential to provide personalized treatment recommendations *via* thoroughly analyzing medical data. There is increasing interest in ML-CDSS in the literature [72]. Much evidence-based research has suggested that ML-CDSS has the potential to enhance diagnostic accuracy, facilitate the selection of the most suitable treatment, and improve patient outcomes by reducing medical errors [73]. It is now an accepted fact that AI increases diagnostic accuracy in radiological imaging [74]. However, integrating AI with CDSSs requires careful evaluation due to various risks [37].

3.2. *Integration with Electronic Health Records*

A surgeon's decision, for example, may be influenced by factors including limited time, inductive reasoning, and biases [75]. Automatic AI models, fed with her data, have the potential to mitigate these uncertainties. When making treatment decisions, surgeons must consider all possible life-threatening or non-life-threatening patient diagnoses and weigh the potential strengths and weaknesses of available tests when forming a differential diagnosis. Ideally, surgeons possess clear judgment that eliminates doubt when confirming a diagnosis. Naturally, these stages are susceptible to error due to high variability [76]. To enhance patient satisfaction and compliance, collaborative decision-making among the doctor, patient, and caregivers is crucial. During this process, patient anxiety and anger may arise, and it can also create pressure on the doctor in emergency surgical situations [75]. Delays in data collection and the intense workload of healthcare professionals can slow down the decision-making process [77].

Using AI models in outpatient clinics, where a large number of patients are evaluated, will positively affect decision-making and patient — doctor relationships [78]. Problems that occur in classical data collection, entry, and evaluation can be overcome by analyzing patient data using AI models supported by real-time preoperative, intraoperative, and postoperative EHR data. In a prospective study, AI models predicted higher rates of postoperative complications. With the increased use of EHR, the time clinicians dedicate to patients has decreased. However, this introduces additional risks, such as the possibility of ML and AI systems presenting incomplete or incorrect data to clinicians [79, 80]. Of the potential difficulties related to the use of ML-CDSS, data confidentiality is paramount. Numerous research studies in the literature have discussed these concerns and proposed solutions on this subject [81]. The weaknesses of the system may be eliminated when AI systems, correctly planned and implemented, are supported by continuous EHR data. This will provide advantages in patient treatment decisions, informing patients, identifying and reducing risks, predicting and managing complications, and optimizing the use of healthcare system resources.

3.3. *Applications in Surgery, Emergency Care, and Chronic Disease Management*

Wijnberge *et al.* demonstrated that intraoperative hypotension could be predicted using ML-CDSS, leading to fewer hypotensive attacks in patients [82]. The FDA has approved an autonomous AI-supported system for diabetic retinopathy screening using retinal fundus photographs [83]. Although the effect of ML-CDSS on clinical decision-making in stroke management is currently limited, appropriate developments could lead to individualized decisions for effective treatments in acute ischemic stroke [84]. In elderly patients, particularly those who are cognitively impaired, ML-CDSS can assist in improving treatment quality [85]. An AI-supported tool developed for sepsis prediction in intensive care units (ICUs) has been associated with shorter ICU stays and lower mortality rates [86]. In diseases such as cervical spondylotic myelopathy and spinal tumors, ML-CDSS has been used to predict patients' functional status and mortality risks [87, 88].

3.4. *Ethical and Legal Considerations in Clinical Decision Support Systems*

It is difficult to predict the future relationship between AI and radiology specialists. The undefined boundaries of this issue do not eliminate the possibility that AI could replace radiology specialists. However, some researchers believe that AI tools can serve as a complement to support and confirm a radiologist's report [89]. This outcome will necessitate radiologists having knowledge of basic AI and related tools. In addition, the cost-effectiveness and ethical evaluation of ML-CDSS are crucial. However, this also raises many ethical issues that need to be discussed. When algorithms are trained with bias, it is possible for the system to make biased decisions. In patients treated with these algorithms, evaluating a possible erroneous decision from a judicial perspective may be challenging. During the design and application of these systems, ethical principles must be adhered to [90].

4. Artificial Intelligence in Personalized and Robotic Treatment Approaches

4.1. *Personalized Medicine with Genetic and Epigenetic Data*

When AI is combined with epigenetic data, it offers groundbreaking potential for personalized treatment approaches in modern medicine. Epigenetics is a branch of science that examines the hereditary mechanisms of gene expression that can change under the influence of environmental factors. By analyzing these complex data, AI-ML models can create epigenetic profiles of individuals, forming a comprehensive database for personalized healthcare services [91]. AI-supported personalized treatment enables the formation of more effective treatment plans by considering the patient's genetic information, medical history, lifestyle, and environmental factors [92]. This method is extremely important in the treatment of complex diseases, particularly conditions such as cancer, cardiovascular diseases, and rare diseases [93]. For example, AI models developed to predict disease activity in systemic lupus erythematosus have achieved success rates of up to 70% [92]. Similarly, studies on single-nucleotide polymorphisms to determine a patient's obesity risk and the use of somatic mutation profile data to identify breast cancer subtypes have demonstrated the potential of AI in these areas [94]. AI-supported systems are used to identify genomic biomarkers in neurodegenerative disorders such as Alzheimer's disease [95]. AI models have also been developed using gene expression and rare variant data to predict common diseases such as hypertension [96].

4.2. *Artificial Intelligence — Assisted Drug Development*

AI also plays a significant role in drug development. AI-supported research has been conducted with the goal of developing more effective treatment options, especially for autoimmune diseases [97]. Using DL models, Stokes *et al.* discovered new molecules with antibacterial activity [98]. By processing a large amount of clinical and genetic data, the most appropriate treatment options for a patient's individual characteristics can be determined. Therefore, while enabling more rapid and effective treatment decisions, treatment processes can also become more reliable by preventing side effects and unnecessary drug use. However, difficulties such as data confidentiality, algorithmic bias, and ethical issues need to be overcome. Nevertheless, it is believed that once these challenges are addressed, personalized treatment will play a greater role in the healthcare services of the future.

4.3. *Robotic Surgery and Orthopedic Applications*

The use of AI in decision support systems for diagnosis and treatment, coupled with the application of robotic surgery in treatment, has led to two major developments in orthopedic surgery as a result of technological advancements [90]. Approximately half of the literature reviews that report on AI in orthopedics have focused on the interpretation of radiological images, with the spine being the most frequently investigated area [99]. The large volume of radiological imaging data and its easy accessibility and evaluation can explain these findings. Spine segmentation became possible using AI-supported algorithms to identify spinal bodies and discs in MRI scans [100]. These developments have facilitated percutaneous vertebroplasty using AI-assisted augmented reality [101]. Due to the availability of arthroplasty records, in orthopedic AI studies, the hip and knee are the most frequently studied areas [99]. Although surgical techniques and implant designs have improved in joint arthroplasty over the years, the surgical outcome is still influenced by the surgeon's level of experience. Technical errors directly affect prosthesis survival and patient satisfaction [102, 103]. Attempts have been made to address these problems with computer-assisted orthopedic surgical procedures. Preoperative planning can be performed using navigation systems, and intraoperative feedback and warnings can be provided to the surgeon. However, this does not prevent intraoperative manual errors by the surgeon [104]. To overcome this, robotic arm — assisted surgical systems have been developed. A mechanical device called a robotic arm is used to physically control the surgical instrument and prosthesis. Its perioperative performance is determined during preoperative procedure planning and through utilizing the operating environment and sensors. Three types of robotic arm — supported systems — active, passive, and semi-active — are the most commonly used [102]. Robotic surgical systems can be categorized into two main types: haptic systems, which require physical intervention from the user (surgeon), and active (autonomous) systems, which follow preoperative planning and do not require surgeon intervention [105]. The ROBODOC system (Curexo Technology, Fremont, CA, USA), an active vision-based robotic system, was the first robotic system used for cementless total hip arthroplasty in 1992 [106]. CASPAR (Ortho-Maquet/URS, Schwerin, Germany) is an image-guided, active (autonomous) robot used for total hip and total knee arthroplasty [107]. The RIO® Robotic Arm Interactive Orthopedic System (MAKO Surgical Corp., Fort Lauderdale, FL, USA) is a haptic robotic system that allows the surgeon to create a 3D preoperative plan, provides perioperative navigation with pins in the surgical field, and enables bone resection with a burr robotic arm [108]. Considering initial investment costs, annual maintenance, and the time and expense required for surgeon training, these new technologies demand significant investments [109]. In the future, AI-assisted robotic surgeries are expected to shorten surgical time and enable more efficient use of resources. Long preoperative preparation time, patient exposure to high amounts of radiation, and problems with the pins used for navigation are challenges that must be overcome in robotic surgery. The literature reports that the perioperative failure rate of surgical robots varies between 0.4% and 4.6% [110, 111]. The shortcomings of AI-assisted robotic surgery include the possibility of robot breakdowns, managing complications, and questions regarding legal liability. In the future, as robotic systems continue to develop, the challenge of managing complications during surgery may be overcome with ML-based AI-supported systems [112].

4.4. *Total Joint Arthroplasty Planning and Outcomes*

Notably, in preoperative arthroplasty planning, MRI and CT imaging with AI-assisted 3D templating shortened surgical time and improved implant size/position compared to traditional radiographic templating [113]. Furthermore, AI-supported radiographic systems that use the CNN technique have demonstrated effectiveness and cost reductions in terms of the design of a total hip replacement [114]. With the preoperative planning required before robotic joint arthroplasty, the operative time is reduced, and the correct positioning of the component is also reported to be improved. This technology has been shown to reduce complication rates and hospital stay, leading to improved patient satisfaction [115]. However, knowledge regarding the long-term outcomes of this technology is limited.

5. Artificial Intelligence in Health Care Management and Administration

5.1. *Health Information Systems and Big Data Analytics*

With technological advancements, paper-based medical records have evolved into electronic medical records [116]. This process has made health information management (HIM) an indispensable component of healthcare institutions. HIM involves the collection, analysis, and management of health data [117]. Information technology requires the collaboration of various scientific and professional branches. The primary aim is to use health informatics to further develop the healthcare services provided to patients [118]. This is proposed to be achieved through access to enormous amounts of data, which, together with the contribution of data scientists, can be analyzed and interpreted with the goal of advancing and delivering improved healthcare services. Health data analytics, which is a methodological approach for the systematic evaluation of health data, has the potential to improve the quality of management, budgeting, and planning of the healthcare system for healthcare professionals [119]. The collection and processing of data originating from health records and the healthcare system are referred to as the health information system [120]. Due to the sheer volume and diversity of data in healthcare services, rapid evaluation using traditional methods has become impossible [121]. The amount of digital health data is continuously increasing, making it difficult to organize, understand, and manage using conventional methods [122].

5.2. *Operational Efficiency and Resource Optimization*

Due to their potential clinical and economic benefits, health informatics technologies have been adopted by policymakers and public institutions in Europe and North America [123]. Hospital managers have invested in both analytical technologies and human resources to implement big data analysis technologies [124]. Research suggests that these investments have led to an increased service quality and productivity, as well as a decrease in costs in healthcare institutions [125, 126].

5.3. *Challenges in Implementation: Education, Cost, and Infrastructure*

Since education in health informatics has not yet been standardized, this further increases the need for health data analysts with the necessary skills and competencies [127, 128]. In addition, the cost-effectiveness and ethical evaluation of ML-CDSS are crucial.

6. Conclusions

The application of AI, ML, and DL in the healthcare sector has initiated a radical transformation in diagnostic and treatment processes. It is anticipated that the productivity of healthcare services will increase, and patient care will be improved by reducing error rates in diagnostic and treatment processes. AI's contributions, particularly to radiological imaging, personalized treatment approaches, and CDSSs, will facilitate the early diagnosis of diseases and the determination of appropriate treatment methods. In radiological imaging, AI-supported systems have begun to be used in image classification and analysis processes. By reducing the risk of human error, this will assist clinicians in diagnosing diseases more rapidly and accurately. AI algorithms in radiological tests such as mammography, MRI, and CT screenings have been shown to reduce the workload of radiology specialists.

6.1. *Potential and Limitations of Artificial Intelligence in Clinical Practice*

However, the areas of potential AI use in surgical procedures have not yet been fully established. This is attributed to the need for a very large number of patient datasets for improved management of the dynamic processes and variables that occur during surgery. AI-supported CDSSs significantly contribute to optimizing a clinician's decision-making process and to forming personalized treatment plans. This will undoubtedly improve patient outcomes, making patient care more effective. Nevertheless, several challenges, such as data confidentiality, ethics, and cost, must be overcome before the widespread implementation of AI-supported systems.

6.2. *Future Directions and Research Needs*

In conclusion, AI technologies have made great strides in the healthcare sector, but further research and development are necessary to realize their full potential. The continuation of studies in this field is of great importance, especially for AI to be routinely used in the clinical environment.

References

1. Pang Z, Yuan H, Zhang YT, Packirisamy M. Guest editorial health engineering driven by the Industry 4.0 for aging society. *IEEE J. Biomed. Health Inform.* 2018 Nov;22(6):1709–10.

2. McCarthy J. Artificial intelligence, logic and formalizing common sense. In: Thomason RH (ed) *Philosophical Logic and Artificial Intelligence*. Dordrecht: Springer, 1989. https://doi.org/10.1007/978-94-009-2448-2_6
3. Turing AM. Computing machinery and intelligence. In: Epstein R, Roberts G, Beber G (ed) *Parsing the Turing Test*. Dordrecht: Springer, 2009. https://doi.org/10.1007/978-1-4020-6710-5_3
4. Jiang F, Jiang Y, Zhi H, Dong Y, Li H, Ma S, et al. Artificial intelligence in healthcare: Past, present and future. *Stroke Vasc. Neurol.* 2017 Jun;2(4):230–43. https://doi.org/10.1136/svn-2017-000101. PMID: 29507784; PMCID: PMC5829945
5. Graham S, Depp C, Lee EE, Nebeker C, Tu X, Kim HC, et al. Artificial intelligence for mental health and mental illnesses: An overview. *Curr. Psychiatry Rep.* 2019 Nov;21(11):116. https://doi.org/10.1007/s11920-019-1094-0. PMID: 31701320; PMCID: PMC7274446.
6. Hamet P, Tremblay J. Artificial intelligence in medicine. *Metabolism.* 2017 Apr;69S:S36–S40. https://doi.org/10.1016/j.metabol.2017.01.011. Epub 2017 Jan 11. PMID: 28126242.
7. Howard J. Artificial intelligence: Implications for the future of work. *Am. J. Ind. Med.* 2019 Nov;62(11):917–26. https://doi.org/10.1002/ajim.23037. Epub 2019 Aug 22. PMID: 31436850
8. Hengstler M, Enkel E, Duelli S. Applied artificial intelligence and trust-the case of autonomous vehicles and medical assistance devices. *Technol. Forecast. Soc. Change.* 2016 Apr;105:105–20.
9. Esteva A, Robicquet A, Ramsundar B, Kuleshov V, DePristo M, Chou K, et al. A guide to deep learning in healthcare. *Nat. Med.* 2019 Jan;25(1): 24–9. https://doi.org/10.1038/s41591-018-0316-z. Epub 2019 Jan 7. PMID: 30617335.
10. LeCun Y, Bengio Y, Hinton G. Deep learning. *Nature.* 2015 May;521(7553): 436–44. https://doi.org/10.1038/nature14539. PMID: 26017442.
11. McKinney SM, Sieniek M, Godbole V, Godwin J, Antropova N, Ashrafian H, et al. International evaluation of an AI system for breast cancer screening. *Nature.* 2020 Jan;577(7788):89–94. Epub 2020 Jan 1. Erratum in: Nature. 2020 Oct;586(7829):E19. https://doi.org/10.1038/s41586-020-2679-9. PMID: 31894144.
12. Arslan A, Alis D, Erdemli S, Seker ME, Zeybel G, Sirolu S, et al. Does deep learning software improve the consistency and performance of radiologists with various levels of experience in assessing bi-parametric prostate MRI? *Insights Imaging.* 2023 Mar;14(1):48. https://doi.org/10.1186/s13244-023-01386-w. PMID: 36939953; PMCID: PMC10027972.

13. Nguyen T, Hermann A-L, Ventre J, Ducarouge A, Pourchot A, Marty V, et al. High performance for bone age estimation with an artificial intelligence solution. *Diagn. Interv. Imaging.* 2023 Jul–Aug;104(7–8):330–6. https://doi.org/10.1016/j.diii.2023.04.003. Epub 2023 Apr 22. PMID: 37095034.
14. Bodenstedt S, Wagner M, Müller-Stich BP, Weitz J, Speidel S. Artificial intelligence-assisted surgery: Potential and challenges. *Visc. Med.* 2020 Dec;36(6):450–5. https://doi.org/10.1159/000511351. Epub 2020 Nov 4. PMID: 33447600; PMCID: PMC7768095.
15. Badillo S, Banfai B, Birzele F, Davydov II, Hutchinson L, Kam-Thong T, et al. An introduction to machine learning. *Clin. Pharmacol. Ther.* 2020 Apr;107(4):871–85. https://doi.org/10.1002/cpt.1796. Epub 2020 Mar 3. PMID: 32128792; PMCID: PMC7189875.
16. Gupta R, Srivastava D, Sahu M, Tiwari S, Ambasta RK, Kumar P. Artificial intelligence to deep learning: Machine intelligence approach for drug discovery. *Mol. Divers.* 2021 Aug;25(3):1315–60. https://doi.org/10.1007/s11030-021-10217-3. Epub 2021 Apr 12. PMID: 33844136; PMCID: PMC8040371.
17. Jiang Y, Luo J, Huang D, Liu Y, Li DD. Machine learning advances in microbiology: A review of methods and applications. *Front. Microbiol.* 2022 May;13:925454.
18. Theodosiou AA, Read RC. Artificial intelligence, machine learning and deep learning: Potential resources for the infection clinician. *J. Infect.* 2023 Oct;87(4):287–94. https://doi.org/10.1016/j.jinf.2023.07.006. Epub 2023 Jul 17. PMID: 37468046.
19. Angermueller C, Pärnamaa T, Parts L, Stegle O. Deep learning for computational biology. *Mol. Syst. Biol.* 2016 Jul;12(7):878. https://doi.org/10.15252/msb.20156651. PMID: 27474269; PMCID: PMC4965871.
20. Sidey-Gibbons JAM, Sidey-Gibbons CJ. Machine learning in medicine: A practical introduction. *BMC Med. Res. Methodol.* 2019 Mar;19(1):64. https://doi.org/10.1186/s12874-019-0681-4. PMID: 30890124; PMCID: PMC6425557.
21. James G, Witten D, Hastie T, Tibshirani R. Introduction. In: *An Introduction to Statistical Learning*. New York: Springer, 2021. https://doi.org/10.1007/978-1-0716-1418-1_1
22. The essential physics of medical imaging. Second edition. 2002. *Eur. J. Nucl. Med. Mol. Imaging.* 2003;30(12):1713. https://doi.org/10.1007/S00259-003-1310-2
23. Hounsfield GN. Computerized transverse axial scanning (tomography). 1. Description of system. *Br. J. Radiol.* 1973 Dec;46(552):1016–22. https://doi.org/10.1259/0007-1285-46-552-1016. PMID: 4757352.

24. Mansfield P. Multi-planar image formation using NMR spin echoes. *J. Phys. C Solid State Phys.* 1977;10(3).
25. Cherry SR, Jones T, Karp JS, Qi J, Moses WW, Badawi RD. Total-body PET: Maximizing sensitivity to create new opportunities for clinical research and patient care. *J. Nucl. Med.* 2018 Jan;59(1):3–12. https://doi.org/10.2967/jnumed.116.184028. Epub 2017 Sep 21. PMID: 28935835; PMCID: PMC5750522.
26. Hutton BF, Buvat I, Beekman FJ. Review and current status of SPECT scatter correction. *Phys. Med. Biol.* 2011 Jul;56(14):R85–112. https://doi.org/10.1088/0031-9155/56/14/R01. Epub 2011 Jun 23. PMID: 21701055.
27. Lorenz JM. Management of malignant biliary obstruction. *Semin. Intervent. Radiol.* 2016 Dec;33(4):259–67. https://doi.org/10.1055/s-0036-1592330. PMID: 27904244; PMCID: PMC5088103.
28. Giardino A, Gupta S, Olson E, Sepulveda K, Lenchik L, Ivanidze J, et al. Role of imaging in the era of precision medicine. *Acad. Radiol.* 2017 May;24(5):639–49. https://doi.org/10.1016/j.acra.2016.11.021. Epub 2017 Jan 25. PMID: 28131497.
29. Buchanan B, Shortliffe E. *Rule Based Expert Systems: The Mycin Experiments of the Stanford Heuristic Programming Project (the Addison-Wesley series in artificial intelligence).* Addison-Wesley, 1984.
30. Pennachin C, Goertzel B. Contemporary approaches to artificial general intelligence. In: Goertzel B, Pennachin C, (eds) *Artificial General Intelligence*. Berlin: Springer, 2007. https://doi.org/10.1007/978-3-540-68677-4_1
31. Jena B, Saxena S, Nayak GK, Saba L, Sharma N, Suri JS. Artificial intelligence-based hybrid deep learning models for image classification: The first narrative review. *Comput. Biol. Med.* 2021 Oct;137:104803. https://doi.org/10.1016/j.compbiomed.2021.104803. Epub 2021 Aug 27. PMID: 34536856.
32. Hosny A, Parmar C, Quackenbush J, Schwartz LH, Aerts HJWL. Artificial intelligence in radiology. *Nat. Rev. Cancer.* 2018 Aug;18(8):500–10. https://doi.org/10.1038/s41568-018-0016-5. PMID: 29777175; PMCID: PMC6268174.
33. Annarumma M, Withey SJ, Bakewell RJ, Pesce E, Goh V, Montana G. Automated triaging of adult chest radiographs with deep artificial neural networks. *Radiology.* 2019 Apr;291(1):196–202. Epub 2019 Jan 22. Erratum in: Radiology. 2019 Apr;291(1):272. https://doi.org/10.1148/radiol.2019194005. PMID: 30667333; PMCID: PMC6438359.

34. van Leeuwen KG, Schalekamp S, Rutten MJCM, van Ginneken B, de Rooij M. Artificial intelligence in radiology: 100 commercially available products and their scientific evidence. *Eur. Radiol.* 2021 Jun;31(6):3797–804. https://doi.org/10.1007/s00330-021-07892-z. Epub 2021 Apr 15. PMID: 33856519; PMCID: PMC8128724.
35. Higuchi M, Nagata T, Iwabuchi K, Sano A, Maekawa H, Idaka T, et al. Development of a novel artificial intelligence algorithm to detect pulmonary nodules on chest radiography. *Fukushima J. Med. Sci.* 2023;69(3):177–83.
36. Treskes K, Sierink JC, Edwards MJR, Beuker BJA, Van Lieshout EMM, Hohmann J, et al. Cost-effectiveness of immediate total-body CT in patients with severe trauma (REACT-2 trial). *Br. J. Surg.* 2021 Apr;108(3): 277–85. https://doi.org/10.1093/bjs/znaa091. PMID: 33793734; PMCID: PMC10364909.
37. Kalmet PHS, Sanduleanu S, Primakov S, Wu G, Jochems A, Refaee T, et al. Deep learning in fracture detection: A narrative review. *Acta Orthop.* 2020 Apr;91(2):215–20. https://doi.org/10.1080/17453674.2019.1711323. Epub 2020 Jan 13. Update in: Acta Orthop. 2020 Jun;91(3):362. https://doi.org/10.1080/17453674.2020.1723292. PMID: 31928116; PMCID: PMC7144272.
38. Mello-Thoms C, Mello CAB. Clinical applications of artificial intelligence in radiology. *Br. J. Radiol.* 2023 Oct;96(1150):20221031. https://doi.org/10.1259/bjr.20221031. Epub 2023 Apr 26. PMID: 37099398; PMCID: PMC10546456.
39. Cau R, Flanders A, Mannelli L, Politi C, Faa G, Suri JS, et al. Artificial intelligence in computed tomography plaque characterization: A review. *Eur. J. Radiol.* 2021 Jul;140:109767. https://doi.org/10.1016/j.ejrad.2021.109767. Epub 2021 May 8. Erratum in: *Eur. J. Radiol.* 2022 Feb;147:110132. https://doi.org/10.1016/j.ejrad.2021.110132. PMID: 34000598.
40. Lin DJ, Walter SS, Fritz J. Artificial intelligence-driven ultra-fast superresolution MRI: 10-fold accelerated musculoskeletal turbo spin echo MRI within reach. *Invest. Radiol.* 2023 Jan;58(1):28–42. https://doi.org/10.1097/RLI.0000000000000928. Epub 2022 Nov 2. PMID: 36355637.
41. Wu J, Xiao P, Huang H, Gou F, Zhou Z, Dai Z. An artificial intelligence multiprocessing scheme for the diagnosis of osteosarcoma MRI images. *IEEE J. Biomed. Health Inform.* 2022 Sep;26(9):4656–67. https://doi.org/10.1109/JBHI.2022.3184930. Epub 2022 Sep 9. PMID: 35727772.
42. Zhao X, Bai JW, Guo Q, Ren K, Zhang GJ. Clinical applications of deep learning in breast MRI. *Biochim. Biophys. Acta Rev. Cancer.* 2023

Mar;1878(2):188864. https://doi.org/10.1016/j.bbcan.2023.188864. Epub 2023 Feb 21. PMID: 36822377.

43. García-Ramó KB, Sanchez-Catasus CA, Winston GP. Deep learning in neuroimaging of epilepsy. *Clin. Neurol. Neurosurg.* 2023 Sep;232:107879. https://doi.org/10.1016/j.clineuro.2023.107879. Epub 2023 Jul 6. PMID: 37473486.
44. Onnis C, van Assen M, Muscogiuri E, Muscogiuri G, Gershon G, Saba L, et al. The role of artificial intelligence in cardiac imaging. *Radiol. Clin. North Am.* 2024 May;62(3):473–88. https://doi.org/10.1016/j.rcl.2024.01.002. Epub 2024 Feb 7. PMID: 38553181.
45. Ringwald FG, Martynova A, Mierisch J, Wielpütz M, Eisenmann U. Explainable artificial intelligence for deep-learning based classification of cystic fibrosis lung changes in MRI. *Stud. Health Technol. Inform.* 2024 Jan;310:921–5. https://doi.org/10.3233/SHTI231099. PMID: 38269943.
46. Ozkaya E, Topal FE, Bulut T, Gursoy M, Ozuysal M, Karakaya Z. Evaluation of an artificial intelligence system for diagnosing scaphoid fracture on direct radiography. *Eur. J. Trauma Emerg. Surg.* 2022 Feb;48(1):585–92. https://doi.org/10.1007/s00068-020-01468-0. Epub 2020 Aug 30. PMID: 32862314.
47. Murata K, Endo K, Aihara T, Suzuki H, Sawaji Y, Matsuoka Y, et al. Artificial intelligence for the detection of vertebral fractures on plain spinal radiography. *Sci. Rep.* 2020;10:20031. https://doi.org/10.1038/s41598-020-76866-w
48. von Schacky CE, Wilhelm NJ, Schäfer VS, Leonhardt Y, Gassert FG, Foreman SC, et al. Multitask deep learning for segmentation and classification of primary bone tumors on radiographs. *Radiology.* 2021 Nov;301(2):398–406. https://doi.org/10.1148/radiol.2021204531. Epub 2021 Sep 7. PMID: 34491126.
49. Beheshtian E, Putman K, Santomartino SM, Parekh VS, Yi PH. Generalizability and bias in a deep learning pediatric bone age prediction model using hand radiographs. *Radiology.* 2023 Feb;306(2):e220505. https://doi.org/10.1148/radiol.220505. Epub 2022 Sep 27. PMID: 36165796.
50. Kim KD, Kyung S, Jang M, Ji S, Lee DH, Yoon HM, et al. Enhancement of non-linear deep learning model by adjusting confounding variables for bone age estimation in pediatric hand X-rays. *J. Digit. Imaging.* 2023 Oct;36(5):2003–14. https://doi.org/10.1007/s10278-023-00849-2. Epub 2023 Jun 2. PMID: 37268839; PMCID: PMC10501988.
51. Huber MB, Lancianese SL, Nagarajan MB, Ikpot IZ, Lerner AL, Wismuller A. Prediction of biomechanical properties of trabecular bone in MR images

with geometric features and support vector regression. *IEEE Trans. Biomed. Eng.* 2011 Jun;58(6):1820–6. https://doi.org/10.1109/TBME.2011.2119484. Epub 2011 Feb 28. PMID: 21356612.

52. Yang CC, Nagarajan MB, Huber MB, Carballido-Gamio J, Bauer JS, Baum T, et al. Improving bone strength prediction in human proximal femur specimens through geometrical characterization of trabecular bone microarchitecture and support vector regression. *J. Electron. Imaging.* 2014 Feb;23(1):013013. https://doi.org/10.1117/1.JEI.23.1.013013. Epub 2014 Jan 9. PMID: 24860245; PMCID: PMC4030629.
53. Regnard NE, Lanseur B, Ventre J, Ducarouge A, Clovis L, Lassalle L, et al. Assessment of performances of a deep learning algorithm for the detection of limbs and pelvic fractures, dislocations, focal bone lesions, and elbow effusions on trauma X-rays. *Eur. J. Radiol.* 2022 Sep;154:110447. https://doi.org/10.1016/j.ejrad.2022.110447. Epub 2022 Jul 22. PMID: 35921795.
54. Lopez CD, Gazgalis A, Boddapati V, Shah RP, Cooper HJ, Geller JA. Artificial learning and machine learning decision guidance applications in total hip and knee arthroplasty: A systematic review. *Arthroplast. Today.* 2021 Sep;11:103–12. https://doi.org/10.1016/j.artd.2021.07.012. PMID: 34522738; PMCID: PMC8426157.
55. Wu H, Bailey C, Rasoulinejad P, Li S. Automated comprehensive adolescent idiopathic scoliosis assessment using MVC-Net. *Med. Image Anal.* 2018 Aug;48:1–11. https://doi.org/10.1016/j.media.2018.05.005. Epub 2018 May 18. PMID: 29803920.
56. Dreizin D, Goldmann F, LeBedis C, Boscak A, Dattwyler M, Bodanapally U, et al. An automated deep learning method for tile AO/OTA pelvic fracture severity grading from trauma whole-body CT. *J. Digit. Imaging.* 2021 Feb;34(1):53–65. https://doi.org/10.1007/s10278-020-00399-x. Epub 2021 Jan 21. PMID: 33479859; PMCID: PMC7886919.
57. Yoon SJ, Kim TH, Joo SB, Oh SE. Automatic multi-class intertrochanteric femur fracture detection from CT images based on AO/OTA classification using faster R-CNN-BO method. *J. Appl. Biomed.* 2020;18(4): 97–105.
58. Pranata YD, Wang KC, Wang JC, Idram I, Lai JY, Liu JW, et al. Deep learning and SURF for automated classification and detection of calcaneus fractures in CT images. *Comput. Methods Programs Biomed.* 2019 Apr;171:27–37. https://doi.org/10.1016/j.cmpb.2019.02.006. Epub 2019 Feb 12. PMID: 30902248.
59. Small JE, Osler P, Paul AB, Kunst M. CT cervical spine fracture detection using a convolutional neural network. *AJNR Am. J. Neuroradiol.* 2021

Jul;42(7):1341–7. https://doi.org/10.3174/ajnr.A7094. Epub 2021 Apr 1. PMID: 34255730; PMCID: PMC8324280.

60. Yacoub B, Kabakus IM, Schoepf UJ, Giovagnoli VM, Fischer AM, Wichmann JL, et al. Performance of an artificial intelligence-based platform against clinical radiology reports for the evaluation of noncontrast chest CT. *Acad. Radiol.* 2022 Feb;29(Suppl 2):S108–S117. https://doi.org/10.1016/j.acra.2021.02.007. Epub 2021 Mar 10. PMID: 33714665.
61. Castro-Zunti R, Chae KJ, Choi Y, Jin GY, Ko SB. Assessing the speed-accuracy trade-offs of popular convolutional neural networks for single-crop rib fracture classification. *Comput. Med. Imaging Graph.* 2021 Jul;91:101937. https://doi.org/10.1016/j.compmedimag.2021.101937. Epub 2021 May 15. PMID: 34087611.
62. Zhang Z, Seeram E. The use of artificial intelligence in computed tomography image reconstruction — A literature review. *J. Med. Imaging Radiat. Sci.* 2020 Dec;51(4):671–7. https://doi.org/10.1016/j.jmir.2020.09.001. Epub 2020 Sep 24. PMID: 32981888.
63. Crombé A, Spinnato P, Italiano A, Brisse HJ, Feydy A, Fadli D, et al. Radiomics and artificial intelligence for soft-tissue sarcomas: Current status and perspectives. *Diagn. Interv. Imaging.* 2023 Dec;104(12):567–83. https://doi.org/10.1016/j.diii.2023.09.005. Epub 2023 Oct 4. PMID: 37802753.
64. Roblot V, Giret Y, Bou Antoun M, Morillot C, Chassin X, Cotten A, et al. Artificial intelligence to diagnose meniscus tears on MRI. *Diagn. Interv. Imaging.* 2019 Apr;100(4):243–9. https://doi.org/10.1016/j.diii.2019.02.007. Epub 2019 Mar 28. PMID: 30928472.
65. Santomartino SM, Kung J, Yi PH. Systematic review of artificial intelligence development and evaluation for MRI diagnosis of knee ligament or meniscus tears. *Skeletal Radiol.* 2024 Mar;53(3):445–54. https://doi.org/10.1007/s00256-023-04416-2. Epub 2023 Aug 16. PMID: 37584757.
66. Schock J, Truhn D, Nürnberger D, Conrad S, Huppertz MS, Keil S, et al. Artificial intelligence-based automatic assessment of lower limb torsion on MRI. *Sci. Rep.* 2021 Dec;11(1):23244. https://doi.org/10.1038/s41598-021-02708-y. PMID: 34853401; PMCID: PMC8636587.
67. Biamonte E, Levi R, Carrone F, Vena W, Brunetti A, Battaglia M, et al. Artificial intelligence-based radiomics on computed tomography of lumbar spine in subjects with fragility vertebral fractures. *J. Endocrinol. Invest.* 2022 Oct;45(10):2007–17. https://doi.org/10.1007/s40618-022-01837-z. Epub 2022 Jun 25. PMID: 35751803.

68. Ferizi U, Honig S, Chang G. Artificial intelligence, osteoporosis and fragility fractures. *Curr. Opin. Rheumatol.* 2019 Jul;31(4):368–75. https://doi.org/10.1097/BOR.0000000000000607. PMID: 31045948; PMCID: PMC7282383.
69. Kahn CE Jr. Artificial intelligence in radiology: Decision support systems. *Radiographics.* 1994 Jul;14(4):849–61. https://doi.org/10.1148/radiographics.14.4.7938772. PMID: 7938772.
70. Sim I, Gorman P, Greenes RA, Haynes RB, Kaplan B, Lehmann H, et al. Clinical decision support systems for the practice of evidence-based medicine. *J. Am. Med. Inform. Assoc.* 2001 Nov–Dec;8(6):527–34. https://doi.org/10.1136/jamia.2001.0080527. PMID: 11687560; PMCID: PMC130063.
71. Beam AL, Kohane IS. Big data and machine learning in health care. *JAMA.* 2018 Apr;319(13):1317–8. https://doi.org/10.1001/jama.2017.18391. PMID: 29532063.
72. Peiffer-Smadja N, Rawson TM, Ahmad R, Buchard A, Georgiou P, Lescure F-X, et al. Machine learning for clinical decision support in infectious diseases: A narrative review of current applications. *Clin. Microbiol. Infect.* 2020 May;26(5):584–95. https://doi.org/10.1016/j.cmi.2019.09.009. Epub 2019 Sep 17. Erratum in: Clin Microbiol Infect. 2020 Aug;26(8):1118. https://doi.org/10.1016/j.cmi.2020.05.020. PMID: 31539636.
73. Ouanes K, Farhah N. Effectiveness of artificial intelligence (AI) in clinical decision support systems and care delivery. *J. Med. Syst.* 2024 Aug;48(1):74. https://doi.org/10.1007/s10916-024-02098-4. PMID: 39133332.
74. Brink JA, Arenson RL, Grist TM, Lewin JS, Enzmann D. Bits and bytes: The future of radiology lies in informatics and information technology. *Eur. Radiol.* 2017 Sep;27(9):3647–51. https://doi.org/10.1007/s00330-016-4688-5. Epub 2017 Mar 9. PMID: 28280932.
75. Loftus TJ, Tighe PJ, Filiberto AC, Efron PA, Brakenridge SC, Mohr AM, et al. Artificial intelligence and surgical decision-making. *JAMA Surg.* 2020 Feb;155(2):148–58. https://doi.org/10.1001/jamasurg.2019.4917. PMID: 31825465; PMCID: PMC7286802.
76. Sacks GD, Dawes AJ, Ettner SL, Brook RH, Fox CR, Maggard-Gibbons M, et al. Surgeon perception of risk and benefit in the decision to operate. *Ann. Surg.* 2016 Dec;264(6):896–903. https://doi.org/10.1097/SLA.0000000000001784. PMID: 27192348.
77. Coleman JJ, Robinson CK, Zarzaur BL, Timsina L, Rozycki GS, Feliciano DV. To sleep, perchance to dream: Acute and chronic sleep deprivation in acute care surgeons. *J. Am. Coll. Surg.* 2019 Aug;229(2):166–74. https://doi.org/10.1016/j.jamcollsurg.2019.03.019. Epub 2019 Apr 6. PMID: 30959105.

78. Brennan M, Puri S, Ozrazgat-Baslanti T, Feng Z, Ruppert M, Hashemighouchani H, et al. Comparing clinical judgment with the MySurgeryRisk algorithm for preoperative risk assessment: A pilot usability study. *Surgery.* 2019 May;165(5):1035–45. https://doi.org/10.1016/j.surg.2019.01.002. Epub 2019 Feb 18. PMID: 30792011; PMCID: PMC6502657.
79. Margalit RS, Roter D, Dunevant MA, Larson S, Reis S. Electronic medical record use and physician-patient communication: An observational study of Israeli primary care encounters. *Patient Educ. Couns.* 2006 Apr;61(1):134–41. https://doi.org/10.1016/j.pec.2005.03.004. PMID: 16533682.
80. Asan O, D Smith P, Montague E. More screen time, less face time — Implications for EHR design. *J. Eval. Clin. Pract.* 2014 Dec;20(6):896–901. https://doi.org/10.1111/jep.12182. Epub 2014 May 19. PMID: 24835678; PMCID: PMC4237676.
81. Price WN 2nd, Cohen IG. Privacy in the age of medical big data. *Nat. Med.* 2019 Jan;25(1):37–43. https://doi.org/10.1038/s41591-018-0272-7. Epub 2019 Jan 7. PMID: 30617331; PMCID: PMC6376961.
82. Wijnberge M, Geerts BF, Hol L, Lemmers N, Mulder MP, Berge P, et al. Effect of a machine learning-derived early warning system for intraoperative hypotension vs standard care on depth and duration of intraoperative hypotension during elective noncardiac surgery: The HYPE randomized clinical trial. *JAMA.* 2020 Mar;323(11):1052–60. https://doi.org/10.1001/jama.2020.0592. PMID: 32065827; PMCID: PMC7078808.
83. Abràmoff MD, Lavin PT, Birch M, Shah N, Folk JC. Pivotal trial of an autonomous AI-based diagnostic system for detection of diabetic retinopathy in primary care offices. *NPJ Digit. Med.* 2018 Aug;1:39. https://doi.org/10.1038/s41746-018-0040-6. PMID: 31304320; PMCID: PMC6550188.
84. Akay EMZ, Hilbert A, Carlisle BG, Madai VI, Mutke MA, Frey D. Artificial intelligence for clinical decision support in acute ischemic stroke: A systematic review. *Stroke.* 2023 Jun;54(6):1505–16. https://doi.org/10.1161/STROKEAHA.122.041442. Epub 2023 May 22. PMID: 37216446.
85. Skuban-Eiseler T, Orzechowski M, Denkinger M, Kocar TD, Leinert C, Steger F. Artificial intelligence-based clinical decision support systems in geriatrics: An ethical analysis. *J. Am. Med. Dir. Assoc.* 2023 Sep;24(9):1271–6.e4. https://doi.org/10.1016/j.jamda.2023.06.008. Epub 2023 Jul 12. PMID: 37453451.
86. Shimabukuro DW, Barton CW, Feldman MD, Mataraso SJ, Das R. Effect of a machine learning-based severe sepsis prediction algorithm on patient

survival and hospital length of stay: A randomised clinical trial. *BMJ Open Respir. Res.* 2017 Nov;4(1):e000234. https://doi.org/10.1136/bmjresp-2017-000234. PMID: 29435343; PMCID: PMC5687546.

87. Khan O, Badhiwala JH, Akbar MA, Fehlings MG. Prediction of worse functional status after surgery for degenerative cervical myelopathy: A machine learning approach. *Neurosurgery.* 2021 Feb;88(3):584–91. https://doi.org/10.1093/neuros/nyaa477. PMID: 33289519.
88. Karhade AV, Thio QCBS, Ogink PT, Shah AA, Bono CM, Oh KS, et al. Development of machine learning algorithms for prediction of 30-day mortality after surgery for spinal metastasis. *Neurosurgery.* 2019 Jul;85(1): E83–91. https://doi.org/10.1093/neuros/nyy469. PMID: 30476188.
89. Liew C. The future of radiology augmented with artificial intelligence: A strategy for success. *Eur. J. Radiol.* 2018 May;102:152–6. https://doi.org/10.1016/j.ejrad.2018.03.019. Epub 2018 Mar 14. PMID: 29685530.
90. Calvert J, Hoffman J, Barton C, Shimabukuro D, Ries M, Chettipally U, et al. Cost and mortality impact of an algorithm-driven sepsis prediction system. *J. Med. Econ.* 2017 Jun;20(6):646–51. https://doi.org/10.1080/13696998.2017.1307203. Epub 2017 Apr 3. PMID: 28294646.
91. De Riso G, Cocozza S. Artificial intelligence for epigenetics: Towards personalized medicine. *Curr. Med. Chem.* 2021;28(32):6654–74. https://doi.org/10.2174/0929867327666201117142006. PMID: 33208060.
92. Kegerreis B, Catalina MD, Bachali P, Geraci NS, Labonte AC, Zeng C, et al. Machine learning approaches to predict lupus disease activity from gene expression data. *Sci. Rep.* 2019 Jul;9(1):9617. https://doi.org/10.1038/s41598-019-45989-0. PMID: 31270349; PMCID: PMC6610624.
93. Vadapalli S, Abdelhalim H, Zeeshan S, Ahmed Z. Artificial intelligence and machine learning approaches using gene expression and variant data for personalized medicine. *Brief. Bioinform.* 2022 Sep;23(5):bbac191. https://doi.org/10.1093/bib/bbac191. PMID: 35595537; PMCID: PMC10233311.
94. Wang H-Y, Chang S-C, Lin W-Y, Chen C-H, Chiang S-H, Huang K-Y, et al. Machine learning-based method for obesity risk evaluation using single-nucleotide polymorphisms derived from next-generation sequencing. *J. Comput. Biol.* 2018 Dec;25(12):1347–60. https://doi.org/10.1089/cmb.2018.0002. Epub 2018 Sep 8. PMID: 30204480.
95. Hampel H, Williams C, Etcheto A, Goodsaid F, Parmentier F, Sallantin J, et al. A precision medicine framework using artificial intelligence for the identification and confirmation of genomic biomarkers of response to an Alzheimer's disease therapy: Analysis of the blarcamesine (ANAVEX2-73)

Phase 2a clinical study. *Alzheimers Dement (N Y).* 2020 Apr;6(1):e12013. https://doi.org/10.1002/trc2.12013.PMID:32318621;PMCID:PMC7167374.

96. Held E, Cape J, Tintle N. Comparing machine learning and logistic regression methods for predicting hypertension using a combination of gene expression and next-generation sequencing data. *BMC Proc.* 2016 Oct; 10(Suppl 7):141–5. https://doi.org/10.1186/s12919-016-0020-2. PMID: 27980626; PMCID: PMC5133520.
97. Moingeon P. Artificial intelligence-driven drug development against autoimmune diseases. *Trends Pharmacol. Sci.* 2023 Jul;44(7):411–24. https://doi.org/10.1016/j.tips.2023.04.005. Epub 2023 May 31. PMID: 37268540.
98. Stokes JM, Yang K, Swanson K, Jin W, Cubillos-Ruiz A, Donghia NM, et al. A deep learning approach to antibiotic discovery. *Cell.* 2020 Feb; 180(4):688–702.e13. https://doi.org/10.1016/j.cell.2020.01.021. Erratum in: Cell. 2020 Apr 16;181(2):475–483. https://doi.org/10.1016/j.cell.2020.04.001. PMID: 32084340; PMCID: PMC8349178.
99. Federer SJ, Jones GG. Artificial intelligence in orthopaedics: A scoping review. *PLoS One.* 2021 Nov;16(11):e0260471. https://doi.org/10.1371/journal.pone.0260471. PMID: 34813611; PMCID: PMC8610245.
100. Zhu X, He X, Wang P, He Q, Gao D, Cheng J, et al. A method of localization and segmentation of intervertebral discs in spine MRI based on Gabor filter bank. *Biomed. Eng. Online.* 2016 Mar;15:32. https://doi.org/10.1186/s12938-016-0146-5. PMID: 27000749; PMCID: PMC4802867.
101. Auloge P, Cazzato RL, Ramamurthy N, de Marini P, Rousseau C, Garnon J, et al. Augmented reality and artificial intelligence-based navigation during percutaneous vertebroplasty: A pilot randomised clinical trial. *Eur. Spine J.* 2020 Jul;29(7):1580–89. https://doi.org/10.1007/s00586-019-06054-6. Epub 2019 Jul 2. PMID: 31270676.
102. Chen X, Deng S, Sun M-L, He R. Robotic arm-assisted arthroplasty: The latest developments. *Chin. J. Traumatol.* 2022 May;25(3):125–31. https://doi.org/10.1016/j.cjtee.2021.09.001. Epub 2021 Sep 2. PMID: 34556374; PMCID: PMC9125720.
103. Mason JB, Fehring TK, Estok R, Banel D, Fahrbach K. Meta-analysis of alignment outcomes in computer-assisted total knee arthroplasty surgery. *J. Arthroplasty.* 2007 Dec;22(8):1097–106. https://doi.org/10.1016/j.arth.2007.08.001. PMID: 18078876.
104. Banerjee S, Cherian JJ, Elmallah RK, Pierce TP, Jauregui JJ, Mont MA. Robot-assisted total hip arthroplasty. *Expert Rev. Med. Devices.* 2016; 13(1):47–56. https://doi.org/10.1586/17434440.2016.1124018. Epub 2015 Dec 21. PMID: 26592900.

105. Stiehl JB. Computer-assisted orthopedic surgery (CAOS): Pros and cons. In: Scuderi GR, Tria AJ, (eds) *Minimally Invasive Surgery in Orthopedics*. New York: Springer, 2009. https://doi.org/10.1007/978-0-387-76608-9_73
106. Mittelstadt B, Paul HA, Kazanzides P, Zuhars J, Williamson B, Pettitt R, et al. Development of a surgical robot for cementless total hip replacement. *Robotica*. 1993;11(6):553–60. https://doi.org/10.1017/S0263574700019408
107. Gourin CG, Terris DJ. History of robotic surgery. In: Faust RA (ed) *Robotic in Surgery History, Current and Future Applications*. New York: Nova Science, 2006.
108. Beyaz S. A brief history of artificial intelligence and robotic surgery in orthopedics & traumatology and future expectations. *Jt. Dis. Relat. Surg.* 2020; 31(3):653–5. https://doi.org/10.5606/ehc.2020.75300. PMID: 32962606; PMCID: PMC7607941.
109. Davies B. Robotic surgery — A personal view of the past, present and future. *Int. J. Adv. Robot. Syst.* 2015;12(5). https://doi.org/10.5772/60118
110. Lavery HJ, Thaly R, Albala D, Ahlering T, Shalhav A, Lee D, et al. Robotic equipment malfunction during robotic prostatectomy: A multi-institutional study. *J. Endourol.* 2008 Sep;22(9):2165–8. https://doi.org/10.1089/end.2007.0407. PMID: 18811574.
111. Kozlowski PM, Porter CR, Corman JM. Mechanical failure rate of davinci robotic system: Implications for pre-op patient counseling. *J. Urol.*2006;4(4): 372–3.
112. Hinterwimmer F, Lazic I, Langer S, Suren C, Charitou F, Hirschmann MT, et al. Prediction of complications and surgery duration in primary TKA with high accuracy using machine learning with arthroplasty-specific data. *Knee Surg. Sports Traumatol. Arthrosc.* 2023 Apr;31(4):1323–33. https://doi.org/10.1007/s00167-022-06957-w. Epub 2022 Apr 8. PMID: 35394135; PMCID: PMC10050062.
113. Velasquez Garcia A, Bukowiec LG, Yang L, Nishikawa H, Fitzsimmons JS, Larson AN, et al. Artificial intelligence-based three-dimensional templating for total joint arthroplasty planning: a scoping review. *Int. Orthop.* 2024 Apr;48(4):997–1010. https://doi.org/10.1007/s00264-024-06088-6. Epub 2024 Jan 15. PMID: 38224400.
114. Borjali A, Chen AF, Muratoglu OK, Morid MA, Varadarajan KM. Detecting total hip replacement prosthesis design on plain radiographs using deep convolutional neural network. *J. Orthop. Res.* 2020 Jul;38(7):1465–71. https://doi.org/10.1002/jor.24617. Epub 2020 Feb 11. PMID: 31997411.
115. Burger JA, Kleeblad LJ, Laas N, Pearle AD. Mid-term survivorship and patient-reported outcomes of robotic-arm assisted partial knee arthroplasty.

Bone Joint J. 2020 Jan;102-B(1):108–16. https://doi.org/10.1302/0301-620X.102B1.BJJ-2019-0510.R1. PMID: 31888356.

116. Fenton SH, Low S, Abrams KJ, Butler-Henderson K. Health Information management: changing with time. *Yearb. Med. Inform.* 2017 Aug;26(1):72–7. https://doi.org/10.15265/IY-2017-021. Epub 2017 Sep 11. PMID: 29063538; PMCID: PMC6239228.
117. Al-dossary H, Alumran A, Al-rayes S, Althumairi A, Aljanoubai H, Alhuseini M, et al. An overview of health information management education in Saudi Arabia. Informatics Med. Unlocked. 2021 Jan 1;23 100530. https://doi.org/10.1016/j.imu.2021.100530.
118. Veinot TC, Ancker JS, Bakken S. Health informatics and health equity: Improving our reach and impact. *J. Am. Med. Inform. Assoc.* 2019 Aug 1;26(8–9):689–95. https://doi.org/10.1093/jamia/ocz132. PMID: 31411692; PMCID: PMC7647232.
119. Raghupathi W, Raghupathi V. Big data analytics in healthcare: Promise and potential. *Health Inf. Sci. Syst.* 2014 Feb 7;2:3. https://doi.org/10.1186/2047-2501-2-3. PMID: 25825667; PMCID: PMC4341817.
120. Nkwanyana A, Mathews V, Zachary I, Bhayani V. Skills and competencies in health data analytics for health professionals: a scoping review protocol. *BMJ Open* 2023;13(11):e070596. https://doi.org/10.1136/bmjopen-2022-070596
121. Dash S, Shakyawar SK, Sharma M, Kaushik S. Big data in healthcare: management, analysis and future prospects. *J. Big Data* 2019;6:54. https://doi.org/10.1186/s40537-019-0217-0
122. Ambigavathi M, Sridharan D. Big data analytics in healthcare. 2018 *Tenth Int. Conf. Adv. Comput*. 2018 Dec 1;269–76. https://doi.org/10.1109/ICoAC44903.2018.8939061
123. Adler-Milstein J, Jha AK. HITECH Act drove large gains in hospital electronic health record adoption. *Health Aff.* 2017 Aug 1;36(8):1416–22. https://doi.org/10.1377/hlthaff.2016.1651. PMID: 28784734.
124. Mehta N, Pandit A, Shukla S. Transforming healthcare with big data analytics and artificial intelligence: A systematic mapping study. *J. Biomed. Inform.* 2019 Dec;100:103311. https://doi.org/10.1016/j.jbi.2019.103311. Epub 2019 Oct 17. PMID: 31629922.
125. Rocchio BJ. Achieving cost reduction through data analytics. *AORN J.* 2016 Oct;104(4):320–5. https://doi.org/10.1016/j.aorn.2016.07.010. PMID: 27692078.

126. Stadler JG, Donlon K, Siewert JD, Franken T, Lewis NE. Improving the efficiency and ease of healthcare analysis through use of data visualization dashboards. *Big Data*. 2016 Jun;4(2):129–35. https://doi.org/10.1089/big.2015.0059. PMID: 27441717.
127. Ibanez-Sanchez G, Fernandez-Llatas C, Martinez-Millana A, Celda A, Mandingorra J, Aparici-Tortajada L, et al. Toward value-based healthcare through ınteractive process mining in emergency rooms: The stroke case. *Int. J. Environ. Res. Public. Health*. 2019 May 20;16(10):1783. https://doi.org/10.3390/ijerph16101783. PMID: 31137557; PMCID: PMC6572362.
128. Ramkumar PN, Karnuta JM, Navarro SM, Haeberle HS, Iorio R, Mont MA, et al. Preoperative prediction of value metrics and a patient-specific payment model for primary total hip arthroplasty: Development and validation of a deep learning model. *J. Arthroplasty*. 2019 Oct;34(10):2228–234.e1. https://doi.org/10.1016/j.arth.2019.04.055. Epub 2019 May 2. PMID: 31122849.
129. Zeeshan S, Xiong R, Liang BT, Ahmed Z. 100 years of evolving gene-disease complexities and scientific debutants. *Brief. Bioinform.* 2020 May;21(3):885–905. https://doi.org/10.1093/bib/bbz038. PMID: 30972412.

https://doi.org/10.1142/9789819819645_0010

Chapter 10

Testing and Assessment Models of Musculoskeletal Disease and Injury

Roberta Blake

Faculty of Science and Engineering, Writtle School of Agriculture, Animal and Environmental Sciences, Writtle University College, ARU Writtle, Lordship Rd, Writtle, Chelmsford CM1 3RR, UK

Chapter Outline

* **Corresponding author:** Roberta Blake, Faculty of Science and Engineering, Writtle School of Agriculture, Animal and Environmental Sciences, Writtle University College, ARU Writtle, Lordship Rd, Writtle, Chelmsford CM1 3RR, UK. E-mail: roberta.blake@aru.ac.uk

Abstract

The ultimate aim of most of the biomedical research conducted within the musculoskeletal (MSK) area is to acquire knowledge about both the health and disease of the tissues and how the interlinked systems affect each other. Further, most MSK research involves studying models rather than the pathology itself. In possession of this knowledge, new therapies can be discovered and tested. However, such knowledge cannot always be attained directly from humans, meaning animal models must be used. Our understanding of pathologies, and the subsequent development of therapies, has been heavily influenced by animal models. In the last four decades, animal models have been extensively used to develop our understanding of several diseases and injuries affecting the MSK system. However, more recently, new models and the use of artificial intelligence (AI) have become increasingly accurate and acceptable, meaning that replacing the use of animals in the understanding of pathologies and development of therapies is more accepted. This chapter will cover both types, animal and nonanimal models, to answer the question, why are models so effective in advancing our understanding of the biology of disease and how to treat it? Models have a very significant place in reducing the ambiguity of experiments because they allow for one thing to be tested repeatedly under controlled conditions. They can be adopted worldwide by different scientists, and when the outcome remains the same, this is a powerful test that a particular discovery is both relevant and robust. Experiments using MSK system models that allow us to repeat the same treatment several times, with positive outcomes, can accelerate progress toward developing new treatments or understanding disease.

1. Why Do We Use Animals as Models?

Understanding of the human musculoskeletal system and common clinical disorders of bones, joints, and soft tissues has been enhanced by the use of experimental animal models [1].

For around the last 50 years, animal models have been critical tools for understanding musculoskeletal (MSK) diseases and injuries, as well as for developing and testing new treatments. These models, ranging from small rodents to large animals, replicate various aspects of human MSK conditions, including bone fractures, osteoarthritis (OA), infections, and surgical interventions such as hip implants, spinal fusion, and ligament repair. The animal model deals with species other than humans, as it can imitate the disease progression, its diagnosis, its and response to treatment similar to humans. The discovery of a drug and/or component, a medical device, and other therapies are studied *in vivo* for future use in humans. Animal models may have the ability to mimic pathologies in humans, which have tremendous importance in the elaboration and development of research associated with medical devices and components/drugs and in tissue repair, regeneration, and engineering. The use of animal models has allowed experiments that would have been impossible to accomplish in humans considering the ethical considerations. For instance, in the orthopedic field, there are many conditions that involve bone pathologies whose treatment requires special care and extensive research using specialized techniques as well as specific animal models. For example, this includes research to investigate fracture healing, bone repair in critical size defects, osteoporosis, osteomyelitis, and osteosarcoma [2]. Likewise, animal models have enormous importance in the study of cartilage repair. *In vitro* models are also widely used for cartilage and other tissue repair studies. However, they cannot completely replace the use of animal models before clinical use [2]. This chapter will provide an overview of the animal models commonly used in MSK research, their applications, advantages, and limitations.

2. The Importance of Choosing the Correct Animal Model

Animal models can come in all sizes, large and small. Selecting an animal model for MSK research is a very intricate process. Not all models are acceptable or suitable for specific research due to limitations such as size and inability to replicate the pathology, among others. Therefore, careful considerations should be taken into account during the selection of an ideal animal model for MSK trials. Several animal species, such as the zebrafish (fish), and mammals, such as mice, rabbits, rats, cats, dogs, pigs, and nonhuman primates, have been accepted worldwide for their phylogenetic resemblance to humans [3]. A deep understanding of the available species is required to ensure that the model is adequate and that the outcome measures closely mirror the human pathology or injury [4]. One of the most important factors involved in choosing an animal model, and one that can limit the outcome metrics, is the ability of the animal to simulate the pathology intended to be studied. For instance, OA occurs spontaneously in domestic animals, including horses, swine, cattle, dogs, and rodents such as mice (e.g., C57BL, STR/1N, NZY/B1, PN, and BLO strains), hamsters, and guinea pigs [5]. Rats, however, except bipedal strains and injury models, are resistant to the development of OA [1].

Small animal models, particularly rodents, are widely used in MSK research due to their cost-effectiveness, ease of handling, and the availability of transgenic manipulation techniques. Despite anatomical and physiological differences from humans, these models provide valuable insights into disease mechanisms and therapeutic responses [4, 6]. Furthermore, through the incorporation of human cells into the recipient animals, researchers can create humanized mice, for instance, as experimental models of OA [7] or for bone research [8, 9]. However, a major drawback of small animal models is the sheer difference in the anatomical sizes compared to humans and the fact that findings from such small animal models may not always translate into human clinical applications. This is another great limitation to be considered when choosing the animal model [10, 11].

Large animal models more closely resemble human physiology, and thus, have been used in extensive preclinical and clinical trials. Large animals also have the advantage of possessing large amounts of tissue, making them ideal for immunohistopathological applications. Their size also allows for the use of loaded models, similar to the loads human tissues would receive, allowing not only for studying new treatment strategies but also pathophysiology and disease prevention. However, compared to small animal models, they pose different limitations regarding genetic modification, dissection of specific signaling pathways, and analyzing cell–cell interactions [12]. Primate models, being a closer mimic of human physiology, would be the obvious choice of model; however, their use in research is extremely limited due to increased ethical concerns [13]. Naturally occurring disease models, particularly for longer-lived large animal species, allow for studying disorders at an advanced age when some diseases, such as OA, are most prevalent. As these diseases are usually a concern in the chosen veterinary species, as in humans, animals alike can also be beneficiaries of newly developed therapies [4]. However, size is not the only translational challenge; there are differences in the bioavailability and toxicity of pharmaceuticals between humans, primates, dogs, and rodents, and whether animals can be used to predict a human response or adverse effects to drugs and other chemicals is still a contentious issue [14]. For example, the painkiller rofecoxib with indications for OA and arthritic pain, among others, was successful during animal testing, but its long-term use by humans led to an increased risk of heart attack and stroke.

As such, issues due to size or an increased knowledge of the dissimilarities between species still pose challenges to the choice of the animal model that is most appropriate. Therefore, the proper selection of an animal model is mainly related to the nature of the disease, the drug, or the medical device under study. However, a key component in selecting and aligning the animal model and research outcomes is a focused consideration of the study objectives, and given the advantages and disadvantages of each model, we can conclude that *not all questions can/will be answered with one model* [15]. In that case, the combination of several models can potentially increase the power of the outcomes.

3. Small Animal Models

Rodents, especially mice and rats, are frequently used to study bone healing and fracture repair, with mice representing 53.5% of the animal models used in the preclinical fracture studies reported over the past decade [16]. The most common model of bone repair used in small animal models is a closed, simple, transverse fracture (usually in the femur or the tibia). The fracture is produced by externally applied blunt trauma and primarily heals through endochondral ossification and the formation of a callus. This model has been used to investigate the stages of bone healing from inflammation and callus formation to remodeling. For example, femoral fracture models in rats are commonly used to study the effects of mechanical stabilization and the role of growth factors in bone healing [17, 18]. Open femoral fracture models in mice have also been used to increase investigation into fracture healing and its disturbance as a delayed union and non-union [19]. Besides endochondral ossification, mice can be used for distraction osteogenesis models, allowing elucidation of mechanisms that translate to clinical treatment of limb length discrepancies and large bone defects. The distraction osteogenesis model is most applicable to studies involving the biological processes that occur in response to mechanical strain applied to the callus during healing and of the cellular and molecular regulators of bone regeneration [20], as well as exploring therapies to enhance bone regeneration [21]. Mice are also a valuable model for age-related research that focuses on bone, such as the osteoporosis/osteopenia pathophysiology and associated therapeutic research [22–25]. Further, the humanized osteosarcoma rat model replicates pathognomonic features of human osteosarcoma [8].

Furthermore, rodent models of OA are crucial for understanding the pathogenesis of the disease [7] and, to a lesser extent, testing potential therapeutics. In comparison with large animal models, small animal models are relatively quicker, cheaper, and easier models to implement and study and can be used as screening models to refine the ideas before the large animal trial, which then precedes the human clinical trial [26]. However, as mentioned before, the drugs, though shown to be efficacious and nontoxic in small animal studies, may not be translatable to humans with the same efficacy and safety. The great disparities between the anatomy, histology, and physiology of small animals and humans are probably the reason for these limitations. For example, the average cartilage thickness in mice is much smaller than that in humans and partial thickness cartilage defects are not recognized [27]. Despite these limitations, small animal OA models account for 77% of the published research in OA animal models since 1964 [27]. The slowly progressing OA in mice and guinea pigs [28] closely simulates the natural progression of human primary OA, and these models are commonly used as naturally occurring OA models for the study of pathophysiology and progression [26, 28, 29]. In addition to this, various transgenic mouse models (e.g., C57BL/6, BALB/c, and STR/ort strains) have been designed to develop OA without intervention. These models, including humanized mice [7], replicate key features of human OA, such as cartilage degradation, subchondral bone sclerosis, and synovitis [30]. OA models used in rodents also include, (i) chemically induced (e.g., *via* mono-iodoacetate injection); (ii) noninvasive (e.g., high-fat diet or obesity-induced); (iii) physical activity and exercise-induced OA; (iv) noninvasive mechanical loading (e.g., repetitive mild loading and single-impact injury); and (v) surgically induced (e.g., meniscectomy or anterior cruciate ligament [ACL] transection). The specific model chosen will depend upon the aim of the study [31–33].

Bone infection, or osteomyelitis, can be studied using rodent models by introducing pathogens such as *Staphylococcus aureus* directly into the bone site or intravenously to generate bone abscesses and reproduce post-traumatic osteomyelitis [34–39], implant-related osteomyelitis [40–44], osteomyelitis secondary to vascular insufficiency [45–48], and hematogenous osteomyelitis [49–52]. While *in vitro* models are useful for initial testing of therapies against *S. aureus* (e.g., biofilm analyses), they may not translate to the infected animal model [53]. Osteomyelitis models are used to investigate the host immune response, the efficacy of antibiotics, and the development of biofilm on bone surfaces. However, and as with any animal model, it has challenges, as the small size of mice and rats makes them inadequate for long bone surgery procedures, but they are unique for quantitative microbiology tests (e.g., cell counting) [35].

Ectopic bone formation models involve the implantation of bone-inducing materials into non-skeletal sites, such as subcutaneously [54, 55], in muscle pouches [56], and within the kidney capsule [57], to study osteogenesis. Virtually any animal model is suitable for this purpose, but rodent models are preferable and most widely used due to their low cost, lax skin (which accommodates large-volume implants), and the availability of immunodeficient rodents for xenograft-based experiments [58]. These models are particularly useful for testing the osteoinductive potential of biomaterials and growth factors.

Rodents can also be a valuable model for ligament and tendon pathophysiology and repair, and rodent models that investigate the ACL have become increasingly prevalent in the past two decades. Despite the ACL in rodents being much less complex than in humans, it has a similar biomechanical function in preventing tibial translation, making this model quite popular [59]. Rodent models of ligament and tendon repair involve surgical transection or nonsurgical rupture, and repair of these structures is followed by the evaluation of healing and functional outcomes. These models are used to study the effects of different surgical techniques, graft materials [60], and biological enhancers for tendon-to-bone healing [61]. However, despite being inexpensive and easy to handle, rodents (rats and mice) also possess challenges due to their small size, which influences the surgical approach, noninvasive imaging techniques, and biomechanical testing [59]. Unloading models, such as hindlimb suspension in rodents, are used to simulate the effects of reduced mechanical loading on bone and muscle. These models are particularly relevant for studying osteoporosis, muscle atrophy, and the effects of prolonged bed rest or spaceflight. Hindlimb suspension in mice has been used to investigate the molecular mechanisms of bone loss and the effectiveness of countermeasures such as mechanical stimulation or pharmacological agents [62–65].

4. Large Animal Models

Large animal models are closer to human physiology and biomechanics, making them more predictive of clinical outcomes. They are particularly valuable for preclinical testing of implants, surgical techniques, and regenerative therapies.

4.1. *Canine Models*

Dogs are used in MSK research due to their size, joint structure, and susceptibility to conditions including OA and ligament injuries. It is important to note that in some countries, such as the UK, the use of this species has special ethical regulations, and therefore their use is extremely limited. Canine models of OA are used to study disease progression and to evaluate new treatments. Naturally occurring OA in dogs, particularly in the hip, elbow, and stifle (human knee) joints, mirrors the human condition, and therefore dogs have been beneficial as natural models in preclinical trials of therapeutic intervention [66–68]. Besides that, their anatomy is markedly similar to that of humans. For instance, the cartilage thickness of dogs is less than half the size of humans [26]. Surgical induction of OA, such as by meniscectomy [69], ligament transection (e.g., cranial cruciate ligament (CCL), the canine equivalent to the ACL) [70], use of the 'groove model' [71], or through the creation of cartilage defect(s) [72], are also used to create controlled models for therapeutic testing. Another advantage in the use of dogs as models for OA is that, differently from small rodents, they tend to express their pain by not being active, and through whining, and licking. Thus, through monitoring these symptoms, changes due to OA in dogs can be more precisely studied than in smaller animals [26]. Nonetheless, dogs are less used than small rodents in OA research due to costs, housing difficulties, and ethical concerns.

Dogs have also been used for bone implant and joint replacement development. The development and testing of hip implants can be conducted in canine models due to the similarities in joint size and loading patterns with humans. These models allow for the assessment of implant stability, wear, and the integration of bone with implant materials. For example, canine hip arthroplasty models have been used to evaluate the long-term performance of various implant designs and materials *in vivo* [73, 74] and also for *ex vivo* biomechanical loading performance tests [75, 76]. Dogs have been used as models for Achilles tendon, flexor tendon, and CCL (ACL) injury and repair. CCL injuries are common in dogs, and the canine stifle (human knee) is remarkably similar to the human joint, making dogs a suitable model for studying ACL repair techniques [77]. Due to naturally occurring ACL rupture in dogs being a common clinical issue, studies performed in these cases are beneficial as they contribute to One Health efforts to advance both companion animal and human health simultaneously [78]. Surgical models, such as tibial plateau leveling osteotomy or extracapsular repair, are used to evaluate the outcomes of different surgical interventions, graft materials, and postoperative rehabilitation protocols.

4.2. *Ovine and Caprine Models*

Sheep and goats are another widely used large animal model in MSK research, particularly for bone and joint studies, due to their size, bone structure, and ability to simulate human orthopedic conditions. Sheep and goats also have adequate cartilage thickness, allowing for cartilage research in loaded models to be performed. Furthermore, the distribution of mechanical loads that act across the joints during load-bearing activities resembles humans, and sheep have a comparable bone healing rate to that of humans [79]. Consequently, the sheep model, in particular, is being increasingly applied to the field of biomedical research and is arguably one of the most influential models of human organ systems [80]. Ovine models are commonly used to study bone fracture healing and the effectiveness of new orthopedic implants. The long bones of sheep, such as the femur or tibia, are similar in size and structure to human bones, making them ideal for testing fixation devices, bone grafts, and biologics. These models have been used to investigate the mechanical and biological factors that influence fracture healing and the performance of novel bone substitutes [81–83]. Hip replacement implant testing often uses sheep as a model, as the size of the femur and acetabulum are suitable to receive human implants [84, 85]. Sheep models have also been valuable in studying intraosseous transcutaneous amputation prostheses implants for both bone integration and soft tissue sealing [86–89].

Sheep are frequently used in spinal fusion research due to the anatomical similarities between the ovine and human spine. Ovine models allow for the evaluation of fusion rates, implant integration, and the biological response to graft materials. These models have been instrumental in testing new spinal fusion techniques, such as the use of growth factors, including bone morphogenetic protein-2, and novel interbody fusion devices [90, 91], as well as the treatment of implant-associated infection [92]. However, caution needs to be taken when sheep are used as the animal model for the functional evaluation of different cervical interbody fusion cages. This is because sheep present exaggerated stresses (up to 3 times more), a range of motion (up to 10 times more), and are very sensitive to variations in prosthetic design [93]. The ovine shoulder model is used to study rotator cuff injuries and repair strategies [94]. The anatomy and biomechanics of the ovine shoulder are comparable to those of humans, making it a valuable model for evaluating surgical techniques, tendon healing, and the efficacy of biological enhancers. Ovine models have been used to assess the mechanical strength and histological outcomes of varying rotator cuff injuries, as well as other ligament and tendon augmentation and repair methods [95–98]. Furthermore, the ovine deep digital flexor partial tendinopathy model has been used to investigate approaches to treat human tendons, such as the Achilles tendon, and in testing several therapies, including regenerative therapies [99] and innovative suture materials [100, 101].

Due to similar stifle anatomy, the sheep and goat stifle (human knee) are interesting models for the study of pathophysiology and therapies for OA [102]. The sizable joint allows for ACL transection, arthroscopic examination, the creation of chondral defect models [103, 104], and serial synovial fluid collection [105]. Although ovine knee cartilage differs in thickness from human cartilage (0.70–1.70 mm and 2.35 mm, respectively), it provides a close match regarding mechanical properties for preclinical research [4]. OA in these models can be simulated by transecting the CCL (ACL), by causing meniscus damage, or by mechanically creating the partial- or full-thickness critical cartilage defect prior to testing therapies such as engineered cartilage [104].

4.3. *Porcine Models*

Pigs are increasingly being used in MSK research due to their physiological and anatomical similarities to humans, including bone density, joint structure, and healing processes. Multiple strains of pigs have been utilized in orthopedic research, including Yorkshire, Red Duroc, and related hybrid breeds [78]. Porcine models are used to study bone healing and the effectiveness of bone grafts and substitutes [106]. The porcine mandible and long bones are commonly used sites for testing the integration and performance of bone scaffolds and growth factors. These models have been valuable for the preclinical testing of new biomaterials intended for use in craniofacial and orthopedic surgery [107, 108]. Similar to sheep, pigs are also used to study spinal fusion due to their comparable vertebral structure and biomechanics. Porcine models allow for the testing of spinal implants, fusion techniques, and growth factors such as FGF2-STAB® and stem cells. These models have been used to investigate the outcome of various interbody fusion devices and the role of bone graft materials in promoting fusion *in vivo* [109, 110], as well as in *ex vivo* studies [111]. Porcine models are also used to study MSK infections, such as osteomyelitis, and particularly implant-associated osteomyelitis, due to their similar immune response and bone structure to humans [112]. Furthermore, pigs are also a good model for studying the normal ACL, as well as ACL injury, repair, and reconstruction [78], with a main limitation being the size of adult pigs, which require larger housing spaces.

5. Emerging Animal Models

In addition to traditional models, new and emerging animal models are being developed to address specific research needs, such as the study of rare diseases, advanced surgical techniques, and personalized medicine.

5.1. *Rabbit Models*

Rabbits are increasingly being used in MSK research due to their manageable size, docile temperament, and well-characterized physiology. Rabbit models are commonly used to study cartilage repair strategies, such as microfracture, autologous chondrocyte implantation, biomaterials, regenerative therapies, and tissue-engineered scaffolds. OA does not occur spontaneously in rabbits but can be induced *via* surgical intervention (e.g., ACL transection [113], collateral ligament transection [114]), mechanical manipulation (e.g., immobilization [115]), or chemical application (e.g., stromal cell-derived factor-1 [116]). These models have been used extensively and continue to offer specific advantages over other models for OA research. The rabbit knee joint is anatomically very similar to that of humans and large enough to enable the collection of adequate amounts of tissue for histopathological analysis. Thus, these models allow for assessment of the quality of cartilage regeneration, integration with surrounding tissue, and the long-term durability of the repair technique. Rabbit models are also used to study the healing of tendons and ligaments, particularly in the context of surgical repair and tissue engineering. In this respect, the model allows for the evaluation of different repair techniques, graft materials, and biological factors that influence tendon-to-bone healing. The most commonly used MSK models in rabbits are the rotator cuff [117–119], the common calcaneal (Achilles) tendon [120, 121], and the patellar tendon [122–124]. In comparison with some other models, the rabbit displays faster skeletal change and bone turnover. As it may be difficult to translate to humans, this therefore limits the use of this species when this type of assessment is necessary. Rabbits, however, are commonly used for screening bone and dental implant materials before testing in a larger animal model [125].

5.2. *Zebrafish Models*

Zebrafish are emerging as a novel model for studying bone biology and regeneration due to their rapid development, genetic tractability, and the ability to observe bone formation and remodeling *in vivo*. Zebrafish models are used to study the mechanisms of bone regeneration and the effects of genetic and pharmacological interventions on bone formation [126–130]. The transparent nature of zebrafish larvae allows for real-time imaging of bone development and the study of osteogenesis.

5.3. *Miniature Pig Models*

Miniature pigs are gaining popularity in MSK research due to their close resemblance to human anatomy and physiology [131], while providing a great opportunity for studying porcine models in institutional environments where a smaller animal size is beneficial. These models are particularly useful for studying joint diseases [132, 133], bone healing [134], and the testing of implants. Miniature pigs are used to model joint diseases such as OA and rheumatoid arthritis, allowing for the study of disease progression and the testing of new treatments. These models provide a more clinically relevant platform for evaluating the efficacy of novel therapies, including biologics and gene therapies.

6. Should We Still Use Animal Models?

Animal models are indispensable tools in MSK research, offering valuable insights into the pathophysiology of diseases and the development of new therapies. While each model has its strengths and limitations, the choice of model depends on the specific research question and the relevance of the model to human conditions. As new technologies and methodologies continue to evolve, the development of more refined and predictive animal models will enhance our ability to translate basic research into clinical applications. Despite animal models being invaluable to advance MSK research, increased ethical concerns and a deeper understanding of the dissimilarities between humans and animals make it difficult to rely exclusively on animal models. Therefore, there is a growing need to develop alternative "humanized" disease models that can recapitulate human pathophysiology with maximum detail [12].

7. Ethics and Future Direction of the Use of Animals as Models

In 2015, 4.1 million experimental procedures were performed in the United Kingdom. Although the annual number of procedures has fallen by a third since 2015 [135], there are still concerns about the number of animals used in experiments globally. To address this, globally, efforts from governmental bodies and institutional review boards are in place, and legislation and ethical approval processes exist to limit the use of animals in research only where all alternatives have been fully considered and animal suffering is minimized. In 1959, the 3Rs of animal research: Replacement, Reduction, and Refinement, were introduced. These three principles are the paramount foundation for animal research and guide the development of future alternatives to the use of animals. However, even these established principles need to be better discussed [136], and the inclusion of a fourth R for "Refusal" of a fruitless, poorly designed protocol, or "Responsibility" to ensure the social and individual welfare of the experimental animal [137], or even the inclusion of two more principles, "Respect" and scientific "Robustness," to create 7Rs of animal research have been suggested [138].

Other concerns around the use of animal models are regarding trial design, analysis, and reporting. To address these, several groups have set out to standardize the collection and reporting of data in animal research (e.g., Animal Research: Reporting of the *In Vivo* Experiments [ARRIVE] guidelines, and NC3Rs), and have encouraged further investigation through systematic review and meta-analysis (e.g., The Collaborative Approach to Meta Analysis and Review of Animal Experimental Studies [CAMARADES], and Systematic Review Center for Laboratory Animal Experimentation [SYRCLE]). Despite this, there remain large amounts of discrepancies within published animal studies, perhaps due in part to the heterogeneity of both animal models and the human conditions they are attempting to replicate, which brings the use of such models into question [139]. Nonetheless, we cannot deny the relevance of animal models providing invaluable information in the advancement of medical knowledge and in the alleviation of human suffering for the improvement of human health. The foundations of our basic understanding of disease pathophysiology and human anatomy can largely be attributed to preclinical investigations using various animal models. Recently, however, the scientific community, citing concerns about animal welfare as well as the validity and applicability of outcomes, has called the use of animals in research into question. These questions about the real validity of using animal models nowadays are constantly raised, and we must re-examine the use of sentient animals in human research, with an eye toward the 3Rs: Reduction, Refinement, and, ultimately, Replacement [139]. Furthermore, the failure rate for the translation of therapies from animal testing to human treatments remains at over 92%, due to unexpected safety issues revealed in human trials that were not apparent in animal tests, or due to lack of efficacy. One example is the recent news that the U.S. Food and Drug Administration is taking a groundbreaking step to advance public health by not requiring animal testing for the development of monoclonal antibody therapies and other drugs where data for human-relevant methods is available [140]. However, despite all limitations, the use of animals in research will, for the foreseeable future, be necessary, even if on a minor scale, to help drive scientific discovery. The use of alternative models in preclinical tests, such as organ-on-a-chip (OoC), can help to predict safety (or lack thereof) and efficacy before a clinical trial [141].

The United Kingdom government's new "Replacing Animals in Science" strategy, announced in November 2025, marks one of the most significant shifts in a country research policy in decades, signalling a concerted effort to phase out animal testing by accelerating the development and regulatory acceptance of non-animal methods. Driven by rapid advances in technologies such as organ-on-a-chip systems, human stem-cell models, AI-enabled drug discovery and complex in-silico simulations, the strategy argues that science is now capable of moving beyond many traditional animal experiments. It sets out a structured plan to achieve this: investing in innovation, establishing a dedicated UK centre for validating alternative methods, reforming regulatory pathways, and encouraging cultural change across industry, academia and publishing. While the approach promises major benefits for both animal welfare and human-relevant science, it also raises important questions about the readiness of these technologies, the feasibility of ambitious timelines, and the challenges of achieving international regulatory alignment. The UK's roadmap therefore represents an ethical commitment that could redefine the future of biomedical research if its aspirations can be matched by sustained investment, rigorous validation and broad cultural uptake.

8. What Are the Alternatives to Animal Models?

It is still claimed that research cannot advance without great reliance on animal models, and this concept may be true to some extent, but only in that, historically, the "options" were limited [141]. Modern replacement techniques and technologies are the core of changing this dogma. Alternatives to animal models aim to overcome translational barriers toward developing needed treatments in a quicker, cheaper, and ethical fashion. As a result, using nonanimal models for research could save the lives of more humans and animals, as well as time, and money. All without sacrificing quality, and safety; alternatives to animal testing could improve the quality of society while improving health outcomes. Alternatives to animal testing, when suitable, are not proposed to hinder scientific progress or put humans at risk. On the contrary, as they evolve, these nonanimal models can be more accurate, cost-effective, and quicker than using animal models. One important example of this change in trend is that in December 2022, U.S. President Joe Biden signed a law allowing researchers to test drug candidates on human tissue or computer models before moving to trials in people. Despite these initial changes in view, and in terms of experimental models, animal studies are still important and often necessary, especially in the latter stages of medical device and drug development. Nonetheless, *in vitro* models are becoming increasingly indispensable tools for studying the cellular and molecular mechanisms underlying MSK health and disease. These models provide controlled environments to investigate cell behavior, tissue formation, and responses to various stimuli, offering valuable insights that can be translated into clinical applications.

Nonanimal models, such as OoC and 3D bioprinting, use human cells to mimic organs and structures to screen treatments before animal testing. This allows researchers to simplify a system, limiting the number of variables, allowing the study of pathophysiology and therapy responses before going to the animal model. Such approaches may never completely replace the animal model, as an organoid or an OoC will never fully substitute for a living being when evaluating, for example, how an experimental drug is absorbed and metabolized throughout the body. However, as mentioned previously, they allow for more initial hypotheses to be based on human-tissue responses to the environment or disease, rather than beginning with observations of the animal model, thereby leading to Refinement, Replacement, and Reduction. We will focus on the diverse range of *in vitro* models used to study MSK cell and tissue responses, including traditional two-dimensional (2D) cell cultures, advanced three-dimensional (3D) models, microfluidic devices, and out-of-chip technologies. Each model is discussed in the context of its application, advantages, and limitations.

8.1. *Cell Culture Models*

2D cell culture has been the cornerstone of *in vitro* research for decades. In MSK research, 2D cultures are widely used to study the behavior of isolated cells, including osteoblasts, chondrocytes, myoblasts, fibroblasts, and stem cells under various conditions. Monolayer cultures, where cells are grown on flat surfaces such as on plastic or glass, are the most common form of 2D cell culture. These models are used to study cell proliferation, differentiation, gene expression, and the response to pharmacological agents. For example, osteoblasts or mesenchymal stem cells cultured in 2D monolayers are frequently used to investigate the effect of mechanical loading, growth factors, and biomaterials on bone formation [142, 143], often followed by *in vivo* studies [144]. Co-culture systems involve growing two or more cell types together, allowing for the study of cell–cell interactions that are crucial for the healthy function of MSK tissues. For instance, co-culturing osteoblasts and osteoclasts in 2D allows researchers to study the dynamics of bone remodeling [142], including the balance between bone formation and resorption. Similarly, chondrocyte-fibroblast co-cultures are used to model cartilage pathophysiological and repair processes [145, 146]. While 2D models are valuable for their simplicity and ease of use, they do not fully replicate the 3D architecture of MSK tissues and may therefore overlook certain important physiological aspects. Cells in 2D cultures often exhibit altered morphology, polarity, and gene expression compared to their *in vivo* counterparts, limiting the applicability of findings from these models to the real world. 3D cell culture models offer a more physiologically relevant environment by resembling more closely the architectural and functional properties of MSK cells and tissues. In these cultures, the cells can be exposed to different concentrations of nutrients, growth factors, oxygen, or cytotoxic agents, depending on their localization and communication, as it would happen in a living animal. The 3D architecture also differentially alters the physiological, biochemical, and biomechanical properties that can affect cell growth, cell survival, differentiation, morphogenesis, cell migration, epithelial–mesenchymal transition properties, mechanical responses, and therapy resistance. This latter point may, in part, explain the failure of current therapies and negatively impact drug research and discovery [147]. Scaffold-based 3D models involve seeding cells onto biocompatible scaffolds made from materials such as collagen, hyaluronic acid, or synthetic polymers. These scaffolds provide structural support, promoting cell adhesion, proliferation, and differentiation. In MSK research, scaffold-based models are used to study bone and cartilage regeneration, tendon and ligament repair, the tendon- and ligament-to-bone interface [148], and even triphasic models such as bone–tendon–muscle interactions [149]. For example, hydrogel scaffolds seeded with chondrocytes have been used to engineer cartilage tissue *in vitro*, providing a platform for testing new therapies for OA [104, 150].

Spheroids and organoids are 3D cultures that self-assemble and regenerate, for instance, from stem cells and tissue progenitor cells. They sit between 2D cultures and *in vivo* models, showing great potential for studying tissue development, responses to changes in the environment, and tissue regeneration [151], but lack the many advantages of a living system [147]. In MSK research, organoids are used successfully to study pathophysiology and therapies for tissues including muscle, cartilage, bone, tendons, and ligaments [152–156]. Despite their advantages, 3D models can be technically challenging and costly to establish and maintain. Additionally, the diffusion of nutrients, oxygen, and waste products is more limited in 3D cultures compared to 2D, which can lead to gradients within the tissue constructs and complicate data interpretation.

8.2. *Microfluidic Devices — Organ-on-a-Chip*

Microfluidic devices, often referred to as OoC technologies, have revolutionized *in vitro* modeling by allowing precise control over the cellular microenvironment. These devices consist of microscale channels that can be used to simulate physiological fluid flow, shear stress, and mechanical loading, which are extremely valuable to MSK research development. The principle behind OoCs is that miniature tissues grown and residing in microfluidic chips can recapitulate one or more tissue-specific functions. These systems can often serve as effective mimics of human physiology and disease, despite being much simpler than the living tissue. OoCs can be considered an advanced *in vitro* technology that enables experimentation using biological cells and tissues outside of the body and in a reasonable semblance of the *in vivo* environment, from a biochemical and physical point of view [157]. The OoC may be regarded as a bridging technology between *in vitro* and *in vivo*, providing information about disease progression, leading to improved prevention, diagnosis, and treatment approaches, particularly in determining how effective or toxic a therapeutic candidate would be in clinical studies [157]. By eliminating toxic or ineffective treatments earlier in development, valuable time and money can be optimized, considerably reducing the number of animals used in research. The benefits of human-specific chips are well recognized, and this method is becoming popular in MSK pathology and injury treatment, discovery, and development.

8.2.1. *Bone-on-a-Chip Models*

Recently, OoC-enabled research on bone physiology has emerged through the creation of the bone-on-a-chip (BoC) device [158, 159]. BoC devices replicate the bone microenvironment by incorporating osteoblasts, osteoclasts, and endothelial cells within microfluidic channels, providing an in-depth view of the development of bone. These features have led to an improvement in the understanding of the bone remodeling process and can aid in the development of therapeutic options for bone-related diseases such as osteoporosis, bone defects, and metastasis [160–164]. It is clear that BoC devices have great potential in translational research, but progress has been compromised by limited availability of biosensing tools for on-chip analysis. Therefore, the new frontier of BoC devices includes the integration of biosensors to provide methods for noninvasive, continuous monitoring.

8.2.2. *Cartilage-on-a-Chip Models*

Cartilage-on-a-chip (CoC) devices can help us understand the pathogenic process by simulating the cartilaginous architecture and mechanical environment [165]. CoC devices are designed to mimic the biomechanical environment of cartilage, including the application of compressive forces and the presence of synovial fluid [166–169]. These models are used to study chondrocyte behavior, cartilage degradation [170], and the efficacy of therapeutic agents for OA. CoC platforms enable high-throughput screening of potential disease-modifying drugs under physiologically relevant conditions. Until recently, the CoC devices would allow only the endpoint detection of biomarkers. However, new models have been enhanced with the integration of sensors that can constantly monitor, for instance, nitric oxide release from chondrocytes under dynamic mechanical loading and/or drug stimulation, demonstrating a synergistic effect of mechanical compression and the inflammatory mediator known as interleukin-1β [165].

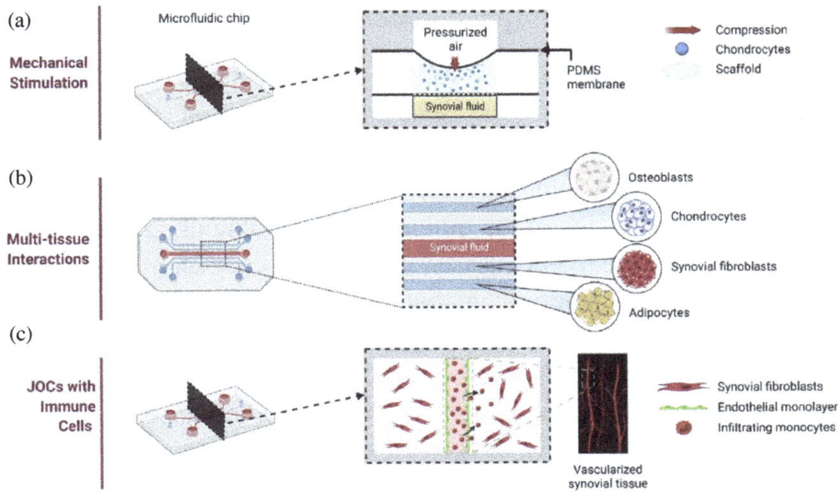

Figure 1. A microfluidic joint-on-a-chip model of knee osteoarthritis. (a) A pneumatic mechanical actuation system using pressurized air to study the compressive forces during motion on the chondrocytes within a scaffold. (b) Multijoint tissue systems in the microfluidic chip to understand the multijoint tissue crosstalk. (c) A microfluidic chip designed to understand the impact of inflammatory conditions on immune cell migration adjacent to the synovium. Adapted from Bahn et al. [171].

Undoubtedly, CoC devices (**Figure 1**) offer a powerful and reliable evaluation platform for cell regulation, tissue engineering, and drug screening.

8.2.3. *Multi-Tissue-on-a-Chip Models*

As mentioned, all tissues in the MSK system affect each other, and as such, OoC devices that can combine more than one MSK organ within a single microfluidic platform, that is, the multi-tissue-on-a-chip device, are emerging in popularity. These models allow the study of the interactions between tissues and the integrated response to mechanical loading, injury, and therapeutic interventions. For example, a bone–muscle–tendon-on-a-chip model can be used to investigate the effects of exercise or immobilization on tissue health, thereby testing the efficacy of combined therapies. Further, a bone-CoC can be used to improve the physiological conditions and pathological changes of the osteochondral unit [172]. Thus, this suggests new opportunities for drug screening and in the development of therapeutically targeted resolution approaches.

8.2.4. *Limitations of Microfluidic Models*

While microfluidic devices offer unprecedented control over the cellular microenvironment, they require specialized equipment and technical expertise to design and operate. Additionally, scaling up these models for high-throughput applications or for simulating large tissue volumes remains a challenge. One of the limitations is that initially, these devices would only allow endpoint measurement of biochemical, biophysical, protein, nucleic acid, and protein content. More recently, the integration of biosensors has been the focus for the refinement of OoC devices. This is considered the most promising solution to monitor the physicochemical environment in the culturing system, through using biosensors that target markers including, pH [173], oxygen pressure [174], glucose [175], alkaline phosphatase [176], nitric oxide [165], BMP [177], and others.

8.3. *Out-of-Chip Technologies*

Out-of-chip technologies involve the use of advanced tools and platforms that extend beyond traditional microfluidics to study MSK cells and tissues. These technologies include dynamic culture systems, bioreactors [178, 179], and engineered tissue scaffolds [180].

8.3.1. *Dynamic Culture Systems and Bioreactors*

Dynamic culture systems, such as rotating wall vessels and perfusion bioreactors, provide continuous mechanical stimulation and improved nutrient exchange for 3D tissue cultures [181]. Bioreactors are specialized devices designed to support the growth and development of engineered tissues under controlled conditions. In MSK research, perfusion and rotating bioreactors are used to cultivate bone, cartilage, and muscle tissues, providing mechanical cues that promote tissue differentiation and maturation [182]. For instance, compression bioreactors are used to apply cyclic loading to cartilage constructs, mimicking the mechanical environment of articular cartilage and enhancing chondrogenesis. These systems are used to study the effects of mechanical loading on bone and cartilage tissues, as well as to enhance the maturation of engineered tissue constructs. For example, perfusion bioreactors have been shown to enhance the mineralization of bone tissue constructs by providing continuous fluid flow and shear stress [183].

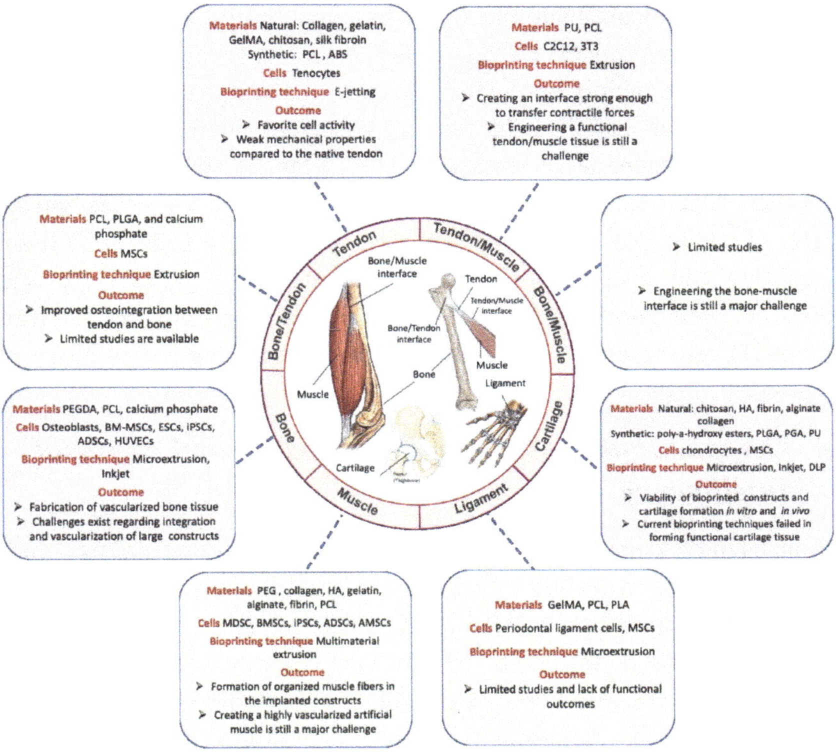

Figure 2. Schematic illustration of the materials and techniques used for the bioprinting of MSK tissues and their interface. Polycaprolactone (PCL), poly(lactide-co-glycolide) (PLGA), mesenchymal stem cells (MSCs), poly(ethylene glycol) diacrylate (PEGDA), bone marrow derived mesenchymal stem cells (BM-MSCs), embryonic stem cells (ESCs), induced pluripotent stem cells (iPSCs), human umbilical vein endothelial cells (HUVECs), adipose-derived stem cells (ADSCs), polyethylene glycol (PEG), hyaluronic acid (HA), mouse-derived stem cells (MDSC), polyglycolide (PGA), photosensitive polyurethane (PU), gelatin methacryloyl (GelMA), polylactide (PLA), and acrylonitrile butadiene styrene (ABS) [188].

8.3.2. *Tissue Bioprinting*

Tissue bioprinting technology (**Figure 2**) allows for the precise placement of cells, biomaterials, and growth factors to create complex 3D tissue constructs that mimic the structure and function of native tissues or organs. The principle behind these constructs is that by precisely placing cells in relation to each other, an environment that encourages physiologically relevant cues can be created, resulting in a tissue construct that mirrors living tissue function. Consequently, the bioprinted constructs could provide more human anatomical and functional similarity to tissues or organs as research models [184]. In MSK research, bioprinted models are used to fabricate mainly bone [185], but with great potential for cartilage and muscle tissue, enabling the study of tissue development, disease progression, and regenerative strategies. For instance, 3D bioprinted bone constructs have been used to study the integration of bone grafts and the effects of mechanical loading on bone regeneration [186, 187]. 3D tissue bioprinting can also produce disease-relevant tissue models that can reduce the predictability gap between the results of therapy options from current 2D cell-based assays and the results from testing in humans.

8.4. *Computational, Mathematical Models, and Artificial Intelligence*

Advances in the capabilities of computers and computer programs benefit a variety of areas in society. For MSK research, it provides the ability to model certain aspects of the MSK system using *in silico* models. Current computer models of the MSK system have been developed to conduct virtual experiments based on existing databases obtained from *in vivo* and *in vitro* experiments. Additionally, data mining tools assist researchers in making predictions about one substance based on existing data from similar substances. There is much excitement about the deployment of artificial intelligence (AI) in healthcare, and the MSK field is no exception. New developments relating to OA, osteoporosis, rheumatoid arthritis (as an example of inflammatory arthritis), and MSK surgical interventions are an exciting new horizon in research [189]. There are a range of applications that utilize machine learning in MSK research. This includes understanding disease pathophysiology, improving diagnosis, and developing treatments. By training AI models using comprehensive datasets of human anatomy, physiology, and molecular interactions, researchers can develop computational models that replicate the behavior of organs, tissues, and biological systems. These virtual models may provide a more accurate representation of human responses to substances, allowing for improved predictions of toxicity and efficacy, which, as discussed before, are great limitations when using animal models. AI can analyze extensive amounts of data and make predictions based on the patterns identified. Additionally, AI algorithms can analyze and interpret experimental data, providing valuable insights and guiding researchers toward more targeted experimental designs and outcome metrics. Several AI projects have been developed globally as an effort to enhance the ability of AI to predict cell and tissue responses to therapies, thereby providing a screening procedure before the need for further research. Some examples include the AnimalGAN, which was developed by the U.S. Food and Drug Administration and can accurately determine how rats would react to any given chemical. Similarly, the Virtual Second Species is creating an AI-powered virtual dog, which is being trained using the data obtained from historic dog test results. More recently, the integration of AI with other emerging technologies, such as OoC models [190] and organoids [191], provide powerful tools that may replace animal testing by offering greater accuracy and higher fidelity. AI algorithms can analyze the complex data generated by these systems, enhancing their predictive capabilities and reducing the reliance on animal testing. Although increasingly promising, *in silico* models face challenges such as regulatory approval and full acceptance, but as new technologies such as it evolve, we would expect a decline in the need for *in vitro* and *in vivo* studies.

9. Emerging Trends and Future Directions

The field of *in vitro* MSK modeling is rapidly evolving, with new technologies and approaches continually being developed. Emerging trends include metallic additive manufacturing [192], the integration of 3D bioprinting with microfluidic devices [193, 194], the use of patient-specific cells for personalized medicine applications [185], and the development of multi-tissue-on-a-chip systems [195] that replicate the interactions between MSK tissues and other organs, such as the immune system or the vascular network.

10. Conclusions

A robust approach to minimize the limitations inherent in MSK discovery should include a staged approach using *in vitro, ex vivo,* and *in silico* models to minimize the need for the use of *in vivo* studies for screening and the early development of studies. This is followed by the use of large animal models, which more closely resemble human disease. *In vitro* models are critical tools for advancing our understanding of MSK health and disease. From traditional 2D cultures to sophisticated microfluidic devices and dynamic culture systems, these models provide valuable insights into the cellular and molecular mechanisms underlying tissue formation, repair, and disease progression. As technology continues to advance, *in vitro* and *in silico* models will play an increasingly important role in the development of new therapies and the translation of basic research into clinical applications.

References

1. Neyt JG, Buckwalter JA, Carroll NC, Professor W. Use of animal models in musculoskeletal research. *Iowa Orthop J.* 1998;18:118–23.
2. Mukherjee P, Roy S, Ghosh D, Nandi SK. Role of animal models in biomedical research: A review. *Lab. Anim. Res.* 2022;38:18. https://doi.org/10.1186/s42826-022-00128-1
3. Andersen ML, Winter LMF. Animal models in biological and biomedical research — experimental and ethical concerns. *An. Acad. Bras. Cienc.* 2019;91(suppl 1):e20170238.
4. Ribitsch I, Baptista PM, Lange-Consiglio A, Melotti L, Patruno M, Jenner F, et al. Large animal models in regenerative medicine and tissue engineering: To do or not to do. *Front. Bioeng. Biotechnol.* 2020;8:972.
5. Moskowitz RW. Experimental models of degenerative joint disease. *Semin. Arthritis Rheum.* 1972;2:95–116.
6. Simmons D. The use of animal models in studying genetic disease: Transgenesis and induced mutation. *Nat. Educ.* 2008;1:70.
7. Bodic B, Boutet MA, Boyer C, Metayer B, Vignes C, Lesoeur J, et al. Development and characterization of a humanized mouse model of osteoarthritis. *Osteoarthr. Cartil.* 2022;30:875–85.
8. Lahr CA, Landgraf M, Wagner F, Cipitria A, Moreno-Jiménez I, Bas O, et al. A humanised rat model of osteosarcoma reveals ultrastructural differences between bone and mineralised tumour tissue. *Bone.* 2022;158:116018.
9. Moreno-Jiménez I, Cipitria A, Sánchez-Herrero A, van Tol AF, Roschger A, Lahr CA, et al. Human and mouse bones physiologically integrate in a humanized mouse model while maintaining species-specific ultrastructure. *Sci. Adv.* 2020;6(44):eabb9265.
10. Prabhakar S. Translational research challenges: Finding the right animal models. *J. Investig. Med.* 2012;60:1141–6.

11. Lorbach O, Baums MH, Kostuj T, Pauly S, Scheibel M, Carr A, et al. Advances in biology and mechanics of rotator cuff repair. *Knee Surg. Sports Traumatol. Arthrosc.* 2015;23(2):530–41.
12. Jain A, Mathur T, Pandian NKR, Selahi A. Organ-on-a-chip and 3D printing as preclinical models for medical research and practice. In: Faintuch J, Faintuch S (eds) *Precision Medicine for Investigators, Practitioners and Providers*. Elsevier; 2019. p. 83–95. https://doi.org/10.1016/B978-0-12-819178-1.00009-5
13. Nakamura T, Fujiwara K, Saitou M, Tsukiyama T. Non-human primates as a model for human development. *Stem Cell Rep.* 2021;16:1093–103.
14. Shanks N, Greek R, Greek J. Are animal models predictive for humans? *Philos. Ethics Humanit. Med.* 2009;4:2.
15. Zaki S, Blaker CL, Little CB. OA foundations — experimental models of osteoarthritis. *Osteoarthr. Cartil.* 2022;30(3):357–80.
16. Gao H, Huang J, Wei Q, He C. Advances in animal models for studying bone fracture healing. *Bioengineering* 2023;10:201.
17. Marsell R, Einhorn TA. The biology of fracture healing. *Injury* 2011;42: 551–55.
18. Lybrand K, Bragdon B, Gerstenfeld L. Mouse models of bone healing: Fracture, marrow ablation, and distraction osteogenesis. *Curr. Protoc. Mouse Biol.* 2015;5:35–49.
19. Collier CD, Hausman BS, Zulqadar SH, Din ES, Anderson JM, Akkus O, et al. Characterization of a reproducible model of fracture healing in mice using an open femoral osteotomy. *Bone Rep.* 2020;12:100250.
20. Tay BK, Le AX, Gould SE, Helms JA. Histochemical and molecular analyses of distraction osteogenesis in a mouse model. *J. Orthop. Res.* 1998;16(5): 636–42.
21. Zhang N, Hua Y, Li Y, Pan J. Sema3A accelerates bone formation during distraction osteogenesis in mice. *Connect. Tissue Res.* 2022;63:382–92.
22. Ballhause TM, Jiang S, Xie W, Sevecke J, Dowling C, Dust T, et al. Fracture healing in a mouse model of Hajdu–Cheney-Syndrome with high turnover osteopenia results in decreased biomechanical stability. *Sci. Rep.* 2023; 13(1):11418.
23. Weiss A, Arbell I, Steinhagen-Thiessen E, Silbermann M. Structural changes in aging bone: Osteopenia in the proximal femurs of female mice. *Bone* 1991;12(3):165–72.
24. Sanghani A, Osagie-Clouard L, Coathup MJ, Briggs T, Bostrom MPG, Blunn GW. CXCR4 has the potential to enhance bone formation in osteopenic rats. *Tissue Eng. Part A* 2018;24(23–24):1775–83.

25. Plotkin LI, Bivi N, Bellido T. A bisphosphonate that does not affect osteoclasts prevents osteoblast and osteocyte apoptosis and the loss of bone strength induced by glucocorticoids in mice. *Bone* 2011;49(1):122–7.
26. Kuyinu EL, Narayanan G, Nair LS, Laurencin CT. Animal models of osteoarthritis: Classification, update, and measurement of outcomes. *J. Orthop. Surg. Res.* 2016;11:19.
27. McCoy AM. Animal models of osteoarthritis. *Vet. Pathol.* 2015;52:803–18.
28. Davis S, Karali A, Zekonyte J, Roldo M, Blunn G. Development of a method to investigate strain distribution across the cartilage-bone interface in guinea pig model of spontaneous osteoarthritis using lab-based contrast enhanced X-ray-computed tomography and digital volume correlation. *J. Mech. Behav. Biomed. Mater.* 2023;144:105999.
29. Drevet S, Favier B, Brun E, Gavazzi G, Lardy B. Mouse models of osteoarthritis: A summary of models and outcomes assessment. *Comp. Med.* 2022;72:3–13.
30. Little CB, Hunter DJ. Post-traumatic osteoarthritis: From mouse models to clinical trials. *Nat. Rev. Rheumatol.* 2013;9:485–97.
31. Malfait AM, Little CB. On the predictive utility of animal models of osteoarthritis. *Arthritis Res. Ther.* 2015;17:225.
32. Wendler A, Wehling M. The translatability of animal models for clinical development: Biomarkers and disease models. *Curr. Opin. Pharmacol.* 2010; 10:601–6.
33. Lampropoulou-Adamidou K, Lelovas P, Karadimas EV, Liakou C, Triantafillopoulos IK, Dontas I, et al. Useful animal models for the research of osteoarthritis. *Eur. J. Orthop. Surg. Traumatol.* 2014;24:263–71.
34. Roux KM, Cobb LH, Seitz MA, Priddy LB. Innovations in osteomyelitis research: A review of animal models. *Anim. Model Exp. Med.* 2021;4:59–70.
35. Meroni G, Tsikopoulos A, Tsikopoulos K, Allemanno F, Martino PA, Filipe JFS. A journey into animal models of human osteomyelitis: A review. *Microorganisms* 2022;10(6):1135.
36. Zelken J, Wanich T, Gardner M, Griffith M, Bostrom M. PMMA is superior to hydroxyapatite for colony reduction in induced osteomyelitis. *Clin. Orthop. Relat. Res.* 2007;462:190–4.
37. Dvorzhinskiy A, Perino G, Chojnowski R, van der Meulen MCH, Bostrom MPG, et al. Ceramic composite with gentamicin decreases persistent infection and increases bone formation in a rat model of debrided osteomyelitis. *J. Bone Jt. Infect.* 2021;6(7):283–93.
38. Fukushima N, Yokoyama K, Sasahara T, Dobashi Y, Itoman M. Establishment of rat model of acute staphylococcal osteomyelitis:

Relationship between inoculation dose and development of osteomyelitis. *Arch. Orthop. Trauma Surg.* 2005;125(3):169–76.
39. Rissing JP, Buxton TB, Fisher J, Harris R, Shockley RK. Arachidonic acid facilitates experimental chronic osteomyelitis in rats. *Infect. Immun.* 1985;49: 141–4.
40. Chen X, Kidder LS, Lew WD. Osteogenic protein-1 induced bone formation in an infected segmental defect in the rat femur. *J. Orthop. Res.* 2002; 20:142–50.
41. Brick KE, Chen X, Lohr J, Schmidt AH, Kidder LS, Lew WD. rhBMP-2 modulation of gene expression in infected segmental bone defects. *Clin. Orthop. Relat. Res.* 2009;467(12):3096–103.
42. Li B, Brown KV, Wenke JC, Guelcher SA. Sustained release of vancomycin from polyurethane scaffolds inhibits infection of bone wounds in a rat femoral segmental defect model. *J. Control. Release.* 2010;145(3):221–30.
43. Chen X, Tsukayama DT, Kidder LS, Bourgeault CA, Schmidt AH, Lew WD. Characterization of a chronic infection in an internally-stabilized segmental defect in the rat femur. *J. Orthop. Res.* 2005;23(4):816–23.
44. Brunotte M, Rupp M, Stötzel S, Sommer U, Mohammed W, Thormann U, et al. A new small animal model for simulating a two-stage-revision procedure in implant-related methicillin-resistant Staphylococcus aureus bone infection. *Injury* 2019;50(11):1921–8.
45. Farnsworth CW, Shehatou CT, Kates SL, Tran NL, Zirkle LG, Squire MW, et al. A humoral immune defect distinguishes the response to Staphylococcus aureus infections in mice with obesity and type 2 diabetes from that in mice with type 1 diabetes. *Infect. Immun.* 2015;83:2264–74.
46. Tian X, Lu Z, Ma C, Wu M, Zhang C, Yuan Y, et al. Antimicrobial hydroxyapatite and its composites for the repair of infected femoral condyle. *Mater. Sci. Eng. C* 2021;121:111807.
47. Soranoglou V, Galanopoulos I, Giamarellos-Bourboulis EJ, Papalois A, Giannitsioti E, Poultsides LA, et al. Efficacy of intramuscular moxifloxacin in the treatment of experimental osteomyelitis caused by methicillin-resistant Staphylococcus aureus. *Int. J. Antimicrob. Agents.* 2017;50: 186–90.
48. Wang Q, Chen C, Liu W, He X, Zhou N, Zhang D, et al. Levofloxacin loaded mesoporous silica microspheres/nano-hydroxyapatite/polyurethane composite scaffold for the treatment of chronic osteomyelitis with bone defects. *Sci. Rep.* 2017;7:41808.
49. Wang Y, Cheng LI, Helfer DR, Ashbaugh AG, Miller RJ, Tzomides AJ, et al. Mouse model of hematogenous implant-related Staphylococcus

aureus biofilm infection reveals therapeutic targets. *Proc. Natl. Acad. Sci. USA* 2017; 114(26):E5094–102.
50. Yoon KS, Fitzgerald RH, Sud S, Song Z, Wooley PH. Experimental acute hematogenous osteomyelitis in mice. II. Influence of Staphylococcus aureus infection on T-cell immunity. *J. Orthop. Res.* 1999;17:382–91.
51. Chadha HS, Fitzgerald RH, Sud S, Song Z, Wooley PH. Experimental acute hematogenous osteomyelitis in mice. I. Histopathological and immunological findings. *J. Orthop. Res.* 1999;17(3):376–81.
52. Elasri MO, Thomas JR, Skinner RA, Blevins JS, Beenken KE, Nelson CL, et al. Staphylococcus aureus collagen adhesin contributes to the pathogenesis of osteomyelitis. *Bone* 2002;30(1):275–80.
53. Huang S, Wen J, Zhang Y, Bai X, Cui Z-K. Choosing the right animal model for osteomyelitis research: Considerations and challenges. *J. Orthop. Translat.* 2023;43:47–65.
54. Kusuma GD, Carthew J, Lim R, Frith JE. Effect of the microenvironment on mesenchymal stem cell paracrine signaling: Opportunities to engineer the therapeutic effect. *Stem Cells Dev.* 2017;26:617–31.
55. Hashimoto K, Kaito T, Furuya M, Seno S, Okuzaki D, Kikuta J, et al. In vivo dynamic analysis of BMP-2-induced ectopic bone formation. *Sci. Rep.* 2020;10(1):4751.
56. Asatrian G, Chang L, James AW. Muscle pouch implantation: An ectopic bone formation model. *Methods Mol. Biol.* 2014;1130:185–91. https://doi.org/10.1007/978-1-4939-1453-1_15
57. Chan CKF, Seo EY, Chen JY, Lo D, McArdle A, Sinha R, et al. Identification and specification of the mouse skeletal stem cell. *Cell* 2015;160(1–2): 285–98.
58. Scott MA, Levi B, Askarinam A, Nguyen A, Rackohn T, Ting K, et al. Brief review of models of ectopic bone formation. *Stem Cells Dev.* 2012;21: 655–67.
59. Bottagisio M, Lovati AB. A review on animal models and treatments for the reconstruction of Achilles and flexor tendons. *J. Mater. Sci. Mater. Med.* 2017;28:45.
60. Willbold E, Wellmann M, Welke B, Angrisani N, Gniesmer S, Kampmann A, et al. Possibilities and limitations of electrospun chitosan-coated polycaprolactone grafts for rotator cuff tear repair. *J. Tissue Eng. Regen. Med.* 2020;14:186–97.
61. Xu B, Wang Y, He G, Tang KL, Guo L, Chen W. A novel and efficient murine model for investigating tendon-to-bone healing. *J. Orthop. Surg. Res.* 2024;19(1):90.

62. Morey-Holton ER, Globus RK. Hindlimb unloading rodent model: Technical aspects. *J. Appl. Physiol.* 2002;92:1367–77.
63. Hawliczek A, Złotkowska D, Carlstedt A, Dey P, Borkowski J. Hind-limb unloading in rodents: Current evidence and perspectives. *Acta Astronaut.* 2022;195:574–82.
64. Kwok AT, Mohamed NS, Plate JF, Yammani RR, Rosas S, Bateman TA, et al. Spaceflight and hind limb unloading induces an arthritic phenotype in knee articular cartilage and menisci of rodents. *Sci. Rep.* 2021;11:10469.
65. Globus RK, Morey-Holton E. Hindlimb unloading: Rodent analog for microgravity. *J. Appl. Physiol.* 2016;120:1196–206.
66. Moreau M, Dupuis J, Bonneau NH, Lécuyer M. Clinical evaluation of a nutraceutical, carprofen and meloxicam for the treatment of dogs with osteoarthritis. *Vet. Rec.* 2003;152:323–9.
67. Moreau M, Pelletier JP, Lussier B, d'Anjou MA, Blond L, Martel-Pelletier J, et al. A posteriori comparison of natural and surgical destabilization models of canine osteoarthritis. *Biomed Res. Int.* 2013;2013:1–12.
68. McDevitt C, Muir H. Biochemical changes in the cartilage of the knee in experimental and natural osteoarthritis in the dog. *J. Bone Joint Surg. Br.* 1976;58-B:94–101.
69. Elliott DM, Guilak F, Parker Vail T, Wang JY, Setton LA. Tensile properties of articular cartilage are altered by meniscectomy in a canine model of osteoarthritis. *J. Orthop. Res.* 1999;17:503–8.
70. Brandt KD. Transection of the anterior cruciate ligament in the dog: A model of osteoarthritis. *Semin. Arthritis Rheum.* 1991;21:22–32.
71. Marijnissen ACA, van Roermund PM, TeKoppele JM, Bijlsma JWJ, Lafeber FPJG. The canine 'groove' model, compared with the ACLT model of osteoarthritis. *Osteoarthr. Cartil.* 2002;10:145–55.
72. Thoma A, Dunlop B, Orr FW, Payk I, Adachi JD. Perichondrial arthroplasty in a canine elbow model. *Plast. Reconstr. Surg.* 1993;91:307–15.
73. Skurla CP, Pluhar GE, Frankel DJ, Egger EL, James SP. Assessing the dog as a model for human total hip replacement. *J. Bone Joint Surg. Br.* 2005; 87-B:120–7.
74. Faria LG de, Silva AF da, Couto AO, Santos MAP dos, Silva MJB da, Ferrigno CRA, et al. Biomechanical evaluation of a new femoral stem design for total hip replacement in a canine model. *Acta Cir. Bras.* 2021;36: e360506.
75. Saban C, Kowaleski MP, Gorse MJ, Breur GJ. Ex vivo postimplantation biomechanical properties of a press-fit cementless femoral stem with transfixation pin for canine total hip replacement. *Am. J. Vet. Res.* 2022;83(11):1–8.

76. Tinga S, Tuyn DD, Kopp RJ, Kim SE. Biomechanical comparison of canine femurs implanted with either cemented (CFX®) or cementless (with lateral bolt) (BFX®+lb) total hip replacement under 4-point bending or torsional loads. *Front. Bioeng. Biotechnol.* 2023;11:999271.
77. Binversie EE, Walczak BE, Cone SG, Baker LA, Scerpella TA, Muir P. Canine ACL rupture: A spontaneous large animal model of human ACL rupture. *BMC Musculoskelet. Disord.* 2022;23(1):116.
78. Little D, Amadio PC, Awad HA, Cone SG, Dyment NA, Fisher MB, et al. Preclinical tendon and ligament models: Beyond the 3Rs (replacement, reduction, and refinement) to 5W1H (why, who, what, where, when, how). *J. Orthop. Res.* 2023;41(10):2133–62.
79. Martini L, Fini M, Giavaresi G, Giardino R. Sheep model in orthopedic research: A literature review. *Comp. Med.* 2001;51:292–9.
80. Banstola A, Reynolds JNJ. The sheep as a large animal model for the investigation and treatment of human disorders. *Biology (Basel)* 2022;11:1251.
81. Coathup M, Blunn G, Flynn N, Williams C, Thomas NP. A comparison of bone remodelling around hydroxyapatite-coated, porous-coated and grit-blasted hip replacements retrieved at post-mortem. *J. Bone Joint Surg. Br.* 2001;83:118–23.
82. Godoy R, Coathup MJ, Blackburn J, Blunn G. Fast plasma sintering delivers functional graded materials components with macroporous structures and osseointegration properties. *Eur. Cell Mater.* 2016;31:250–63.
83. Kent NW, Blunn G, Karpukhina N, Davis G, de Godoy RF, Wilson RM, et al. In vitro and in vivo study of commercial calcium phosphate cement HydroSet™. *J. Biomed. Mater. Res. B Appl. Biomater.* 2018;106(1):21–30.
84. Melanie C, Coathup MJ, Meswania JM, Blunn GW. A novel ceramic coating for reduced metal ion release in metal-on-metal hip surgery. *Front. Bioeng. Biotechnol.* 2016;4.
85. Blunn GW, De Godoy RF, Meswania J, Briggs TWR, Tyler P, Hargunani R, et al. A novel ceramic coating for reduced metal ion release in metal-on-metal hip surgery. *J. Biomed. Mater. Res. B Appl. Biomater.* 2019;107(6):1760–71.
86. Chimutengwende-Gordon M, Pendegrass C, Blunn G. Enhancing the soft tissue seal around intraosseous transcutaneous amputation prostheses using silanized fibronectin titanium alloy. *Biomed. Mater.* 2011;6(2):025008.
87. Chimutengwende-Gordon M, Pendegrass C, Blunn G. The *in vivo* effect of a porous titanium alloy flange with hydroxyapatite, silver and fibronectin coatings on soft-tissue integration of intraosseous transcutaneous amputation prostheses. *Bone Joint J.* 2017;99-B(3):393–400.

88. Pendegrass CJ, Goodship AE, Blunn GW. Development of a soft tissue seal around bone-anchored transcutaneous amputation prostheses. *Biomaterials.* 2006;27(23):4183–91.
89. Giusto E, Blunn G, de Godoy RF, Liu C, Pendegrass C. Optimising soft tissue in-growth in vivo in additive layer manufactured osseointegrated transcutaneous implants. *Biomater. Transl.* 2022;3:243–9.
90. Lindley EM, Barton C, Blount T, Burger EL, Cain CMJ, Seim HB, et al. An analysis of spine fusion outcomes in sheep pre-clinical models. *Eur. Spine J.* 2017;26:228–39.
91. Fredericks DC, Gandhi AA, Grosland NM, Smucker JD. Assessment of BioPlex interbody fusion device in a sheep lumbar fusion model. *Iowa Orthop. J.* 2013;33:33–9.
92. Shaw JD, Bailey TL, Ong J, Brodke DS, Williams DL, Wawrose RA, et al. Development and validation of a large animal ovine model for implant-associated spine infection using biofilm based inocula. *Biofilm* 2023;6:100138.
93. Wang L, Wang Y, Shi L, Liu P, Kang J, He J, et al. Can the sheep model fully represent the human model for the functional evaluation of cervical interbody fusion cages? *Biomech. Model. Mechanobiol.* 2019;18:607–16.
94. Lovric V, Ledger M, Goldberg J, Harper W, Bertollo N, Pelletier MH, et al. The effects of Low-intensity Pulsed Ultrasound on tendon-bone healing in a transosseous-equivalent sheep rotator cuff model. *Knee Surg. Sports Traumatol. Arthrosc.* 2013;21:466–75.
95. Sundar S, Pendegrass CJ, Blunn GW. Tendon bone healing can be enhanced by demineralized bone matrix: A functional and histological study. *J. Biomed. Mater. Res. B Appl. Biomater.* 2009;88B:115–22.
96. Thangarajah T, Sanghani-Kerai A, Henshaw F, Lambert SM, Pendegrass CJ, Blunn GW. Tendon reattachment to bone in an ovine tendon defect model of retraction using allogenic and xenogenic demineralised bone matrix incorporated with mesenchymal stem cells. *PLoS One.* 2016;11(9):e0161473.
97. Elnikety S, Pendegrass CJ, de Godoy RF, Holden C, Blunn GW. Augmentation and repair of tendons using demineralised cortical bone. *BMC Musculoskelet. Disord.* 2016;17(1):483.
98. Hexter AT, Thangarajah T, Blunn G, Haddad FS. Mesenchymal stromal cells and platelet-rich plasma promote tendon allograft healing in ovine anterior cruciate ligament reconstruction. *Knee Surg. Sports Traumatol. Arthrosc.* 2021;29:3678–88.
99. Khan MR, Smith RK, David F, Lam R, Hughes G, De Godoy R, et al. Evaluation of the effects of synovial multipotent cells on deep digital flexor

tendon repair in a large animal model of intra-synovial tendinopathy. *J. Orthop. Res.* 2020;38:128–38.
100. Rashid M, Dudhia J, Dakin SG, Snelling SJB, Smith RKW, Blunn GW. Histopathological and immunohistochemical evaluation of cellular response to a woven and electrospun polydioxanone (PDO) and polycaprolactone (PCL) patch for tendon repair. *Sci. Rep.* 2020;10:4754.
101. Rashid M, Dudhia J, Dakin SG, Snelling SJB, Smith RKW, Blunn GW. Histological evaluation of cellular response to a multifilament electrospun suture for tendon repair. *PLoS One.* 2020;15:e0234982.
102. Proffen BL, McElfresh M, Fleming BC, Murray MM. A comparative anatomical study of the human knee and six animal species. *Knee.* 2012;19: 493–9.
103. Music E, Futrega K, Doran MR. Sheep as a model for evaluating mesenchymal stem/stromal cell (MSC)-based chondral defect repair. *Osteoarthr. Cartil.* 2018;26:730–40.
104. Dickinson SC, Sutton CA, Brady K, Salerno A, Katopodi T, Williams RL, et al. The Wnt5a receptor, receptor tyrosine kinase-like orphan receptor 2, is a predictive cell surface marker of human mesenchymal stem cells with an enhanced capacity for chondrogenic differentiation. *Stem Cells* 2017;35:2280–91.
105. Mickiewicz B, Heard BJ, Chau JK, Chung M, Hart DA, Shrive NG, et al. Metabolic profiling of synovial fluid in a unilateral ovine model of anterior cruciate ligament reconstruction of the knee suggests biomarkers for early osteoarthritis. *J. Orthop. Res.* 2015;33(1):71–7.
106. Li Y, Chen SK, Li L, Qin L, Wang XL, Lai YX. Bone defect animal models for testing efficacy of bone substitute biomaterials. *J. Orthop. Translat.* 2015;3:95–104.
107. Shanbhag S, Mohamed-Ahmed S, Lyngstadaas SP, Reseland JE, Haugen HJ. Regeneration of alveolar bone defects in the experimental pig model: A systematic review and meta-analysis. *Clin. Oral Implants Res.* 2024;35:467–86.
108. Erdoğan Ö, Üstün Y, Tatli U, Damlar I, Dağlıoğlu K. A pig model for the histomorphometric evaluation of hard tissue around dental implants. *J. Oral Implantol.* 2013;39:551–7.
109. Hildebrandt U, Pistorius G, Olinger A, Menger MD. First experience with laparoscopic spine fusion in an experimental model in the pig. *Surg. Endosc.* 1996;10:143–6.
110. Krticka M, Planka L, Vojtova L, Nekuda V, Stastny P, Sedlacek R, et al. Lumbar interbody fusion conducted on a porcine model with a

bioresorbable ceramic/biopolymer hybrid implant enriched with hypersta-ble fibroblast growth factor 2. *Biomedicines.* 2021;9:733.

111. Laznovsky J, Brinek A, Zikmund T, Boudova M, Vojtova L, Dorazilova J, et al. Automatic 3D analysis of the ex-vivo porcine lumbar interbody fusion based on X-ray micro computed tomography data. *Comput. Biol. Med.* 2022;145:105438.
112. Jensen LK, Koch J, Dich-Jorgensen K, Aalbaek B, Petersen A, Fuursted K, et al. Novel porcine model of implant-associated osteomyelitis: A comprehensive analysis of local, regional, and systemic response. *J. Orthop. Res.* 2017;35:2211–21.
113. Yoshioka M, Coutts RD, Amiel D, Hacker SA. Characterization of a model of osteoarthritis in the rabbit knee. *Osteoarthr. Cartil.* 1996;4(2):87–98.
114. Liu Z, Hu X, Man Z, Zhang J, Jiang Y, Ao Y. A novel rabbit model of early osteoarthritis exhibits gradual cartilage degeneration after medial collateral ligament transection outside the joint capsule. *Sci. Rep.* 2016;6:34423.
115. Zhou Q, Wei B, Liu S, Mao F, Zhang X, Hu J, et al. Cartilage matrix changes in contralateral mobile knees in a rabbit model of osteoarthritis induced by immobilization. *BMC Musculoskelet. Disord.* 2015;16:224.
116. Li C, He Y, Li Y, Wang G, Liu D, Cai G, et al. A novel method to establish the rabbit model of knee osteoarthritis: Intra-articular injection of SDF-1 induces OA. *BMC Musculoskelet. Disord.* 2021;22:329.
117. Gurger M, Once G, Yilmaz E, Demir S, Calik I, Say Y, et al. The effect of the platelet-rich plasma and ozone therapy on tendon-to-bone healing in the rabbit rotator cuff repair model. *J. Orthop. Surg. Res.* 2021;16:202.
118. Yildiz F, Bilsel K, Pulatkan A, Kapicioglu M, Uzer G, Çetindamar T, et al. Comparison of two different superior capsule reconstruction methods in the treatment of chronic irreparable rotator cuff tears: A biomechanical and histologic study in rabbit models. *J. Shoulder Elbow Surg.* 2019;28:530–8.
119. Xu J, Li Y, Zhang X, Han K, Ye Z, Wu C, et al. The biomechanical and histological processes of rerouting biceps to treat chronic irreparable rotator cuff tears in a rabbit model. *Am. J. Sports Med.* 2022;50:347–61.
120. Meier Bürgisser G, Calcagni M, Bachmann E, Fessel G, Snedeker JG, Giovanoli P, et al. Rabbit Achilles tendon full transection model — wound healing, adhesion formation and biomechanics at 3, 6 and 12 weeks post-surgery. *Biol. Open* 2016;5(5):1324–33.
121. de Cesar Netto C, Godoy-Santos AL, Pontin PA, Natalino RJM, Pereira CAM, de Oliveira Lima FD, et al. Novel animal model for Achilles

tendinopathy: Controlled experimental study of serial injections of collagenase in rabbits. *PLoS One* 2018;13:e0192769.
122. Lyras DN, Kazakos K, Tilkeridis K, Kokka A, Ververidis A, Botaitis S, et al. Temporal and spatial expression of TGF-b1 in the early phase of patellar tendon healing after application of platelet rich plasma. *Arch. Bone Jt. Surg.* 2016;4(2):156–60.
123. Kim DK, Ahn J, Kim SA, Go EJ, Lee DH, Park SC, et al. Improved healing of rabbit patellar tendon defects after an atelocollagen injection. *Am. J. Sports Med.* 2021;49(11):2924–32.
124. Xu D, Zhang T, Qu J, Hu J, Lu H. Enhanced patella–patellar tendon healing using combined magnetic fields in a rabbit model. *Am. J. Sports Med.* 2014;42(10):2495–501.
125. Thomas BS, Bhat KM, Mapara M. Rabbit as an animal model for experimental research. *Dent. Res. J.* 2012;9:111.
126. Marí-Beffa M, Mesa-Román AB, Duran I. Zebrafish models for human skeletal disorders. *Front. Genet.* 2021;12:675331.
127. Dietrich K, Fiedler IA, Kurzyukova A, López-Delgado AC, McGowan LM, Geurtzen K, et al. Skeletal biology and disease modeling in zebrafish. *J. Bone Miner. Res.* 2021;36(3):436–58.
128. Busse B, Galloway JL, Gray RS, Harris MP, Kwon RY. Zebrafish: An emerging model for orthopedic research. *J. Orthop. Res.* 2020;38(5):925–36.
129. Kaliya-Perumal A-K, Ingham PW. Musculoskeletal regeneration: A zebrafish perspective. *Biochimie* 2022;196:171–81.
130. Tonelli F, Bek JW, Besio R, De Clercq A, Leoni L, Salmon P, et al. Zebrafish: A resourceful vertebrate model to investigate skeletal disorders. *Front. Endocrinol.* 2020;11:489.
131. Schulze-Tanzil G, Silawal S, Hoyer M. Anatomical feature of knee joint in Aachen minipig as a novel miniature pig line for experimental research in orthopaedics. *Ann. Anat.* 2020;227:151411.
132. Chevalier JM, Pearson GB, Nixon N, Flannery CR, Campoy L, Fortier LA. Destabilization of the medial meniscus to induce post-traumatic osteoarthritis in domestic pigs. *J. Cartil. Joint Preserv.* 2023;3(4):100139.
133. Schwarz ML, Reisig G, Schütte A, Becker K, Serba S, Forsch E, et al. Report on a large animal study with Göttingen minipigs where regenerates and controls for articular cartilage were created in a large number. Focus on the conditions of the operated stifle joints and suggestions for standardized procedures. *PLoS One* 2019;14(12):e0224996.

134. Ruehe B, Niehues S, Heberer S, Nelson K. Miniature pigs as an animal model for implant research: Bone regeneration in critical-size defects. *Oral Surg. Oral Med. Oral Pathol. Oral Radiol. Endod.* 2009;108(5):699–706.
135. Sturge G. Animal experiment statistics. 2023.
136. Tannenbaum J, Bennett BT. Russell and Burch's 3Rs then and now: The need for clarity in definition and purpose. *J. Am. Assoc. Lab. Anim. Sci.* 2015;54(2):120–32.
137. Lee KH, Lee DW, Kang BC. The 'R' principles in laboratory animal experiments. *Lab. Anim. Res.* 2020;36:45.
138. Crespi-Abril AC, Rubilar T. Moving forward in the ethical consideration of invertebrates in experimentation: Beyond the Three R's principle. *Rev. Biol. Trop.* 2021;69(Suppl 1):S346–57.
139. Robinson NB, Krieger K, Khan FM, Huffman W, Chang M, Naik A, et al. The current state of animal models in research: A review. *Int. J. Surg.* 2019; 72:9–13.
140. FDA. FDA announces plan to phase out animal testing requirement for monoclonal antibodies and other drugs. https://www.fda.gov/news-events/press-announcements/fda-announces-plan-phase-out-animal-testing-requirement-monoclonal-antibodies-and-other-drugs
141. Marshall LJ, Bailey J, Cassotta M, Herrmann K, Pistollato F. Poor translatability of biomedical research using animals-a narrative review. *Altern. Lab. Anim.* 2023;51(2):102–35. https://doi.org/10.1177/02611929231157756
142. Shah R, Thomas R, Gowda TM, Baron TKA, Vemanaradhya GG, Bhagat S. In vitro evaluation of osteoblast response to the effect of injectable platelet-rich fibrin coating on titanium disks. *J. Contemp. Dent. Pract.* 2021;22(2):107–10.
143. Subramani K, Pandruvada SN, Puleo DA, Hartsfield JK, Huja SS. In vitro evaluation of osteoblast responses to carbon nanotube-coated titanium surfaces. *Prog. Orthod.* 2016;17:23.
144. Lee JH, Jang HL, Lee KM, Baek H-R, Jin K, Hong KS, et al. In vitro and in vivo evaluation of the bioactivity of hydroxyapatite-coated polyetheretherketone biocomposites created by cold spray technology. *Acta Biomater.* 2013;9(4):6177–87.
145. Huh YH, Lee G, Song W-H, Koh J-T, Ryu J-H. Crosstalk between FLS and chondrocytes is regulated by HIF-2α-mediated cytokines in arthritis. *Exp. Mol. Med.* 2015;47(12):e197.
146. Huch K, Stöve J, Günther KP, Puhl W. Interactions between human osteoarthritic chondrocytes and synovial fibroblasts in co-culture. *Clin. Exp. Rheumatol.* 2001;19(1):27–33.

147. Suarez-Martinez E, Suazo-Sanchez I, Celis-Romero M, Carnero A. 3D and organoid culture in research: Physiology, hereditary genetic diseases and cancer. *Cell Biosci.* 2022;12(1):39.
148. Lei T, Zhang T, Ju W, Chen X, Heng BC, Shen W, et al. Biomimetic strategies for tendon/ligament-to-bone interface regeneration. *Bioact. Mater.* 2021;6(8):2491–510.
149. Balestri W, Hickman GJ, Morris RH, Hunt JA, Reinwald Y. Triphasic 3D in vitro model of bone-tendon-muscle interfaces to study their regeneration. *Cells* 2023;12(3):313.
150. Kafienah W, Mistry S, Dickinson SC, Sims TJ, Learmonth I, Hollander AP. Three-dimensional cartilage tissue engineering using adult stem cells from osteoarthritis patients. *Arthritis Rheum.* 2007;56:177–87.
151. Yousafzai MS, Hammer JA. Using biosensors to study organoids, spheroids and organs-on-a-chip: A mechanobiology perspective. *Biosensors.* 2023; 13:905.
152. Wang Y, Jin S, Luo D, He D, Shi C, Zhu L, et al. Functional regeneration and repair of tendons using biomimetic scaffolds loaded with recombinant periostin. *Nat. Commun.* 2021;12:1293.
153. Mizuno S, Takada E, Fukai N. Spheroidal organoids reproduce characteristics of longitudinal depth zones in bovine articular cartilage. *Cells Tissues Organs.* 2016;202:382–92.
154. Yu Y, Wang J, Li Y, Chen Y, Cui W. Cartilaginous organoids: Advances, applications, and perspectives. *Adv. Nanobiomed. Res.* 2023;3(1):2200114.
155. Lin W, Wang M, Xu L, Tortorella M, Li G. Cartilage organoids for cartilage development and cartilage-associated disease modeling. *Front. Cell Dev. Biol.* 2023;11:1125405.
156. Johnson N, Filler AC, Sethi A, Smith LR, Leach JK. Skeletal muscle spheroids as building blocks for engineered muscle tissue. *ACS Biomater. Sci. Eng.* 2024;10:497–506.
157. Leung CM, de Haan P, Ronaldson-Bouchard K, Kim GA, Ko J, Rho HS, et al. A guide to the organ-on-a-chip. *Nat. Rev. Methods Primers.* 2022;2:33. https://doi.org/10.1038/s43586-022-00118-6
158. Mansoorifar A, Gordon R, Bergan RC, Bertassoni LE. Bone-on-a-chip: Microfluidic technologies and microphysiologic models of bone tissue. *Adv. Funct. Mater.* 2021;31(6):2006796.
159. Nasello G, Cóndor M, Vaughan T, Schiavi J. Designing hydrogel-based bone-on-chips for personalized medicine. *Appl. Sci.* 2021;11:4495.
160. Lee S, Kim YG, Jung HI, Lim JS, Nam KC, Choi HS, et al. Bone-on-a-chip simulating bone metastasis in osteoporosis. *Biofabrication* 2024;16:045025.

161. Yang J, Duan P, Liu Q, Yu H, Fang F, Liu X. Microfluidic bone chip to study osteogenesis of porous substrate topographies in normal and osteoporotic microenvironments. *Eur. Cell Mater.* 2024;47:238–52.
162. Mansoorifar A, Gordon R, Bergan RC, Bertassoni LE. Bone-on-a-chip: Microfluidic technologies and microphysiologic models of bone tissue. *Adv. Funct. Mater.* 2021;31(6):2006796.
163. Phillips R. Progress toward 'bone-on-a-chip'. *Nat. Rev. Rheumatol.* 2023; 19:463.
164. Kim MK, Paek K, Woo SM, Kim JA. Bone-on-a-chip: Biomimetic models based on microfluidic technologies for biomedical applications. *ACS Biomater. Sci. Eng.* 2023;9:3058–73.
165. Qin Y, Li J-X, Cai W, Fan W-T, Duan B, Zhao Y, et al. A cartilage-on-a-chip for recapitulating cell microenvironment and real-time nitric oxide monitoring. *Device* 2024;2(6):100410.
166. Paggi C, Hendriks J, van Leeuwen A, Karperien M, van Apeldoorn A, Le Gac S. Cartilage-on-chip: A multi-modal platform to study human chondrocyte's response to mechanical stimuli. *Osteoarthr. Cartil.* 2020;28:S176–7.
167. Occhetta P, Mainardi A, Votta E, Vallmajo-Martin Q, Ehrbar M, Martin I, et al. Hyperphysiological compression of articular cartilage induces an osteoarthritic phenotype in a cartilage-on-a-chip model. *Nat. Biomed. Eng.* 2019;3(7):545–57.
168. Paggi CA, Hendriks J, Karperien M, Le Gac S. Emulating the chondrocyte microenvironment using multi-directional mechanical stimulation in a cartilage-on-chip. *Lab Chip* 2022;22:1815–28.
169. Liu H, Wu X, Liu R, Wang W, Zhang D, Jiang Q. Cartilage-on-a-chip with magneto-mechanical transformation for osteoarthritis recruitment. *Bioact. Mater.* 2024;33:61–8.
170. Mainardi A, Occhetta P, Rasponi M. Mechanical induction of osteoarthritis traits in a cartilage-on-a-chip model. *Methods Mol. Biol.* 2022;2422:231–51. https://doi.org/10.1007/978-1-0716-1693-2_14
171. Banh L, Cheung KK, Chan MWY, Young EWK, Viswanathan S. Advances in organ-on-a-chip systems for modelling joint tissue and osteoarthritic diseases. *Osteoarthr. Cartil.* 2022;30:1050–61.
172. Hu Y, Zhang H, Wang S, Cao L, Zhou F, Jing Y, et al. Bone/cartilage organoid on-chip: Construction strategy and application. *Bioact. Mater.* 2023;25:29–41.
173. Rupprecht C, Wingen M, Potzkei J, Gensch T, Jaeger KE, Drepper T. A novel FbFP-based biosensor toolbox for sensitive in vivo determination of intracellular pH. *J. Biotechnol.* 2017;258:25–32.

174. Rivera KR, Pozdin VA, Young AT, Erb PD, Wisniewski NA, Magness ST, et al. Integrated phosphorescence-based photonic biosensor (iPOB) for monitoring oxygen levels in 3D cell culture systems. *Biosens. Bioelectron.* 2019;123:131–40.
175. Liang Z, Zhang J, Wu C, Hu X, Lu Y, Wang G, et al. Flexible and self-healing electrochemical hydrogel sensor with high efficiency toward glucose monitoring. *Biosens. Bioelectron.* 2020;155:112105.
176. Balbaied T, Moore E. Overview of optical and electrochemical alkaline phosphatase (ALP) biosensors: Recent approaches in cells culture techniques. *Biosensors* 2019;9:102.
177. Aykul S, Martinez-Hackert E. High-throughput, biosensor-based approach to examine bone morphogenetic protein (BMP)–receptor interactions. *Methods Mol. Biol.* 2019;1891:37–49. https://doi.org/10.1007/978-1-4939-8904-1_5
178. Oragui E. The role of bioreactors in tissue engineering for musculoskeletal applications. *Open Orthop. J.* 2011;5:267–70.
179. Wong TY, Chang CH, Yu CH, Huang SF. Closer to nature through dynamic culture systems. *Cells.* 2019;8:942.
180. Jenkins TL, Little D. Synthetic scaffolds for musculoskeletal tissue engineering: Cellular responses to fiber parameters. *NPJ Regen. Med.* 2019;4:15.
181. Wong TY, Chang CH, Yu CH, Huang SF. Closer to nature through dynamic culture systems. *Cells.* 2019;8:942.
182. Kazimierczak P, Kalisz G, Sroka-Bartnicka A, Przekora A. Effectiveness of the production of tissue-engineered living bone graft: A comparative study using perfusion and rotating bioreactor systems. *Sci. Rep.* 2023;13:13737.
183. Zhao F, van Rietbergen B, Ito K, Hofmann S. Flow rates in perfusion bioreactors to maximise mineralisation in bone tissue engineering in vitro. *J. Biomech.* 2018;79:232–7.
184. Kengla C, Atala A, Lee SJ. Bioprinting of organoids. In: *Essentials of 3D Biofabrication and Translation.* Elsevier; 2015:271–82. https://doi.org/10.1016/B978-0-12-800972-7.00015-3
185. Persaud A, Maus A, Strait L, Zhu D. 3D bioprinting with live cells. *Eng. Regen.* 2022;3:292–309.
186. Wei Q, Peng Y, Chen W, Duan Y, Chua G, Hu J, et al. Three-dimensional bioprinting for musculoskeletal regeneration and disease modeling. *Int. J. Bioprinting* 2024;10:1037.
187. Burdis R, Kelly DJ. Biofabrication and bioprinting using cellular aggregates, microtissues and organoids for the engineering of musculoskeletal tissues. *Acta Biomater.* 2021;126:1–14.

188. Potyondy T, Uquillas JA, Tebon PJ, Byambaa B, Hasan A, Tavafoghi M, et al. Recent advances in 3D bioprinting of musculoskeletal tissues. *Biofabrication* 2021;13(2):022001.
189. Cooray S, Omaar A, Goel V, Wood J, Kelly-Morland C, Chari A, et al. Artificial intelligence in musculoskeletal medicine: A scoping review. *touchREV. RMD* 2024;3:15–23.
190. Deng S, Wang Y, Chen KG, Ward A, Chen W. Organ-on-a-chip meets artificial intelligence in drug evaluation. *Theranostics* 2023;13:4526–58.
191. Bai L, Wu Y, Li G, Zhang W, Zhang H, Su J. AI-enabled organoids: Construction, analysis, and application. *Bioact. Mater.* 2024;31:525–48.
192. Shaikh M, Kahwash F, Lu Z, Alkhreisat M, Mohammad A, Shyha I. Revolutionising orthopaedic implants — a comprehensive review on metal 3D printing with materials, design strategies, manufacturing technologies, and post-process machining advancements. *Int. J. Adv. Manuf. Technol.* 2024; 134:1043–76.
193. Wu X, Shi W, Liu X, Gu Z. Recent advances in 3D-printing-based organ-on-a-chip. *EngMedicine* 2024;1(1):100003.
194. De Spirito M, Palmieri V, Perini G, Papi M. Bridging the gap: Integrating 3D bioprinting and microfluidics for advanced multi-organ models in biomedical research. *Bioengineering* 2024;11:664.
195. Picollet-D'hahan N, Zuchowska A, Lemeunier I, Le Gac S. Multiorgan-on-a-chip: A systemic approach to model and decipher inter-organ communication. *Trends Biotechnol.* 2021;39(8):788–810.

https://doi.org/10.1142/9789819819645_0011

Chapter 11

CRISPR Technology

Elif Durasi, Esra Kuscu, Nurseda Surgit, Hilal Calik, Rabia Cakir*

Department of Bioengineering, Faculty of Chemical and Metallurgical Engineering, Yıldız Technical University, Istanbul, Turkey

Chapter Outline

Abstract

CRISPR technology stands out as a promising strategy in gene modification, base editing, and epigenetic modification, representing a novel approach to treating a wide range of disorders. The simple and efficient mechanism of CRISPR provides editing opportunities for a wide range of applications, such as drug development, agriculture, animal models, medical treatments, gene therapy development, and infectious diseases.

***Corresponding author:** Rabia Cakir, Department of Bioengineering, Faculty of Chemical and Metallurgical Engineering, Yıldız Technical University, Istanbul, Turkey. E-mail: rabiacakir@gmail.com

Although CRISPR technology is a targeted, accurate, easy-to-use, and multipotent strategy, there are still limitations and concerns to address. These include immune responses to CRISPR-based therapeutics, problems based on the transporting of CRISPR-Cas components to particular cells, tissues, and organs for precise targeted genome editing, and the high frequency of off-target effects. CRISPR-based technologies can be utilized to study musculoskeletal diseases, especially in modeling *in vitro* and *in vivo* disease-causing mutations, as well as to investigate musculoskeletal malignancies and develop new therapy alternatives. While there are no clinical trials yet investigating the use of CRISPR technologies for the treatment of musculoskeletal disease, research in this area is currently being improved. This chapter discusses published studies that report on the various CRISPR strategies used in the treatment of musculoskeletal disease, the moral, ethical, safety, and technical concerns associated with the increasing use of CRISPR, and future perspectives on CRISPR technology and its use in the treatment of musculoskeletal disease.

1. Introduction

First discovered in *Escherichia coli* in 1987 [1], clustered regularly interspaced short palindromic repeats (CRISPR) are a unique part of the prokaryotic immune system. Regarded as one of the most reliable gene editing and engineering techniques available today, the CRISPR-Cas-based bacterial immune response can be dissected into three steps. The first step, known as the adaptive phase, begins when a plasmid or viral threat is present; bacteria and archaea carrying at least one CRISPR region integrate small segments of foreign sequence (also called protospacers) into the host chromosome at the proximal end of the CRISPR array [2, 3]. The second step, the expression phase, involves the host organism transcribing the CRISPR element (pre-crRNA) and modifying it through enzymatic cleavage to generate short CRISPR RNAs (crRNAs) compatible with the invading organism's protospacers [4–6]. In the final step, the CRISPR-associated protein (Cas), working in conjunction with the crRNAs, recognizes the foreign sequences and inactivates them by cutting the target DNA [7–10]. The most recent classification of CRISPR-Cas systems divides it into two groups based on the encoded effector proteins: Class 1 and Class 2 [11].

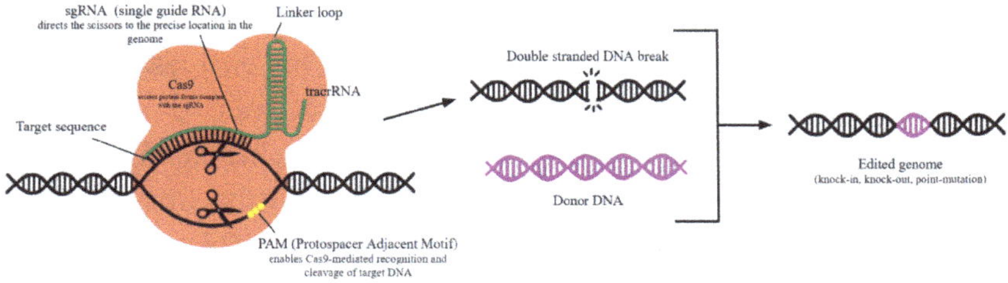

Figure 1. Schematic of the CRISPR-Cas9 genome editing system.

Multisubunit effector complexes containing four to seven Cas proteins present in a differing stoichiometry are used in Class I CRISPR-Cas systems. Class I is prevalent in prokaryotes and accounts for over 90% of all known CRISPR-Cas loci. The remaining 10% are categorized as Class 2, which are virtually exclusively present in bacteria and employ a single multidomain effector protein [12]. As of right now, each class has three types: Class 1 consists of types I, III, and IV, and Class 2 consists of types II, V, and VI. Because of the straightforward construction of the effector complex, Class 2 CRISPR-Cas systems are a desirable option for creating a new generation of genome editing tools. There are many unique Class 2 effectors, including Cas9 (type II), Cas12a (type V), Cas12b (type V), Cas13a (type VI), and Cas13b (type VI) [13]. Cas9 is a crRNA-dependent endonuclease that is the most commonly used and extensively researched multidomain effector protein. It is composed of RuvC and HNH nuclease domains, which cleave the target and nontarget (displaced) DNA strands in the crRNA-target DNA complex, respectively [14].

Originally evolved as an adaptive defense system in prokaryotic organisms to prevent harm from invading viruses and plasmids, CRISPR-Cas systems are currently used as a genetic engineering tool in many fields, from plant biotechnology to genomic medicine [15]. How CRISPR-Cas systems work as a genetic editing tool is fairly simple. CRISPR's guided RNA, single guided RNA or sgRNA, has a target location in the DNA, which it finds and binds to while using protospacer adjacent motifs (PAMs) for recognition. Then, the Cas enzyme creates a double-stranded break at the region where sgRNA is bound. It initiates DNA repair processes that integrate the foreign DNA to complete the host DNA by ligating the two DNA pieces by their compatible ends. This technique utilizes the host cell's established primitive immune system whereby it is able to integrate foreign DNA into its genetic material. This enables the cell to recognize previously encountered threats and activate a subsequent immune response [9]. There are (as of writing this chapter) 57 ongoing clinical trials employing CRISPR-Cas systems, and the first CRISPR-based therapy was approved by the FDA in January 2024 to treat sickle cell disease (Casgevy™). Out of the 57 ongoing clinical trials, there are 24 that are cancer-targeted, 16 related to hematologic diseases, 4 viral disease-related, 4 eye disease-related, 5 targeted toward rare genetic disorders, and finally, 2 targeted toward diabetes and infectious diseases, respectively. As of writing this chapter, there are no clinical trial phase studies employing CRISPR technologies for the treatment of musculoskeletal disease. However, there are plenty of studies still being improved, and with CRISPR still being a young and developing technology, an increase in the number of preclinical and clinical trials using CRISPR-based therapies to target musculoskeletal diseases is expected in the future.

2. CRISPR-Based Musculoskeletal Therapies

The broad application of CRISPR, including gene modification, base editing, and epigenetic modification, represents a novel approach to treating many diseases, including those related to the musculoskeletal system [16]. In this section, examples of various CRISPR techniques used in the therapy of various musculoskeletal diseases will be presented.

Osteoarthritis (OA) is a degenerative joint disease that causes articular cartilage loss, synovial hyperplasia, joint space narrowing, subchondral bone sclerosis, and osteophyte formation [17]. Abnormal overexpression of many proteins such as matrix metalloproteinase 13 (MMP13), interleukin-1β (IL-1β), and nerve growth factor (NGF) is associated with OA. It is incurable, and clinical research targeting OA-associated variables such as MMPs, inflammatory cytokines, and growth factors produced inconsistent results in terms of treatment effectiveness and safety [18]. Current therapies provide short-term relief of symptoms, do not prevent the degenerative process, and can have considerable side effects when used in the long term. Joint replacement and surgery are costly and painful. Conversely, CRISPR is a potentially beneficial treatment for OA sufferers in the long term [19]. A study by Zhao et al. employed an adeno-associated virus to deliver CRISPR/Cas9 components that targeted MMP13, IL-1β, and NGF genes in murine models with OA. CRISPR-mediated knockout of these genes proved beneficial for joint structure preservation and pain management [20]. A study performed by Liang et al. in 2022 used chondrocyte-targeting exosomes (CAP-Exo) to encapsulate CRISPR-Cas9 plasmids, which were used to suppress the expression of MMP13. The study was carried out *in vivo* in arthritic rats, and CAP-Exo was given intra-articularly. The results showed promise to reduce OA by inhibiting cartilage degeneration [19]. Bonato et al. used the CRISPR knockout mechanism in polydactyl human chondrocyte models (both *in vivo* and *in vitro*) to regulate the transforming growth factor-β-activated kinase 1 (TAK1) gene to engineer a more inflammation-resistant cartilage tissue. They found that following inflammatory stimulation, TAK1 knockout chondrocytes showed increased incorporation into cartilage [21].

Osteogenesis imperfecta (OI) is a hereditary disorder defined by bone fragility and recurrent fractures. OI-related bone fragility occurs due to a deficiency in collagen production induced by a collagen type I alpha 1 chain (COL1A1) or collagen type I alpha 2 chain (COL1A2) mutation. Several treatments have been tested; however, they have not resulted in total recovery [22]. Current therapies involve surgical procedures, the use of prostheses, intramedullary stabilization, and pharmaceutical drugs derived mostly from those used to treat osteoporosis or osteolytic bone metastases, and their consequences. However, because these medications cannot modify the source of the collagen alterations, they have had limited clinical success [23]. Gene therapy includes suppressing unfavorable or damaging transcripts, increasing healthy allele expression, or repairing genetic defects, either temporarily or permanently. Also, CRISPR/Cas9 gene editing offers the potential for fixing mutated alleles [24]. The rarity of the disease, combined with the fundamental genetic defect, has hindered the development of an effective treatment [22]. Yang et al. devised a genome-editing technique to rectify a COL1A2 mutation in a murine model that mimicked OI's type III in humans. A genetically modified adeno-associated virus carrying a promoterless partial mouse COL1A2 complementary DNA sequence was used by the researchers to introduce CRISPR-Cas9 into osteoblast-lineage cells in the skeleton, and homology-directed repair

(HDR)-mediated gene editing efficacy in these cells was enhanced. Results showed that the COL1A2 mutation-induced dysregulation of osteogenic differentiation was successfully corrected *in vitro* [23]. Another study by Jung et al. used blood cells from an OI patient with a COL1A1 gene mutation to create induced pluripotent stem cells (iPSCs) with CRISPR-Cas9-mediated COL1A1 gene correction. This experiment helped prove the relation between type I collagen production and mutation of the COL1A1 gene. After correcting the mutation with the CRISPR-Cas9 method, type I collagen expression and cell osteogenic capacity were effectively restored [22].

Duchenne muscular dystrophy (DMD) is a disease caused by mutations in the dystrophin gene, and genetically transmitted by the X chromosome, which encodes a protein necessary for muscle fiber integrity. There is no curative treatment for DMD [25]. At the moment, both antisense oligonucleotide and corticosteroid treatments are available to alleviate the symptoms of this disease, but the current therapeutic approaches are primarily focused on alleviating DMD symptoms such as inflammation, fibrosis, mitochondrial dysfunction, impaired angiogenesis, or calcium dyshomeostasis. Long-term corticosteroid use has numerous negative consequences, including growth delay and bone fragility [26]. CRISPR technology provides a promising therapeutic option for restoring the expression of dystrophin and muscle function in DMD patients by removing pathogenic mutations at the genomic level [27]. In 2014, Long et al. applied the first *in vivo* CRISPR-mediated gene editing approach to target DMD. The authors used *mdx* mice zygotes injected with SpCas9, synthetic short guide RNA (sgRNA), and an exogenous DNA template for HDR and thus created mosaic mice with corrected dystrophin levels differing between 2% and 100%. The results of the study pointed out that the gene editing technique does not need to be 100% to restore average dystrophin levels, instead ~15% was adequate [25]. Moretti et al. also investigated somatic gene editing that reconstructed the DMD gene's reading frame using CRISPR-Cas9 exon excision in a pig model *in vivo* and a patient-derived iPSC model *in vitro*. The study aimed to improve skeletal integrity and reduce the possibility of cardiac muscle failure, which succeeded by inducing the expression of a shorter than naturally occurring, albeit functioning dystrophin [28]. Zhang et al. conducted a study using human-derived iPSCs and CRISPR-CPF1 to facilitate DMD in *mdx* mice and to regulate dystrophin expression and muscle contraction performance in cardiomyocytes. They employed two approaches: reframing and exon skipping, to reinstate the original reading frame of the DMD gene. Their results showed that even though the achieved dystrophin was not the same as the wild type, the outcome was still remarkably improved [29]. By focusing on the DMD mutational hotspot at exons between 45 and 55 and altering or deleting one or more exons, Ousterout et al. created sgRNAs and used them in conjunction with SpCas9 nuclease to restore the dystrophin reading frame. This study showed that by removing exons 45–55 of the dystrophin gene, a replicable single genome-editing technique can be utilized to correct over half of the deletions found in DMD patients [30].

Chen et al. aimed to create a novel treatment option for calvarial bone defects *via* regulating vascular endothelial growth factor-A (VEGF-A) and transforming growth factor ß1 (TGF-ß1) genes using CRISPR. In this study, they found that using co-activated TGF-ß1 and VEGF-A genes within a tunable dual-crosslinked hydrogel synergistically promoted bone regeneration [31]. Hsu et al. used a synergistic activation mediator-based CRISPRa system to induce Wnt10b and forkhead box protein C2 (FOXC2) genes in bone marrow-derived mesenchymal stem cells to achieve calvarial bone regeneration in Sprague–Dawley rats. Constructing an efficient baculovirus vector, Bac-CRISPRa facilitated CRISPRa delivery and potently activated endogenous Wnt10b and FOXC2 expression in stem cells. Coactivated Wnt10b and FOXC2 showed promising results both *in vivo* and *in vitro* [32]. Nguyen et al. investigated the use of CRISPR activation technology to enhance calvarial bone repair in rats and induce rat chondrogenesis from adipose-derived stem cells by activating differentiation antagonizing non-protein coding RNA (DANCR). The outcomes demonstrated that the *Staphylococcus aureus*-derived Cas9 effectively enhanced calvarial bone repair [33].

3. Challenges and Opportunities in CRISPR

CRISPR/Cas systems are genome editing techniques that have shown promise for detecting, imaging, manipulating, and annotating specific DNA and RNA sequences in single cells or entire organisms. Genome editing includes sequence deletions, insertions, substitutions, integrations, and the regulation of epigenetic genes [34, 35]. The simple and efficient method of CRISPR provides editing opportunities for many different applications, such as drug development, agriculture, animal models, medical treatments, gene therapy development, and infectious diseases [36]. The CRISPR-Cas9 system consists of a programmable Cas9 nuclease and sgRNA. The guide RNA determines the specificity of DNA targets. Consequently, the CRISPR-Cas9 system is significantly simpler to create than Zinc finger or TALENs; it is simple, efficient, low in cost, and can target several genes at once [37, 38].

Over the past years, advances in CRISPR/Cas technologies have demonstrated that CRISPR technology has significant potential in many different areas of life science research. Although CRISPR technology is more targeted, more accurate, easy to use, and multipotential, limitations and issues still need to be addressed [35]. Humans can develop strong innate immunity and/or adaptive immunity (cellular and humoral immunity) in response to foreign elements when CRISPR systems are delivered *in vivo* [39]. According to research, immunological responses can be triggered by pre-exposure to comparable antigens of CRISPR system constituents, including Cas9, guide RNAs, and delivery vectors (such as adenoviral vectors), which could prevent effective genome editing [40, 41]. Multiple approaches have been proposed to solve this issue, consisting of the use of phosphatase to treat *in vitro*-transcribed guide RNAs, the development of special Cas proteins and delivery vectors that decrease the probability of previous exposure in humans, and the monitoring and assessment of immune responses to the CRISPR system components both before and during clinical studies [42].

Another main challenge in gene therapy is efficiently transporting CRISPR-Cas components to specific cells, tissues, and organs for precisely targeted genome editing. Non-toxicity, excellent targeting capability, superior effectiveness, cost-effectiveness, and biodegradability should be the characteristics of ideal delivery vectors [43, 44]. There are three main techniques for the delivery of CRISPR/Cas components: Physical (microinjection, electroporation, and hydrodynamic delivery), viral (e.g., an adeno-associated virus, adenovirus [AdV], lentivirus [LV]), and nonviral (extracellular vesicle-based systems [liposomes and peptide nanoparticles] techniques) [42]. Physical methods such as microinjection and electroporation are simple, efficient, low-cost, and virus-free ways to deliver CRISPR-Cas components [41, 44]. However, physical methods can cause mechanical deformation and trauma to cells, tissues, and the body [41, 43]. Furthermore, viral vectors are also frequently utilized because of their excellent delivery effectiveness for both *in vivo* and *in vitro/ex vivo* delivery. Although viral vectors can be utilized both *in vivo* and *in vitro*, they have limitations, including immunological reaction and insertional restriction [44]. A viral vector is exposed for a considerable amount of time after being introduced *in vivo*, which increases the mutations and off-targeting possibilities [45]. In response to the safety concerns with viral vectors, nonviral vectors such as liposomes, polymers, and nanoparticles are given attention due to their advantages, including safety, accessibility, and affordability [44]. Besides these advantages, there are a few concerns, such as complex design and production in high quantities for clinical usage, potential toxicity, and efficacy issues [42, 46]. In addition, off-target effects are unexpected gene mutations caused by nontarget DNA sequence mismatch with the designed sgRNA. The high frequency of off-target effects is one of the major concerns when applying CRISPR/Cas9 for gene therapy because that causes genome instability and introduces unwanted mutations in off-target regions, thereby causing important functional loss and disruption of essential human genes, leading to a variety of physiological or signaling abnormalities [47, 48]. However, there are numerous techniques for reducing off-target effects. The specific binding of sgRNA with the target sequence is the fundamental issue of CRISPR-Cas systems. Using highly specific sgRNAs with a rational design can reduce off-target effects [44]. Also, Cas enzyme inhibition is a useful strategy for minimizing off-target effects. Small molecule Cas inhibitors, anti-CRISPR (Acr) proteins, and small nucleic acid-based CRISPR inhibitors are three types of inhibitor techniques that have been developed [41]. In addition to providing short-term inhibition of Cas enzyme activity for precise temporal control, small molecule inhibitors offer several advantageous properties, including cell permeability, reversibility, proteolytic stability, and low immunogenicity. Small inhibitor screening is still difficult since sensitive, low-cost, high-throughput assays are currently unavailable [41, 49].

4. Ethical and Practical Considerations

The application of CRISPR-based methods in preclinical and clinical research in musculoskeletal disease, as well as in many other diseases, has accelerated with the recent development of the CRISPR system. However, the increase in the application areas of CRISPR has raised various moral, ethical, safety, and technical concerns [16, 50]. Ethical concerns with CRISPR applications arise mainly for three reasons. The first is related to the technical limitations of the CRISPR system and caused by limited targeting efficiency, incomplete editing (mosaicism), and incorrect or off-target editing. The second is that it is unclear whether the genes edited in the modified organism can be transferred to future generations. The last is that even if the genome is edited as desired, the potential risks and benefits cannot be determined in the long term due to the lack of a complete understanding of the relationship between genetic information and biological phenotypes [51–53]. Current treatment strategies involve editing at the somatic cell level, where changes will be limited to the treated individual. However, the potential for CRISPR-based treatments to edit germ cells continues to generate debate in the scientific and public arena. Although the goal of CRISPR is to treat or prevent diseases, the application of advancements in this field for other goals, such as enhancing intelligence, physical attributes, and appearance, as well as the fact that these attributes can be passed on to future generations, can result in social inequality and discrimination. In addition, transferring gene editing tools to future generations and potentially altering the course of human evolution may lead to unexpected results. Additionally, advancements in CRISPR could lead to a decrease in or even the eradication of genetic illnesses, which could have detrimental socioeconomic effects on communities. All of the ethical concerns mentioned regarding CRISPR are also valid for the application of the technology in musculoskeletal disease. International standards for the ethical, practical, and accessible application of CRISPR-based technologies in the clinical and research settings must be developed immediately. Although some regions have procedures to assess and manage the ethical aspects of the technology, there is a need for a comprehensive evaluation of ethical issues at the global level [54, 55]. Therefore, the development and oversight of global standards for the ethical use of

CRISPR by the scientific and medical communities will contribute to the elimination of existing concerns.

5. The Future of CRISPR in Treating Musculoskeletal Diseases

CRISPR-based technologies stand out as a promising strategy to prevent and treat musculoskeletal disease, especially in modeling *in vitro* and *in vivo* disease-causing mutations, investigating musculoskeletal malignancies, and developing new treatment methods for these diseases. However, some difficulties prevent the development and clinical phase of CRISPR-based treatments for musculoskeletal diseases. One of the biggest challenges to the use of CRISPR-based technologies, as it is in many other fields, is the potential for off-target consequences from the CRISPR system. The main reason for off-target mutations in the CRISPR/Cas9 system, which is the most commonly used among CRISPR-based technologies, is that the Cas9-sgRNA has a sequence mismatch tolerance against the target DNA. The human genome contains DNA sequences that are either identical or comparable. This results in the binding of Cas9-sgRNA to off-target areas, which introduces undesired mutations [42]. However, there are studies in which the Cas9 protein is artificially modified or new sgRNAs are designed to increase the sensitivity and specificity of the CRISPR/Cas9 system [56]. Future developments in CRISPR technology are expected to benefit the treatment of musculoskeletal diseases and many other diseases by reducing off-target effects. A further barrier to the application of CRISPR technology in musculoskeletal disease is the lack of efficient delivery methods for tissues such as bone and cartilage and the transfection resistance of some cell types, including chondrocytes. In order to overcome the delivery difficulties, viral vectors, lentiviruses, and adenoviruses are frequently preferred in current studies. However, these systems have serious immunogenicity and safety problems [16]. Therefore, in order to effectively use CRISPR technology for musculoskeletal diseases, new delivery mechanisms are required. Nanoparticle carrier systems stand out as a promising area in the delivery of CRISPR-based methods to the relevant region. The fact that models and treatment strategies produced in animals cannot be applied to humans is another factor that limits the use of CRISPR-based treatments. Although the human and mouse genomes are quite similar in terms of exon composition and amino acid sequence, there are differences at the genomic level. Therefore, sgRNAs designed specifically for humans cannot target the mouse genome [57]. It is expected that the deployment of humanized models, in which the important gene areas are replaced with human autologous genes in model animals, will be beneficial in overcoming the genetic disparities between the created models and people. Despite the difficulties encountered, CRISPR technology continues to be a promising method for modeling musculoskeletal diseases, understanding the genetic causes underlying these diseases, and treating them. For example, cellular aging, DNA damage, telomere shortening, oxidative stress, mitochondrial dysfunction, and continuous cytokine activation are the most important factors affecting the development of OA. CRISPR technology is ideal for effectively verifying the relevant pathways and efficiently and precisely reversing cellular aging. In addition, it requires less effort to slow down or prevent aging compared to traditional gene therapy methods [58]. Another common musculoskeletal disease is DMD. Current treatment methods for DMD are limited to improving a patient's quality of life and slowing down the progression of the disease. However, developments in CRISPR technology allow for the targeting and correction of genetic mutations responsible for DMD, which not only alleviates symptoms but also holds promise for the development of curative treatments [55]. The advancement of CRISPR technology, its demonstrated safety in clinical trials, and its long-term viability will make it feasible to create individualized treatment plans for musculoskeletal disorders, particularly those linked to single nucleotide polymorphisms. Therefore, new approaches that can overcome the mentioned disadvantages need to be investigated in order to use the CRISPR-based approach to target the treatment of musculoskeletal disease and translate them into clinical practice.

References

1. Ishino Y, Shinagawa H, Makino K, Amemura M, Nakata A. Nucleotide sequence of the iap gene, responsible for alkaline phosphatase isozyme

conversion in Escherichia coli, and identification of the gene product. *J. Bacteriol.* 1987;169(12):5429–33.

2. Bhaya D, Davison M, Barrangou R. CRISPR-Cas systems in bacteria and archaea: Versatile small RNAs for adaptive defense and regulation. *Annu. Rev. Genet.* 2011;45(1):273–97.
3. Wiedenheft B, Sternberg SH, Doudna JA. RNA-guided genetic silencing systems in bacteria and archaea. *Nature.* 2012;482(7385):331–8.
4. Deltcheva E, Chylinski K, Sharma CM, Gonzales K, Chao Y, Pirzada ZA, et al. CRISPR RNA maturation by trans-encoded small RNA and host factor RNase III. *Nature.* 2011;471(7340):602–7.
5. Haurwitz RE, Jinek M, Wiedenheft B, Zhou K, Doudna JA. Sequence-and structure-specific RNA processing by a CRISPR endonuclease. *Science.* 2010;329(5997):1355–8.
6. Sashital DG, Jinek M, Doudna JA. An RNA-induced conformational change required for CRISPR RNA cleavage by the endoribonuclease Cse3. *Nat. Struct. Mol. Biol.* 2011;18(6):680–7.
7. Brouns SJ, Jore MM, Lundgren M, Westra ER, Slijkhuis RJ, Snijders AP, et al. Small CRISPR RNAs guide antiviral defense in prokaryotes. *Science.* 2008;321(5891):960–4.
8. Hale CR, Majumdar S, Elmore J, Pfister N, Compton M, Olson S, et al. Essential features and rational design of CRISPR RNAs that function with the Cas RAMP module complex to cleave RNAs. *Mol. Cell.* 2012;45(3): 292–302.
9. Westra ER, van Erp PB, Künne T, Wong SP, Staals RH, Seegers CL, et al. CRISPR immunity relies on the consecutive binding and degradation of negatively supercoiled invader DNA by Cascade and Cas3. *Mol. Cell.* 2012; 46(5):595–605.
10. Zhang J, Rouillon C, Kerou M, Reeks J, Brugger K, Graham S, et al. Structure and mechanism of the CMR complex for CRISPR-mediated antiviral immunity. *Mol. Cell.* 2012;45(3):303–13.
11. Shmakov S, Smargon A, Scott D, Cox D, Pyzocha N, Yan W, et al. Diversity and evolution of class 2 CRISPR–Cas systems. *Nat. Rev. Microbiol.* 2017; 15(3):169–82.
12. Burstein D, Harrington LB, Strutt SC, Probst AJ, Anantharaman K, Thomas BC, et al. New CRISPR–Cas systems from uncultivated microbes. *Nature.* 2017;542(7640):237–41.
13. Koonin EV, Makarova KS, Zhang F. Diversity, classification and evolution of CRISPR-Cas systems. *Curr. Opin. Microbiol.* 2017;37:67–78.

14. Ishino Y, Krupovic M, Forterre P. History of CRISPR-Cas from encounter with a mysterious repeated sequence to genome editing technology. *J. Bacteriol.* 2018;200(7): e00580–17.
15. Jinek M, Chylinski K, Fonfara I, Hauer M, Doudna JA, Charpentier E. A programmable dual-RNA–guided DNA endonuclease in adaptive bacterial immunity. *Science.* 2012;337(6096):816–21.
16. Fitzgerald JJ. Applications of CRISPR for musculoskeletal research. *Bone Joint Res.* 2020;9(7):351–9.
17. Goldring SR, Goldring MB. Changes in the osteochondral unit during osteoarthritis: Structure, function and cartilage-bone crosstalk. *Nat. Rev. Rheumatol.* 2016;12:632–44.
18. Chevalier X, Eymard F, Richette P. Biologic agents in osteoarthritis: Hopes and disappointments. *Nat. Rev. Rheumatol.* 2013;9:400–10.
19. Liang Y, Xu X, Xu L, Iqbal Z, Ouyang K, Zhang H, et al. Chondrocyte-specific genomic editing enabled by hybrid exosomes for osteoarthritis treatment. *Theranostics.* 2022;12(11):4866.
20. Zhao L, Huang J, Fan Y, Li J, You T, He S, et al. Exploration of CRISPR/Cas9-based gene editing as therapy for osteoarthritis. *Ann. Rheum. Dis.* 2019;78(5):676–82.
21. Bonato A, Fisch P, Ponta S, Fercher D, Manninen M, Weber D, et al. Engineering inflammation-resistant cartilage: Bridging gene therapy and tissue engineering. *Adv. Healthc. Mater.* 2023;12(17):2202271.
22. Jung H, Rim YA, Park N, Nam Y, Ju JH. Restoration of osteogenesis by CRISPR/Cas9 genome editing of the mutated COL1A1 gene in osteogenesis imperfecta. *J. Clin. Med.* 2021;10(14):3141.
23. Yang Y-S, Sato T, Chaugule S, Ma H, Xie J, Gao G, et al. AAV-based gene editing of type 1 collagen mutation to treat osteogenesis imperfecta. *Nat. Commun.* 2024;35(1):102111.
24. Schindeler A, Lee LR, O'Donohue AK, Ginn SL, Munns CF. Curative cell and gene therapy for osteogenesis imperfecta. *J. Bone Miner. Res.* 2020; 37(5):826–36.
25. Long C, McAnally JR, Shelton JM, Mireault AA, Bassel-Duby R, Olson EN. Prevention of muscular dystrophy in mice by CRISPR/Cas9–mediated editing of germline DNA. *Science.* 2014;345(6201):1184–8.
26. Chen G, Wei T, Yang H, Li G, Li H. CRISPR-based therapeutic gene editing for Duchenne muscular dystrophy: Advances, challenges and perspectives. *Cells.* 2022;11(19):2964. https://doi.org/10.3390/cells11192964

27. Nelson CE, Robinson-Hamm JN, Gersbach CA. Genome engineering: A new approach to gene therapy for neuromuscular disorders. *Nat. Rev. Neurol.* 2017;13:647–61.
28. Moretti A, Fonteyne L, Giesert F, Hoppmann P, Meier A, Bozoglu T, et al. Somatic gene editing ameliorates skeletal and cardiac muscle failure in pig and human models of Duchenne muscular dystrophy. *Nat. Med.* 2020;26(2): 207–14.
29. Zhang Y, Long C, Li H, McAnally JR, Baskin KK, Shelton JM, et al. CRISPR-Cpf1 correction of muscular dystrophy mutations in human cardiomyocytes and mice. *Sci. Adv.* 2017;3(4):e1602814.
30. Ousterout DG, Kabadi AM, Thakore PI, Majoros WH, Reddy TE, Gersbach CA. Multiplex CRISPR/Cas9-based genome editing for correction of dystrophin mutations that cause Duchenne muscular dystrophy. *Nat. Commun.* 2015;6(1):6244.
31. Chen G, Deng S, Zuo M, Wang J, Cheng D, Chen B. Non-viral CRISPR activation system targeting VEGF-A and TGF-β1 for enhanced osteogenesis of pre-osteoblasts implanted with dual-crosslinked hydrogel. *Mol. Ther. Biotechnol.* 2022;16:100356.
32. Hsu M-N, Huang K-L, Yu F-J, Lai P-L, Truong AV, Lin M-W, et al. Coactivation of endogenous Wnt10b and Foxc2 by CRISPR activation enhances BMSC osteogenesis and promotes calvarial bone regeneration. *Biomaterials.* 2020;28(2):441–51.
33. Nguyen NTK, Chang Y-H, Truong VA, Hsu M-N, Pham NN, Chang C-W, et al. CRISPR activation of long non-coding RNA DANCR promotes bone regeneration. *Biomaterials.* 2021;275:120965.
34. Barrangou R, Doudna JA. Applications of CRISPR technologies in research and beyond. *Nat. Biotechnol.* 2016;34(9):933–41.
35. Yang Y, Xu J, Ge S, Lai L. CRISPR/Cas: Advances, limitations, and applications for precision cancer research. *Front. Immunol.* 2021;8:649896.
36. Hsu PD, Lander ES, Zhang F. Development and applications of CRISPR-Cas9 for genome engineering. *Cell.* 2014;157(6):1262–78.
37. Cong L, Ran FA, Cox D, Lin S, Barretto R, Habib N, et al. Multiplex genome engineering using CRISPR/Cas systems. *Science.* 2013;339(6121): 819–23.
38. Mali P, Yang L, Esvelt KM, Aach J, Guell M, DiCarlo JE, et al. RNA-guided human genome engineering via Cas9. *Science.* 2013;339(6121): 823–6.

39. Chew WL. Immunity to CRISPR Cas9 and Cas12a therapeutics. *Wiley Interdiscip. Rev. Syst. Biol. Med.* 2018;10(1):e1408.
40. Crudele JM, Chamberlain JS. Cas9 immunity creates challenges for CRISPR gene editing therapies. *Nat. Commun.* 2018;9(1):3497.
41. Liu W, Li L, Jiang J, Wu M, Lin P. Applications and challenges of CRISPR-Cas gene-editing to disease treatment in clinics. *Precis. Clin. Med.* 2021; 4(3):179–91.
42. Liu W, Wang S, Lin B, Zhang W, Ji G. Applications of CRISPR/Cas9 in the research of malignant musculoskeletal tumors. *Bone Marrow Dis.* 2021; 22:1–12.
43. Uddin F, Rudin CM, Sen T. CRISPR gene therapy: Applications, limitations, and implications for the future. *Front. Oncol.* 2020;10:1387.
44. Xu Y, Li Z. CRISPR-Cas systems: Overview, innovations and applications in human disease research and gene therapy. *Comput. Struct. Biotechnol. J.* 2020;18:2401–15.
45. Morshedzadeh F, Ghanei M, Lotfi M, Ghasemi M, Ahmadi M, Najari-Hanjani P, et al. An update on the application of CRISPR technology in clinical practice. *Exp. Mol. Med.* 2024;66(2):179–97.
46. van Haasteren J, Li J, Scheideler OJ, Murthy N, Schaffer DV. The delivery challenge: Fulfilling the promise of therapeutic genome editing. *Nat. Biotechnol.* 2020;38(7):845–55.
47. Kuscu C, Arslan S, Singh R, Thorpe J, Adli M. Genome-wide analysis reveals characteristics of off-target sites bound by the Cas9 endonuclease. *Nat. Biotechnol.* 2014;32(7):677–83.
48. Zhang X-H, Tee LY, Wang X-G, Huang Q-S, Yang S-H. Off-target effects in CRISPR/Cas9-mediated genome engineering. *Mol. Ther. Nucleic Acids.* 2015;4:e264.
49. Weiss WA, Taylor SS, Shokat KM. Recognizing and exploiting differences between RNAi and small-molecule inhibitors. *Nat. Chem. Biol.* 2007;3(12): 739–44.
50. Brokowski C, Adli M. CRISPR ethics: Moral considerations for applications of a powerful tool. *J. Mol. Biol.* 2019;431(1):88–101.
51. Gostimskaya I. CRISPR–cas9: A history of its discovery and ethical considerations of its use in genome editing. *Biochemistry.* 2022;87(8):777–88.
52. Schaefer KA, Wu W-H, Colgan DF, Tsang SH, Bassuk AG, Mahajan VB. Unexpected mutations after CRISPR–Cas9 editing in vivo. *Nat. Methods.* 2017;14(6):547–8.

53. Tu Z, Yang W, Yan S, Yin A, Gao J, Liu X, et al. Promoting Cas9 degradation reduces mosaic mutations in non-human primate embryos. *Sci. Rep.* 2017;7(1):42081.
54. Zhang D, Hussain A, Manghwar H, Xie K, Xie S, Zhao S, et al. Genome editing with the CRISPR-Cas system: An art, ethics and global regulatory perspective. *Plant Biotechnol. J.* 2020;18(8):1651–69.
55. Ali A, Rahman MY, Sheikh D. The role of CRISPR/Cas9 in revolutionizing Duchenne's muscular dystrophy treatment: Opportunities and obstacles. *Glob. Med. Genet.* 2024;11(04):349–57.
56. Moon SB, Ko J-H, Kim J-S, Kim Y-S. Improving CRISPR genome editing by engineering guide RNAs. *Trends Biotechnol.* 2019;37(8):870–81.
57. Zhang Y, Nishiyama T, Olson EN, Bassel-Duby R. CRISPR/Cas correction of muscular dystrophies. *Exp. Cell Res.* 2021;408(1):112844.
58. Jia S, Liang R, Chen J, Liao S, Lin J, Li W. Emerging technology has a brilliant future: The CRISPR-Cas system for senescence, inflammation, and cartilage repair in osteoarthritis. *Cell. Mol. Biol. Lett.* 2024;29(1):64.
59. Pferdehirt L, Ross AK, Brunger JM, Guilak F. A synthetic gene circuit for self-regulating delivery of biologic drugs in engineered tissues. *Tissue Eng. Part A.* 2019;25(9–10):809–20.
60. Truong VA, Lin Y-H, Nguyen NTK, Hsu M-N, Pham NN, Chang Y-H, et al. Bi-directional gene activation and repression promote ASC differentiation and enhance bone healing in osteoporotic rats. *Biomaterials.* 2022;30(1):92–104.
61. Rauch F, Geng Y, Lamplugh L, Hekmatnejad B, Gaumond M-H, Penney J, et al. Crispr-Cas9 engineered osteogenesis imperfecta type V leads to severe skeletal deformities and perinatal lethality in mice. *Bone.* 2018;107:131–42.
62. Perrin A, Rousseau J, Tremblay JP. Increased expression of laminin subunit alpha 1 chain by dCas9-VP160. *Mol. Ther. Nucleic Acids.* 2017;6:68–79.
63. Li M, Tang X, You W, Wang Y, Chen Y, Liu Y, et al. HMEJ-mediated site-specific integration of a myostatin inhibitor increases skeletal muscle mass in porcine. *Mol. Ther.* 2021;26:49–62.
64. Przymuszała M, Martyniak A, Kwiatkowska J, Meyer-Szary J, Śledzińska K, Wierzba J, et al. Generation of human induced pluripotent stem cell line derived from Becker muscular dystrophy patient with CRISPR/Cas9-mediated correction of DMD gene mutation. *Stem Cell Res.* 2024;76:103327.

65. Pini V, Mariot V, Dumonceaux J, Counsell J, O'Neill HC, Farmer S, et al. Transiently expressed CRISPR/Cas9 induces wild-type dystrophin in vitro in DMD patient myoblasts carrying duplications. *Sci. Rep.* 2022;12(1):3756.
66. Loeser RF, Goldring SR, Scanzello CR, Goldring MB. Osteoarthritis: A disease of the joint as an organ. *Arthritis Rheum.* 2012;64:1697–707.
67. Hellio Le Graverand-Gastineau M-P. OA clinical trials: Current targets and trials for OA. Choosing molecular targets: What have we learned and where we are headed? *Osteoarthritis Cartilage.* 2009;17:1393–401.

https://doi.org/10.1142/9789819819645_bmatter

Index

www.ingramcontent.com/pod-product-compliance
Lightning Source LLC
Chambersburg PA
CBHW070726150426
42667CB00011B/5
* 9 7 8 9 8 1 9 8 1 9 6 3 8 *